Accessing the E-book edition

Using the VitalSource® ebook

Access to the VitalBook™ ebook accompanying this book is via VitalSource® Bookshelf – an ebook reader which allows you to make and share notes and highlights on your ebooks and search across all of the ebooks that you hold on your VitalSource Bookshelf. You can access the ebook online or offline on your smartphone, tablet or PC/Mac and your notes and highlights will automatically stay in sync no matter where you make them.

1. **Create a VitalSource Bookshelf account at** *https://online.vitalsource.com/user/new* or log into your existing account if you already have one.

2. **Redeem the code provided in the panel below to get online access to the ebook.**
   Log in to Bookshelf and select **Redeem** at the top right of the screen. Enter the redemption code shown on the scratch-off panel below in the **Redeem Code** pop-up and press **Redeem**. Once the code has been redeemed your ebook will download and appear in your library.

No returns if this code has been revealed.

DOWNLOAD AND READ OFFLINE

To use your ebook offline, download BookShelf to your PC, Mac, iOS device, Android device or Kindle Fire, and log in to your Bookshelf account to access your ebook:

On your PC/Mac

Go to *https://support.vitalsource.com/hc/en-us* and follow the instructions to download the free **VitalSource Bookshelf** app to your PC or Mac and log into your Bookshelf account.

On your iPhone/iPod Touch/iPad

Download the free **VitalSource Bookshelf** App available via the iTunes App Store and log into your Bookshelf account. You can find more information at *https://support.vitalsource.com/hc/en-us/categories/200134217-Bookshelf-for-iOS*

On your Android™ smartphone or tablet

Download the free **VitalSource Bookshelf** App available via Google Play and log into your Bookshelf account. You can find more information at *https://support.vitalsource.com/hc/en-us/categories/200139976-Bookshelf-for-Android-and-Kindle-Fire*

On your Kindle Fire

Download the free **VitalSource Bookshelf** App available from Amazon and log into your Bookshelf account. You can find more information at *https://support.vitalsource.com/hc/en-us/categories/200139976-Bookshelf-for-Android-and-Kindle-Fire*

N.B. The code in the scratch-off panel can only be used once. When you have created a Bookshelf account and redeemed the code you will be able to access the ebook online or offline on your smartphone, tablet or PC/Mac.

SUPPORT

If you have any questions about downloading Bookshelf, creating your account, or accessing and using your ebook edition, please visit *http://support.vitalsource.com/*

Laparoscopic Colorectal Surgery

Laparoscopic Colorectal Surgery

A Step by Step Guide with Video Atlas

Edited by

Sanjiv Haribhakti

Chairman, Department of Surgical Gastroenterology
Kaizen Hospital
Ahmedabad, Gujarat, India

CRC Press
Taylor & Francis Group
Boca Raton London New York

CRC Press is an imprint of the
Taylor & Francis Group, an **informa** business

First edition published 2021
by CRC Press
6000 Broken Sound Parkway NW, Suite 300, Boca Raton, FL 33487-2742

and by CRC Press
2 Park Square, Milton Park, Abingdon, Oxon, OX14 4RN

© 2021 Taylor & Francis Group, LLC

CRC Press is an imprint of Taylor & Francis Group, LLC

Library of Congress Cataloging–in–Publication Data
Names: Haribhakti, Sanjiv, editor.
Title: Laparoscopic colorectal surgery : a step by step guide with video atlas / Sanjiv Haribhakti.
Other titles: Laparoscopic colorectal surgery (Haribhakti)
Description: First edition. | Boca Raton, FL : CRC Press, 2020. | Includes bibliographical references and index. |
    Summary: "This comprehensive book provides the reader a perspective of the current evidence based management
    of Laparoscopic Colorectal Surgery. It covers sections on benign surgery for IBD, diverticulitis, rectal prolapse etc.
    along with the procedures for colon and rectal cancers, including laparoscopic TME"-- Provided by publisher.
Identifiers: LCCN 2020037689 (print) | LCCN 2020037690 (ebook) | ISBN
    9780367352844 (hardback) | ISBN 9780429330377 (ebook)
Subjects: MESH: Colon--surgery | Rectum--surgery | Colonic
    Diseases--surgery | Rectal Diseases--surgery | Laparoscopy--methods
Classification: LCC RC804.C64 (print) | LCC RC804.C64 (ebook) | NLM WI 650 | DDC 617.5/5470597--dc23
LC record available at https://lccn.loc.gov/2020037689
LC ebook record available at https://lccn.loc.gov/2020037690

ISBN: 9780367352844 (hbk)
ISBN: 9780429330377 (ebk)

Typeset in Warnock Pro
by Nova Techset Private Limited, Bengaluru & Chennai, India

CONTENTS

Video Atlas of Laparoscopic Colorectal Surgery..vii

Foreword..ix

Preface...x

Acknowledgments...xi

Editor..xii

Contributors..xiii

SECTION I: INTRODUCTION AND BASIC CONCEPTS

1 History, Evolution, and Current Scenario of Laparoscopic Colorectal Surgery..2
   Jitendra Mistry

2 Training for Laparoscopic Colorectal Surgery...8
   Prakash Kumar Sasmal

3 Clinical Anatomy Related to Laparoscopic Colorectal Surgery...12
   David N. Naumann, Mark Dilworth, and Sharad Karandikar

4 Basic Principles and Techniques of Laparoscopic Colorectal Surgery..17
   Sanjiv Haribhakti and Shobhit Sengar

5 Patient Selection..27
   Harsh Shah

6 Stoma and Its Complications..29
   Ankur Tiwari

SECTION II: PERIOPERATIVE CARE OF PATIENT

7 Bowel Preparation in Colorectal Surgery...35
   Harshad Soni and Benjamin Perakath

8 ERAS in Colorectal Surgery..38
   Harsh Shah and Kantilal S Patel

9 Anesthetic Management of Laproscopic Colorectal Surgery...44
   Raxesh Desai and Nisarg Patel

10 Complications in Laparoscopic Colorectal Surgery...48
   Sanjiv Haribhakti and Shobhit Sengar

SECTION III: LAPAROSCOPY IN BENIGN COLORECTAL DISEASES

11 Laparoscopic Ileocecal Resection...59
   Vismit Joshipura

12 Laparoscopic Appendectomy...62
   Atul Shah and Rajat Srivastava

13 Laparoscopic Sigmoid Colectomy for Diverticulitis...68
   Paul Trinity Stephen and Rohin Mittal

14 Laparoscopic Rectopexy for Rectal Prolapse...75
   Sanjiv Haribhakti and Jitender Singh Chauhan

15 Laparoscopic-Assisted Stomas and Stoma Reversal..85
   Fazl Q Parray and Zamir A Shah

16 Laparoscopic Restorative Proctocolectomy and Ileal Pouch Anal Anastomosis..90
   Sanjiv Haribhakti and Rajat Srivastava

17 Parastomal Hernias..109
   Arun Prasad and Sanjiv Haribhakti

SECTION IV: LAPAROSCOPY COLORECTAL CANCER SURGERY

18 Laparoscopic versus Open Colorectal Resection: An Evidence-Based Review..117
   Anish Nagpal

19 Laparoscopic Right Hemicolectomy for Right Colon Cancer..123
   Harshad Soni and Jitender Singh Chauhan

20 Laparoscopic Transverse Colectomy for Transverse Colon Cancer 128
    Prajesh Bhuta

21 Laparoscopic Hemicolectomy for Left Colon Cancer 131
    Ashwin deSouza and Shankar Malpangudi

22 Laparoscopic Anterior Resection and Total Mesorectal Excision for Rectosigmoid Cancer 139
    Avanish Saklani, S Barath Raj Kumar, and Sanket Bankar

23 Techniques for Laparoscopic Low Anterior Resection, Ultra Low Anterior Resection,
    and Inter Sphincteric Resection (ISR) 146
    S Rajapandian, R Parthasarathy, Raghavendra Gupta, Sunil Kumar Nayak, and C Palanivelu

24 Laparoscopic Conventional Abdominoperineal (CAPE) and Extra-Levator Abdominoperineal Resection (ELAPE) 154
    Sanjiv Haribhakti and Deepak Govil

25 Laparoscopic Subtotal/Total/Proctocolectomy 160
    Sanjiv Haribhakti

26 Laparoscopic Management of T4 Tumor and Pelvic Exenteration for Locally Advanced Tumors 165
    Ajay Punpale

27 Laparoscopic Surgery in Obstructed and Recurrent Tumors...172
    Ramraj Vemala Nagendra Gupta and Govind Nandakumar

28 Resection for Colorectal Liver Metastasis...179
    Palanisamy Senthilnathan, Srivatsan Gurumurthy Sivakumar, Srinivasan Muthukrishnan, and C Palanivelu

29 Specimen Retrieval after Laparoscopic Colectomy and NOSE..185
    Deep Goel, Ravindra Vats, Luv Gupta, Vipin Pal Singh, and Virandera Pal Bhalla

SECTION V: ROBOTIC COLORECTAL SURGERY

30 Robotic Colonic Cancer Surgery 190
    Varun Madaan, Rigved Gupta, Supreet Kumar, and Deepak Govil

31 Robotic Rectal Cancer Surgery 196
    Somashekhar SP and Ashwin K Rajagopal

SECTION VI: TRANSANAL SURGERY

32 Transanal Minimally Invasive Surgery (TAMIS)...203
    Sanjeev Patil and Shrikant Makam

33 Transanal Total Mesorectal Excision for Rectal Cancer...211
    Daniel Peyser and Patricia Sylla

34 Combined Endoscopic-Laparoscopic Surgery (CELS) for Colorectal Polypectomy..................................224
    Miguel E Gomez and Parul J Shukla

SECTION VII: HAND-ASSISTED AND SINGLE-INCISION LAPAROSCOPIC COLORECTAL SURGERY

35 Hand-Assisted Laparoscopic Colorectal Surgery...230
    Deeksha Kapoor, Amanjeet Singh, and Adarsh Chaudhary

36 Single-Incision Laparoscopic Colorectal Surgery..236
    Muralidhar Kathlagiri

Index 241

VIDEO ATLAS OF LAPAROSCOPIC COLORECTAL SURGERY

General Principles

Video 1   Basic Principles and Techniques of Laparoscopic Colorectal Surgery – Part 1 (**Chapter 4**)
Sanjiv Haribhakti

Video 2   Basic Principles and Techniques of Laparoscopic Colorectal Surgery – Part 2 (**Chapter 4**)
Sanjiv Haribhakti

Video 3   Principles of GI Stapling – Open and Laparoscopic (**Chapter 4**)
Harshad Soni

Video 4   Stoma Creation (**Chapter 6**)
Harsh Shah

Video 5   Restoration of Loop Ileostomy – Part 1 (**Chapter 15**)
Sanjiv Haribhakti

Video 6   Restoration of Loop Ileostomy – Part 2 (**Chapter 15**)
Sanjiv Haribhakti

Laparoscopy in Benign Diseases

Video 7   Laparoscopic Ileocecal Resection (**Chapter 11**)
Sanjiv Haribhakti

Video 8   Laparoscopic Appendectomy (**Chapter 12**)
Atul Shah

Video 9   Laparoscopic Sigmoid Colectomy for Diverticulitis (**Chapter 13**)
Sanjiv Haribhakti

Video 10   Laparoscopic Suture Rectopexy (**Chapter 14**)
Sanjiv Haribhakti

Video 11   Laparoscopic Ventral Rectopexy (**Chapter 14**)
Sanjiv Haribhakti

Video 12   Laparoscopic Resection Rectopexy (**Chapter 14**)
Sanjiv Haribhakti

Video 13   Laparoscopic Restorative Proctocolectomy and Ileal Pouch for Ulcerative Colitis – Part 1 (**Chapter 16**)
Sanjiv Haribhakti

Video 14   Laparoscopic Restorative Proctocolectomy and Ileal Pouch for Ulcerative Colitis – Part 2 (**Chapter 16**)
Sanjiv Haribhakti

Video 15   Lap Sugarbaker Hernioplasty for Parastomal Hernias (**Chapter 17**)
Sanjiv Haribhakti

Video 16   Robotic Parastomal Hernioplasty for Parastomal Hernias (**Chapter 17**)
Arun Prasad

Video 17   Laparoscopic Adhesiolysis for Intestinal Obstruction (**Chapter 10**)
Harshad Soni

Laparoscopic Colorectal Cancer Surgery

Video 18   Laparoscopic Extended Right Hemicolectomy for Right Colon Cancer – Part 1 (**Chapter 19**)
Sanjiv Haribhakti

Video 19   Laparoscopic Extended Right Hemicolectomy for Right Colon Cancer – Part 2 (**Chapter 19**)
Sanjiv Haribhakti

Video 20   Laparoscopic Anterior Resection and TME for Rectosigmoid Cancer (**Chapter 22**)
Avanish Saklani

Video 21   Ultralow Resections and Coloanal Anastomosis for Low Rectal Cancers – Part 1 (**Chapter 23**)
Govind Nandakumar

Video 22   Ultralow Resections and Coloanal Anastomosis for Low Rectal Cancers – Part 2 (**Chapter 23**)
Govind Nandakumar

Video 23   Laparoscopic APE (**Chapter 24**)
Harshad Soni

Video 24   Anterior Resection and TME – Part 1 (**Chapter 22**)
Ramakrishnan AS

Video 25   Anterior Resection and TME – Part 2 (**Chapter 22**)
Ramakrishnan AS

Video 26   Extralevator APE (**Chapter 24**)
Ramakrishnan AS

Video 27   Laparoscopic Pelvic Exenteration for Locally Advanced Rectal Tumours (**Chapter 26**)
Ajay Punpale

Video 28   Management of Locally Advanced Colon Cancer (**Chapter 26**)
Rajat Srivastava

Video 29   Specimen Extraction – Trans-abdominal and Natural Orifice (**Chapter 29**)
Rajat Srivastava

Video 30   Peritonectomy + HIPEC for Colorectal Cancer (**Chapter 27**)
Shivendra Singh, Shaifali Goel

Video 31   Laparoscopic Left Segmental Colectomy (**Chapter 21**)
Ashwin deSouza

Recent Advances in Laparoscopic Colorectal Surgery

Video 32   Robotic LAR (**Chapter 31**)
Somashekhar SP

Video 33   Robotic LAR (**Chapter 31**)
Deepak Govil

Video 34   Transanal Full Thickness Resections (**Chapter 32**)
Sanjeev Patil

Video 35   Transanal TME for Rectal Cancers (**Chapter 33**)
Patricia Sylla

Video 36   Hand Assisted Laparoscopic TME (**Chapter 35**)
Amanjeet Singh

Video 37   Single Access laparoscopic and Transanal TME (**Chapter 33**)
Giovanni Dapri

Video 38   SILS Right hemicolectomy – Part 1 (**Chapter 36**)
Giovanni Dapri

Video 39   SILS Right hemicolectomy – Part 2 (**Chapter 36**)
Giovanni Dapri

FOREWORD

It is my great honor to contribute a foreword to this wonderful book on laparoscopic colorectal surgery. It has been a long time since I met Dr Sanjiv Haribhakti, during the dawning period of laparoscopic surgery. He has been actively performing laparoscopic colorectal surgeries and has devoted himself to disseminating these techniques all over India, organizing many didactic courses, as well as writing a book, the third edition of the textbook *Surgical Gastroenterology*, which was recently published. I would like to congratulate him for successfully accomplishing the mammoth task of editing and writing this book on laparoscopic colorectal surgery. This book has been written by him and many renowned experts to cover every important aspect in the field of laparoscopic colorectal surgery.

Laparoscopic colorectal surgery has rapidly evolved over the last three decades, now to be a routine clinical practice in treating benign and malignant diseases of colon and rectum with little debate. However, for the beginners – even experienced surgeons – it still seems difficult to learn and to reach a level of high competency. I am sure that this book, along with the accompanying online video atlas, will provide a valuable window on all the necessary laparoscopic techniques in detail, on a proper use of instruments, and also towards a better understanding of colorectal diseases.

Once again, I would like to express special thanks to Dr Sanjiv Haribhakti for his enormous efforts in editing this book, and I wish all the best to the readers.

Gyu-Seog Choi, MD, Phd
Professor
Colorectal Cancer Center, Kyungpook National University
Chilgok Hospital
School of Medicine, Kyungpook National University
Daegu, Korea

PREFACE

Colorectal surgery, as a specialty, has developed significantly in the United States and Europe, while it is still in its infancy in developing countries. Laparoscopic – or minimally invasive surgery, started in the early 1990s, and soon became a gold standard for many common abdominal operations, particularly cholecystectomy, fundoplication, and bariatric surgery to name a few. Laparoscopic colorectal surgery (LCRS) started in the late 1990s; however, due to a few scary reports of port-site metastasis, it did not become popular in the early part of the new millennium. Fortunately, these reports inspired a few prospective randomized trials, which then firmly established the early benefits of LCRS and the noninferiority of long-term outcomes in colorectal cancers. These trials firmly established the place of LCRS in the management of colorectal diseases. However, several issues resulted in the low worldwide usage of LCRS during the last decade. Amongst the prominent ones were the lack of standardization and a significant learning curve – resulting from difficulties in manipulation of the highly mobile colon, and dissection in the small confines of the pelvis for rectal surgery.

The purpose of writing this book on laparoscopic colorectal surgery was to specifically address and overcome these issues related to LCRS, so that more surgeons can venture into this field, and overcome the early hurdles of LCRS. This book is aimed at general surgeons with a special interest in LCRS, surgical gastroenterologists who commonly perform LCRS, and surgical oncologists who may not have the learning experience of performing other more common benign laparoscopic operations. LCRS has a rather long learning curve, and unfortunately there are very few residencies, or fellowship programs, addressing the need for learning LCRS. Thus, this book intends to fill this void, providing help for surgeons wanting to become proficient in LCRS.

This book focuses on basic understanding of the surgical embryology and anatomy, which forms the foundation of the surgical principles of LCRS, and outlines the important principles of laparoscopy in benign and cancer patients. It succinctly enumerates the indications and selection of patients for various procedures, outlines the importance of preoperative preparation and postoperative care, and highlights the importance of preventing and managing the postoperative complications.

This book is accompanied by an online video atlas consisting of teaching videos, which supplement the knowledge and understanding gained from this book through the learning of surgical skills and techniques. The accompanying teaching videos demonstrate the surgical steps and techniques in a step-wise format, for easy understanding, along with the audio narration focusing on important surgical landmarks and the correct planes of dissection. The importance of teamwork and coordination is abundantly clear from the various teaching videos. The appropriate use of various surgical technologies such as energy devices, clips, staplers, and so on are highlighted throughout the surgical demonstration. Also included are chapters and videos on new and emerging technologies such as SILS, robotics, and transanal surgery that help illustrate the future of LCRS.

I am sure the efforts made in creating this book and video atlas will help you, the aspirant, learn and master the skills of LCRS. Mostly, we hope this work will eventually help patients at large benefit from the appropriate utilization of these modern technologies.

I will be happy to receive your feedback at sharibhakti@gmail.com

Dedicated to...

'The Almighty'
Who bestows us with this body, energy, mind and intellect
to perform what we are supposed to do,
Who has given us this opportunity to practice this noble profession,
Who makes all circumstances conducive for us to treat our patients,
Who gives us the appropriate fruits of our actions; and
Who constantly inspires us to learn and grow, more and more...
to attain the final goal of our life...
My Parents, who brought me to this world, nurtured me,
and educated me to become what I am today
My Family, who has been a constant source of strength and support
for all my academic endeavours,
My Guru, who shows me the light of knowledge
All my Teachers who were compassionate to teach me the nuances of our profession
All my Colleagues, who stand by me day in and out
Finally, **All my Patients**, who were kind enough to trust me,
For myself being instrumental, in taking care of them....

ACKNOWLEDGMENTS

First and the foremost, I would like to thank all the contributors to this book and teaching video atlas for their timely inputs, without which this book would have not seen the light of day.

I would like to thank my wife, Dr Neebha, and my daughter, Pranali, for their constant support and encouragement towards my academic ambitions.

I sincerely thank Ms Ronnie Stephen, editorial secretary, for putting in a massive effort in collating, compiling, and coordinating all the chapters for the creation of this book. I thank my colleagues, Dr KS Patel, Dr Atul Shah, Dr Harshad Soni, Dr Harsh Shah, and Dr Disha Chawla for sharing my clinical work so as to allow me to complete this project on time. I thank my fellow trainee surgeons Dr Rajat Srivastava, Dr Jitendra Chauhan, and Dr Shobhit Sengar for reading the proofs and helping with the figures. I thank the video editorial team Harsh Vataliya, Sandip Bhatia, Hiren Bhatia, and Dr Ankur Tiwari for the crisply edited teaching videos. I would especially like to thank Dr Vismit Joshipura for contributing the sketches used in this book.

Finally, I would like to thank the editorial team at Taylor & Francis group, Ms Shivangi Pramanik and Ms Himani Dwivedi, for coordinating this project.

I thank one and all who made this project feasible.

Dr Sanjiv Haribhakti

EDITOR

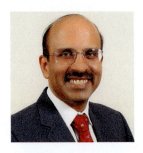

Dr Sanjiv Haribhakti is a surgical gastroenterologist practicing in Ahmedabad, India, since 1997. Currently, he is the chairman of the department of surgical gastroenterology at Kaizen Hospital, Institute of GE in Ahmedabad, India. After completing his basic medical education in Gujarat University, he was a Gold medalist at both his final MBBS and MS (general surgery). He then did diplomate of the National Board (DNB) (surgery) and undertook training in GI surgery at India's premier institute, AIIMS, in New Delhi. He later completed his specialty training MCh (surgical GE) from SGPGIMS, Lucknow, a state-of-art super specialty training center in 1996.

Dr Haribhakti is keenly involved in academic activities. He is passionate about training young surgeons in GI and laparoscopic surgery, and has been as a course director for 'Lap Skill' courses since 1997. He has organized more than 20 conferences in the field of surgical GE, and is an invited faculty in more than 100 national and over 10 international meetings. Dr Haribhakti also has to his credit 28 publications in indexed journals. He performs a wide spectrum of advanced laparoscopic and open GI surgery; however, his special interest is in the field of laparoscopic ileal pouch surgery for ulcerative colitis, laparoscopic colorectal cancer surgery, and minimally invasive surgery for pancreatic necrosis.

His significant contribution has been the development of an indigenous table mounted 'Haribhakti's' abdominal self-retaining retractor system, which is used routinely by many Indian institutions and practicing surgeons. Dr Haribhakti has also innovated a scarless retractor, the 'Hammock Retractor' for atraumatic retraction of the left lobe of the liver in laparoscopic UGI surgery. His latest innovations have been in the field of natural orifice surgery – ports for transoral UGI surgery, transanal surgery, SILS ports for single incision laparoscopic surgery, and VARD port for retroperitoneal pancreatic necrosectomy.

He is an editor of the comprehensive state-of-the-art textbook *Surgical Gastroenterology, 3rd ed.*, which was released recently in two volumes of 188 chapters and includes the works of several contributors across the globe. To accompany this book, Dr Haribhakti has also created an online educational video, the *Atlas of GI Surgery*, featuring more than 100 teaching videos exploring surgical gastroenterology with audio narration, step-by-step demonstrations, and important anatomical landmarks – with contributions from many international experts, available on www.gisurgery.info.

www.gisurgery.info, an educational website, initiated by Dr Haribhakti, is a virtual repository that regularly provides state-of-the-art learning videos of GI surgical techniques, presentations, journal articles, photographs, news, classifications of diseases, score calculators, and many recent advances on surgical gastroenterology. This website also includes a patient portal for patient awareness in field of GI surgery.

CONTRIBUTORS

Sanket Bankar
Division of Colorectal Oncology
Department of Surgical Oncology
Tata Memorial Centre
Mumbai, India

Virandera Pal Bhalla
Surgical Gastroenterology
Institute for Digestive & Liver Diseases
B L Kapur Superspeciality Hospital
New Delhi, India

Prajesh Bhuta
Department of Surgery
Jaslok Hospital
Maharashtra, India

Adarsh Chaudhary
Department of GI Surgery, GI Oncology,
   Minimally Invasive & Bariatric
   Surgery
Medanta, The Medicity
Gurugram, India

Jitender Singh Chauhan
Department of Surgical Gastroenterology
Kaizen Hospital
Memnagar, India

Raxesh Desai
Department of Surgical Gastroenterology
Kaizen Hospital
Ahmedabad, India

Ashwin deSouza
Minimally Invasive, Liver
   Transplantation & HPB Surgery
Tata Memorial Centre
Homi Bhabha National University
Mumbai, India

Mark Dilworth
Institute of Inflammation & Ageing
University of Birmingham
Edgbaston, United Kingdom

Deep Goel
Deptartment of Surgical Gastroentero
   Oncology, Bariatric & Minimal Access
   Surgery
B L Kapur Superspeciality Hospital
New Delhi, India

Miguel E Gomez
Colon & Rectal Surgery
Weill Cornell Medicine
New York City, New York

Deepak Govil
Department of Surgical Gastroenterology
   & GI Oncology
Indraprastha Apollo Hospital
New Delhi, India

Luv Gupta
Department of Surgical
   Gastroenterology, Bariatric &
   Minimal Access Surgery
B L Kapur Superspeciality Hospital
New Delhi, India

Ramraj Vemala Nagendra Gupta
Minimal Invasive, Bariatric and
   Metabolic
BR LIFE-SSNMC Super Speciality
   Hospital
Karnataka, India

Raghavendra Gupta
Department of Colorectal Surgery
GEM Hospital & Research Centre
Chennai, India

Rigved Gupta
Department of Surgical Gastroenterology
   & GI Oncology
Indraprastha Apollo Hospital
New Delhi, India

Sanjiv Haribhakti
Department of Surgical
   Gastroenterology
Kaizen Hospital
Ahmedabad, India

Vismit Joshipura
Department of Surgical Gastroenterology
Vivaan Clinic
Ahmedabad, India

Deeksha Kapoor
Institute of Digestive and Hepatobiliary
   Science
Medanta, The Medicity
Gurugram, India

Sharad Karandikar
Department of General Surgery
Heartlands Hospital
University Hospitals Birmingham
   NHS Foundation Trust
Birmingham, United Kingdom

Muralidhar Kathlagiri
Department of Minimal Access Surgery
Fortis Hospital
Bangalore, India

S Barath Raj Kumar
Division of Colorectal Oncology
Department of Surgical Oncology
Tata Memorial Centre
Mumbai, India

Supreet Kumar
Department of Surgical Gastroenterology
   & GI surgery
Indraprastha Apollo Hospital
New Delhi, India

Varun Madaan
Department of Surgical Gastroenterology
   & GI surgery
Indraprastha Apollo Hospital
New Delhi, India

Shrikant Makam
Asian Institute of Gastroenterology
Hyderabad, India

Shankar Malpangudi
Department of GI and HPB Oncology
Tata Memorial Centre
Mumbai, India

Jitendra Mistry
Mission Gastrocare
Gujarat, India

Rohin Mittal
Department of Surgery
Christian Medical College
Tamil Nadu, India

Srinivasan Muthukrishnan
Minimally Invasive, Liver
   Transplantation & HPB Surgery
Tata Memorial Centre
Mumbai, India
and
GEM Hospital
Chennai, India

Anish Nagpal
Department of Gastrointestinal Surgery
HCG Hospitals
Gujarat, India

Govind Nandakumar
Gastrointestinal, HPB and Colorectal
   Surgery
Columbia Asia Hospitals
Bangalore, India
and
Weill Cornell Medical College
New York City, New York

David N. Naumann
Institute of Inflammation & Ageing
University of Birmingham
Edgbaston, United Kingdom

Sunil Kumar Nayak
Department of Colorectal Surgery
GEM Hospital & Research Centre
Chennai, India

C Palanivelu
Institute of Gastroenterology & Minimal
    Access Surgery
GEM Hospital & Research Centre
Chennai, India

R Parthasarathy
Department of Upper GI Surgery
GEM Hospital & Research Centre
Chennai, India

Fazl Q Parray
Department of General & Minimal
    Invasive Surgery
Sher-i-Kashmir Institute of Medical
    Sciences
Srinagar, India

Kantilal S Patel
Department of Surgical
    Gastroenterology
Kaizen Hospital
Ahmedabad, India

Nisarg Patel
Department of Surgical Gastroenterology
Kaizen Hospital
Ahmedabad, India

Sanjeev Patil
Asian Institute of Gastroenterology
Hyderabad, India

Benjamin Perakath
Department of Surgery
Dr Gray's Hospital
Elgin, United Kingdom

Daniel Peyser
Department of Surgery
The Mount Sinai Medical Center
New York City, New York

Arun Prasad
Department of Surgery
Manipal Hospitals
New Delhi, India

Ajay Punpale
Latur Cancer & Laparoscopy Centre
Latur, India

Ashwin K Rajagopal
Manipal Comprehensive Cancer Center
Manipal Hospitals
Bengaluru, India

S Rajapandian
Department of Colorectal Surgery
GEM Hospital & Research Centre
Chennai, India

Avanish Saklani
Division of Colorectal Oncology
Department of Surgical Oncology
Tata Memorial Centre
Mumbai, India

Prakash Kumar Sasmal
Deptartment of Surgery
All India Institute of Medical Sciences
    (AIIMS)
Odisha, India

Shobhit Sengar
Department of Surgical Gastroenterology
Kaizen Hospital
Ahmedabad, India

Palanisamy Senthilnathan
Division of Minimally Invasive, Liver
    Transplantation & HPB surgery
GEM Centre for Liver & Pancreas
GEM Hospital & Research Centre
Coimbatore, India

Atul Shah
Department of Surgical Gastroenterology
Kaizen Hospital
Ahmedabad, India

Harsh Shah
Department of Surgical Gastroenterology
Kaizen Hospital
Ahmedabad, India

Zamir A Shah
Department of General & Minimal
    Invasive Surgery
Sher-i-Kashmir Institute of Medical
    Sciences
Srinagar, India

Parul J Shukla
Colon & Rectal Surgery
Weill Cornell Medicine
New York City, New York

Amanjeet Singh
Department of GI Surgery, GI Oncology,
    Minimal Access & Bariatric Surgery
Medanta, The Medicity
Gurugram, India

Vipin Pal Singh
Department of Surgical
    Gastroenterology, Bariatric &
    Minimal Access Surgery
B L Kapur Superspeciality Hospital
New Delhi, India

Srivatsan Gurumurthy Sivakumar
Minimally Invasive, Liver
    Transplantation & HPB surgery
GEM Hospital
Chennai, India

Somashekhar SP
Department of Surgical Oncology
Manipal Hospital
Bengaluru, India

Harshad Soni
Department of Surgical
    Gastroenterology
Kaizen Hospital
Ahmedabad, India

Rajat Srivastava
Department of Surgical Gastroenterology
Kaizen Hospital
Ahmedabad, India

Paul Trinity Stephen
Department of Surgery
Christian Medical College
Vellore, India

Patricia Sylla
Department of Colorectal Surgery
Icahn School of Medicine at
    Mount Sinai
New York City, New York

Ankur Tiwari
Department of Surgical
    Gastroenterology
Sterling Hospitals
Gujarat, India

Ravindra Vats
Department of Surgical
    Gastroenterology, Bariatric &
    Minimal Access Surgery
B L Kapur Superspeciality Hospital
New Delhi, India

Section I
Introduction and Basic Concepts

1 History, Evolution, and Current Scenario of Laparoscopic Colorectal Surgery. 2
2 Training for Laparoscopic Colorectal Surgery 8
3 Clinical Anatomy Related to Laparoscopic Colorectal Surgery 12
4 Basic Principles and Techniques of Laparoscopic Colorectal Surgery. 17
5 Patient Selection 27
6 Stoma and Its Complications 29

Chapter 1

HISTORY, EVOLUTION, AND CURRENT SCENARIO OF LAPAROSCOPIC COLORECTAL SURGERY

Jitendra Mistry

Contents

Learning objectives 2
Introduction 2
Evolution of laparoscopic surgery 2
    Technological evolution 2
    Evolution of laparoscopic surgery in general 2
Technical evolution of rectal cancer surgery 4
Evolution of laparoscopy for colorectal cancers 4
Evolution of laparoscopic surgery for benign colorectal condition 4
    Rectal prolapse 4
    Inflammatory bowel disease 4
    Diverticular disease 5
Laparoscopic colorectal surgery in emergency situations 5
Future of laparoscopic colorectal surgery 5
Summary 6
Key points 6
References 6

'The patient is the center of the medical universe around which all our works revolve and towards which all our efforts tend'

– John Benjamin Murphy (1857–1916)

Learning objectives

- The technical evolution of rectal cancer surgery
- The evolution of laparoscopy for colorectal cancers
- The evolution of laparoscopic surgery for benign colorectal condition
- Laparoscopic colorectal surgery in emergency situations
- The future of laparoscopic colorectal surgery

Introduction

Evolution of any surgical procedure, or technique, is mainly aimed at improving the outcomes and quality of life of the patient. Laparoscopic surgery has come a long way after an initial resistance from conventional doctrine. It began with diagnostic laparoscopy and has grown into currently complex procedures such as laparoscopic colorectal surgery and pancreatoduodenectomy. As any new procedure or innovation comes into the market, it follows an evolution process (Figure 1.1) and is initially considered as an experimental procedure; once safety has been proven and it gives reasonable results compared to existing procedures, it then becomes an acceptable procedure and an alternative option. As time passes, if new procedures consistently produce better results than existing ones, then it becomes the standard of care, the procedure of choice. There are many laparoscopic procedures which are at different phases of this evolution cycle. We think laparoscopic colorectal surgery is an acceptable procedure at present – if not the standard of care.

We will describe the history, evolution, and current situation of laparoscopic colorectal surgery in this chapter. We will also briefly discuss its history, its technological evolution, as well as laparoscopy in general, as it cannot be separated from evolution of laparoscopic colorectal surgery.

Evolution of laparoscopic surgery

Technological evolution

Along with the history and evolution of laparoscopic surgery, we must recognize that laparoscopic surgery has a very close and never seen before association with technology. Technological advancements must be given a due acknowledgement here, as thinking about further progress could not have been possible without these early era technological advancements. These technological advancements include light sources, optical systems, computer chip video cameras, laparoscopic longer hand instruments, and energy devices. A majority of these developments occurred between the 1960s and 1980s, which fueled advancements in laparoscopy over the next decade. Collectively, these made advanced laparoscopic surgery possible today. The light bulb was invented during the 1870s and 1880s, but the real spark was given by the invention of professor Harold Hopkins in 1954, when he invented the glass rod system which allowed the transmission of light from an external source to the area of interest. In 1960, Dr Karl Storz developed cold light source, where the light is generated outside and passes through optical fibers which minimize the heat at the tip of instrument. The laparoscopic HD chip-based camera came into vogue in the 1980s, improving vision and allowing to perform complex surgeries. Three-dimension (3D) camera system and robotic platform have also entered the field, and the benefits of these advancements are presently under evaluation.

Evolution of laparoscopic surgery in general

Laparoscopic surgery came in vogue in the 1990s [1]; it is one of the significant revolutions in the history of surgery, and has

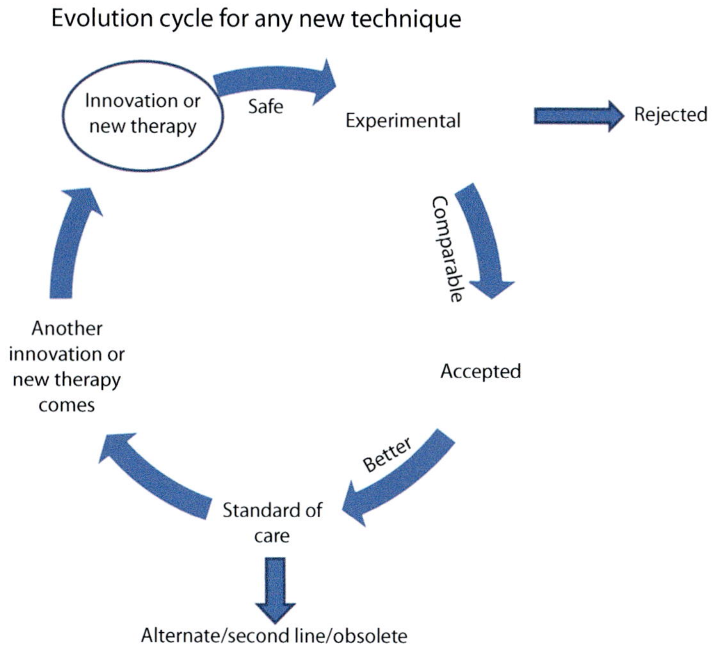

Evolution cycle for any new technique

FIGURE 1.1   Evolution cycle of any new procedure or technique.

changed the face of gastrointestinal and many other surgeries. Although the history of the use of the speculum for examining the rectum and vagina goes way back to the era of Hippocrates (460–375 BC), George Kelling was the one who performed the first experimental celioscopy on a dog in 1901, where he insufflated air into the abdomen. Dr Hans-Christian Jacobaeus performed the first human celioscopy in 1910 to evaluate patients with ascites. One major breakthrough in laparoscopy was claimed, in 1920, by Zollikofer when he suggested using CO_2 for insufflations for faster absorption and to avoid complications of other gases. The Veress needle was introduced in 1938 by Janos Veress. In 1953, Harold Hopkins introduced the rod lens system which allowed better illumination and thus clearer vision to work. In 1960, Karl Storz introduced the cold light system in which light from an external source passes through optical fires to the area of interest to reduce the temperature at the tip of the scope. We must compliment Kurt Semm, a German gynaecologist, for his contributions. He introduced automatic insufflators, thermocoagulation, endoloops, and irrigation devices. He performed not only gynaecological procedures but he also popularized many general surgical procedures in that era; he performed the first incidental appendectomy in 1983, when even surgeons were hesitant to venture into laparoscopic surgery. In 1974, Harith Hasson proposed an open technique for introducing a trocar under direct vision, using minilaparotomy incision. The first laparoscopic cholecystectomy was performed by Dr Erich Muhe in 1985, while the first human laparoscopic cholecystectomy was performed by Philip Mouret, and has become the gold standard treatment since. Until 1986, the vision of camera systems was a limitation, which was overcome by the invention of computer chip camera systems which improved vision significantly and allowed surgeons to become comfortable using laparoscopy. From 1990 onward, various surgeons across the globe started using laparoscopy for various gastrointestinal surgeries, urological surgeries, general surgeries, and gynaecological surgeries. It is worth mentioning names of stalwarts (Figures 1.2–1.4) from India, such as Prof. T.E. Udwadia who performed the first laparoscopic cholecystectomy in India, Prof. C. Palanivelu who popularized advanced laparoscopic surgeries in India, and

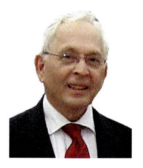

FIGURE 1.2   Professor T.E. Udwadia.

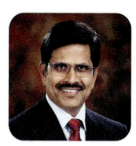

FIGURE 1.3   Professor C. Palanivelu.

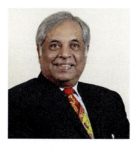

FIGURE 1.4   Dr Pradeep Chowbey.

Dr Pradeep Chowbey who popularized laparoscopic cholecystectomy in northern India. There are other advances, which have yet to gain a hold in laparoscopic surgeries, such as natural orifice transluminal endoscopic surgery (NOTES) and single port laparoscopic surgery (SILS). Robotic surgery is the latest to be introduced, and is currently under process to prove its benefits over traditional laparoscopic surgery.

Technical evolution of rectal cancer surgery

Before 1907, the intent for any rectal cancer surgery was symptomatic palliation; in the year 1907, Sir William Ernest Miles performed the first rectal resection with curative intent [2]. Moynihan introduced the concept of high ligation of the inferior mesenteric artery with the intent of better lymphadenectomy [3], although the benefits of the concept are still not clear. Leg rests were designed by Sir Huge Devine in 1937, up to then the perineal part of the procedure was performed by changing the position of the patient to either prone or lateral [4]. The morbidity and mortality of abdomino-perineal resection (APR) was very high, and in order to reduce it, Sir Henri Albert Hartmann introduced the concept of Hartmann's procedure where perineal dissection is avoided for upper and middle third rectal cancer [5]. Although this procedure reduced the morbidity and mortality of APR, it still required permanent stoma. Claude F. Dixon initiated restorative procedures and published research showing a 64% 5-years survival rate in 1948 [6]; people started accepting the procedure for sigmoid and upper rectal cancers. Further evolution took place for the distal margin: Golligher found that only 2% of patient have a positive margin beyond a 2 cm margin [7], so initially a 5 cm margin was accepted which reduced over a period of time to 2 cm; even today, in selected cases, a 1 cm margin is also well accepted [4]. So, eventually, more and more rectal cancer cases underwent restorative procedures. Hand sewn low colorectal anastomosis was the difficult procedure, and the use of the stapler in 1975 made a remarkable difference and allowed even lower rectal cancers to have the possibility of restorative procedure [8]. Introduction of the double stapler technique, in 1980, further made the procedure easier and comfortable [9]. Coloanal anastomosis and intersphincteric resection were the further developments that allowed restorative resection in very low rectal cancer, while colonic pouch formation was an attempt to improve the functional outcomes of such a low anastomosis [10,11]. Until the 1980s, dissection for rectal cancer was blunt with finger dissection, which produced high local recurrence. In 1982, Heald suggested the importance of an intact mesorectum using a sharp dissection for better local recurrence; thus, the concept of total mesorectal excision (TME) was born [12]. He published his results in 1998, showing a 80% 5-year survival and a 4% local recurrence [13]. TME also preserves the hypogastric nerves and reduces urogenital complications. Transanal endoscopic microsurgery (TEM) was introduced in 1983 for local resection of rectal tumors in selected cases [14]. Transanal TME (TaTME) and transanal minimally invasive surgery are also new frontiers in the field.

Evolution of laparoscopy for colorectal cancers

In general, laparoscopic surgery has advantages over its open counterpart in terms of smaller scars, lesser pain, shorter hospitalizations, and earlier returns to work. As a result, the first laparoscopic-assisted colonic surgery was performed by Jacobs et al. in 1991 [15]. If we look at other laparoscopic surgeries performed in the 1990s, such as cholecystectomy and fundoplication, the development of laparoscopic colorectal surgery has lagged behind. The probable reasons are that colorectal surgeries are multiquadrant surgeries; require retraction of mobile small bowels; require ligation of major vascular pedicles; need safeguarding of important structures present such as the ureter, duodenum, and many vessels as well; and of course, require a longer learning curve. Recognition of the role of laparoscopic surgery for colorectal malignancy took a bit longer. Apart from technical hurdles, issues such as safety, specimen removal, port site recurrence, and oncological outcomes were initial concerns. In the 1990s, oncological concerns were overriding the benefits of minimal access surgery. From 1991 until the early 21st century, laparoscopic colorectal surgery was limited to rectal prolapses because for malignancy, oncological concerns were high and for benign inflammatory conditions like diverticulitis, technical concerns were prevailing.

Port site recurrence has been thoroughly evaluated and it has been confirmed that it is close to 1%, which is as good as wound site recurrence in open surgery [16–19]. The data suggests that the wound/port site metastasis can be reduced with the use of wound protection devices during specimen removal [20].

Despite early reports on the safety of laparoscopic colorectal surgery for malignancy, it was predominantly used for benign conditions, most notably for rectal prolapses. It was from 2001 onward, when many randomized controlled trials and larger experiences started appearing, that laparoscopic colorectal surgery took its next step (Table 1.1). Multiple RCTs and meta-analyses confirmed the noninferiority of laparoscopic surgery for colorectal cancers, and it appears that laparoscopic colorectal surgery has taken further steps ahead over the last five years.

Evolution of laparoscopic surgery for benign colorectal condition

Rectal prolapse
Laparoscopic surgery for benign colorectal surgery mainly involves surgery for rectal prolapses. As per the guidelines, in any patient with rectal prolapse, the preferred treatment is transabdominal fixation of the rectum [29]. Open surgery has its own morbidity, while laparoscopic surgery has definitive advantages like smaller scars, lesser pain, shorter hospitalizations, and early returns to work. Laparoscopic surgery has been rapidly accepted for rectal prolapses, and has become a kind of standard of care – it does not involve much handling of the small bowel, and it does not involve anastomosis unless it is a resection rectopexy. A laparoscopic rectopexy is either a suture or a mesh rectopexy, and in patients presenting significant constipation, resection rectopexy is preferred. D'Hoore, in 2004, described anterior rectopexy to prevent injury to the nerves [30]. The procedure involves only an anterior dissection in the rectovaginal septum and avoids a posterior dissection altogether and prevents nerve injury. Although the procedure has gotten some acceptance, it is important to note that no high-level evidence is available yet and morbidities as high as 36% [31], as well as 4% mesh complications [32], have been reported.

Inflammatory bowel disease
Total proctocolectomy and ileal pouch anal anastomosis (TPC-IPAA) for ulcerative colitis is the standard of care when surgery is indicated. Laparoscopic TPC-IPAA has slightly lagged behind other laparoscopic procedures due to many challenges such as fragile bowels, multiquadrant surgery, difficulties in mobile small

TABLE 1.1: Randomized Control Trials Comparing Laparoscopy versus Open Surgery for Colorectal Cancers

Name of The Study	Published Year	Study Details	Number of Patients	Follow-Up	Primary End Points	Secondary End Points	Outcomes	Comments
Barcelona group (RCT) [21]	2002	Lap assisted vs. open colon cancer, single center	219	3.5 years	Cancer related survival		Benefits in terms of perioperative outcomes, better recurrence rate and disease-free survival for laparoscopic-assisted group.	The study was criticized for 12% recurrence rate in open group and poor lymphnode harvest in open group
COST (RCT) [22]	2004	Lap vs. open colon cancer, multicenter	872	3 years	Time to recurrence		Shorter hosptial stay in lap group, no difference in morbidity. Equivalent recurrence and disease-free survival at 3 years. Equal wound site recurrence than 1% in both groups.	
CLASSIC (RCT) [23,24]	2005, 2010 (5 years follow-up)	Conventional vs. lap assisted colon and rectal cancer	794	3 years, 5 years	Overall survival, disease-free survival, recurrence		Similar overall survival, disease-free survival, recurrence	
COLOR (RCT) (10 years results) [25]	2017	European muulticenter, lap vs. open colon cancer (10 years results)	1248	10 years	Disease-free survival	Overall survival and recurrence	Similar results in terms of recurrence, disease-free and overall survival	
COLOR II (RCT) [26]	2013	Lap vs. open for rectal cancer	1044	3 years	Recurrence	Disease free and overall survival	Similar results in terms of recurrence, disease-free and overall survival	
COREAN (RCT) [27]	2014	Lap vs. open for rectal cancer	340	3 years	Disease-free survival		Similar disease-free survival	
ACOSOG (RCT) [28]	2015	Lap assisted vs. open surgery for stage II and III rectal cancer	486	NA	Circumferential, distal margin and completeness of TME		Failed to meet noninferiority criteria	

bowel retraction, technical difficulties, complexity of the procedure, and a significant longer learning curve to cite a few. The first published report describing the role of laparoscopic surgery for IBD was in 1992 [33]. Although there are no randomized controlled trials for IBD, apart from the general benefits of laparoscopic surgery, there is a trend towards the additional benefits in case of TPC-IPAA in ulcerative colitis (UC), which are lesser adhesions and fertility advantages. As the surgery for UC involves multiple operations, lesser adhesions mean easier subsequent surgery. The disease involves a younger population, and in these cases there are potential benefits regarding fertility after laparoscopic surgery, probably due to fewer adhesions.

Segmental resection or limited ileocaecal resection in Crohn's disease are good indications for laparoscopic surgery, although fistulizing and structure in Crohn's disease may pose a challenge due to inflammation and adhesions.

Diverticular disease
The main concern in diverticular disease is linked to technical difficulties due to inflammations and adhesions. In 2017, Cochrane's review suggests that evidence is insufficient to support or refute the safety and effectiveness of laparoscopic surgery for colonic diverticular disease [34], although many smaller and retrospective studies have shown its safety and effectiveness [35].

Laparoscopic colorectal surgery in emergency situations

Although laparoscopic colorectal surgery progress has lagged behind due to its complexity, it is being increasingly performed across the globe. There are centers where laparoscopic surgery for elective colorectal operations are being routinely performed, and it is even being increasingly used for emergency colorectal surgeries. The data for emergency laparoscopic colorectal surgery is inadequate; however, in selected patients it may yield the benefits of minimal invasive surgery [36,37].

Future of laparoscopic colorectal surgery

Conventional laparoscopic surgery is spreading very well across the globe, and it has come very far from its beginnings in the last decades. In many diseases, there are many advantages of minimal access surgery over its open counterpart; some of them are well established while others are under investigation. Technology and medicine are progressing day-by-day, and now the time has arrived where we can start thinking about the disadvantages of laparoscopic surgery, and how to progress further.

The disadvantages, or limitations, of conventional laparoscopic surgery are the lack of tactile feedbacks, 2D view, and a limited degree of freedom offered by conventional laparoscopic instruments. The learning curve of conventional laparoscopic surgery is quite high for many complex surgeries. Conventional laparoscopic surgery has also resulted in many musculoskeletal professional hazards to the surgeon. Surgeons are also trying to reduce the size and number of ports, thus imparting further cosmetic benefits.

To overcome these limitations, options being explored are natural orifice transluminal endoscopic surgery (NOTES), single incision laparoscopic surgery (SILS), 3D laparoscopy camera systems, and robotic platforms capable of performing laparoscopic surgery.

NOTES was developed to avoid or reduce scars over the abdomen, but as of now it has not gained much success for a variety of reasons, and for colorectal surgery it appears to be far away from becoming a option of the treatment. NOTES' relative failure led to the development of SILS, although few surgeries are being performed with this technique and it has not become very popular as a result of inadequate instrumentations, lack of triangulation, and technical difficulties [38]. Better instrumentation is the need of the hour in order to make the SILS technique more acceptable. 3D camera systems have improved the quality of vision through better depth perception. A few surgeons feel dizziness and headache when working on 3D laparoscopy, which is an issue that needs to be considered. There is more evidence suggesting its advantages over conventional 2D camera systems, but we need more data for long-term benefits [39]. It may be beneficial for a few procedures and may not be beneficial for others, as it adds to the costs of the procedure as well. Surgical robots enhance the surgeon's skills and comfort, and in certain areas, like in the deep pelvis, they definitely make life more comfortable but clinical outcome improvements have yet to be decided upon as the technology needs further refinement. Robotic rectal surgery deep in the pelvis, especially in male pelvis and large rectal mass, does help in few situations. As of now, it adds much to the cost of the procedure, but once these go down, robotic platforms definitely have a future in laparoscopic colorectal surgery.

Summary

Laparoscopic colorectal surgery is undoubtedly here to stay. At present, although not the standard of care except for rectal prolapse, it is definitely an alternative option for colorectal diseases including colorectal cancers. There are centers where laparoscopic surgery is routinely offered for uncomplicated colorectal diseases. It should be performed by a surgeon experienced in advanced laparoscopic surgery. Robotic surgery provides assistance to the surgeon and helps in operating more comfortably in the narrow pelvis area, although definitive benefits have yet to be established.

Key points

- The invention of the computer chip camera system and other technologies improve vision significantly, allowing surgeons to become comfortable using the laparoscope.
- Wound/port site metastasis can be reduced with the use of wound protection devices.
- Recognition of the role of laparoscopic surgery for colorectal malignancy has been established.
- The concept of laparoscopic total mesorectal excision (TME) has also been established.
- The disadvantages, or limitations, of conventional laparoscopic surgery are the lack of tactile feedbacks, 2D view, and a limited degree of freedom offered by conventional laparoscopic instruments.
- Conventional laparoscopic surgery has also created many musculoskeletal professional hazards to the surgeon.

References

1. Kaiser AM. Evolution and future of laparoscopic colorectal surgery. *World J Gastroenterol* 2014;20(41):15119–24.
2. Miles WE. A method of performing abdomino-perineal excision for carcinoma of the rectum and of the terminal portion of the pelvic colon (1908). *CA Cancer J Clin* 1971;21:361–4.
3. Moynihan BGA. The surgical treatment of cancer of the sigmoid flexure and rectum. *Surg Gynecol Obstet* 1908;6:463–8.
4. Lirici MM, Hüscher CGS. Techniques and technology evolution of rectal cancer surgery: A history of more than a hundred years. *Minim Invasive Ther Allied Technol* 2016;25:DOI: 10.1080/13645706.2016.1198381
5. Ronel D, Hardy M. Henri Albert Hartmann: Labor and discipline. *Curr Surg* 2002;59:59–64.
6. Dixon CL. Anterior resection for malignant lesions of the upper part of the rectum and lower part of the sigmoid. *Ann Surg* 1948;128:425–42.
7. Golligher JC, Dukes CE, Bussey HJR. Local recurrences after sphincter saving excisions for carcinoma of the rectum and rectosigmoid. *Br J Surg* 1951;39:199–211.
8. Fain SN, Patin CS, Morgenstern L. Use of a mechanical suturing apparatus in low colorectal anastomosis. *Arch Surg* 1975;110:1079–82.
9. Knight CD, Griffen FD. An improved technique for low anterior resection of the rectum using the EEA stapler. *Surgery* 1980;88:710–14.
10. Reguero JL, Longo WE. The evolving treatment of rectal cancer. In: Longo WEM Reddy V, Audisio RA (Eds.), *Modern Management of Cancer of the Rectum.* New York: Springer, 2015; 1–12.
11. Lange MM, Rutten HJ, van de Velde CJ. One hundred years of curative surgery for rectal cancer: 1908–2008. *Eur J Surg Oncol* 2009;35:456–63.
12. Heald RJ, Husband EM, Ryall RD. The mesorectum in rectal cancer surgery-the clue to pelvic recurrence? *Br J Surg* 1982;69:613–16.
13. Heald RJ, Moran BJ, Ryall RD, Sexton R, MacFarlane JK. Rectal cancer: The Basingstoke experience of total mesorectal excision, 1978–1997. *Arch Surg* 1998;133:894–9.
14. Buess G, Theiss B, Hutterer F et al. Transanal endoscopic surgery of the rectum – testing a new method in animal experiments. *Leber Magen Darm* 1983;13:73–7.
15. Jacobs M, Verdeja JC, Goldstein HS. Minimally invasive colon resection (laparoscopic colectomy). *Surg Laparos Endosc Percut Tech* 1991;1:144–50.
16. Reilly WT, Nelson H, Schroeder G, Wieand HS, Bolton J, O'Connell MJ. Wound recurrence following conventional treatment of colorectal cancer. A rare but perhaps underestimated problem. *Dis Colon Rectum* 1996;39:200–7 [PMID: 8620788 DOI: 10.1007/BF02068076]
17. Hughes ES, McDermott FT, Polglase AL, Johnson WR. Tumor recurrence in the abdominal wall scar tissue after large bowel cancer surgery. *Dis Colon Rectum* 1983;26:571–2 [PMID: 6223795 DOI: 10.1007/BF02552962]
18. Fleshman JW, Nelson H, Peters WR et al. Early results of laparoscopic surgery for colorectal cancer. Retrospective analysis of 372 patients treated by clinical outcomes of surgical therapy (COST) study group. *Dis Colon Rectum* 1996;39:S53–8 [PMID: 8831547 DOI: 10.1007/BF02053806]
19. Allardyce RA. Is the port site really at risk? Biology, mechanisms and prevention: A critical view. *Aust N Z J Surg* 1999;69:479–85 [PMID: 10442917 DOI: 10.1046/j.1440-1622.1999.01606]
20. Jacobs M, Misiakos L, Pelaez-Echevarria G, Plasencia G. Single center experience in laparoscopic colectomy for cancer. *Ann Gastroenterol* 2001;14:303–9.
21. Lacy AM, García-Valdecasas JC, Delgado S, Castells A, Taurá P, Piqué JM, Visa J. Laparoscopy-assisted colectomy versus open colectomy for treatment of non-metastatic colon cancer: A randomised trial. *Lancet* 2002;359:2224–9 [PMID:12103285]
22. Clinical Outcomes of Surgical Therapy Study Group. Nelson H, Sargent DJ, Wieand HS et al. A comparison of laparoscopically assisted and open colecto- my for colon cancer. *N Engl J Med* 2004;350:2050–9 [PMID:15141043]

23. Guillou PJ, Quirke P, Thorpe H, Walker J, Jayne DG, Smith AM, Heath RM, Brown JM. Short-term endpoints of conventional versus laparoscopic-assisted surgery in patients with colorectal cancer (MRC CLASICC trial): Multicentre, randomised controlled trial. *Lancet* 2005;365:1718–26 [PMID: 15894098]

24. Jayne DG, Thorpe HC, Copeland J, Quirke P, Brown JM, Guillou PJ. Five-year follow-up of the Medical Research Council CLASICC trial of laparoscopically assisted versus open surgery for colorectal cancer. *Br J Surg* 2010; 97: 1638–45 [PMID: 20629110 DOI: 10.1002/bjs.7160]

25. Deijen CL, Vasmel JE, de Lange-de Klerk ESM et al. Ten-year outcomes of a randomised trial of laparoscopic versus open surgery for colon cancer. *Surg Endosc* 2017;31(6):2607–15.

26. Bonjer HJ, Deijen CL, Haglind E. COLOR II Study Group. A Randomized Trial of Laparoscopic versus Open Surgery for Rectal Cancer. *N Engl J Med.* 2015 Jul 9;373(2):194.

27. Kang SB, Park JW, Jeong SY et al. Open vs. Laparoscopic surgery for mid or low rectal cancer after neoadjuvant chemoradiotherapy (COREAN trial): Short-term outcomes of an open-label randomised controlled trial. *Lancet Oncol* 2010;11:637–45.

28. Fleshman J, Branda M, Sargent DJ et al. Effect of Laparoscopic-Assisted resection vs open resection of stage II or III rectal cancer on pathologic outcomes: The ACOSOG Z6051 randomized clinical trial. *JAMA* 2015;314:1346–55.

29. Bordeianou L, Paquette I, Johnson E, Holubar SD, Gaertner W, Feingold DL, Steele SR, Clinical practice guidelines for the treatment of rectal prolapse. *Dis Colon Rectum* 2017;60:1121–31.

30. D'Hoore A, Cadoni R, Penninckx F. Long-term outcome of laparoscopic ventral rectopexy for total rectal prolapse. *Br J Surg* 2004;91:1500–5.

31. Naeem M, Anwer M, Qureshi MS. Short term outcome of laparoscopic ventral rectopexy for rectal prolapse. *Pak J Med Sci* 2016;32:875–9.

32. Rickert A, Kienle P. Laparoscopic surgery for rectal prolapse and pelvic floor disorders. *World J Gastrointest Endosc* 2015;7:1045–54.

33. Sardinha TC, Wexner SD. Laparoscopy for inflammatory bowel disease: Pros and cons. *World J Surg* 1998;22:370–4.

34. Abraha I, Binda GA, Montedori A, Arezzo A, Cirocchi R. Laparoscopic versus open resection for sigmoid diverticulitis. *Cochrane Database Syst Rev* 2017; 11(11):CD009277. DOI: 10.1002/14651858.CD009277.pub2.

35. Royds J, O'Riordan JM, Eguare E, O'Riordan D, Neary PC. Laparoscopic surgery for complicated diverticular disease: A single-centre experience. *Colorectal Dis* 2012 Oct;14(10):1248–54.

36. Vallance AE, Deborah SK, James H, Michael B, Angela K, van der Meulen J, Kate W, Manish C. Role of Emergency Laparoscopic Colectomy for Colorectal Cancer - A Population-based study in England. *Ann Surg* 2019;270(1):172–9.

37. Chand M, Siddiqui MRS, Gupta A, Rasheed S, Tekkis P, Parvaiz A, Mirnezami AH, Qureshi T. Systematic review of emergent laparoscopic colorectal surgery for benign and malignant disease. *World J Gastroenterol* 2014 December 7;20(45):16956–63.

38. Rao PP, Rao PP, Bhagwat S. Single-incision laparoscopic surgery – current status and constrovorsies. *J Minim Access Surg* 2011;7(1):6–16.

39. Yim C, Lo CH, Lau MH et al. Three-dimenstion laparoscopy: Is it as good as it looks? – a review of the literature. *Ann Laparosc Endosc Surg* 2017;2:131.

Chapter 2

TRAINING FOR LAPAROSCOPIC COLORECTAL SURGERY

Prakash Kumar Sasmal

Contents

Learning objectives 8
Introduction 8
Laparoscopic surgery in colorectal diseases 8
Knowledge of basic laparoscopic surgical skills 9
Learning tools, techniques and methodologies 9
    Animal and human cadaver training models.. 9
    Endotrainer box 9
    Virtual reality simulators... 9
    Training in a specialized colorectal unit.. 9
Standard training models for teaching advanced laparoscopic skills in colorectal surgery 10
    General surgery apprenticeship and traineeship programmes.. 10
    Fellowships in MAS or advanced laparoscopy 10
    Master class or dedicated fellowship courses 10
    Preceptorship and proctorship... 10
    Highly structured training courses 10
        LAPCO programme... 10
Training of a laparoscopic colorectal surgeon... 10
Summary 11
Key points 11
References 11

Learning objectives

- Knowledge of basic skills of laparoscopic surgery
- Factors playing a role in the acquisition of skills in laparoscopic surgery
- Learning tools, techniques, and methodologies for acquiring the skills of laparoscopic colorectal surgery (LCS)
- Various evidence-based structured learning methods to perform LCS
- Planning an optimal training environment with a structured module to train aspiring surgeons

Introduction

The evolution of the field of surgical science has undergone a sea of changes over the decades, moving from open surgery through minimal access surgery (MAS) to robotic surgery. However, over decades, the teaching and training of the budding future surgeons have still been following the apprenticeship model of graded responsibility by hospital-based surgical training programs supervised by mentors, which was introduced by Dr William Stewart Halsted [1].

Following the introduction and increasing use of laparoscopic surgery in the late 20th century, until today MAS is the procedure of choice in nearly all major surgical diseases. The early part of the 21st century experienced a renaissance in technologically driven MAS, with the global performance of advanced surgical procedures for various diseases, including colorectal.

However, the teaching and training modules prevailing in medical schools are lagging behind the pace of advancements in the field of MAS. Due to public and professional expectations, the inadequately trained surgeon gets compelled to adopt the improvements in MAS with increasing compromises on patient's safety. Hence, it is the need of the hour to introduce an optimal training environment with a structured module to train aspiring surgeons. Also, it is not acceptable that the trainees acquire experience at the cost of the patient's safety – and there shouldn't be a compromise regarding this when various other training modalities are available to learn laparoscopic skills [2].

Laparoscopic surgery in colorectal diseases

The advantages of MAS in colorectal surgery for patients in terms of early recovery, lower rates of surgical site infections (SSIs), decreased postoperative pain, and shorter duration of hospital stay are very well known [3]. It comes at the cost of procuring advanced gadgets by the hospital, increased operating room (OR) time, and the requirement of trained and skillful surgeons. An inadequate and unstructured MAS training program during a surgical residency curriculum is likely to place patients at additional risk of injury, thereby offsetting the benefits of MAS. Nevertheless, adequately trained surgeons working with experienced trainers in specialized centers, routinely performing laparoscopic colorectal surgeries, can perform major colorectal resections without compromising the outcome [4].

The various factors playing a role in the acquisition of skills in laparoscopic surgery are: use of long hand instruments, perception of haptic feedback, proper hand–eye coordination, following the basics of ergonomics, and ambidexterity at times. However, the training curriculum during residency programs is insufficient to meet the standard due to various reasons including the lack of adequately trained trainers, stipulated duty hours for surgical residents with less time in the OR [5], and lack of a structured training module for MAS.

The ultimate goal of the training should be to groom safe and competent laparoscopic colorectal surgeons, who should be mature enough to utilise their clinical acumen and judgement at times of difficulty [6].

Knowledge of basic laparoscopic surgical skills

It is worth reiterating; the trainee needs to be proficient in necessary laparoscopic surgical skills before advancing to training in LCS. The trainee can acquire the fundamental skills of laparoscopy by practising alone in the endotrainers, the virtual simulation labs, before performing laparoscopic cholecystectomy, appendectomy and diagnostic laparoscopy, or adhesiolysis independently in patients. It is needless to stress upon the practicing of essential skills such as bowel walking, knotting and endosuturing which is crucial for LCS. Moreover, handling the small intestine in diagnostic laparoscopy with ambidexterity and taking verbal feedback from experts will be of utmost help in proceeding to learn LCS [7].

Learning tools, techniques and methodologies

Time and again, it is imperative to state that adequate and structured training for the laparoscopic colorectal surgeons is the most essential way to prevent and reduce potential complications of the complex procedure [8]. The different learning tools adapted for training in laparoscopic cholecystectomy may not be sufficient for conducting LCS.

Advanced simulation training is required in place of simple box endotrainers due to the need to operate in multiple quadrants of the abdominal cavity, dissect the hollow viscera from vital structures in confined spaces, and restore the continuity of the bowel [2]. The different types of learning tools utilised for imparting training in LCS – which have demonstrated advantages – are listed in Figure 2.1.

Animal and human cadaver training models
This method of simulation is the best way to improve the orientation of surgical anatomy, tissue handling, and demonstrating surgical dissections instead of exposing the patients directly to the threat of complications [9,10]. The models using embalmed human anatomical specimens have the advantages of enabling the practice of laparoscopic colorectal surgical procedures using standard laparoscopic hand instruments on actual human anatomy and near-normal tissue handling conditions [11], which provide a more realistic simulation than animal models [12]. A study comparing human cadaver and augmented reality simulator models, using a ProMIS simulator (http://www.haptica.com) for colorectal skills acquisition training, found the human cadaver

model to be more challenging to work with, but better appreciated [13]. The authors recommended the use of augmented simulator training, followed by cadaver training for optimal learning.

However, the difficulties faced when using live animal models (porcine) are due to anatomical differences along with strict ethical issues put in place in many countries relating to the handling of live animals, the requirement for appropriate operating rooms with facilities to anaesthetize, and the proper disposal of specimens after use. Furthermore, the availability of human cadavers (with necessary arrangements for training in LCS) is problematic and they are expensive. Also, a trainee can practice less often using these types of models, which is a hindrance.

Endotrainer box
These box simulators are readily available, economical, and can be used a number of times by multiple users. Standard laparoscopic hand instruments are used to practice basic laparoscopic surgical skills such as hand–eye coordination, ambidexterity, cutting, knotting, and suturing with good tactile feedback – usually under the observation of a trainer [2]. Training with this basic fundamental simulator, which is available in the surgical residency curriculum, improves the trainees' performance in the OR [14].

However, these basic box simulators are not sufficient to practice LCS due to the lack of tissue handling and anatomical recognition.

Virtual reality simulators
These models use various computer-based environments with advanced software to provide a virtual operating field for different basic and advanced surgical procedures such as cholecystectomy, gastrectomy, colectomy, and so on. Virtual simulators provide minor sensory feedback, a performance score with a recording of the skills for critical appraisal by a trainer, but come at a high cost for the initial set up. The motor skill acquisition occurs in three stages, as stated by Fitts and Posner. The first two stages, that is the cognitive and associative phase, can be accomplished outside the operation theatre through the various skill-based curricula carried out in simulation labs [15]. However, the automation phase is learnt in the OR directly by operating on patients under the supervision of trainers.

The virtual simulators provide pretask tutorials as well as posttask scoring of various criteria such as the movement of instruments and the duration to complete the task among others, along with the safety guidance during the procedure. It includes the identification of errors with management by the simulator aids in the execution of safe surgical practices [16]. The simulator also provides tactile sensations with constant feedback while handling the virtual tissues and can be used repeatedly during one's free time, without the requirement of assistants. The actual basic surgical skills performance of the residents in the real OR improves among those who practice in virtual simulators, as has been shown during laparoscopic cholecystectomy [17,18].

A dedicated tailored program offering a competency-based curriculum – to practice skills of different complexity in a step-by-step approach, may be used to perform laparoscopic colectomy [2,18].

Training in a specialized colorectal unit
The trainees in dedicated colorectal units running structured training programs under a mentor, who is proficient in performing LCS, can perform laparoscopic procedures with good clinical outcomes and without oncological compromises [4,19,20]. Also, video analysis of the recorded surgical procedures along with the trainer can be of immense help in grading and evaluating the trainees' progress. The residents should have some basic experience in laparoscopic surgery before proceeding to learn advanced colorectal procedures.

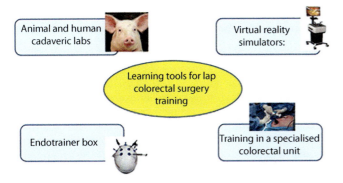

FIGURE 2.1 Different types of learning tools for learning LCS.

Standard training models for teaching advanced laparoscopic skills in colorectal surgery

The acquisition of the knowledge and skill of LCS is basically through graded exposure to the field during the various phases of learning. It is needless to emphasise that without proper knowledge and training in basic surgical procedures, venturing into advanced colorectal surgeries may be detrimental.

General surgery apprenticeship and traineeship programmes

The general surgery training system is based on a graded responsibility model, with an additional rotation schedule in various subspecialties. The duration of the training with the apprenticeship model varies between three years in India, to two to three years in western countries. During a short period, the trainee is expected to observe and assist during laparoscopic colorectal procedures as they are demonstrated by qualified trainers. The trainee is expected to learn only the basics of a safe laparoscopic colorectal procedure. However, additional training in LCS can be obtained through a structured fellowship program in colorectal surgery, or through pursuing higher studies in surgical gastroenterology.

Fellowships in MAS or advanced laparoscopy

The ideal and most comprehensive way to be proficient in acquiring the knowledge and skill of LCS is to undergo a fellowship training in MAS, or a dedicated fellowship training in colorectal surgery. These structured fellowship programs of one to two years duration exposes a trainee to observing and assisting various basic and advanced laparoscopic procedures, including colorectal surgeries performed by mentors. During the last part of this apprenticeship model of training, the fellow is allowed to perform colorectal procedures under supervision, including intracorporeal anastomosis and total mesorectal excision.

Master class or dedicated fellowship courses

These dedicated short courses in exclusive LCS are covered in three to seven days and are a combination of didactic lectures, live demonstrations of operative procedures, and hands-on training sessions in the skill lab or animal laboratory. Most of the courses focus on colectomies, which is possible to practice hands on using laparoscopy in porcine models. The rectal procedures are usually demonstrated step-by-step either by live surgery, or operative video presentations made by experts. Some of the well-known fellowship programs dedicated to training in the west are the laparoscopic colectomy courses offered by the American Society of Colon and Rectal Surgeons (ASCRS) and the Society of American Gastrointestinal and Endoscopic Surgeons (SAGES) [21]; in India, courses are offered by the Association of Colon and Rectal Surgeons of India (Fellow of ACRSI) [www.acrsi.com].

Preceptorship and proctorship

Although both terms used interchangeably, precepting is the process through which a surgeon gains experience – and/or training on new skills and knowledge, by visiting a dedicated colorectal training center. Usually, the less experienced surgeons in a surgical group are supervised and trained by an experienced surgeon in the unit (in-house preceptorship) [22].

Whereas proctorship is provided by an expert surgeon in laparoscopic colorectal procedures, who offers on-site training, assisting the trainee during the first few procedures at the trainees' hospital. This form of exercise is beneficial to the trainee to build considerable confidence, as the proctor can intervene during difficult times and will supervise the steps with constructive criticism. Most often, the proctor assists the trainee by operating the camera and orchestrating the procedure. Meta-analysis of outcome data from 6064 patients concluded that trainees performing procedures under proctorship had similar rates of complication, conversion, and mortality as done by expert laparoscopic colorectal surgeons [20].

Highly structured training courses

A structured and supervised training program in a high volume center is quite essential for the acquisition of advanced laparoscopic colorectal surgical skills. Many countries have designed their highly structured training programs to train budding surgeons in the skills of advanced laparoscopic surgery, including colorectal procedures.

In India, it is through the Fellow of National Board in MAS, under the National Board of Examinations – a certified two-year structured course – that the trainee is exposed to basic and advanced MAS by expert consultants. In the West, similar courses are available like the National Training Programme for LCS in England, and the Focus Group on Laparoscopic Colectomy Education in the USA [21].

LAPCO programme

The National Training Programme (NTP) for laparoscopic colonic surgery was introduced in England in 2007, funded by the Cancer Action Team, to train the existing consultant laparoscopic colorectal surgeons to a level of competence within five years [www.lapco.nhs.uk]. The program intended to provide all patients diagnosed with colorectal cancer in England access to a trained laparoscopic colorectal surgeon. The program was highly structured and integrated, focusing on cadaveric training and hands-on training in the operating room, all the while under supervision and preceptorship by an experienced laparoscopic colorectal specialist and providing the formative assessment after each training case [23,24].

The NTP also stressed on enhanced recovery after surgery, provide proctorship to outreach trainees' own hospital and audit the entire learning process to adjudge the improvement of skills in LCS [12].

At the end of the training, the trainee had to submit an electronically validated task-specific self-assessment form (GAS-Global Assessment Score). The Competency Assessment Tool (CAT) was formulated and implemented in the Lapco programme to demonstrate differences in levels of skill and competency [25]. An average minimum number of 20 cases completed was required by each surgeon to meet the level of competence demanded by the training. These supervised training programs have been effective in training laparoscopic colorectal surgeons without compromising the patient's safety [23,26].

Training of a laparoscopic colorectal surgeon

The components of the training of a laparoscopic colorectal surgeon should also include ensuring the necessary safety measures such as proper patient positioning on the operating table, providing adequate padding at pressure points, strapping the patient securely to the operating table for avoiding slippage during steep positions, and introducing the primary port after pneumoperitoneum.

The knowledge of the safe and practical application of electrosurgical devices and other energy sources should be a must in the training module. The principles of hemostasis and the modes of controlling bleeding from different vessels should also be an essential aspect of training for the execution of safe and effective LCS.

A stepwise approach towards the training of a laparoscopic colorectal surgeon is prudent to allow the trainee to be proficient in each stage. Also, different approaches to the same surgical procedures (like medial to lateral or lateral to medial approaches to colectomy) should be stressed upon. Last, a structured and dedicated colorectal training program is the pillar stone in producing safe and expert laparoscopic colorectal surgeons.

Summary

Since the introduction and increasing use of laparoscopic surgery in the late 20th century, minimally invasive surgery (MIS) has become the procedure of choice in nearly all major abdominal diseases. The ultimate goal of the training should be to groom safe and competent laparoscopic colorectal surgeons mature enough to utilise their clinical acumen and judgement with surgical skills at times of difficulty. The teaching and training modules prevailing at this time in medical schools are lagging behind the pace of advancements in the field of MAS. Advanced simulation training is required in place of simple box endotrainers to train in LCS. This is mainly due to the need to operate in multiple quadrants of the abdominal cavity, dissect the hollow viscera from vital structures in confined spaces, and restore the continuity of the bowel. The components of training of a laparoscopic colorectal surgeon should also include ensuring the necessary safety measures such as proper patient positioning on the operating table, providing adequate padding at pressure points, strapping the patient securely to the operating table for avoiding slippage during steep positions, and introducing the primary port after pneumoperitoneum.

Key points

- The ultimate goal of the training should be to groom safe and competent laparoscopic colorectal surgeon.
- Self-practicing in the endotrainers, virtual simulation labs, and at least performing laparoscopic cholecystectomy, appendectomy, and diagnostic laparoscopy or adhesiolysis independently in patients before starting LCS.
- Advanced simulation training is preferable in place of simple box endotrainers to train in LCS.
- Animal and human cadaver training models are beneficial if available.
- Three stages of learning: cognitive, associative, and automation stages.
- Dedicated fellowship courses, preceptorship, and proctorship.

References

1. Cameron JL. William Stewart Halsted. Our surgical heritage. *Ann Surg* 1997;225(5):445–58.
2. Celentano V. Need for simulation in laparoscopic colorectal surgery training. *World J Gastrointest Surg* 2015;7(9):185–9.
3. Guillou PJ, Quirke P, Thorpe H, Walker J, Jayne DG, Smith AM, Heath RM, Brown JM. MRC CLASICC trial group. Short-term endpoints of conventional versus laparoscopic-assisted surgery in patients with colorectal cancer (MRC CLASICC trial): Multicentre randomised controlled trial. *Lancet* 2005;365:1718–26.
4. Engledow AH, Thiruppathy K, Arulampalam T, Motson RW. Training in laparoscopic colorectal surgery – experience of training in a specialist unit. *Ann R Coll Surg Engl* 2010;92:395–7.
5. Varley I, Keir J, Fagg P. Changes in caseload and the potential impact on surgical training: A retrospective review of one hospital's experience. *BMC Med Educ* 2006;6:6.
6. Schlachta CM, Sorsdahl AK, Lefebvre KL, McCune ML, Jayaraman S. A model for longitudinal mentoring and telementoring of laparoscopic colon surgery. *Surg Endosc* 2009;23(7):1634–8. Epub 2008 Dec 6.
7. Porte MC, Xeroulis G, Reznick RK, Dubrowski A. Verbal feedback from an expert is more effective than self-accessed feedback about motion efficiency in learning new surgical skills. *Am J Surg* 2007;193(1):105–10.
8. Moore MJ, Bennett CL. The learning curve for laparoscopic cholecystectomy. The Southern Surgeons Club. *Am J Surg* 1995;170:55–9.
9. Ross HM, Simmang CL, Fleshman JW, Marcello PW. Adoption of laparoscopic colectomy: Results and implications of ASCRS hands-on course participation. *Surg Innov* 2008;15:179–83.
10. Katz R, Hoznek A, Antiphon P, Van Velthoven R, Delmas V, Abbou CC. Cadaveric versus porcine models in urological laparoscopic training. *Urol Int* 2003;71:310–5.
11. Slieker JC, Theeuwes HP, van Rooijen GL, Lange JF, Kleinrensink GJ. Training in laparoscopic colorectal surgery: A new educational model using specially embalmed human anatomical specimen. *Surg Endosc* 2012 Aug;26(8):2189–94.
12. Wyles SM, Miskovic D, Ni Z et al. Analysis of laboratory-based laparoscopic colorectal surgery workshops within the English National Training Programme. *Surg Endosc* 2011;25(5):1559–66.
13. Leblanc F, Champagne BJ, Augestad KM et al. A comparison of human cadaver and augmented reality simulator models for straight laparoscopic colorectal skills acquisition training. *J Am Coll Surg* 211(2):250–5.
14. Sroka G, Feldman LS, Vassiliou MC, Kaneva PA, Fayez R, Fried GM. Fundamentals of laparoscopic surgery simulator training to proficiency improves laparoscopic performance in the operating room – a randomized controlled trial. *Am J Surg* 2010;199(1):115–20.
15. Reznick RK, MacRae H. Teaching surgical skills–changes in the wind. *N Engl J Med* 2006;355(25):2664–9.
16. Satava RM. Identification and reduction of surgical error using simulation. *Minim Invasive Ther Allied Technol* 2005;14(4):257–61.
17. Seymour NE, Gallagher AG, Roman SA, O'Brien MK, Bansal VK, Andersen DK, Satava RM. Virtual reality training improves operating room performance: Results of a randomized, double-blinded study. *Ann Surg* 2002 Oct;236(4):458–63; discussion 463–4.
18. Beyer-Berjot L, Berdah S, Hashimoto DA, Darzi A, Aggarwal RA. Virtual reality training curriculum for laparoscopic colorectal surgery. *J Surg Educ* 2016 Nov - Dec;73(6):932–41.
19. de Campos Lobato LL, Ferreira PCA, de Oliveira PG et al. Laparoscopic training in colorectal surgery: Can we do it safely? *J Coloproctol (Rio J.)* 2013 Apr;33(1):3–8.
20. Miskovic D, Wyles SM, Ni M, Darzi AW, Hanna GB. Systematic review on mentoring and simulation in laparoscopic colorectal surgery. *Ann Surg* 2010 Dec;252(6):943–51.
21. Fleshman J, Marcello P, Stamos MJ, Wexner SD. American Society of Colon and Rectal Surgeons (ASCRS); Society of American Gastrointestinal and Endoscopic Surgeons (SAGES). Focus group on laparoscopic colectomy education as endorsed by American Society of Colon and Rectal Surgeons (ASCRS) and the Society of American Gastrointestinal and Endoscopic Surgeons (SAGES). *Dis Colon Rectum* 2006 Jul;49(7):945–9.
22. Chikkappa MG, Jagger S, Griffith JP, Ausobsky JR, Steward MA, Davies JB. In-house colorectal laparoscopic preceptorship: A model for changing a unit's practice safely and efficiently. *Int J Colorectal Dis* 2009;24(7):771–6.
23. Coleman M, Rockall T. Teaching of laparoscopic surgery colorectal. *The Lapco Model Cir Esp* 2013 May;91(5):27.
24. Coleman M. Lapco: National training programme for laparoscopic colorectal surgery. *Ann R Coll Surg Engl (Suppl)* 2009; 91:274–5.
25. Miskovic D, Wyles SM, Francis NK, Rockall TA, Kennedy RH, Hanna GB. On behalf of the National training programme in laparoscopic colorectal surgery. Laparoscopic colorectal competency assessment tool (LCAT) for the National training programme in England. *Ann Surg* 2013;257(3):476–82.
26. Mackenzie H, Miskovic D, Ni M, Parvaiz A, Acheson AG, Jenkins JT, Griffith J, Coleman MG, Hanna GB. Clinical and educational proficiency gain of supervised laparoscopic colorectal surgical trainees. *Surg Endosc* 2013;27(8):2704–11.

Chapter 3

CLINICAL ANATOMY RELATED TO LAPAROSCOPIC COLORECTAL SURGERY

David N. Naumann, Mark Dilworth, and Sharad Karandikar

Contents

Learning objectives 12
Introduction 12
Embryological development of the colon and rectum. 12
Vascular anatomy of colon and rectum 13
    Arterial supply. 13
    Venous drainage 14
Lymphatic drainage of the colon and rectum 14
Fascias of colon and rectum 14
Posterior relationships of colon 16
Summary 16
Key points 16
References 16

Learning objectives

- Understand the embryological development of the colon and rectum from the primitive midgut, hindgut, and cloaca
- Recognize how the lymphovascular supply to the colon and rectum affects colorectal resection
- Appreciate the fascial planes of the colon and rectum that are exploited during colorectal resection surgery

Introduction

A laparoscopic colorectal surgeon must correctly identify and develop planes of dissection, choose the correct margins of resection (including lymphatic drainage), and ligate the appropriate vessels, while avoiding the surgical pitfalls of bleeding and iatrogenic injury to the mesenteries and retroperitoneum. These objectives require a detailed understanding of the anatomy of the colon and rectum, and their embryological origin. This knowledge will allow the surgeon to develop bloodless planes of dissection as well as 'ideal' margins of resection. In this chapter, we will summarize the embryological development of the colon and rectum, then discuss the vascular and lymphatic supply, fascial layers, and posterior relationships. Throughout our discussion we will summarize how the choice and performance of key laparoscopic colorectal techniques are affected by the application of this important anatomical knowledge.

Embryological development of the colon and rectum

One of the best ways to understand the blood supply and anatomical planes of dissection in the colon and rectum is to consider how the midgut and hindgut formed and migrated into their final resting positions during embryological development. The midgut and hindgut are the final two thirds of the gut from mouth to anus, distal to the foregut. They therefore take their main blood supply from the lower two of the three anterior branches to the gut from the aorta – the superior mesenteric artery (SMA) and inferior mesenteric artery (IMA) respectively, along with their corresponding venous and lymphatic supplies. Running with these structures are the parasympathetic nerves from S2, 3, and 4 and the sympathetic nerves from T5 to L2 via the splanchnic nerves and autonomic plexuses. It is useful to conceptualize that the entire adult gut with its many twists and turns is really a midline structure suspended on a single mesentery, which has simply folded in various ways during embryological development. These arteries, veins, lymphatic vessels, and nerves can also be considered as midline structures that have 'followed' the gut during its developmental migration.

The rotation of the hindgut is normally considered in three distinct stages during embryological development. First, the primitive midline 'tube' structure elongates at the SMA and herniates into the umbilical cord, and this herniated portion of gut rotates anticlockwise 90° (Figure 3.1a,b). Then, the gut returns into the abdominal cavity while rotating a further 180° anticlockwise. Importantly during this stage, the gut proximal to the superior mesenteric artery reenters the abdomen first, followed by the more distal segments, meaning that sequentially the duodenum ends up being most posterior, with the SMA anterior to it, and then the distal (hindgut) ends up lying in front of the SMA (Figure 3.1c,d). This is ultimately why the duodenal–jejunal flexure lies posteriorly to the colon, and the colon has rotated in an anticlockwise direction around the SMA axis. In the final stage of development, there is further rotation so that the caecum descends into the right iliac fossa, and the rest of the colon continues to rotate into the position we are accustomed to seeing in the adult abdomen (Figure 3.1e). We can now understand from the embryological development of the colon and rectum that these structures were originally all suspended on their own common primitive mesentery. This is the case until the end of the first trimester, when the entire gut comes to rest in its final position. At this point the small bowel, transverse colon, and sigmoid colon remain suspended on their mesenteries, but the duodenum and the ascending and descending colon fuse with the posterior abdominal wall (i.e., the retroperitoneum).

The rectum is derived embryologically from the cloaca, which is the enlarged part of the distal gut, which curls forward and communicates with the allantois. The mesoderm between the cloaca and allantois (also known as the urorectal septum)

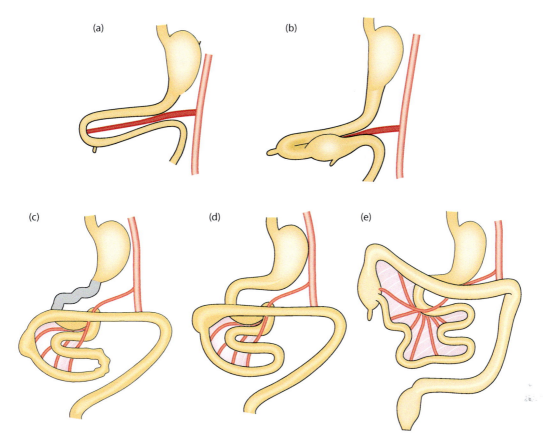

FIGURE 3.1 Embryological development of the gut: (a) the primitive gut elongates at the superior mesenteric artery (SMA) and herniates into the umbilical cord; (b) the herniated portion of gut rotates anticlockwise 90°; (c) the gut travels back into the abdominal cavity while rotating a further 180° anticlockwise; (d) the gut now lies within the abdominal cavity with the duodenum most posteriorly, followed by the SMA and then the hindgut anteriorly; (e) The gut continues to rotate until it ends in its final position.

pushes caudally until it divides the ventral and dorsal segments of this 'curled tube'; the allantois becomes the bladder and urogenital sinus, and the cloaca becomes the rectum and anus (Figure 3.2). These structures, now separated, fuse with the genital and anal tubercles respectively, with the perineal body in between them.

Vascular anatomy of colon and rectum

Arterial supply

As we have discussed, the colon derives its blood supply from the lower two arteries of the gut – the SMA and IMA. These correspond to their original embryological segments during

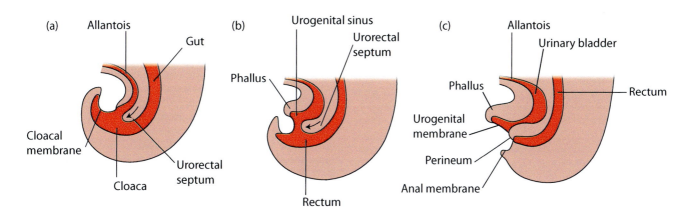

FIGURE 3.2 Embryological division of the urogenital sinus and rectum: (a) the urorectal septum moves caudally; (b) movement of the urorectal septum divides the cloaca into ventral and dorsal segments; (c) the ventral segment becomes the urinary tract and the dorsal segment becomes the rectum and anus.

development, with a transition between arterial supply occurring approximately two thirds of the way along the transverse colon, approximating the division of the midgut and hindgut – at the marginal artery of Drummond. There are rare occasions when there are variations to this conventional anatomical distribution, making preoperative cross-sectional imaging particularly important. For example, a common celiaco-mesenteric trunk has been reported (coeliac artery and SMA arising from the same trunk) [1]. For the purposes of the descriptions herein, we will assume common anatomical distribution of the main branches of the aorta, with the caveat that preoperative imaging is prudent.

The right colon is supplied by branches of the SMA, including the ileocolic artery (ICA), right colic artery (RCA), and middle colic artery (MCA). During a right hemicolectomy, the ICA is usually ligated along with the RCA, and right branch of the MCA (or the main MCA for an extended right hemicolectomy). Further branches of the ICA include the colic branch to the ascending colon, the anterior and posterior caecal branches, and the ileal branch (all providing blood to their namesake segments of ileum and colon). Some variation has been reported in the distribution of the three main arteries of the SMA (ICA, RCA, and MCA). The ICA and MCA are always present, but there is considerably variability in the RCA, which is often absent [2,3]. The following patterns of distribution have been described: (a) each artery arises independently; (b) there is a common trunk for RCA and MCA, and ICA arises independently; (c) RCA and ICA have a common trunk and MCA arises independently; (d) all three branches arise from a common trunk; (e) absence of RCA; and (f) multiple (accessory) right colic arteries are present [4]. The surgeon must therefore anticipate these variations when planning and undertaking right-sided surgery, while aiming for high ligation on the relevant branches of the SMA and minimizing bleeding during laparoscopic surgery.

The left colon is supplied by the IMA, from which the branches include the left colic artery supplying the descending colon, the sigmoid branches to the sigmoid colon, and the superior rectal artery to the upper third of the rectum. For left-sided cancer resections, the IMA is usually ligated as a 'high tie' (i.e., as close to its origin on the aorta as possible). Since the branches of the IMA arise at variable distances from its origin, a high tie is the only approach to ensure standardization of approach while ensuring adequate lymph node clearance [5]. The IMA high tie will take away the main blood supply from the distal third of the transverse colon to the upper third of the rectum, with the remaining colon and rectum reliant on branches of the SMA and internal iliac arteries from above and below, respectively. As described earlier, anatomical variations exist, and rare (but clinically relevant) variations in the vascular cascade have been reported [6]. The surgeon must be able to anticipate and make adjustments on operative planning with the aid of cross-sectional and contrast-enhanced imaging.

The rectum takes its blood supply in approximate thirds from the superior, middle, and inferior rectal arteries (also known as haemorrhoidal arteries). The first of these is a branch of the IMA, and the distal two are branches of the internal iliac arteries. There is therefore an anastomosis between IMA and internal iliac arteries at the junction between the upper and lower two thirds of the rectum between the superior and middle rectal arteries.

Venous drainage
The venous drainage of the colon largely follows the arterial supply; the ileocolic, right colic, and middle colic veins drain into the superior mesenteric vein (SMV). However, similar to the RCA, the right colic vein is also often absent [2]. The left colic and

sigmoid veins drain into the inferior mesenteric vein (IMV). The SMV and IMV ultimately drain into the hepatic portal vein, the latter via the splenic vein.

Venous drainage of the rectum corresponds to the arterial supply in thirds; the superior rectal vein drains into the inferior mesenteric vein, whereas the middle and inferior rectal veins drain into the internal iliac vein (the latter via the internal pudendal vein).

Lymphatic drainage of the colon and rectum

The lymphatic drainage to the colon and rectum tend to follow the arterial supply to the relevant segments. The choice of curative resections for colorectal cancer are often determined by which lymph nodes – and therefore which arteries – must be taken with the colonic specimen, since these are the first sites of metastasis. The first lymph nodes to drain the colon are present at the colonic wall (named the epicolic lymph nodes). These then drain into the paracolic lymph nodes, which then drain into the intermediate colic lymph nodes, which tend to follow the 'named' arteries mentioned earlier. Ultimately, the final lymph nodes of the colon are situated on the trunks of the SMA and IMA. Colonic cancer resections should therefore take the highest level of lymph node as possible that drains the relevant segment of bowel. In the case of a left-sided cancer, this would be the IMA, in order to include the final lymph nodes. On the right side, it would not be practical to ligate the SMA since this would also take away the blood supply to a large portion of the small bowel. Therefore, the intermediate lymph nodes are taken at the ICA, RCA, and MCA (as described earlier).

The main lymph nodes of the rectum are found in the mesorectum – the fatty tissue surrounding the rectum in its entire length that is enclosed within the perirectal fascia. These lymph nodes then drain into those around the IMA via the superior rectal artery. This means that during a rectal tumor resection (e.g., a low anterior resection), as well as taking the IMA and associated lymph nodes, the entire mesorectum may also be taken with the specimen (including the mesorectum distal to the tumor), to ensure the maximum number of local lymph nodes that drain the rectum are also harvested.

Fascias of colon and rectum

As we have discussed, the primitive colon and rectum began as a midline tubular structure suspended on a mesentery that included its blood supply and lymphatic drainage, and then rotated and rested in its final position. This resulted in some of the mesenteries fusing with the posterior abdominal wall. It is the exploitation of these fascial planes that allows the colorectal surgeon to resect a segment of colon or rectum along with its lymphovascular supply and visceral peritoneum. Such 'complete' resections have shown evidence of improved outcomes for the colon (complete mesocolic excision [CME]) [7] and the rectum (total mesorectal excision [TME]) [8].

For both left- and right-sided laparoscopic colonic resections, the surgeon must develop the bloodless embryological plane between the mesentery and the posterior abdominal wall that has previously been discussed. The ascending and descending colonic mesenteries can be separated from the retroperitoneum and restored to their 'midline' embryological positions during medial-to-lateral dissection. For example, during a right hemicolectomy, a plane is developed between the intersection of the ileocolic pedicle and the SMV (appearing as

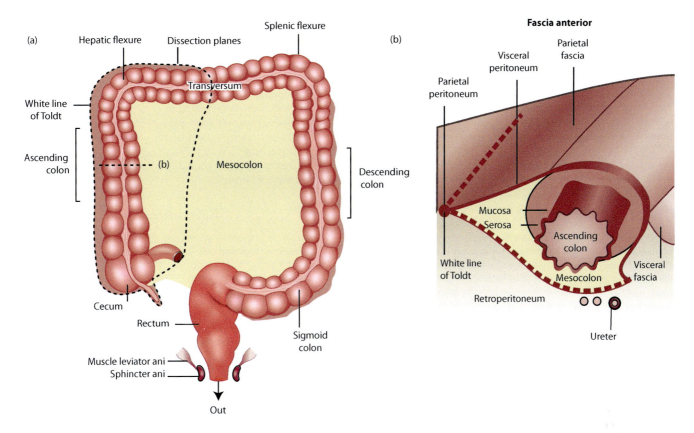

FIGURE 3.3   Relationship between the visceral and parietal peritoneum, and the white line of Toldt: (a) anterior view of colon and rectum; (b) cross sectional view of ascending colon.

a blue bulge), opening up this embryological space [9]. On the lateral sides of the ascending and descending colon, the visible white line of Toldt represents the lateral fusion points of the primitive mesentery to the posterior abdominal wall (i.e., the point at which the visceral peritoneum of the colon fuses with the parietal peritoneum of the retroperitoneum) (Figure 3.3). Once these segments of colon are mobilized during surgery, they are returned to their primitive state of being suspended on their mesentery, at which point their lymphovascular supply can be addressed as described earlier.

The transverse colon is suspended on its mesentery and therefore this must also be mobilized when performing left or right hemicolectomies. The root of this mesentery lies in front of the pancreas and is fused with the dorsal mesentery of the stomach during embryological development, forming the transverse mesocolon. This is directly posterior to the segment of greater omentum just inferior to the stomach (Figure 3.4). If the surgeon were to divide this part of the omentum, they would enter the lesser sac and the transverse colon would remain suspended on the transverse mesocolon, ready for ligation of appropriate vessels.

The mesorectum completely surrounds the rectum, and is itself surrounded by fascia propria (perirectal fascia) that causes it to be fixed in the pelvis. This layer of perirectal fascia is actually an extension of the retroperitoneal visceral fascia lying posteriorly to the inferior mesenteric vessels. It forms a sheath-like encapsulation of the mesorectum, and marks the surgeon's point of dissection to completely excise the mesorectum. As the mesorectum tapers at its most caudal part of the rectum, the perirectal fascia joins the rectum as it heads towards the anorectal junction, marking the lower border of the TME.

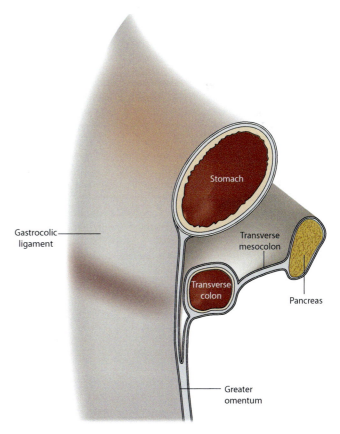

FIGURE 3.4   Access to the transverse mesocolon via the greater omentum.

Posterior relationships of colon

Most colorectal surgery requires the mobilization of the colon away from its retroperitoneal attachments, or fusion points, so that it can be resected or manipulated into a tension-free position for anastomosis or stoma. It is therefore essential that surgeons have an in-depth understanding of the posterior relationships within the retroperitoneum. In particular these include the right ureter and duodenum for right-sided surgery, and the left ureter for left-sided surgery, as well as the kidneys, pancreas, large vessels, and nerves for all resections.

For right-sided colonic mobilization, the ascending colon is effectively 'lifted' away from its right-sided position towards the midline by developing the embryological plane discussed earlier. During this maneuver, the duodenum and head of the pancreas will be encountered as they lie directly posterior to the transverse colon. It is important to develop the plane between the mobilized colon and duodenum while protecting them both from iatrogenic injury. This is usually done using blunt dissection, and when correctly applied, should develop a relatively bloodless plane. Similarly, the right kidney, ureter, and gonadal vessels lie just posterior to the embryological plane that is being exploited by the surgeon, and must remain posterior and protected. If these structures are lifted with the ascending colon then this is a sign that the surgeon is not within the correct plane.

For left-sided colonic mobilization, the left kidney, ureter, and gonadal vessels that lie directly posterior must be similarly protected from iatrogenic injury, or from being pulled upwards with the colonic dissection. For mobilization of the splenic flexure, attention must be paid to the careful manipulation of the splenocolic ligament that attaches the transverse colon to the splenic capsule. Both the ligament itself and the splenic capsule may bleed heavily if improperly handled.

Summary

Laparoscopic resection of a diseased segment of colon or rectum depends on the appropriate isolation and ligation of key lymphovascular structures that lie within the relevant mesenteries, while protecting any surrounding structures from inadvertent iatrogenic injury. This requires understanding of the optimal anatomical pathways to access these structures, using knowledge of the embryological development of the mid- and hindgut, and the resultant fascial relationships of interest. Furthermore, preoperative planning requires knowledge of the variability of anatomy, and thorough preoperative imaging so that variations are anticipated and addressed. We have discussed the relevant lymphatic, arterial, and venous considerations for laparoscopic colorectal resection, as well as summarizing the fascial planes of interest, and how these relate to access and mobilization of the relevant mesenteries

Key points

- Identification and exploitation of the embryological layers allows the surgeon to develop bloodless dissection planes
- Lymphovascular supply to the diseased segment must be considered when undertaking complete mesocolic excision and total mesorectal excision
- Preoperative cross-sectional and contrast enhanced imaging helps the surgeon to plan the optimal operative strategy
- Retroperitoneal structures must be protected from iatrogenic injury, and should not be lifted upwards with the colonic mobilization

References

1. Sangster G, Ramirez S, Previgliano C, Al Asfari A, Hamidian Jahromi A, Simoncini A. Celiacomesenteric trunk: A rare anatomical variation with potential clinical and surgical implications. *J La State Med Soc* 2014;166:53–5.
2. Alsabilah J, Kim WR, Kim NK. Vascular structures of the right colon: Incidence and variations with their clinical implications. SJS: Official organ for the Finnish Surgical Society and the Scandinavian Surgical Society *Scand J Surg* 2017;106:107–15.
3. Haywood M, Molyneux C, Mahadevan V, Lloyd J, Srinivasaiah N. The right colic artery: An anatomical demonstration and its relevance in the laparoscopic era. *Ann R Coll Surg Engl* 2016;98:560–3.
4. Gamo E, Jimenez C, Pallares E et al. The superior mesenteric artery and the variations of the colic patterns. A new anatomical and radiological classification of the colic arteries. *Surg Radiol Anat* 2016;38:519–27.
5. Bertrand MM, Delmond L, Mazars R, Ripoche J, Macri F, Prudhomme M. Is low tie ligation truly reproducible in colorectal cancer surgery? Anatomical study of the inferior mesenteric artery division branches. *Surg Radiol Anat* 2014;36:1057–62.
6. Hansdak R, Pakhiddey R, Thakur A, Mehta V, Rath G. Anatomical description and clinical relevance of a rare variation in the mesenteric arterial arcade pattern. *J Clin Diagn Res: JCDR* 2015;9:Ad01–2.
7. Bertelsen CA, Neuenschwander AU, Jansen JE et al. Disease-free survival after complete mesocolic excision compared with conventional colon cancer surgery: A retrospective, population-based study. *Lancet Oncol* 2015;16:161–8.
8. Quirke P, Steele R, Monson J et al. Effect of the plane of surgery achieved on local recurrence in patients with operable rectal cancer: A prospective study using data from the MRC CR07 and NCIC-CTG CO16 randomised clinical trial. *Lancet* 2009;373:821–8.
9. Ye K, Lin J, Sun Y, Wu Y, Xu J, He S. Variation and treatment of vessels in laparoscopic right hemicolectomy. *Surg Endosc* 2018;32:1583–4.
10. Danowitz M, Solounias N. Embryology, comparative anatomy, and congenital malformations of the gastrointestinal tract. *Edorium J Anat Embryo* 2016;3:39–50.
11. Development of the Digestive System. In: *Reference Module in Biomedical Sciences*. Elsevier, 2014.
12. Kuipers EJ, Grady WM, Lieberman D. Colorectal cancer. *Nature Reviews Disease Primers* 2015;1:15065.

Chapter 4

BASIC PRINCIPLES AND TECHNIQUES OF LAPAROSCOPIC COLORECTAL SURGERY

Sanjiv Haribhakti and Shobhit Sengar

Contents

Learning objectives 17
Introduction 17
Potential benefits of laparoscopic colorectal surgery. 18
Training in laparoscopic colorectal surgery. 18
Basic principles of laparoscopic colorectal surgery 18
Patient preparation. 20
OR setup. 20
Standard port placements. 20
Initial entry and initial assessment 20
Instrumentation 21
Energy sources 22
Staplers and accessories. 22
Standard operative steps 22
    Laparoscopic ileocaecal resection or right hemicolectomy for ileocaecal tuberculosis 22
    Laparoscopic suture rectopexy for rectal prolapse. 22
    Laparoscopic sigmoid colectomy for sigmoid colon cancer 22
    Laparoscopic APR for ultra-low rectal cancers. 22
    Laparoscopic anterior resection and low anterior resection for rectal cancers 23
    Laparoscopic left hemicolectomy for descending colon cancer. 23
    Laparoscopic right hemicolectomy for right colon cancer 23
    Laparoscopic transverse colectomy. 23
    Laparoscopic restorative proctocolectomy and ileal pouch anal anastomosis 23
    Laparoscopic total colectomy and ileorectal anastomosis 24
    Laparoscopic total proctocolectomy and ileostomy. 24
    Laparoscopic reversal of Hartmann's operation 24
    Laparoscopic colon replacement for corrosive strictures 24
Newer techniques and adjuncts. 24
    Intersphincteric dissection and coloanal anastomosis. 24
    Transvaginal/transanal specimen removal. 24
    Proximal diversion 24
    Neoadjuvant chemoradiation. 24
    Adjuvant chemotherapy 24
Conversion in laparoscopic colorectal surgery 24
Complications of laparoscopic colorectal surgery 25
Summary 25
Key points 25
Videos. 25
References 25

Learning objectives

- Understand the basic principles behind laparoscopic colorectal resections including its development, selection of patients, preoperative preparation, operative plan, operative techniques, postoperative care, and complications.
- Understand the basic surgical principles of exposure, OR setup, port placements, retraction and counter traction, dissection, stapling, and other anastomotic techniques in commonly employed laparoscopic colorectal procedures.
- Understand the principles of oncology such as the no touch technique, central vascular control, complete mesocolic excision (CME) and total mesorectal excision (TME), wound protection, and early adjuvant therapy for better outcomes in colorectal cancers.
- Apply these basic principles in the conduct of commonly employed laparoscopic colorectal surgeries.

Introduction

The last decade has seen a meteoric rise and standardization of laparoscopic colorectal surgery. Almost all colorectal surgeries have been performed with the laparoscopic method. However, the learning curve is longer than laparoscopic upper gastrointestinal (UGI) surgeries such as laparoscopic fundoplication and laparoscopic bariatric surgery primarily because handling the large mobile viscus is more difficult, and colonic surgery frequently involves operating in multiple quadrants. Thus, laparoscopic colorectal surgery is at a more advanced stage of laparoscopic surgery in the overall learning curve of the surgeon. However, the benefits it offers patients and surgeons make it a first choice for management of colorectal diseases. The benefits of laparoscopic colorectal surgery have been substantiated by numerous prospective randomized trials and have proven beneficial through evidence-based studies [1–3].

Potential benefits of laparoscopic colorectal surgery

The potential benefits for laparoscopic colorectal surgery to the patients and to the surgeons can be summarized as:

1. *Early postoperative recovery*: Due to a smaller wound and less pain, the patients can be mobilized much earlier, reducing the risks of thromboembolism and hastening the recovery of patients undergoing major resections. The hospital stay is also reduced [4] and they can get back to adjuvant therapy or their work faster than they would after open surgery. However, with the fast track protocols, the recovery from open surgeries has also been expedited [5,6].
2. *Better cosmesis*: The smaller scar required for laparoscopic colorectal resection improves the cosmetic appearance [6,8]. This would be more of a benefit in benign disease; however, even in malignancy and in young patients, this can also be beneficial.
3. *Less intraoperative bleed and need for blood transfusion (BT)*: Laparoscopic surgery typically utilizes energy sources and a clear field of vision for proper tissue dissection, which results in minimal blood loss and rarely the need for BT. Prospective randomized trials have shown that BT adversely affects long term survival in colorectal resections [9,10]. Thus, minimizing the blood loss and BT would be beneficial for patients.
4. *Less immunosuppression*: Performing a laparoscopic resection means that the bowel is in their natural environment during the surgery, handling of bowel is minimized, trauma of large wound and retraction is also minimized, which minimizes the tissue trauma overall. This would translate to lesser immune-suppression and less immune response, which may be beneficial for a patient with malignancy [11,12].
5. *Early adjuvant therapy*: It is well established that early adjuvant therapy after colon cancer resection significantly reduces the recurrence rates in loco-regionally advanced tumors. Early recovery after laparoscopic surgery and reduced wound complications allows patients to get early adjuvant therapy, and may become one of the main advantages for long-term outcomes in the future [13].

Training in laparoscopic colorectal surgery

Training in laparoscopic colorectal surgery requires understanding of the principles of colorectal surgery. Some experience in open colorectal resections and experience in advanced laparoscopic surgery is highly desirable. Understanding the principles of laparoscopic port placements, mechanisms of traction and countertraction, understanding the anatomical tissue planes, and developing a good team and adequate instrumentation would go a long way in mastering laparoscopic colorectal surgery. One should

select patients well in the early part of the learning curve. The learning curve for laparoscopic colorectal surgery would be anywhere between 25 and 50 cases depending on the surgeon [14,15].

Basic principles of laparoscopic colorectal surgery (see Videos 1 and 2)

Like all procedures, techniques for laparoscopic colorectal surgeries should be standardized to obtain a consistent outcome.

1. *Exposure and vision*: As in any surgery, the exposure and the clarity of vision is of paramount importance in laparoscopic colorectal surgery. Although not a must, a HD camera with a xenon light source and large flat panel LED monitor improves the quality of vision and dissection, and the ability to identify anatomical structures and prevent complications. Recently 3D laparoscopic systems have also become popular to get better depth perception; however, their use has not shown to significantly reduce the risk of complications.
2. *Team work*: Laparoscopic colorectal surgery is not for an individual surgeon. There is a need for a camera surgeon and an assistant surgeon for performing laparoscopic colorectal surgery. The entire team should fully understand the principles of surgery and work in coordination with each other for the smooth conduct of the operation.
3. *Ergonomics*: The surgeon's comfort plays an important role, as these resections are time consuming and take anywhere between 2 and 4 hrs of surgical time depending on the procedure. We have adopted an ergonomic technique where both the surgeon's left and right trocar are on one side, i.e., for a left colon resection, both surgeon's trocars are in the right abdomen and both the assistant trocars are in the left abdomen. Although theoretically this does not provide a perfect triangulation for laparoscopic surgery, most of the dissection can be easily performed with this technique.
4. *Bowel handling*: Gentle bowel handling with laparoscopic instruments is of paramount importance in bowel surgery. The small bowel can be manipulated with gentle atraumatic instruments (Figure 4.1) and patient positioning to keep them out of pelvis during the pelvic dissection. However, the traction on the colon should only be given by holding the taenia, epiploicae, or mesocolon (Figure 4.2). The colon should never be retracted by holding its wall as it can easily be traumatized due to the thin wall and excessive traction necessary to keep them out of the surgical field.
5. *Traction and countertraction*: Adequate traction of the colon to keep them out of the way and countertraction by

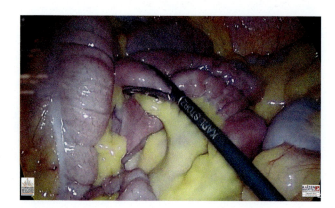

FIGURE 4.1   Small bowel handling.

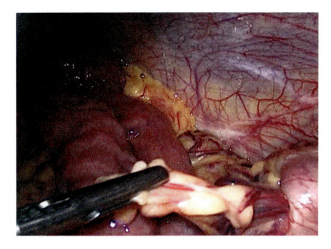

FIGURE 4.2 Colon handling by epiploicae.

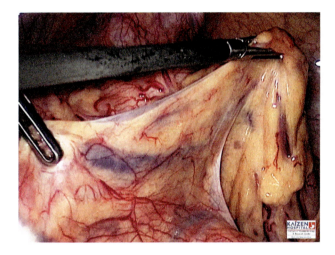

FIGURE 4.3 Traction.

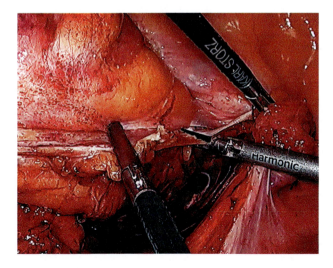

FIGURE 4.4 Countertraction.

another grasper at the site of dissection is an extremely important principle of laparoscopic colorectal surgery. The traction is given by an assistant grasper (either one or two graspers) (Figure 4.3) and the countertraction is done by the surgeon's left-hand grasper (Figure 4.4). We prefer to

use two assistant graspers for the purpose of traction – the first one keeps the colon or rectum away and is out of the surgical field, whereas the second one provides traction in the area of surgical dissection.

6. *Dissection and hemostasis*: Most of the dissection in colorectal surgery happens in the avascular tissue planes along the planes of embryonic fusion. This plane contains only the areolar tissue and is easily accentuated with the pneumoperitoneum. Dissection along this plane is bloodless and can avoid complications, and should be the goal in colorectal surgery whether it is medial to lateral colonic dissection or TME. Most of this dissection can be done with monopolar energy without the need for special energy sources. Hemostasis should be meticulous during the dissection to keep the planes clear and avoid the red glow.

7. *Principles of vascular control*: In colon cancer surgery, one of the important principle of vascular control at the root of the vascular pedicle is well honored in laparoscopic surgery. For a left colon resection, the ligation of IMA is done at the root to procure the LN at the root of IMA. For a right colon resection, the ligation of ileocolic, right colic, and middle colic pedicles is done at the root of these vessels for adequate LN clearance and to obtain at least 12 LN, which is considered a minimum for colorectal cancer surgery.

8. *No touch technique*: The principle of the 'no touch technique' is well honored in laparoscopic colorectal surgery as the tumor handling is minimal by laparoscopic instrumentation. Later, while tumor handling is performed for specimen extraction, the vascular pedicles are already ligated and the risk of tumor cell dissemination or embolization is minimized.

9. *Principles of splenic flexure mobilization*: The complete mobilization of the splenic flexure is the most important step in low anterior resection to reduce any tension on the anastomosis to prevent an anastomotic breakdown. The adequate mobilization is determined when the entire splenic flexure and distal transverse colon is separated from its peritoneal attachments and perinephric fascia and can be turned downward completely.

10. *Principles of wound protection in laparoscopic colorectal cancer surgery*: Certain precautions during a tumor extraction from a mini-laparotomy are necessary to prevent tumor cell implantation at the wound sites. The deflation of the pneumoperitoneum should be gradual at the end of the procedure, as it is envisaged that tumor cells circulating in the peritoneum can implant at the wound sites when a rapid release of pneumoperitoneum occurs by creating turbulence at the wound site. All tumor extractions from a minilaparotomy should always be done by protecting the wound edges with a wound protector [16,17] (Figure 4.5).

11. *Principles of anastomosis and checking its integrity*: For most left-sided laparoscopic colonic resections and rectal resections, an intracorporeal double-stapled anastomosis is employed. For right colectomies, there is an option of hand sewn anastomosis through periumbilical mini-laparotomy incision or a stapled/hand sewn intracorporeal anastomosis, when the specimen can be removed from a Pfannenstiel incision or a natural orifice such as anus or vagina. An attempt should be made to check the anastomotic vascularity by using ICG (Figure 4.6). The integrity of the anastomosis should be checked whenever possible by air leak test or saline leak test.

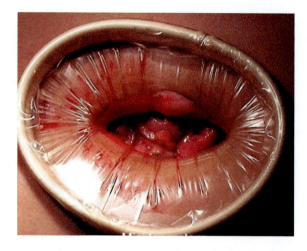

FIGURE 4.5 Wound protector.

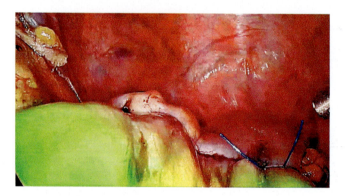

FIGURE 4.6 ICG showing ileorectal anastomosis.

Patient preparation

The patient is prepared in the same manner as in open surgery. The preoperative laboratory workup is done for any patient having to undergo a general anesthetic. The colon preparation is done similarly to open surgery. We do not believe in local antibiotic preparation; however, despite controversies in literature regarding mechanical bowel preparation, it is our routine to prepare our patients with a mechanical bowel lavage on the day before surgery for left-sided and rectal resections. We would also give them IV antibiotics starting 12 hrs before surgery as well as DVT prophylaxis with low molecular weight heparin starting 12 hrs before surgery. Clear liquids are allowed to patients after mechanical lavage until 3 hours before the procedure. Local preparation is done in the same way as for any major abdominal surgery. For patients undergoing a stoma, counselling is done with stoma appliances, and a stoma marking is done on the day before surgery.

OR setup

The OR setup is like any advanced laparoscopic surgery. The LED monitors are placed on the side of the tumor or on the opposite side of the surgeon. For proctocolectomy, it is mandatory to have monitors on both the sides of the patients. After induction of general anesthesia, both the arms of the patients are placed on the side of the body tucked in, with extension lines for IV support for IV access. An indwelling urinary catheter is placed for all colorectal procedures.

Standard port placements

For a left colonic resection, the surgeon stands on the right side of the patient facing the monitor, and the camera surgeon is to the left of the surgeon. The first surgical assistant is on the left of the patient, opposite to the surgeon.

The standard port placement for any left-sided colonic resection, including a rectal resection, is to have two surgeons working ports in the right abdomen – a 12 mm port in the RIF and a 5 mm port in the right upper abdomen. The RIF port is slightly lateral to the midaxillary line and lower than the McBurneys point so as to achieve a good angle for low rectal mobilization and firing of the stapler. The left surgeon 5 mm port is slightly medial to the midaxillary line to achieve a comfortable angle and triangulation for the surgeon.

For a left-sided resection, two assistant grasper 5 mm ports are placed in the left abdomen, both in the midaxillary line, one in the LIF and the other in the left upper abdomen. An endoclinch type of bowel grasper is used for both these ports to achieve colon mobilization by the assistant (Figure 4.7). An additional 5 mm grasper may be necessary in the suprapubic region or in epigastrium occasionally, for difficulty in retraction of the splenic flexure or for uterine retraction in females. Alternatively, the uterus can be hitched up with a suture with the anterior abdominal wall to give sustained traction.

For a right colon resection, the surgeon is standing on to the left of the patient, whereas the assistant is on the right side of the patient, and the camera surgeon is to the left of the surgeon. The port placements are similar to the left sided resection, except that a 12 mm port is not needed for a right hemicolectomy, as we prefer to perform the anastomosis extracorporeally after complete mobilization of the right colon and intracorporeal division of the major vascular pedicles.

For a total proctocolectomy, the port placements are essentially similar, with surgeon and the entire team rotating to the other side after completing the colectomy on one side.

Initial entry and initial assessment

We use the Verres needle-sharp trocar insertion technique for creating the first access after the pneumo-peritoneum. Alternatively, a blunt or Hasson trocars can be inserted by an open technique. The skin incision for the first 10 mm trocar is a infraumbilical vertical incision, so as to extend it during the minilaparotomy required later for specimen extraction (Figure 4.8). All skin incisions should be such that trocars snugly fit the incision, so that during a long procedure the trocars don't keep moving while the instruments are being exchanged. In patients with prior surgery,

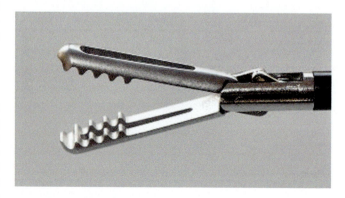

FIGURE 4.7 Atraumatic endoclinch grasper.

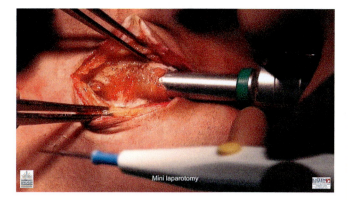

FIGURE 4.8 Ten mm port converting to vertical mini laparotomy.

initial entry should be away from the scar. Most likely the initial entry would be a 5 mm trocar from the left Palmar's point, 2 cm below the left midclavicular line.

After initial entry, an initial inspection of the abdominal cavity is performed, especially for all malignant or suspected malignant cases. The right and left liver is seen in anti-Trendelenburg position, the peritoneal cavity is carefully inspected especially in the pelvis, also the omentum and the local tumor with LN are inspected and noted. Any suspicious areas are sent for frozen section and any fluid is also collected for cytology.

Instrumentation

Apart from the routine instrumentation needed for any laparoscopic surgery, the special instrumentation required for laparoscopic colorectal resections is:

1. *Atraumatic bowel graspers*: For small bowel handling and to keep them out of the way from the pelvis along with a steep Trendelenburg position.
2. *Two Endoclinch type graspers*: For colonic traction by assistant graspers.
3. *Monopolar Hook or spatula*: For dissection along the tissue planes.

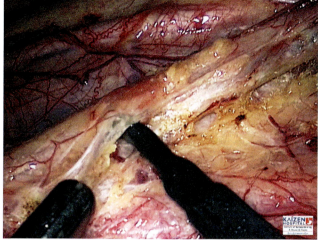

FIGURE 4.10 IMA ligation after ureter visualization.

4. Atraumatic grapser or a Maryland dissector for the surgeons left hand to provide countertraction during the dissection.
5. A 10-mm right angled instrument is used to dissect and encircle the IMA pedicle before clipping (Figure 4.9). The IMA is ligated only after the left ureter is visualized (Figure 4.10).
6. A suction and a bipolar is useful if any bleed occurs and to control the bleed and keep the field clean.
7. IMA pedicle can be ligated with locking polymer clips (Haemolock), standard metallic clips, ligature, or firing with endovascular staplers. We prefer to use the locking clips on the IMA.
8. Endoscopic roticulating staplers are very useful for low anterior resections, whereas straight staplers are sufficient for high resections at the promontory. We prefer a 45 mm cartridge, and generally two firings are needed for low anterior resections. If the pelvis is capacious and adequate space is available, a single firing of a 60 mm stapler would also be sufficient in some patients.

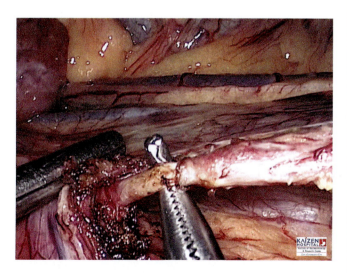

FIGURE 4.9 Ten mm right angled instrument is used to dissect and encircle the IMA pedicle.

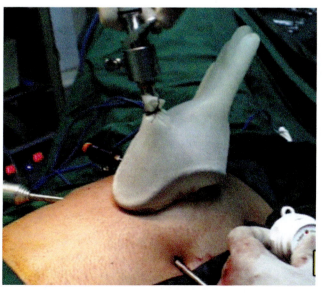

FIGURE 4.11 Recreation of pneumoperitoneum by glove.

9. *Wound protector*: To protect the wound during specimen extraction.
10. *Devices for recreating pneumoperitoneum*: For a left-sided resection and a double-stapled anastomosis, pneumoperitoneum needs to be recreated after specimen extraction from minilaparotomy. Several methods used are temporary suture closures, clip closures, using wound retractors and a glove (Figure 4.11), or using a handport device. Even permanent closure of the wound can be achieved if the trocars are not to be used from the incision.
11. End-to-end anastomosis stapler for left-sided resection for intracorporeal anastomosis.

Energy sources

1. *Monopolar energy*: We use it most often for most of the dissection in laparoscopic colorectal surgery. This is done using the spatula or the hook electrode. Minor ooze from small unnamed vessels of diameter 1–2 mm can easily be controlled with monopolar diathermy. The advantages of monopolar energy are its ease of use, minimal smoke generated, and that it preserves the tissue planes in the areolar tissue and helps the surgeon to maintain the tissue planes during CME and TME.
2. *Bipolar energy*: It is used most often for hemostasis from vessels larger than can be controlled by monopolar vessels (3–5 mm), and when there is a brisk bleed. In our opinion, bipolar is best to control even major bleeds and achieve a temporary control before clipping can be done. It is superior to ultracision from a hemostatic point of view for vessels 3–5 mm diameter.
3. *Ultrasonic energy*: It is useful for selected use in laparoscopic colorectal surgery. We use it mainly for the lateral rectal mobilization and for the mobilization of splenic and hepatic flexure. The entire colorectal resection can be safely performed without the use of any special energy sources. Some surgeons routinely perform the entire dissection with the help of a Harmonic scalpel™; however, we do not advocate this practice, as it generates more particles in the environment, smogs the camera more often, destroys the tissue planes during dissection, and slows down the surgical dissection times.
4. *Vessel sealing devices*: These are useful for major vessel pedicles, and mesocolic vessels of diameter 5–7 mm. These special devices, although useful, are not a must for performing laparoscopic colorectal resections.

Staplers and accessories (see Video 3)

Staplers are mainly necessary for a left colonic or anterior resection of the rectum. For a right-sided colonic lesion, we prefer an extracorporeal hand sewn anastomosis, avoiding the use of staplers.

For division of the rectum for high or low anterior resection, an endo GIA/Linear cutting stapler is necessary. For high division at the promontory or above the peritoneal reflection, a straight stapler 60 mm is sufficient after adequate mobilization. For low anterior resection, a roticulating stapler is necessary and generally we prefer two firing of endoGIA/Linear cutter 45 mm, as the space available in the low pelvis is reduced, especially in the male pelvis. In female patients with a capacious pelvis, a single firing of 60 mm roticulator stapler would be sufficient to perform the transection of rectum on the pelvic floor.

Standard operative steps

Laparoscopic ileocaecal resection or right hemicolectomy for ileocaecal tuberculosis
This can be a beginning point for venturing into laparoscopic colorectal surgery. With the standard port placement, the ileocaecal junction is lifted up by the two assistant graspers and the surgeon standing on the left side of the patient divides the lateral attachments of the caecum, right colon, and the root of the mesentery from DJ flexure to hepatic flexure of the colon. Once the complete mobilization of the lateral attachments of the right colon is done, the hepatic flexure is mobilized if a right hemicolectomy is necessary. A midline minilaparotomy of approximately 5–6 cm incision is made skirting around the umbilicus on the right side. The mobilized right colon is delivered from the wound and extracorporeal resection and anastomosis is performed. After the replacing of the bowel, abdominal wall closure is performed.

Laparoscopic suture rectopexy for rectal prolapse
We prefer to perform a laparoscopic suture rectopexy rather than mesh rectopexy due to the equivalent results of both the techniques and to avoid the rare, albeit serious complications of mesh implant close to the bowel. After standard port placements, the mesorectal dissection plane is entered at the sacral promontory. The posterior rectal mobilization is performed down to the pelvis. The lateral ligaments are preserved and not divided to preserve the pelvic splanchnic nerves. The anterior mobilization is also limited to divide just the peritoneum, so that the mobilized rectum can be pulled up to hitch it up to the sacral promontory. After complete rectal mobilization, one assistant grasper pulls out the rectum, and the rectum is sutured to the sacral promontory. We prefer to use two interrupted Ethibond™ 2-0 sutures on one side of the rectum with the seromuscular rectum and the sacral fascia, so as to avoid the hypogastric nerve, ureters, and the presacral vessels. No drain is left at the end of the procedure.

Laparoscopic sigmoid colectomy for sigmoid colon cancer
The medial to lateral dissection is performed on the left colon. The root of the IMA pedicle is divided, and lateral attachments of the colon are divided. Extensive splenic flexure mobilization is not necessary in such patients, as the rectum is divided at the sacral promontory or above the peritoneal reflection. The site of rectal division is decided upon and the mesorectum is divided at this point. A 60-mm straight Endo-GIA stapler is used to divide the rectum. Subsequently, a minilaparotomy is done at approximately 5–7 cm, depending on the tumor's bulk. We prefer a midline incision; however, a Pfannensteil, or a left iliac fossa muscle splitting incision can also be used. The mobilized colon is extracted with adequate wound protection. The proximal division is performed, and the anvil of the EEA stapler no. 31 is placed and a pursestring suture of no 1 Prolene™ is tied around the anvil. The proximal colon is then placed back into the abdomen. Pneumoperitoneum is recreated, and under laparoscopic vision, end-to-end anastomosis is performed with a stapler. The anastomosis is checked for any leaks. No proximal stoma is used if the colon is not obstructed.

Laparoscopic APR for ultra-low rectal cancers
Laparoscopic APR is now infrequently performed as better techniques of sphincter preservation are used such as low, ultralow, or inter-sphincteric resections to achieve sphincter preservation.

However, laparoscopic APR is an ideal laparoscopic surgery to begin learning rectal resections and TME. In such cases, there is no tumor in the pelvic rectum, and no anastomosis is necessary. Furthermore, the specimen removal is also done from the perineal route, so Minilaparotomy is not needed for specimen removal. After ligation of the IMA, medial to lateral dissection of the left colon is performed. The rectum is mobilized in the avascular holy plane between the visceral and the presacral fascia posteriorly, down to the pelvis. The lateral dissection is also performed dividing the inconsistent middle rectal vessels. The anterior peritoneum is incised and anterior dissection is performed by preserving the Denonvilliers fascia in males to avoid injury to the pelvic autonomic nerves. The ureters have to be safeguarded on both sides. The rectum is divided intracorporeally after complete mobilization, the specimen is then delivered from the perineum. The perineum is closed by apposing the pelvic floor muscles and the skin is closed. Reperitonealisation of the peritoneum is done and an end colostomy is performed at the previously marked stoma site in LIF.

Laparoscopic anterior resection and low anterior resection for rectal cancers

This surgery is a more advanced surgery requiring skills of complete splenic flexure mobilization, TME, and low rectal division. After the standard port placements, the peritoneum is incised at the promontory, and the incision is extended cranially up to the root of the IMA. The IMA is divided at the root taking care as not to injure the sympathetic nerves. Subsequently, medial to lateral dissection of the left colon is performed, so that the mesocolon and its vessels are separated from the retroperitoneal structures, and the ureters and the gonadal vessels are safeguarded and kept posteriorly. This lateral dissection is continued up to the white line of Toldt. Superiorly, the splenic flexure is separated from the left kidney and the perinephric fascia as far as the body of the pancreas superiorly and the spleen superio-laterally. This mobilization is crucial for adequate mobilization of the splenic flexure. Next, the lateral attachment of the sigmoid colon is divided extending the same dissection up to the splenic flexure. The entire splenic flexure is completely mobilized, and the omentum is detached from the distal transverse colon. The lesser sac is entered, the mesenteric attachments to the body and tail of pancreas are divided to ensure that the splenic flexure and the distal transverse colon are completely free and would reach down low into the pelvis without any tension on the anastomosis.

Subsequently, the rectal dissection (TME) is started, initially posteriorly, then laterally, anteriorly going down into the pelvic floor along the avascular plane of dissection. The low division of the rectum is decided based on the tumor location, confirmed intraoperatively by rectal digital palpation. The rectum is divided by roticulating endo-GIA staplers using 45 or 60 mm cartridges based on tumor and pelvis characteristics. Next, through a minilaparotomy, the mobilized rectum is extracted, the proximal level of colon divided, and the anvil is placed with application of a purse-string. The colon is placed back into the abdomen, pneumoperitoneum is recreated under vision, and stapled end-to-end anastomosis is performed. A proximal stoma may be created based on the surgeon's preference.

Laparoscopic left hemicolectomy for descending colon cancer

Most of the dissection would be similar to that performed in sigmoid colon cancer. However, mobilization of the entire descending colon and splenic flexure would be essential to achieve colorectal anastomosis.

Laparoscopic right hemicolectomy for right colon cancer

This is one of the difficult operations, as compared to other laparoscopic colorectal surgeries, as it involves dissecting very close to the SMV. After standard port placements, with the surgeon on the left of the patient, all the small bowels are folded up in a steep Trendelenburg position. The root of the mesentery is identified and is held up with two graspers, one near the DJ flexure and another at the IC junction. An incision in the root of mesentery is placed on the peritoneum, and dissection is extended medial to lateral and inferiorly towards superiorly on the right side to separate the right mesocolon from the retroperitoneal structures, including the duodenal second part, ureters, gonadals, and the right kidney. Once this is achieved, the right colic vessels, starting from the ileocolic vessels are clipped and divided at the base, extending to the right colic and the right branch of the middle colic vessels for a standard right hemicolectomy. For an extended right hemicolectomy, the middle colic vessels are divided at the base and the splenic flexure may need to be mobilized. The vascular division at the root ensures maximal clearance of the lymph nodes. Next, the lateral attachments of the right colon are divided, and the hepatic flexure is completely mobilized from above. The right colon is completely freed except the luminal continuity. A midline minilaparotomy is then performed, the mobilized colon is exteriorized with adequate wound protection, and resection and anastomosis is performed, after which the colon is replaced back and abdominal closure is performed.

Laparoscopic transverse colectomy

Laparoscopic transverse colectomy is one of the more difficult and uncommonly performed procedures for transverse colon malignancy. For tumors in the right half of transverse colon, an extended right hemicolectomy may be better choice. For tumors in the central or left half of transverse colon, a laparoscopic transverse colectomy is necessary. The middle colic vessels are divided at the root, and both the splenic and hepatic flexures are mobilized. After complete mobilization, through a small periumbilical skin incision, after adequate wound protection, exteriorization and extracorporeal colocolic anastomosis is performed.

Laparoscopic restorative proctocolectomy and ileal pouch anal anastomosis

Laparoscopic restorative proctocolectomy and ileal pouch anal anastomosis has become a standard procedure at our center. With standard ports and monitors on both sides of the patients, with the patient in a low lithotomy Trendelenburg position, the left colectomy is first started with the surgeon on the right side of the patient. The medial to lateral dissection of the left colon is followed by division of the lateral attachments of the left colon. Subsequently, complete mobilization of the splenic flexure is performed. Then, the rectum is mobilized with dissection in the avascular tissue plane of TME. Low rectal division at the pelvic floor is done with roticulating staplers. Then the entire surgical team shifts to the left of the patient, and the mobilization of the right colon is commenced with peritoneal incision at the root of the mesentery. The medial to lateral and inferior to superior dissection of the right colon is performed. Subsequently, lateral attachments of the right colon are taken, and complete mobilization of the hepatic flexure is performed. At this point, a minilaparotomy approximately 5–6 cm is done skirting around the umbilicus in the midline, and the mobilized colon is exteriorized. The vascular division of the colon can be done close to the colonic wall intracorporealy (at laparoscopy) or extracorporealy and the specimen is removed. A 15 cm ileal J pouch is created by folding the terminal ileum and double firing of GIA/Linear Cutter 75/80 stapler. The anvil of EEA 28/29 stapler is applied with a purse string and the pouch is replaced into the peritoneum. Pneumoperitoneum is recreated, and under laparoscopic guidance, circular double stapled J pouch anal anastomosis is performed. A drain and covering loop ileostomy is done in most cases.

Laparoscopic total colectomy and ileorectal anastomosis

Steps of colonic dissection, and both flexures mobilization is similar to Lap RPC. However, rectal mobilization is avoided and colorectal division is done with a straight stapler 60 at the sacral promontory and ileo-rectal anastomosis, with the help of EEA stapler 31/33, is then performed.

Laparoscopic total proctocolectomy and ileostomy

Steps are similar to Lap RPC; however, the rectum is completely dissected and the specimen can be delivered transperinealy. The colonic vascular division can be done with laparoscopy, to avoid any incision on the abdomen. This surgery, however, is rarely done nowadays with the universal application of sphincter preservation in ulcerative colitis. This procedure may be needed in patients with low rectal cancers in ulcerative colitis, for those elderly who have a poor sphincter tone or patients with severe Crohn's colitis.

Laparoscopic reversal of Hartmann's operation

There are two techniques. One is initial laparoscopic adhesiolysis, mobilization of the sigmoid colon, and subsequent taking down of the colostomy after placing the anvil and tying the purse-string over anvil of No. 33 EEA stapler. The abdomen is closed and under laparoscopic vision, and the EEA stapler is fired to create the anastomosis. Another technique is to take down the colostomy after placing the anvil and application of the purse-string. Subsequent laparoscopic adhesiolysis and colorectal stapled anastomosis is then carried out. A single incision port can also be used at the stoma incision to perform the procedure.

Laparoscopic colon replacement for corrosive strictures

Port placements are similar to standard colorectal resection. Mobilization of left colon, splenic flexure mobilization, and the subsequent mobilization of the right colon and hepatic flexure is then performed. The retrosternal tunnel is developed under laparoscopic vision. Due to triangulation, care must be taken to avoid pleural puncture via a minilaparotomy, then, the mobilized colon is delivered, the middle colic is ligated at the root, the vascularity of the marginal artery is confirmed, and the subsequent colonic conduit is fashioned. The colo-colic anastomosis is performed extracorporeally with minilaparotomy. Neck dissection through the left neck is then carried out, to divide the cervical esophagus. The colonic conduit is pulled up through the retrosternal tunnel, and cervical as well as abdominal anastomosis is performed.

Newer techniques and adjuncts

Intersphincteric dissection and coloanal anastomosis

For very low rectal tumors, laparoscopic intersphincteric resection, as well as perineal dissection, can be performed to achieve sphincter preservation, and a subsequent coloanal hand sewn anastomosis is performed through the perineal route with a Lonestar™ retractor.

Transvaginal/transanal specimen removal

In selected situations, with prior consent, transvaginal or transanal delivery of colonic specimens may be possible. This would avoid any incision or scars on the abdominal wall and also an exclusively laparoscopic surgery is feasible rather than laparoscopic-assisted surgery.

Proximal diversion

Proximal diversion is done in selected patients with low anterior resection. This may be in form of loop ileostomy or loop colostomy depending on the surgeon's preference. More details on stoma is discussed in a separate chapter.

> *Hand assisted and SILS Colorectal surgery* – discussed in separate chapter
> *Robotic Laparoscopic Coloectal Surgery* – discussed in separate chapter
> *Transanal tumour excision or transanal TME* – discussed in separate chapter.

Neoadjuvant chemoradiation

Nowadays, a majority of locoregionally advanced rectal tumors are subjected to neoadjuvant chemoradiation [18,19] before undergoing a laparoscopic resection. Studies have shown that even after chemoradiation, laparoscopic resection can be safely performed.

Adjuvant chemotherapy

Most patients with locoregionally advanced colonic cancers receive early adjuvant chemotherapy to reduce their risk of recurrence [20,21].

Conversion in laparoscopic colorectal surgery

The conversion rate of laparoscopic colorectal resection for cancer is an average of 5%–25% [22,23]. In centers where more advanced tumors are being treated, the conversion rates would be higher, whereas in centers of excellence and who deal with early tumors, the conversion rates would be less than 5%. Conversion rates for benign cases are very low in the range of 1%–2%. Most common causes for conversion would be difficulty in access and dissection in the pelvis in a rectal tumor due to the bulk of the tumor, bowel rupture, local adhesion of the rectal tumor to structures such as pelvic sidewall, ureters or bladder, which cannot be safely dissected; unexpected bleeding, which cannot be controlled at laparoscopy; and extensive bowel adhesions due to previous surgery or irradiation. There is some evidence from the literature that patients who have been converted do poorly in terms of long-term survival [7,24]. Most probably this appears to be due to the advanced nature and stage of the disease, which increases the risk of local and distant metastasis. However, technical factors and risk of tumor rupture and dissemination should also be considered. One should always counsel all the patients undergoing laparoscopic colorectal surgery for a possible conversion. A timely conversion should be considered an extension of the procedure and a safe surgical practice rather than a complication. Methods to reduce this risk would be to select patients and tumors in the early part of the 'learning curve', and accept a slightly higher conversion rate in the best interest of the patient.

Complications of laparoscopic colorectal surgery

All the complications that can occur in open colorectal surgery are possible with laparoscopic colorectal surgery. These would include injuries to ureters, duodenum, small bowel, as well as intraoperative bleeds, postoperative intra-abdominal sepsis, anastomotic leaks, and intestinal obstruction secondary to adhesion or persistent ileus. Later in the postoperative period, urinary and sexual dysfunction may occur secondary to autonomic nerve injury or neuropraxia. Especially in laparoscopic surgery, one should be more cautious about the thermal injuries due to excessive or unintended use of energy sources. These are discussed in details in another chapter.

Summary

Laparoscopic colonic and rectal surgery has demonstrated benefits, which have been substantiated with randomized controlled trials. One should carefully select patients for those undergoing laparoscopic colorectal resection, especially in the early learning curve. Laparoscopic colonic surgery and laparoscopic TME for rectal cancer are here to stay. Training in laparoscopic colorectal surgery is possible using a step-by-step method, and a proper understanding of the principles of anatomy, surgical techniques, and procedures.

Key points

- Laparoscopic colorectal surgery has been firmly established as a procedure of choice for treating benign and malignant colorectal diseases.
- Laparoscopic colorectal surgery has a higher learning curve; however, it can be learned by understanding the basic principles and techniques related to these procedures, as outlined in this chapter.
- Standardization of the port placement and the surgical procedures will go a long way in reducing the learning curve and the OR time, and to optimize the outcomes.
- Laparoscopic colorectal surgery is teamwork, an effort between surgeons and the paramedical staff understanding the procedure and having good team coordination.
- Laparoscopic surgery can be safely applied to the care of colorectal diseases provided surgical principles of oncology such as radical resection, safe dissection, timely conversion, and wound protection is utilized to reduce unwarranted complications, and to optimize long-term outcomes.
- Laparoscopic colorectal surgery has distinct short-term benefits for outcomes in benign and cancer patients pertaining to reduced pain, better cosmesis, early return of bowel function, and early recovery – many prospective trials have shown equivalent long-term results in terms of 5-year survivals and recurrences when compared to open surgery.

Videos

VIDEO 1   https://youtu.be/NrRIX7yNoyU

Basic Principles and Techniques of Laparoscopic Colorectal Surgery – Part 1.

VIDEO 2   https://youtu.be/sQOx3X-VDmU

Basic Principles and Techniques of Laparoscopic Colorectal Surgery – Part 2.

VIDEO 3   https://youtu.be/o-T8y2tN3p4

Principles of GI stapling – Open and Laparoscopic.

References

1. Heroor A, Panjwani G, Chaskar R. A Study of 101 laparoscopic colorectal surgeries: A single surgeon experience. How important is the learning curve?. *Indian J Surg* 2015 Dec;77(S3):1275–9.
2. Akiyoshi T, Kuroyanagi H, Ueno M et al. Learning curve for standardized laparoscopic surgery for colorectal cancer under supervision: A single-center experience. *Surg Endosc* 2011 May;25(5):1409–14.
3. Moirangthem G. Laparoscopic colorectal surgery: An update (with special reference to Indian scenario). *J Clin Diagn Res.* 2014;8(4):NE01-NE6. doi:10.7860/JCDR/2014/8269.4285
4. Attaallah W, Babayev H, Yardimci S, Cingi A, Ugurlu MU, Gunal O. Laparoscopic resection for colorectal diseases: Short-term outcomes of a single center. *UCD* 2016 Jul 28;32(3):199–202.
5. Khoury W, Dakwar A, Sivkovits K, Mahajna A. Fast-track rehabilitation accelerates recovery after laparoscopic colorectal surgery. *JSLS* 2014;18(4):e2014.00076.
6. Kehlet H, Wilmore DW. Evidence-based surgical care and the evolution of fast-track surgery. *Ann Surg* 2008 Aug;248(2):189–98.
7. Allaix ME, Furnée EJ, Mistrangelo M, Arezzo A, Morino M. Conversion of laparoscopic colorectal resection for cancer: What is the impact on short-term outcomes and survival. *World J Gastroenterol* 2016 Oct 7;22(37):8304–13.
8. Dunker MS, Stiggelbout AM, van Hogezand RA, Ringers J, Griffioen G, Bemelman WA. Cosmesis and body image after laparoscopic-assisted and open ileocolic resection for Crohn's disease. *Surg Endosc* 1998 Nov;12(11):1334–40.
9. Gunka I, Dostalik J, Martinek L, Gunkova P, Mazur M. Impact of blood transfusions on survival and recurrence in colorectal cancer surgery. *Indian J Surg* 2013 Apr;75(2):94–101.
10. Pang Q, An R, Liu H. Perioperative transfusion and the prognosis of colorectal cancer surgery: A systematic review and meta-analysis. *World J Surg Onc* 2019 Dec;17(1).
11. Novitsky YW, Litwin DEM, Callery MP. The net immunologic advantage of laparoscopic surgery. *Surg Endosc* 2004 Oct;18(10):1411–9.
12. Veenhof AAFA, Vlug MS, van der Pas MHGM et al. Surgical stress response and postoperative immune function after laparoscopy or open surgery with fast track or standard perioperative care. *Ann Surg* 2012 Feb;255(2):216–21.
13. Veenhof AAFA, Engel AF, Craanen ME, Meijer S, de Lange-de Klerk ESM, Van der Peet DL, Meijerink WJHJ, Cuesta MA. Laparoscopic versus open total mesorectal excision: A comparative study on short-term outcomes. *Dig Surg* 2007;24: 367–74.
14. Son G, Kim J, Lee J et al. Multidimensional analysis of the learning curve for laparoscopic rectal cancer surgery. *J Laparoendosc Adv Surg Tech* 2010 Sep;20(7):609–17.
15. Chen G, Liu Z, Han P, Li J, Cui B. The learning curve for the laparoscopic approach for colorectal cancer: A single institution's experience. *J Laparoendosc Adv Surg Tech* 2013 Jan;23(1): 17–21.
16. Nakagoe T, Sawai T, Tsuji T et al. A new device that protects from Minilaparotomy wound infection in minimally-invasive approaches to colon cancer. *Acta Med Nagasaki* 2001;46:55–60.

17. Horiuchi T, Tanishima H, Tamagawa K et al. A wound protector shields incision sites from bacterial invasion. *Surg Infect (Larchmt)* 2010 Dec;11(6):501–3.

18. Bernier L, Balyasnikova S, Tait D, Brown G. Watch-and-wait as a therapeutic strategy in rectal cancer. *Curr Colorectal Cancer Rep* 2018 Apr;14(2):37–55.

19. Lai C, Lai M, Wu C, Jao S, Hsiao C. Rectal cancer with complete clinical response after neoadjuvant chemoradiotherapy, surgery, or 'watch and wait'. *Int J Colorectal Dis* 2016 Feb;31(2):413–9.

20. Milinis K. Adjuvant chemotherapy for rectal cancer: Is it needed?. *WJCO* 2015;6(6):225.

21. You KY, Peng HH, Gao YH et al. [Value of postoperative adjuvant chemotherapy in locally advanced rectal cancer patients with ypT1-4N0 after neo-adjuvant chemoradiotherapy]. *Zhonghua Zhong Liu Za Zhi* 2013 Sep;35(9):708–13.

22. de Neree tot Babberich MPM, van Groningen JT, Dekker E et al. Laparoscopic conversion in colorectal cancer surgery; is there any improvement over time at a population level?. *Surg Endosc* 2018 Jul;32(7):3234–46.

23. Tekkis PP, Senagore AJ, Delaney CP. Conversion rates in laparoscopic colorectal surgery: A predictive model with 1253 patients. *Surg Endosc* 2005;19:47–54.

24. Yamamoto S, Fukunaga M, Miyajima N, Okuda J, Konishi F, Watanabe M. Impact of conversion on surgical outcomes after laparoscopic operation for rectal carcinoma: A Retrospective Study of 1,073 patients. *J Am Coll Surg* 2009 Mar;208(3):383–9.

Chapter 5

PATIENT SELECTION

Harsh Shah

Contents

Learning objectives 27
Introduction 27
Why selection of patient is essential? 27
Summary 28
Key points 28
References 28

Learning objectives

- To select patients based on their demographic and tumor characteristics for laparoscopic colorectal surgeries.

Introduction

Laparoscopic resection of colorectal cancer is a routine procedure for many expert centers today. It has passed through a lot skepticism in the beginning; however, since randomized controlled trials have shown its noninferiority over open surgery [1,2], it has now found its way into the mainstream.

Why selection of patient is essential?

Selecting your patients wisely has many advantages. First of all, a clear expectation with regard to surgical procedure and the scar can be conveyed to the patient preoperatively. The operation theater timings and staffing can be better managed when an open surgery is performed upfront rather than converting to open surgery after prolonged laparoscopic surgery. However, the biggest advantage is the lower complication rate in open surgical patients, in comparison to those who have been converted to open surgery after failure of a laparoscopic procedure [3].

Selecting patients who are suitable for laparoscopic resection is vital for safe completion of the procedure. Since there are relatively few surgeons even today who possess the required skill and expertise to successfully complete such complex procedures, this chapter will outline patient selection from both the perspective of an experienced and inexperienced surgeon. Thus, a broad categorization will be as follows:

A. Patient selection for experienced surgeons
B. Patient selection for relatively inexperienced surgeons

A) Patient selection for experienced laparoscopic colorectal surgeon:

There is no universally accepted definition of an experienced surgeon. Different studies define an experienced surgeon as one who has successfully completed anywhere between 30 to 70 laparoscopic colorectal surgeries [4,5]. The higher number of procedures may be required to master left-sided colonic procedures, as compared to the right side.

a. *Pathology*:
   i. *Diverticulitis and severe active inflammatory bowel disease*: It poses a challenge to the operating surgeon. Extensive adhesions, a bulky and sometimes friable colon can be difficult to manage laparoscopically. Most of the experienced surgeons will be able to safeguard ureter during a sigmoid resection, even in the presence of extensive adhesions. Preoperative ureteric stent placement can be of great help in such scenarios. However, when the CT scan shows hydronephrosis and possible involvement of the ureter within the inflammatory process, it deserves an open surgical procedure, as ureteric reconstruction is always required.

   ii. *Locally advanced colorectal tumors (T4)*: Margin positive resections are never acceptable and surgeons should be able to identify such tumors from preoperative imaging, as they would better be removed by open surgery. Advanced hepatic flexure tumors may infiltrate the duodenum and the head of the pancreas. Similarly, advanced sigmoid tumors may infiltrate the ureter, the urinary bladder, and sometimes the small bowel. Knowing the extent of the tumor preoperatively will spare the agony of nonproductive laparoscopic dissection efforts. Also, the patient can be well prepared for the radical surgery in advance, e.g., neo-adjuvant chemotherapy, or ureteric stent placement.

b. *Obstructed bowel*: Dilated bowel secondary to complete luminal compromise is a common presentation of colorectal malignancies. Many such patients will require emergency exploration. In such scenarios, laparoscopic procedures are contraindicated.

c. *Obesity*: The studies have shown mixed results, with regard to short-term outcomes in obese individuals [6,7]. The unfavorable results of laparoscopic surgery may be attributable to longer operating time and higher conversion rate, all of which can be mitigated with proper training.

d. *Elderly patients*: Laparoscopic surgeries are safe and even better when compared to open surgeries in elderly individuals [8] and should be carried out by an experienced surgeon.

B) Patient selection for a relatively inexperienced surgeon:

Surgeons who have not performed large numbers of laparoscopic colorectal surgeries should select their patient wisely. Doing so can have advantages to both patient and the surgeon.

a. *Pathology*:
   i. *Diverticulitis and severe inflammatory bowel disease*: Recurrent attacks of diverticulitis leads to extensive pericolonic adhesions, which can be a hindrance for a novice surgeon. Pericolonic abscess or phlegmon are better served by open surgery with proper preoperative preparation. Bulky and occasionally friable colon, in cases of sever inflammatory bowel disease, should not be operated laparoscopically.
   ii. *Tumors*: Locally advanced tumors (T4), as mentioned previously, are challenging for an experienced operator. They should not attempted by a relatively inexperienced surgeon.

b. *Tumor location*:
   i. *Left-sided tumors*: Left-sided, sigmoid, and rectal tumors invariably requires splenic flexure mobilization. The take down of the splenic flexure requires extensive experience, which may be a hindrance for a beginner.
   ii. *Low rectal tumors*: Performing a complete mesorectal excision with autonomic nerve preservation, along with obtaining adequate distal margin, is essential for rectal tumors. Taking the vascular pedicles at the origin along with lymph node dissection is a skill that is mastered only after adequate training. Neoadjuvant chemoradiotherapy for rectal cancer does not usually increase the operative difficulty, and they should not be considered a contraindication as such.

c. *Patient demographics*
   i. *Elderly*: As mentioned previously, laparoscopic surgery can be a boon to elderly individuals. However, prolongation of the procedure beyond the desired time period is detrimental to the ultimate outcome.
   ii. *Obesity*: As already mentioned, obese individuals are better served by laparoscopic surgery. Presence of excess mesorectal and omental fat poses a challenge to a novice surgeon during mobilization of flexures and division of vascular pedicles.
   iii. *Narrow pelvis*: Males have a narrow pelvis, which may be a limiting factor for safe rectal mobilization. Similar difficulty is encountered in females with large fibroids in the uterus.

Summary

- Locally advanced tumors and extensive pericolonic inflammatory processes are contraindications to laparoscopic surgeries.

- In experienced hands, laparoscopic surgery can be offered to the elderly and obese patients.
- A relatively inexperienced surgeon should proceed cautiously with left-sided and low rectal tumors.

Key points

- In locally advanced tumors, involvement of the ureter, duodenum, urinary bladder, and small bowel by the tumor should be diagnosed preoperatively; as such, patients should be excluded from laparoscopic resection attempts.
- Patient selection can be generous for an experienced surgeon; however, a novice surgeon should consider the pathology and extent of the disease prior to attempting laparoscopic surgery.

References

1. Bonjer HJ, Hop WC, Nelson H et al. Laparoscopically assisted versus open colectomy for colon cancer: A meta-analysis. *Arch Surg* 2007;142(3):298–303.
2. Fleshman J, Sargent DJ, Green E, Anvari M, Stryker SJ, Beart Jr RW, Hellinger M, Flanagan Jr R, Peters W, and Nelson H, Clinical Outcomes of Surgical Therapy Study Group. Laparoscopic colectomy for cancer is not inferior to open surgery based on 5–year data from the COST Study Group trial. *Ann Surg* 2007 Oct 1;246(4):655–64.
3. Marusch F, Gastinger I, Schneider C et al. Importance of conversion for results obtained with laparoscopic colorectal surgery. *Dis Colon Rectum* 2001;44:207–14.
4. Schlachta CM, Mamazza J, Seshadri PA et al. Defining a learning curve for laparoscopic colorectal resections. *Dis Colon Rectum* 2001;44:217–22.
5. Dincler S, Koller MT, Steurer J et al. Multidimensional analysis of learning curves in laparoscopic sigmoid resection: Eight-year results. *Dis Colon Rectum* 2003;46:1371–8.
6. Hotouras A, Ribas Y, Zakeri SA, Nunes QM, Murphy J, Bhan C, and Wexner SD. The influence of obesity and body mass index on the outcome of laparoscopic colorectal surgery: A systematic literature review. *Colorectal Dis* 2016 Oct;18(10):O337–66.
7. Bell S, Kong JC, Wale R, Staples M, Oliva K, Wilkins S, Mc Murrick P, and Warrier SK. The effect of increasing body mass index on laparoscopic surgery for colon and rectal cancer. *Colorectal Dis* 2018 Sep;20(9):778–88.
8. Devoto L, Celentano V, Cohen R, Khan J, and Chand M. Colorectal cancer surgery in the very elderly patient: A systematic review of laparoscopic versus open colorectal resection. *Int J Colorectal Dis* 2017 Sep 1;32(9):1237–42.

Chapter 6

STOMA AND ITS COMPLICATIONS

Ankur Tiwari

Contents

Learning objectives 29
Introduction 29
Stoma marking, counseling, and consenting. 29
Indications for temporary stoma. 30
   Ileostomy versus colostomy 30
Preoperative oral antibiotics and mechanical bowel preparation 30
Anastomotic leak 30
Role of rectal drains to prevent stoma 31
Stoma care 31
   Stoma complications 31
      Mucocutaneous separation. 31
      Retraction/flush stoma. 31
      Bowel obstruction. 31
      Stenosis. 31
      Prolapse. 31
      Parastomal hernia 32
      Granulomas 32
      Pancaking 32
      High-output ileostomy. 32
      Peristomal skin excoriations and infections. 32
Stoma closure and its complications. 32
Summary 32
Key points 32
Video. 33
References 33

Learning objectives

- Study the indications, types, and preference of diversion stoma along with associated advantages and disadvantages.
- Study the morbidities and complications associated with stoma creation and reversal of stoma.
- Study special techniques to avoid creation of stoma, and detect high-risk anastomosis.
- Study the optimum time interval between creation of stoma and reversal of stoma (ileostomy vs. colostomy).

Introduction

The word stoma (or ostomy) is derived from Greek and means 'mouth'. It is created by a surgical procedure consisting of forming an aperture in the intestine and placing it on the anterior abdominal wall. This aperture allows the patient to eliminate feces and urine out of the body, and to administer nutritional and therapeutic substances. The stoma can be either intestinal or urinary. Intestinal stoma are either an ileostomy or colostomy. There are both advantages and disadvantages of ileostomies and colostomies, and the choice of stoma is based on the nature of the disease and the morbidities associated with a particular type of stoma. Several predictors of high-risk stomas are studied here, as well as a few techniques – such as identifying compromised vascularity and transanal rectal tube drainage – are described for reducing anastomotic leak rates

and thus avoiding the creation of diversion stoma. It is important to understand the appropriate time for reversal of stoma. It depends on disease and treatment factors, and reversal of stoma cannot be attempted too early nor can it be delayed too late.

Stoma marking, counseling, and consenting

For stoma formation on the anterior abdominal wall, it is essential to select a proper site. Usually, it is preferred to create the stoma on the spino-umbilical line, either midway or just lateral to midline, taking into consideration that the stoma should not be depressed into the belly while sitting or standing, causing compression of the stoma site, or making visualization of the stoma difficult for the patient.

Preoperative counseling, in terms of discussing the creation of a diversion stoma, should be done in detail, and include information on its most probable type and nature, the probable duration for stoma reversal, the key points for stoma care, and the most commonly anticipated complications such as bleeding, peristomal skin excoriations, retraction of stoma, and parastomal herniation.

It is very important to obtain informed, written consent from patient and relatives preoperatively. If consent is not obtained preoperatively, and during surgery it is decided that stomal diversion is mandatory, relatives should then be counseled and consent should be obtained during surgery.

Indications for temporary stoma

An indication for colorectal anastomosis is most often for cancer, but is also done for other conditions like diverticulitis, polyps, volvulus, trauma, and so on. Irrespective of the pathology of disease, colorectal resection followed by anastomosis carries a risk of anastomosis dehiscence with severe consequences that can endanger a patient's life. Staplers provide a clear-cut advantage in low rectal anastomosis, in a male pelvis with narrow basin, and in obese individuals.

Risk of anastomotic dehiscence and its fatal outcome is the reason many surgeons prefer a defunctioning stoma. But unfortunately, these stomas are not free from complications and can even endanger the patient's life sometimes. The decision for creating a covering stoma should depend upon the risk factors associated with a high incidence of anastomotic fistula [1]. These are classified as follows:

- *Host-related factors*: Diabetes, anemia, hypoprotinemia, bowel inflammation, smoking, chronic obstructive pulmonary disease, corticosteroid use, and male gender.
- *Disease related factors*: Tumor features, location and level of anastomosis.
- *Surgery related factors*: Anastomosis under tension and poor blood supply, prolonged operative time, large volume of blood loss and blood transfusion, and contamination of operative field.
- *Preoperative pelvic radiotherapy*: The highest rate of leakage was reported by Oprescu C et al. in cases of preoperative radiotherapy patients: 64.7% for mechanical anastomosis vs. 35.3% for manual anastomosis.

Recently, systematic reviews and a meta-analysis have concluded that low-level anastomosis, male gender, preoperative radiotherapy and malnutrition, and smoking are the most crucial risk factors associated with anastomotic leaks. Whereas bowel preparation, drain use, tumor stage, type of anastomosis (manual or mechanical), and type of approach (open or laparoscopic) do not seem to affect the leakage rate.

Ileostomy versus colostomy

On this debate, most of the authors agree that an ileostomy is associated with few definite advantages over colostomy, as it can be performed and repaired easily (Table 6.1).

There appears to be no difference between a loop ileostomy and a loop colostomy in overall morbidity, after stoma creation, and closure. Morbidity rates following creation of a loop ileostomy were significantly decreased at the cost of a risk for dehydration (Table 6.1).

Creation of a stoma in colorectal surgery can be prevented or avoided if the chances of anastomotic leak are predicted to be low. Though the literature suggests that stoma formation does

TABLE 6.1: Comparison of Stoma-Related Complications Rates of Loop Ileostomy and Loop Colostomy

Stoma Related Complications		Loop Ileostomy (%)	Loop Colostomy (%)
1	Overall morbidity (Stoma creation to closure)	15.6	20.4
2	Morbidity after stoma creation	18.2	30.6
3	Dehydration rate	3.1	0
4	Ileus rate	5.2	1.7

not prevent anastomotic leak, it definitely reduces the morbidity and mortality associated with anastomotic leak. Anastomotic leak not only prolongs the course of recovery, but also increases the chances of revision surgery and delays, or avoids, adjuvant chemotherapy. Hence, the factors promoting anastomotic leak should be considered carefully, and accordingly the formation of a diversion stoma should be considered.

Patient-related factors are male gender, smoking, obesity, alcohol, steroid and nonsteroidal anti-inflammatory drugs, operative time, transfusion contamination of the operative field, and emergency surgery.

Preoperative oral antibiotics and mechanical bowel preparation

Multiple publications have demonstrated a lack of benefit associated with the use of preoperative oral antibiotics and mechanical bowel preparation in decreasing anastomotic leak in elective colorectal surgery. Scarborough et al. postulated that mechanical bowel preparation (MBP) allowed improved delivery of an oral antibiotic preparation to the bowel mucosa. This study showed that MBP and preoperative oral antibiotics lower anastomotic leak (AL) rates, from 5.7% to 2.8%, in colorectal surgery when compared with patients not receiving any kind of preparation.

Anastomotic leak

Recent evidence has supported the hypothesis of the occurrence of AL secondary to local infection, resulting in local increase in collagenous activity [2]. The outcomes of surgery performed by laparoscopic or using an open approach remains similar for colorectal surgery in elective surgeries [3]. Recent systematic reviews and meta analyses, which includes 10 RCTs (1969 patients), found similar outcomes in patients with hand sewn or stapled anastomosis.

Many methods have been developed to assess the integrity of anastomosis perioperatively. Air leak tests have been demonstrated to identify anastomotic leaks during surgery, which could be repaired to decrease the rate of anastomotic leak. Another technique such as intraoperative endoscopy allows identifying intra-op leaks and bleeds which may endanger anastomosis.

Newly developed methods rely upon the assessment of blood supply to the anastomosis. Previous methods included relying on the color of the bowel or observing the pulsatile flow at the cut section [4]. More recently, fluorescence perfusion angiography has been widely used and is more reliable. Here, a fluorophore is injected intravenously, and then excited by a specific wavelength to emit in another specific wavelength (usually infrared) just after the vessel division at the anastomotic site, thus helping the surgeon to identify any defect in vascularization at the anastomotic level. Jafari et al. reported that fluorescence perfusion angiography reduced AL from 18% to 6% after robotic-assisted anterior resection.

A recent systematic review and meta-analysis of 1302 patients confirmed the role of fluorescence perfusion angiography in reducing the incidence of AL in colorectal cancer [5]. Another systematic review and meta-analysis of 1772 patients undergoing anterior resection, showing transanal tube decompression, has demonstrated a reduction of anastomotic leak risk [5]. Thus, prophylactic transanal tube decompression could reduce anastomotic leak in high risk patients without causing complications related to diverting stoma. However, a well conducted large-scale RCT, comparing the two techniques, remains to be conducted.

Role of rectal drains to prevent stoma

Stoma-related complications can be avoided by avoiding the creation of a stoma and managing instead with a transanal drainage tube. Some authors have reported lesser leak rates associated with transanal tube drainage. Combination of a defunctioning ileostomy with a transanal tube drainage is associated with less infection rates in low rectal anastomosis, whereas some author have reported higher rates of anastomotic leaks related to transanal drainage compared to an ileostomy (15.1% v/s 4.9%) [1].

Stoma care

A stoma needs to be taken good care of as it may otherwise lead to serious complications. There are dedicated stoma nurses who teach and help in taking care of a stoma, but in many developing countries, the patient has to manage stoma care alone, and the onus of educating the patient lies on the treating surgeons.

Ostomates can withdraw themselves from society, as they might feel stigmatized by their stoma. They become accustomed to living with a stoma and manage it on their own with help of paramedic staff; however, it is a gradual process and requires regular encouragement and support from healthcare professionals, family members, and society as well.

Various types of appliances are available but there is nothing ideally suited for them. In the end, the one which suits the patient best and is manageable for him or her should be used. There are various complications associated with stomas as discussed further, and the healthcare providers and the patient themselves should be vigilant enough to care and avoid developing them, and the ones that do develop should be diagnosed and managed at the earliest.

Patient should be adequately educated to be observant about the nature of the effluent from stoma and its quantity. Any alteration in its nature, character, or quantity should be taken seriously and be examined by a specialist in time. A stoma care ostomy research (SCOR) assessment tool allows the monitoring of the peristomal skin condition (Table 6.2).

Stoma complications

There are various complications associated with stoma, and their treatment options need to be known in order to reduce stoma-related morbidities.

Mucocutaneous separation

This complication can develop within days after stoma creation where stoma separates from skin leaving a visible gap of tissue. This may result from tension in bowel, infection, malnutrition, or steroid use. For superficial mucocutaneous separation, protective powder and seals, or paste, can be used while deeper wounds may require alginate dressings.

Retraction/flush stoma

This complication arises when the stoma is created flush to the abdomen, or when it retracts into the abdomen. In such condition, the spout is not created or disappears, resulting in the drain of the stoma not draining directly into the bag and touching the skin, thus causing local complications.

This can be caused by variations in the size or shape of the stoma, which is associated with a patient's weight loss or gain, and with ischemia or tension in the bowel. Refraction of stoma may cause leakage, spillage, and skin irritation as well as difficulty in adhering appliances to the skin. Convexity of the stoma pouch can help in assuring a good seal and preventing leaks. But extra pressure exerted on to the abdomen by the convex shape of the appliance may cause ulceration and does require close regular observation.

Bowel obstruction

Partial obstruction of the bowel may occur resulting in abdominal pain, watery output with foul odor, abdominal distension, and swelling of the stoma. Whereas complete bowel obstruction is associated with no output from the stoma, accompanied by severe cramping, abdominal distension, and nausea or vomiting. In either condition, patients should be advised to avoid eating and increase fluid intake, and take hot baths and massage their abdomen to reduce pain. If the pain increases in intensity and the patient starts vomiting, then he should be taken to an emergency department.

Stenosis

It is the condition where the opening of the stoma becomes narrow, which is caused by ischemia, stoma retraction, Crohn's disease, or exposure of the intestine to radiation. Management for stenosis of the stoma consists of dilatation or surgical refashioning.

Prolapse

A prolapse is a stoma that essentially telescopes out through itself, leading to abnormal lengthening. Prolapsed stoma may be due to weakened abdominal muscles, obesity, ongoing constipation, or chronic coughing. If the prolapsed stoma is functioning normally without any color change, no surgical intervention is required. Measurement of the aperture can accommodate the changing size of the stoma, as a prolapse can increase in size throughout the day. A barrier ring may be required to accommodate the stoma, patient can also wear supportive clothing which will support the prolapse and the weakened muscles.

TABLE 6.2: **Comparison of Stoma-Related Complications Rates Between Ileostomy and Colostomy [6]**

| | Ileostomy Group (n = 33) | | | | | Colostomy Group (n = 49) | | | | |
| | C-D Classification | | | | | C-D Classification | | | | |
	I	II	III	IV	Total (%)	I	II	III	IV	Total (%)
Irritation	3	2	0	0	5 (15.2)	1	2	0	0	3 (6.1)
Dehiscence	2	0	0	0	2 (6.1)	4	1	0	0	5 (10.2)
High output	1	5	0	0	6 (18.2)	0	2	0	0	2 (4.1)
Necrosis	0	1	0	0	1 (3.0)	0	1	0	0	1 (2.0)
Prolapse	0	0	1	0	1 (3.0)	0	0	0	0	0 (0)
Fistula	0	1	0	0	1 (3.0)	0	0	0	0	0 (0)
Total	6	9	1	0	16* (48.5)	5	6	0	0	11* (22.4)

Source: dx.doi.org/10.23922/jarc.2018-018 http://journal-arc.jp
*$p = 0.014$, C-D classification = the Clavien-Dindo classification

Parastomal hernia

It is a very common complication which can arise at any time after the creation of a stoma, ranging from weeks to years. Patients complain of a dragging sensation, which is usually painless and associated with a sudden increase in size and shape of the stomach. The risk factors associated are being overweight, postoperative complications, and heavy lifting. If a parastomal hernia is obstructed or associated with other complications, then surgical repair should considered.

Granulomas

It is a condition where red nodules occur around the edge of a stoma, which are usually not painful but may become irritable and can bleed. It may be caused by improperly fitting stoma devices. Silver nitrate ointment, barrier powder, and a seal/ring used to protect the stoma are the most common treatments to reduce granulomas.

Pancaking

It is a common occurrence in a colostomy where the bowel contents stick around the stoma. Patients should be encouraged to increase fluid intake and use a bowel softener. A vacuum must be prevented from forming inside the pouch and the presence of air inside the pouch will prevent pancaking. Pancaking can also be prevented by using a cover over the filter, and using oil-based products such as vaseline or baby oil inside the pouch.

High-output ileostomy

Ileostomy output should not be greater than 2000 mL in a 24-hour period. There are several factors contributing to high output stoma and its treatment may be required to prevent the complications arising from a high output.

Peristomal skin excoriations and infections

It is very important to maintain the hygiene of the peristomal skin to avoid complications. Contact dermatitis, candida, peristomal pyoderma gangrenosum, skin stripping, psoriasis, infections, and ulcerations are a few of the complications associated with peristomal skin, which would require prompt treatment to avoid further dreadful complications.

Stoma closure and its complications

The overall total complication rate from stoma creation to closure is 36.4%, whereas the same rate related to closure is 36%. An ileostomy leads to a greater incidence of renal insufficiency than a colostomy, and leads to increased admission rates. A multivariate analysis showed that closure of ≤ 109 days was an independent risk factor for developing complications [7].

Thus, the optimal timing after stoma construction in rectal cancer patients, receiving concurrent chemoradiotherapy, is at least 109 days. The reference total complication rate from stoma creation to closure was 36.4%, and electrolyte imbalance occurred in 30.3%, followed by renal insufficiency in 21.2%. The total complication rate was significantly higher in ileostomy patients, 50.0%, versus colostomy, 26.3%. Also, a colostomy yielded a lower readmission rate (5.4% vs. 35.7%) compared to ileostomy. Electrolyte imbalance was 42.9% versus 21.1% in ileostomy versus colostomy patients. Stoma prolapse rates after a colostomy are much lower compared to ileostomy (Table 6.3).

Summary

Stoma is an intestinal aperture created on the anterior abdominal wall. The most common indication is for colorectal cancers,

TABLE 6.3: Factors Related to Time for Stoma Reversal [7]

	Time to Reversal, Days (SD)	p value
Age		0.479
<70	157.5 (67.1)	
≥70	143.5 (65.6)	
Sex		0.384
Male	145.1 (55.6)	
Female	163.8 (80.6)	
Metastatic disease		0.653
Yes	162.5 (41.2)	
No	151.5 (68.3)	
Locally advanced disease		0.071
Yes	173.8 (79.6)	
No	136.5 (50.0)	
Distance from anal verge		0.011*
≤5 cm	157.6 (68.6)	
>5 cm	115.0 (25.7)	
Complication during defunctioning period		0.406
Yes	141.8 (67.1)	
No	158.5 (66.0)	
Renal insufficiency during defunctioning period		0.003*
Yes	113.8 (36.3)	
No	163.5 (69.0)	
Electrolyte imbalance during defunctioning period		0.562
Yes	163.6 (73.4)	
No	149.1 (64.7)	
Iles during defunctioning period		<0.001*
Yes	187.5 (3.5)	
No	150.9 (67.2)	
Readmission during defunctioning period		0.032*
Yes	122.5 (42.1)	
No	161.0 (69.8)	

Source: Yin et al. *World J Surg Oncol* 2017;15:80, DOI 10.1186/s12957-017-1149-9.
*p < 0.05

especially those treated by low rectal resections and anastomosis to cover as a diversion stoma. Essentially, intestinal stomas are either an ileostomy or colostomy, and an ileostomy is associated with more morbidity than colostomy. A colostomy is associated with relatively less stoma-related complications and readmission rates compared to an ileostomy, whereas surgically it is easier to create and reverse an ileostomy. Overall morbidity from stoma creation to reversal in various studies have shown that a colostomy is better than an ileostomy. Stoma care and patient education plays a vital role in the early detection and prompt treatment of stoma-related complications. Various techniques or markers are used to predict high-risk anastomosis and it is advisable to cover the high risk-anastomosis with a diversion stoma. Early reversal of stoma is considered an independent risk factor for complications arising after reversal, while the appropriate time interval between stoma reversal and chemo-radiotherapy is also an essential factor to be considered in order to avoid complications after stoma reversal.

Key points

- Diversion stoma are most commonly created in colorectal cancers, low rectal cancers, suspected high-risk primary anastomosis, and emergency colon/small bowel surgeries.

- A colostomy is better than an ileostomy, and is associated with a lower overall complication rate and readmission rate in case of permanent stoma or palliative stoma; whereas an ileostomy is associated with lower infection rates and higher rates of dehydration.
- Transanal rectal tube drainage is an effective technique in preventing infections associated with low rectal anastomosis; however, they are not of great advantage in the prevention of stoma creation. Fluorescence perfusion angiography is an excellent technique to assess vascularity of the anastomosis and thus alerting the surgeon concerning the high risk of anastomotic dehiscence, which shall be always covered with a diversion stoma.
- The optimum time interval before stoma closure depends upon patient recovery and the administration of adjuvant chemo-radiotherapy. The closure of stoma within 109 days is an independent risk factor for stoma closure.

See Video 4.

Video

VIDEO 4   https://youtu.be/4fRgo7NBrgE

Stoma Creation.

References

1. Meyer J et al. Reducing anastomotic leak in colorectal surgery: The old dogmas and the new challenges. *World J Gastroeneterol* 2019;25(34):5017–25.
2. Shogan BD et al. Collagen degradation and MMP9 activation by Enterococcus fecalis contribute to intestinal anastomotic leak. *Sci Transl Med* 2015;7:286ra68.
3. Juo YY et al. Is minimally invasive colon resection better than traditional approaches? First comprehensive national examination with propensity score matching. *JAMA Surg* 2014;149:177–84.
4. Goligher JC et al. The blood supply to the sigmoid colon and rectum with reference to the technique of rectal resection with restoration of continuity. *Br J Surg* 1949;37:157–62.
5. Novell JR et al. Peroperative observation of marginal artery bleeding: A predictor of anastomotic leakage. *Br J Surg* 1990;77:137–8.
6. Blanco-Colino R et al. Intraoperative use of ICGfluorescence imaging to reduce the risk of anastomotic leakage in colorectal surgery: A systematic review and metaanalysis. *Tech Coloproctol* 2018;22:15–23.
7. Yasuo N et al. Comparative outcomes between palliative ileostomy and colostomy in patients with malignant large bowel obstruction. *J Anus Rectum Colon* 2019;3(2):73–7.
8. Tzu-Chieh Yin et al. Early closure of defunctioning stoma increases complications related to stoma closure after concurrent chemoradiotherapy and low anterior resection in patients with rectal cancer. *World J Surg Oncol* 2017;15:80.

Section II
Perioperative Care of Patient

7   Bowel Preparation in Colorectal Surgery...35
8   ERAS in Colorectal Surgery 38
9   Anesthetic Management of Laproscopic Colorectal Surgery 44
10 Complications in Laparoscopic Colorectal Surgery...................................48

Chapter 7

BOWEL PREPARATION IN COLORECTAL SURGERY

Harshad Soni and Benjamin Perakath

Contents

Learning objectives 35
Introduction 35
The evidence 35
History of bowel preparation in colorectal surgery 35
Guidelines 36
Types of bowel preparation 36
    Mechanical bowel preparation... 36
    Mechanical bowel preparation and oral antibiotic prophylaxis.................. 36
    Oral antibiotics alone.. 36
    MOABP with IV antibiotics 36
    Phosphate enemas 36
    Contraindications for bowel preparation 36
Summary 36
Key points 36
References 36

Learning objectives

- Review the evidence for and against bowel preparation
- Understand the history of bowel preparation
- Understand the pros and cons of bowel preparation

Introduction

Infectious complications due to colorectal surgery continue to present a significant burden to both patients and healthcare providers. Complications such as surgical site infection (SSI) and anastomotic leak (AL) cause considerable morbidity and mortality, cost, prolonged length of stay (LOS), and impaired quality of life (QOL) [1]. It is well recognized that rates of SSI can be significantly reduced by using infection control bundles. Combined mechanical bowel preparation and preoperative oral antibiotic preparation (MBP/OAP) are common in such bundles [2].

There has been an increasing volume of recent evidence suggesting that the preoperative use of combined mechanical bowel preparation and oral antibiotics is associated with a significant reduction in the incidence of infectious complications of elective colorectal surgery [3]. The use of combined MBP and OABP is supported by randomized controlled trial data, especially for reducing SSI; however, much of the support for the use of combined MBP/OABP is from large North American cohort studies, including the data from the American College of Surgery National Surgical Quality Improvement Program (ACS NSQIP) [4].

The evidence

The best data come from the targeted colectomy data of three large retrospective cohort studies of the ACS-NSQIP [9,10]. In the largest study, 45,724 elective colectomies with anastomosis were performed from 2012 to 2015. Thirty-seven percent of these procedures used both mechanical bowel preparation and oral antibiotics, 33% used mechanical bowel preparation only, 4% used oral antibiotics only, and 25% used no bowel preparation. Compared to other bowel prep strategies, the combination of mechanical bowel preparation and oral antibiotics was associated with lower rates of surgical site infection (2.9% vs. 4.6% with oral antibiotics only, 5.9% with mechanical bowel preparation only, and 6.7% with no preparation), anastomotic leaks (2.2% vs. 2.9%, 3.5%, and 4.2%), overall complications (10% versus 13.2%, 15%, and 17.3%), and 30-day mortality (0.4% versus 0.8%, 0.7%, and 1.4%).

Similarly, a 2016 meta-analysis of seven randomized trials showed that, compared with patients who received mechanical bowel preparation, patients who received oral antibiotics plus a mechanical bowel preparation had a significantly lower rate of overall surgical site infection (7% vs. 16%) and superficial surgical site infection (5% vs. 12%), but not deep surgical site infection (4% versus 5%) [9].

In most studies, oral antibiotics were coadministered with mechanical bowel preparation. Given the existing data, oral antibiotics are best administered in conjunction with mechanical bowel preparation for bowel preparation before elective colorectal surgery. This recommendation is consistent with the World Health Organization's global guidelines for the prevention of surgical site infection [1]. In a network meta-analysis of 38 randomized trials, mechanical bowel preparation with oral antibiotics was associated with the lowest risk of surgical site infection. Oral antibiotics only were ranked as the second best; however, this is based on limited data. There was no difference in surgical site infection rate between mechanical bowel preparation only and no preparation [10,11].

History of bowel preparation in colorectal surgery

Perhaps no subject has raised as much interest in colorectal surgery as the controversies surrounding the use of bowel preparation.

With the advent of microbiological techniques – to grow and quantify bacteria in the early 1900s – it was recognized that the colon has a heavy bacterial load. As surgery became safer and more bowel resections were undertaken, it became clear that the high rate of infective complications in colonic resections was related to contamination by these bacteria at the time of operation.

In the late 1930s and early 1940s, Poth [1] and others demonstrated a reduction in bacterial load with mechanical bowel preparation and also showed that MBP was necessary to allow antimicrobials to act effectively.

Nicholls [2] then showed in elegant studies that the rate of surgical site infections and anastomotic leaks could be reduced from 39% to 9% and 10% to 0%, respectively, with the combined use of oral and mechanical bowel preparation (MOABP).

MOABP became the accepted modality of preoperative bowel preparation for decades. Intravenous antibiotic prophylaxis was introduced later and was universally adopted. Numerous studies have shown that MBP alone does not reduce the rate of infective complications [3,4].

MOABP required patients to be admitted a few days preoperatively. With a worldwide move to reduce hospital stay, and the introduction of ERAS programs, MBP was increasingly self-administered at home. More studies demonstrated that MBP was not necessary, or even harmful before colorectal surgery, and MBP gradually fell out of favor, particularly in Europe, and with it, the use of oral antibiotics.

Practice varied widely in the 2000s, with evidence for and against bowel preparation. In 2011, a Cochrane systematic review [5] seemed to lay the issue to rest by categorically stating that MBP was unnecessary. Opinion seemed to be divided between the evidence from large (American) cohort studies [6,7] (including meta-analyses in favor of MOABP) and studies opposing MBP [3,4].

After 2010, oral antibiotics began to make a comeback and American guidelines recommended MOABP. Since, MOABP began to be reintroduced gradually around the world.

Guidelines

The use of MBP and OAP in elective colorectal surgery remains the subject of considerable debate, reflected in the discrepancy observed between the guidelines issued by various authorities around the world [6].

Present guidelines by bodies worldwide are outlined below:

- American Society of Colon and Rectal Surgeons (ASCRS): MOABP recommended
- Society of American Gastrointestinal and Endoscopic Surgeons (SAGES): MOABP recommended
- American Society for Enhanced Recovery (ASER): MOABP
- Perioperative Quality Initiative: MOABP
- National Institue for Health and Care Excellence (NICE): Avoid MBP
- European Society of Coloproctology (ESCP): No specific recommendations, but published a paper in favor of MOABP
- Société Française de Chirurgie Digestive (SFCD): No MBP for colon
- Scottish Intercollegiate Guidelines Network (SIGN): MBP for rectal, IV prophylaxis for all, no MBP for colon

Types of bowel preparation

Mechanical bowel preparation

This involves the patient consuming an osmotic laxative on the day prior to the operation. The aim is to have a colon free of feces, collapsed, and easy to handle during the operation.

Mechanical bowel preparation and oral antibiotic prophylaxis

The addition of oral intraluminally acting antibiotics reduces the bacterial load in the colon, and current evidence seems to suggest that this combination leads to the lowest rates of SSI.

Oral antibiotics alone

This is rarely used these days. Oral neomycin and metronidazole are commonly used.

MOABP with IV antibiotics

In practice, this is widely used. Intravenous prophylaxis prior to the incision is almost universally practiced.

Phosphate enemas

Often used alone or in combination, for rectal and left-sided resections.

Benefits of MBP: If effective, the advantage of MBP is that the large bowel is free from solid feces and bowel gas intraoperatively. Bowel handling is said to be better, and fecal spillage and contamination is reduced. This could translate into less SSI and AL [7,8].

Disadvantage of MBP: Osmotic cathartics can cause marked fluid and electrolyte imbalance in the perioperative period, and this is a consideration in the frail and elderly. There is also concern that bowel preparation liquefies the feces, thereby increasing the risk of spillage and contamination intraoperatively.

Contraindications for bowel preparation

MBP is contraindicated in patients with obstruction. It is also contraindicated in patients with electrolyte imbalance, renal disease, and cardiac unstable patients.

Summary

While current recommendations suggest MOABP results in the lowest SSI rates, practice still varies around the world. MPB is contraindicated in case of obstruction, electrolyte imbalance, renal disease, and cardiac instability. However, more randomized data is required.

Key points

- Mechanical bowel preparation
- Mechanical bowel preparation and oral antibiotic prophylaxis (MBP +OAP/MOABP)
- Oral antibiotics alone
- MOABP with IV antibiotics

References

1. Artinyan A, Orcutt ST, Anaya DA, Richardson P, Chen GJ, Berger DH. Infectious postoperative complications decrease long-term survival in patients undergoing curative surgery for colorectal cancer: A study of 12,075 patients. *Ann Surg* 2015;261(3):497–505.
2. Harris J. Success of a Colorectal Surgical Site Infection Prevention Bundle in a Multihospital System. *AORN J* 2018;107(5):592–600.
3. Cannon JA, Altom LK, Deierhoi RJ et al. Preoperative oral antibiotics reduce surgical site infection following elective colorectal resections. *Dis Colon Rectum* 2012;55(11):1160–6.
4. McSorley ST, Steele CW, McMahon AJ. Meta-analysis of oral antibiotics, in combination with preoperative intravenous antibiotics and mechanical bowel preparation the day before surgery, compared with intravenous antibiotics and mechanical bowel preparation alone to reduce surgical-site infections in elective colorectal surgery. *BJS Open* 2018;2(4):185–94.

5. Guenaga KF, Matos D, Wille-Jorgensen P. Mechanical bowel preparation for elective colorectal surgery. *Cochrane Database of Syst Rev* 2011; 2011(9):Cd001544. doi:10.1002/14651858.CD001544.pub4

6. Slim K, Kartheuser A. Mechanical Bowel Preparation Before Colorectal Surgery in Enhanced Recovery Programs: Discrepancy Between the American and European Guidelines. *Dis Colon Rectum* 2018;61(2):e13–4.

7. Jung B, Matthiessen P, Smedh K, Nilsson E, Ransjö U, Påhlman L. Mechanical bowel preparation does not affect the intramucosal bacterial colony count. *Int J Colorectal Dis* 2010;25:439–42 [PMID: 20012296 DOI: 10.1007/s00384-009-0863-3]

8. Mahajna A, Krausz M, Rosin D, Shabtai M, Hershko D, Ayalon A, Zmora O. Bowel preparation is associated with spillage of bowel contents in colorectal surgery. *Dis Colon Rectum* 2005;48:1626–31 [PMID: 15981063 DOI: 10.1007/s10350-005-0073-1]

9. Midura EF, Jung AD, Hanseman DJ et al. Combination oral and mechanical bowel preparations decreases complications in both right and left colectomy. *Surgery* 2018;163:528.

10. Klinger AL, Green H, Monlezun DJ et al. The role of bowel preparation in colorectal surgery: Results of the 2012–2015 ACS-NSQIP data. *Ann Surg* 2019;269:671.

11. Chen M, Song X, Chen LZ et al. Comparing mechanical bowel preparation with both oral and systemic antibiotics versus mechanical bowel preparation and systemic antibiotics alone for the prevention of surgical site infection after elective colorectal surgery: A meta-analysis of randomized controlled clinical trials. *Dis Colon Rectum* 2016;59:70.

Chapter 8

ERAS IN COLORECTAL SURGERY

Harsh Shah and Kantilal S Patel

Contents

Learning objectives 38
Introduction 38
Components of ERAS protocols and current recommendations 38
Summary 41
Key points 41
References 41

Learning objectives

- Learn the perioperative components of the 'Enhanced Recovery' pathway.
- To provide the latest evidence on the outcomes of various components of the 'Enhanced Recovery' pathway.

Introduction

The enhanced recovery after surgery (ERAS) program, also known as 'fast-track surgery', is a combination of evidence-based perioperative strategies that work synergistically to expedite recovery after surgery.

Factors such as wound infection, anastomosis leak, malnutrition, pain, pulmonary complications, venous thrombosis, and so on delay the recovery of surgical patients. Guidelines are frequently published by surgical societies for their effective management. The ERAS program is a thoughtful amalgamation of all such guidelines to improve patient care and expedite recovery. Although each of these individual strategies are beneficial to some extent on their own to achieve maximum benefit, they have to be used together in the form of a package. The underlying mechanism of ERAS protocol is thought to be an attenuation of the perioperative stress response [1], although there is increasing evidence to suggest that the benefits of ERAS are actually mediated by the return of organ – particularly gut – function [2].

ERAS protocols are usually applied for all colorectal surgeries performed under general anesthesia. Emergency surgeries, malnourished patients, and patients with chronic liver disease (Childs B & C) should not be included as ERAS may not be beneficial in them.

Components of ERAS protocols and current recommendations

ERAS protocols typically include 15–20 elements or components combined to form a multimodal pathway. Components of ERAS protocols can be broadly categorized into preoperative, perioperative, and postoperative interventions.

PREOPERATIVE COMPONENTS (Includes following policies):

1. *Preoperative counselling and training*: The process involves the surgical team as well as physiotherapists, dietitians, and stoma nurses. A dedicated ERAS nurse is essential for the success of the program.

Information discussed should include:
- What enhanced recovery involves, its core components, and envisaged benefits.
- Smoking and alcohol cessation. At least 3 weeks of smoking cessation is essential to recover function of the respiratory epithelium.
- Exercise schedule, which includes daily walking, deep breathing, aerobic exercises, spirometry, etc.
- Patients who may require a stoma should be identified and appropriately trained such that they are proficient at stoma care, ideally prior to surgery. The stoma site should be marked a day prior to surgery and the patient is shown the videos/photographs of various stoma appliances and their handling.

2. *Risk evaluation*: Medical comorbidities, including cardiovascular, respiratory, and/or renal disease should be evaluated and optimized similarly to any routine surgeries.

3. *Bowel preparation*: We suggest performing mechanical bowel preparation combined with oral antibiotics for all patients undergoing elective colorectal resection, based on the preponderance of data [3]. Others choose to omit bowel preparation [4]. We use mechanical bowel preparation for left-sided colonic and rectal surgeries. We typically use antibiotics, e.g., ciprofloxacin or Ofloxacin with Metronidazole or Ornidazole for 48 hours prior to any bowel surgery.

4. *Fasting guidelines*: Preoperative fasting guidelines have been established by the American Society of Anesthesiologists (ASA) and are based upon randomized trials and nonrandomized comparative studies [5].

   A. *Clear liquids*: The ASA guidelines recommend fasting for at least **2** hours from clear liquids and all other intake, including medicines [6]. Patients may consume clear liquids including nonalcoholic beverages such as water, juices without pulp, coffee or tea without milk, and carbohydrate drinks up until 2 hours before surgery. This approach to fasting helps avoid symptoms of dehydration, hypoglycemia, and caffeine withdrawal. Intravenous fluids are withheld, even in patients prescribed mechanical bowel preparation.

   B. *Solid foods and milk*:
   - Fried or fatty foods or meat: ASA guidelines recommend that patients fast **8** hours or more following intake of fried or fatty foods or meat due to a prolonged gastric emptying time.

– Light meal or milk: ASA guidelines recommend that patients fast **6** hours or more following ingestion of a light meal (e.g., toast and tea) or milk.

C. *Carbohydrate-rich drink*: This practice has been suggested as a method to convert the patient from the 'fasted' to the 'fed' state, reducing postoperative insulin resistance and postoperative weight loss [7]. Evidence to support carbohydrate-rich drinks before elective colon surgery is limited [7]. Carbohydrate loading involves the administration of carbohydrate drinks the night before surgery and 3 hours prior to surgery. We typically use a a dose of 6 tablespoons full of glucose, which provides approximately 350 kCal. Any commercially available preparation may be used. However, care should be taken that the formulation used is clear and residue free. It is generally agreed upon to avoid glucose solutions for diabetic patients.

5. *Alvimopan*: Prolonged postoperative ileus is a main cause of delayed patient recovery, and reducing this complication is a specific objective of ERAS protocols. Alvimopan, an oral peripherally acting mu-opioid receptor antagonist, that has a limited ability to cross the blood–brain barrier, appears to reduce prolonged ileus after bowel surgery [8]. The benefits of alvimopan are questionable when nonopioid analgesics and other perioperative opioid-sparing techniques are employed. When administration is planned, Alvimopan should be started preoperatively to be effective.

6. *Deep vein thrombosis prophylaxis*: A single daily dose of low molecular weight heparin (LMWH) is recommended for deep vein thrombosis prophylaxis because of its ease of administration and lower risk of bleeding complications [9]. The use of LMWH in conjunction with graduated compression stockings was found to be the most effective thromboprophylaxis in a Cochrane review [10]. There is an increased risk of thrombotic complications up to one month after surgery, due to a hypercoagulable state, and prolonged (up to 1 month after discharge) antithrombotic prophylaxis with low molecular weight heparin confers significant benefit in terms of reduction of thrombotic complications [11]. We give the first dose of LMWH 12 hours prior to surgery, along with fitting graduated compression stocking for all colorectal surgeries. This will be continued for 3–5 days postoperatively until the patient becomes satisfactorily ambulant.

7. *Antibiotic prophylaxis*: Antibiotic prophylaxis is used to reduce the rates of wound infection after surgery. Multiple doses have not been found to confer additional advantages and result in increased costs and risk of infections (e.g., Clostridium difficile). For this reason, a single dose of antibiotics, covering both aerobic and anaerobic organisms, should be administered just prior to incising the skin in all clean procedures which do not involve the insertion of prosthetic materials. When deciding on the type of antibiotic used, local resistance patterns should be considered.

INTRAOPERATIVE COMPONENTS (Intraoperative strategies in ERAS protocols include the selection of anesthetic agents and techniques, lung-protective ventilation, fluid management, temperature regulation, and the choice of the surgical approach):

1. *Selection of anesthetic agents*:
   • Use of only short-acting anesthetic agents (e.g., propofol, inhaled anesthetics such as sevoflurane or desflurane) that are administered at the lowest possible doses.

• Avoidance of premedication with midazolam to reduce the risk of dose-dependent postoperative sedation and respiratory depression, particularly if opioids are administered [12].

• Avoidance of long-acting opioids and reduction of total intraoperative opioid doses. We use Diclofenac suppositories at the induction of anesthesia for sustained pain relief.

2. *Lung-protective ventilation*: The primary goals for intraoperative ventilation are to provide nonharmful ventilation that opens the lungs and keeps them open into the postoperative period. For most patients, we suggest low tidal volumes of 6–8 mL/kg, with an initial positive end-expiratory pressure (PEEP) of 5 cm H_2O (10 cm H_2O during laparoscopy), and plateau pressures of ≤ 16 mmHg.

3. *Intraoperative fluid management*: Intraoperative fluid management is aimed at restoring and maintaining euvolemia.
   • Restrictive fluid therapy (i.e., zero-balance approach) avoids fluid overload by replacing only the fluid that is lost during surgery [13]. Given that the ERAS goals for perioperative fluid management include avoidance of either hypovolemia or excessive fluid administration that may result in pulmonary complications, we typically use restrictive fluid therapy to minimize fluid administration, rather than the other two strategies, e.g., goal directed, fixed volume fluid therapy [14]. In one randomized multicenter trial of 150 patients undergoing elective colorectal surgery, equivalent postoperative outcomes were noted with a zero-balance (restrictive) approach compared to a goal-directed approach to fluid therapy [15].
   • If preoperative dehydration is avoided and early postoperative alimentation is emphasized as part of an ERAS protocol, then goal-directed fluid therapy may be unnecessary because of the low risk of perioperative fluid imbalance [16]. A 2016 meta-analysis of randomized controlled trials of patients undergoing elective major abdominal surgery (2099 patients; 23 studies) noted no benefit when goal-directed fluid therapy was used within the setting of an ERAS protocol, compared with a fixed-volume regimen [17].

4. *High inspired oxygen concentrations*: Molecular oxygen is required by polymorphonuclear cells to produce free radicals which form an important line of defense against pathogens [18]. Higher tissue oxygenation levels in the immediate postoperative period, as a result of 80% inspired oxygen, have been shown to improve perfusion at the anastomotic site and reduce the risk of surgical site infections [19]. In addition, there is some evidence that it may also reduce postoperative nausea and vomiting, although this is contentious [20].

5. *Prevention of hypothermia*: General anesthesia can disrupt the normal thermoregulatory processes and result in hypothermia. In addition, exposure of the patient to the cold theater environment also contributes. Hypothermia (core temperature less than 36°C) can, in turn, lead to an increase in the incidence of surgical site infections, thought to be due to peripheral vasoconstriction induced hypoxia [21] and an altered immune response. Other undesirable effects of hypothermia include coagulopathy [22], increased cardiac morbidity [23], and increased levels of circulating catecholamines with a resultant exaggerated catabolic

response [24]. Active prevention of hypothermia during the perioperative period has been shown to reduce blood loss and prevent infective [25] and cardiac complications [26]. For these reasons, hypothermia should be actively prevented using warm-air blankets. Warming should be continued for as long as the patient is in recovery. If the procedure is expected to last for more than two hours, then dual temperature monitoring and warmed intravenous fluids should be used [27]. An esophageal probe should be used during the procedure for measurement of core body temperature.

6. *Laparosopic surgery*: Minimaly invasive techniques are central to ERAS protocols because they decrease inflammatory mediator release, improve pulmonary function, expedite return of bowel function, and reduce the length of hospital stay [28]. Several randomized trials have compared laparoscopic and open colorectal surgery with the utilization of an ERAS protocol. A meta-analysis of these trials concluded that laparoscopic surgery reduced both the length of hospital stay and the rate of complications [29].

7. *Peritoneal drains*: Drains versus no drains have been a topic of debate. Drains do not prevent complications, but may facilitate identification of an anastomotic leak earlier. However, due to the significant pain related to its mere existence, it may prolong recovery. So, it is our policy to put drains on a selective basis, e.g., for low rectal anastomosis.

8. *Avoidance of nasogastric tubes*: Nasogastric tubes, once a mainstay of colon and rectal surgery, are associated with patient discomfort and a delay in time for oral intake, and are not included in the ERAS protocols for elective patients [30].

POSTOPERATIVE COMPONENTS (Postoperative goals in ERAS protocols include prevention and relief of pain or nausea and vomiting, and facilitation of early nutrition and mobilization):

1. *Supplemental Oxygen*: Adequate tissue oxygenation is essential for tissue healing. We recommend supplemental oxygen to all patients for 2 hours. The duration should be increased up to 12 hours for patients undergoing major surgeries, e.g., for restorative proctocolectomy.

2. *Pain management*: Optimal perioperative pain management enhances recovery after surgery by facilitating postoperative ambulation and rehabilitation. Procedure-specific multimodal analgesia that minimizes opioid use is ideal [31]. Opioids are potential cause of postoperative ileus. For patients undergoing laparoscopic colorectal procedures, we use nonopioid analgesics (e.g., nonsteroidal anti-inflammatory drug [NSAID] or cyclooxygenase [COX]-2 specific inhibitor) in combination with local anesthetic infiltration at the port sites [32]. In a nonrandomized study of laparoscopic colorectal surgery, local infiltration with a long-acting local anesthetic (liposomal bupivacaine) was associated with reduced opioid use, a shorter length of stay (mean 3 vs. 4 days), and lower overall cost [33].

Acetaminophen, ibuprofen, and ketorolac are available in intravenous forms for patients who do not yet tolerate oral formulations. It remains controversial whether perioperative use of NSAIDs increases the risk of anastomotic leak. Thoracic epidural analgesia is no longer recommended after laparoscopic surgery because it could potentially delay ambulation and hospital discharge without providing any additional benefit in pain control [32].

For patients undergoing open procedures, if an epidural catheter is not placed, we typically use a transversus abdominis plane block (TAP block), or surgical site infiltration, in combination with nonopioid analgesic agents [31].

3. *Prophylactic antiemetic*: Antiemetics helps counter the side effects of surgery as well as anaesthetic agents and improves patient well-being. We recommend prophylactic antiemetics for first 24 hours.

4. *Fluid management*: Intravenous fluid administration should be discontinued as soon as the patient can tolerate oral liquids. Before oral intake is allowed, patients typically receive an infusion of a balanced salt solution (e.g., Lactated Ringers) at 50 mL/hour, with boluses of 100 mL if necessary to treat hemodynamic instability and/or inadequate urine output (UO). Although maintenance of a minimum hourly UO of 0.5 mL/kg is a common goal, limited data support this practice. In one randomized trial in 40 patients without significant risk factors for kidney injury, fluid was administered to maintain a minimum UO of either 0.2 or 0.5 mL/kg per hour during and after major abdominal surgery (from the time of anesthetic induction until the second postoperative day) [34]. While patients in the low-target UO group received less fluid than the high-target UO group (3170 versus 5490 mL), laboratory measurements of kidney function and other outcomes were not different. Thus, patients without risk factors for acute kidney injury may be managed with less postoperative fluid, but it is not known whether this practice can reduce postoperative complications or length of hospital stay.

5. *Diet*: ERAS programs incorporate resumption of a diet within a few hours after surgery and can be supplemented with high-calorie drinks to minimize the negative protein balance after surgery. This is in contrast to the traditional approach where oral feedings were withheld until signs of bowel activity (e.g., bowel sounds, flatus, bowel movement) were evident. In one study, the presence of bowel sounds, flatus, or bowel movement after major abdominal surgery was not predictive of tolerance of oral intake [35]. We start liquids through FJ/oral within 24 hours of surgeries.

6. *Early mobilization and chest physiotherapy*: Early mobilization is a key element of ERAS protocols for all postoperative patients capable of ambulation [36]. Early mobilization is essential to reducing the risk of postoperative pneumonia [37] and venous thromboembolism. Involving hospital personnel resources such as physiotherapists can help achieve the goal of early mobilization. It is measured in terms of hours out of bed. We typically advise 2 hours out of bed on POD-1, and 4 hours out of bed on POD-2.

7. *Early urinary catheter removal*: To aid with early mobilization, urinary catheters should be removed as early as possible, a process that also reduces the incidence of urinary tract infection after surgery. We prefer to remove it on POD-2 for all major surgeries.

8. *Chewing gum* – Use of chewing gum hastens recovery of bowel function after colorectal surgery [38]. We use sugar free chewing gum for all cases of bowel resection until the return of peristalsis.

9. *Predicting infective complication*: C-reactive protein (CRP) is effective as an early predictor of infective complications after colorectal surgery. Postoperative day 3 CRP >150 mg/L or persistent elevation of CRP should increase

suspicion of an infective complication. Conversely, CRP levels below this threshold are highly predictive of an uncomplicated recovery and are commonly used in ERAS protocols to guide discharge [39]. We do not routinely use this parameter.

10. *Early discharge*: The goal of ERAS programs is an accelerated recovery and return to normal activity. Hospital stay (typically ≤5 days) is often used as a surrogate marker of recovery, but is not the only focus of the protocol [40].

OUTCOMES: Data from observational studies and randomized trials show that ERAS protocols are associated with a reduced hospital length of stay (LOS) and morbidity, faster recovery, comparable or reduced readmission rate, and cost savings compared with traditional care in both older and young adults [41].

- *Length of stay and morbidity*: Contemporary series of colorectal surgery using ERAS protocols report hospital LOS ranging from 3 to 5 days [43–49]. In a 2014 systematic review and meta-analysis of 16 randomized trials of elective colorectal surgery, those managed with versus those without an ERAS program had a significantly reduced LOS and reduced overall morbidity and nonsurgical complications, but not a higher readmission rate [51]. A 2014 meta-analysis of 38 trials across all surgical specialties, including but not limited to colorectal surgery, reached a very similar conclusion that ERAS reduced both complications and LOS [52].
- *Faster recovery*: In addition to shorter hospital LOS and lower morbidity, several other favorable postoperative outcomes of 'enhanced' or faster recovery have been attributed to ERAS protocols in observational studies:
  - Reduced duration of an ileus [53].
  - Preservation of lean body mass and exercise performance [54].
  - Improved grip strength suggesting overall improvement in muscle function [45].
  - Earlier resumption of normal activities, reduced need for daytime sleep, and no increased use of primary care services [55].
- *Readmission rates*: Early discharge (LOS ≤5 days) is the goal of ERAS protocols, but the benefit of early discharge may be offset by a higher rate of hospital readmissions [43,51]. Early studies suggested that patients managed with ERAS programs had an increased readmission rate compared with traditional practice [42]. However, a meta-analysis of six later randomized trials and prospective studies found that the rate of readmission was not significantly different after ERAS versus traditional recovery programs [43].
- *Cost*: For an ERAS protocol to be financially justified, the cost (e.g., from a laparoscopic procedure) must be balanced with savings from a shorter hospital admission, with fewer readmissions and complications. Prospective trials to analyze the costs and benefits of ERAS programs are in progress, with the initial data suggesting an overall cost benefit [50].

Summary

ERAS programs are evidence-based protocols designed to standardize medical care, improve outcomes, and lower health care costs. The elements of an ERAS protocol include:

- Preoperative strategies (e.g., medical risk evaluation, patient education including stoma management, mechanical bowel preparation plus oral antibiotics, and appropriate fasting guidelines).
- Intraoperative strategies (e.g., selection of short-acting anesthetic agents, lung-protective ventilation, restrictive fluid therapy, temperature regulation, and laparoscopic surgery).
- Postoperative strategies (e.g., multimodal analgesia with an emphasis on nonopioid pain management, appropriate fluid management, early oral feeding and mobilization, avoidance of nasogastric tubes, early removal of urinary catheter, and early discharge).
- The use of ERAS protocols is associated with reduced hospital length of stay and morbidity, faster recovery, comparable or reduced readmission rate, and cost savings compared with traditional care in both old and young patients.

Key points

- Each individual component of ERAS is helpful by itself, but they are synergistic when used together.
- Institutes should develop dedicated ERAS teams.
- The data on both adherence to ERAS strategy and patient outcome should be audited regularly.

References

1. Kehlet H, Wilmore DW. Multimodal strategies to improve surgical outcome. *Am J Surg* 2002 Jun;183(6):630–41.
2. Gatt M, Anderson AD, Reddy BS, Hayward-Sampson P, Tring IC, MacFie J. Randomized clinical trial of multimodal optimization of surgical care in patients undergoing major colonic resection. *Br J Surg* 2005;92:1354–1362.
3. Scarborough JE, Mantyh CR, Sun Z, Migaly J. Combined mechanical and oral antibiotic bowel preparation reduces incisional surgical site infection and anastomotic leak rates after elective colorectal resection: an analysis of colectomy-targeted ACS NSQIP. *Ann Surg* 2015;262:331.
4. Güenaga KF, Matos D, Wille-Jørgensen P. Mechanical bowel preparation for elective colorectal surgery. *Cochrane Database Syst Rev* 2011; 2011(9):CD001544. doi:10.1002/14651858.CD001544. pub4
5. Practice Guidelines for Preoperative Fasting and the Use of Pharmacologic Agents to Reduce the Risk of Pulmonary Aspiration: Application to Healthy Patients Undergoing Elective Procedures: An Updated Report by the American Society of Anesthesiologists Task Force on Preoperative Fasting and the Use of Pharmacologic Agents to Reduce the Risk of Pulmonary Aspiration. *Anesthesiology* 2017;126:376.
6. American Society of Anesthesiologists Committee. Practice guidelines for preoperative fasting and the use of pharmacologic agents to reduce the risk of pulmonary aspiration: Application to healthy patients undergoing elective procedures: An updated report by the American Society of Anesthesiologists Committee on Standards and Practice Parameters. *Anesthesiology* 2011;114:495.
7. Gillis C, Carli F. Promoting Perioperative Metabolic and Nutritional Care. *Anesthesiology* 2015;123:1455.
8. Adam MA, Lee LM, Kim J et al. Alvimopan provides additional improvement in outcomes and cost savings in enhanced recovery colorectal surgery. *Ann Surg* 2016;264:141.
9. Levine MN, Raskob G, Landefeld S, Kearon C. Hemorrhagic complications of anticoagulant treatment. *Chest* 2001 Jan;119(1 Suppl):108S–121S.

10. Gould MK, Dembitzer AD, Doyle RL, Hastie TJ, Garber AM. Low-molecularweight heparins compared with unfractionated heparin for treatment of acute deep venous thrombosis. A meta-analysis of randomized, controlled trials. *Ann Intern Med* 1999 May 18;130(10):800–9.

11. Rasmussen MS, Jørgensen LN, Wille-Jørgensen P. Prolonged thromboprophylaxis with Low Molecular Weight heparin for abdominal or pelvic surgery. *Cochrane Database of Syst Rev* 2009;1(1). Art. No.:CD004318. DOI: 10.1002/14651858.CD004318.pub2.

12. Feldheiser A, Aziz O, Baldini G et al. Enhanced Recovery After Surgery (ERAS) for gastrointestinal surgery, part 2: Consensus statement for anaesthesia practice. *Acta Anaesthesiol Scand* 2016;60:289.

13. Maurice-Szamburski A, Auquier P, Viarre-Oreal V et al. Effect of sedative premedication on patient experience after general anesthesia: A randomized clinical trial. *JAMA* 2015;313:916.

14. Brandstrup B. Fluid therapy for the surgical patient. *Best Pract Res Clin Anaesthesiol* 2006;20:265.

15. Brandstrup B, Svendsen PE, Rasmussen M et al. Which goal for fluid therapy during colorectal surgery is followed by the best outcome: Near-maximal stroke volume or zero fluid balance? *Br J Anaesth* 2012;109:191.

16. Joshi GP, Kehlet H. CON: Perioperative Goal-Directed Fluid Therapy Is an Essential Element of an Enhanced Recovery Protocol? *Anesth Analg* 2016;122:1261.

17. Rollins KE, Lobo DN. Intraoperative Goal-directed Fluid Therapy in Elective Major Abdominal Surgery: A Meta-analysis of Randomized Controlled Trials. *Ann Surg* 2016;263:465.

18. Babior BM. Oxygen-dependent microbial killing by phagocytes. *N Engl J Med* 1978;298:659–68.

19. Qadan M, Akça O, Mahid SS, Hornung CA, Polk HC Jr. Perioperative supplemental oxygen therapy and surgical site infection: A meta-analysis of randomized controlled trials. *Arch Surg* 2009 Apr;144(4):359–66; discussion 366–7.

20. Greif R, Laciny S, Rapf B, Hickle RS, Sessler DI. S upplemental oxygen reduces the incidence of postoperative nausea and vomiting. *Anesthesiology* 1999;91:1246–1252.

21. Ozaki M, Sessler D I, Suzuki H, Ozaki K, Tsunoda C, Atarashi K. Nitrous oxide decreases the threshold for vasoconstriction less than sevoflurane or isoflurane. *Anesth Analg* 1995 Jun;80(6):1212–6.

22. Schmied H, Kurz A, Sessler DI, Kozek S, Reiter A. Mild hypothermia increases blood loss and transfusion requirements during total hip arthroplasty. *Lancet* 1996 Feb 3;347(8997):289–92.

23. Frank SM, Fleisher LA, Breslow MJ, Higgins MS, Olson KF, Kelly S, Beattie C. Perioperative maintenance of normothermia reduces the incidence of morbid cardiac events. A randomized clinical trial. *JAMA* 1997 Apr 9;277(14):1127–34.

24. Frank SM, Higgins MS, Breslow MJ, Fleisher LA, Gorman RB, Sitzmann JV, Raff H, Beattie C. The catecholamine, cortisol, and hemodynamic responses to mild perioperative hypothermia. A randomized clinical trial. *Anesthesiology* 1995 Jan;82(1):83–93.

25. Wong P F, Kumar S, Bohra A, Whetter D, Leaper D J. Randomized clinical trial of perioperative systemic warming in major elective abdominal surgery. *Br J Surg* 2007 Apr;94(4):421–6.

26. Elmore JR, Franklin DP, Youkey JR, Oren JW, Frey CM. Normothermia is protective during infrarenal aortic surgery. *J Vasc Surg* 1998 Dec;28(6):984–94.

27. Smith CE, Gerdes E, Sweda S, Myles C, Punjabi A, Pinchak AC, Hagen JF. Warming intravenous fluids reduces perioperative hypothermia in women undergoing ambulatory gynecological surgery. *Anesth Analg* 1998 Jul;87(1):37–41

28. Lourenco T, Murray A, Grant A et al. Laparoscopic surgery for colorectal cancer: Safe and effective? - A systematic review. *Surg Endosc* 2008;22:1146.

29. Lei QC, Wang XY, Zheng HZ et al. Laparoscopic Versus Open Colorectal Resection Within Fast Track Programs: An Update Meta-Analysis Based on Randomized Controlled Trials. *J Clin Med Res* 2015;7:594.

30. Nelson R, Tse B, Edwards S. Systematic review of prophylactic nasogastric decompression after abdominal operations. *Br J Surg* 2005;92:673.

31. Joshi GP, Schug SA, Kehlet H. Procedure-specific pain management and outcome strategies. *Best Pract Res Clin Anaesthesiol* 2014;28:191.

32. Joshi GP, Bonnet F, Kehlet H, PROSPECT collaboration. Evidence-based postoperative pain management after laparoscopic colorectal surgery. *Colorectal Dis* 2013;15:146.

33. Keller DS, Pedraza R, Tahilramani RN et al. Impact of long-acting local anesthesia on clinical and financial outcomes in laparoscopic colorectal surgery. *Am J Surg* 2017;214:53.

34. Puckett JR, Pickering JW, Palmer SC et al. Low Versus Standard Urine Output Targets in Patients Undergoing Major Abdominal Surgery: A Randomized Noninferiority Trial. *Ann Surg* 2017;265:874.

35. Read TE, Brozovich M, Andujar JE et al. Bowel Sounds Are Not Associated With Flatus, Bowel Movement, or Tolerance of Oral Intake in Patients After Major Abdominal Surgery. *Dis Colon Rectum* 2017;60:608.

36. Zutshi M, Delaney CP, Senagore AJ, Fazio VW. Shorter hospital stay associated with fastrack postoperative care pathways and laparoscopic intestinal resection are not associated with increased physical activity. *Colorectal Dis* 2004;6:477.

37. Kamel HK, Iqbal MA, Mogallapu R et al. Time to ambulation after hip fracture surgery: Relation to hospitalization outcomes. *J Gerontol A Biol Sci Med Sci* 2003;58:1042.

38. Song GM, Deng YH, Jin YH, Zhou JG, Tian X. Meta-analysis comparing chewing gum versus standard postoperative care after colorectal resection. *Oncotarget* 2016 Oct 25;7(43):70066.

39. MacKay GJ, Molloy RG, O'Dwyer PJ. C-reactive protein as a predictor of postoperative infective complications following elective colorectal resection. *Colorectal Dis* 2011;13:583.

40. Hendren S, Morris AM, Zhang W, Dimick J. Early discharge and hospital readmission after colectomy for cancer. *Dis Colon Rectum* 2011;54:1362.

41. Delaney CP, Fazio VW, Senagore AJ et al. 'Fast track' postoperative management protocol for patients with high co-morbidity undergoing complex abdominal and pelvic colorectal surgery. *Br J Surg* 2001;88:1533.

42. Basse L, Hjort Jakobsen D, Billesbølle P et al. A clinical pathway to accelerate recovery after colonic resection. *Ann Surg* 2000;232:51.

43. Wind J, Polle SW, Fung Kon Jin PH et al. Systematic review of enhanced recovery programmes in colonic surgery. *Br J Surg* 2006;93:800.

44. Proske JM, Raue W, Neudecker J et al. [Fast track rehabilitation in colonic surgery: Results of a prospective trial]. *Ann Chir* 2005;130:152.

45. Delaney CP, Zutshi M, Senagore AJ et al. Prospective, randomized, controlled trial between a pathway of controlled rehabilitation with early ambulation and diet and traditional postoperative care after laparotomy and intestinal resection. *Dis Colon Rectum* 2003;46:851.

46. Anderson AD, McNaught CE, MacFie J et al. Randomized clinical trial of multimodal optimization and standard perioperative surgical care. *Br J Surg* 2003;90:1497.

47. Kremer M, Ulrich A, Büchler MW, Uhl W. Fast-track surgery: The Heidelberg experience. *Recent Results Cancer Res* 2005;165:14.

48. Susa A, Roveran A, Bocchi A et al. [FastTrack approach to major colorectal surgery]. *Chir Ital* 2004;56:817.

49. Smedh K, Strand E, Jansson P et al. [Rapid recovery after colonic resection. Multimodal rehabilitation by means of Kehlet's method practiced in Vasteras]. *Lakartidningen* 2001;98:2568.

50. Wind J, Hofland J, Preckel B et al. Perioperative strategy in colonic surgery; LAparoscopy and/or FAst track multimodal management versus standard care (LAFA trial). *BMC Surg* 2006;6:16.;

51. Greco M, Capretti G, Beretta L et al. Enhanced recovery program in colorectal surgery: A meta-analysis of randomized controlled trials. *World J Surg* 2014;38:1531.

52. Nicholson A, Lowe MC, Parker J et al. Systematic review and meta-analysis of enhanced recovery programmes in surgical patients. *Br J Surg* 2014;101:172.

53. Basse L, Madsen JL, Kehlet H. Normal gastrointestinal transit after colonic resection using epidural analgesia, enforced oral nutrition and laxative. *Br J Surg* 2001;88:1498.

54. Basse L, Raskov HH, Hjort Jakobsen D et al. Accelerated postoperative recovery programme after colonic resection improves physical performance, pulmonary function and body composition. *Br J Surg* 2002;89:446.

55. Jakobsen DH, Sonne E, Andreasen J, Kehlet H. Convalescence after colonic surgery with fast-track vs conventional care. *Colorectal Dis* 2006;8:683.

Chapter 9

ANESTHETIC MANAGEMENT OF LAPROSCOPIC COLORECTAL SURGERY

Raxesh Desai and Nisarg Patel

Contents

Learning objectives 44
Introduction 44
Preoperative assessment and optimization 44
Preoperative preparation. 44
Physiological changes occurring during laparoscopic surgery. 45
    Effect on respiratory system 45
    Effect on cardiovascular system. 45
    Renal and metabolic effect 45
    Gastrointestinal effect 45
Anesthetic techniques and intraoperative monitoring 45
    Goal-directed fluid therapy. 46
    Blood transfusion 46
Recovery. 46
Pain control 46
Morbidity and mortality 46
Summary 46
Key points 47
References 47

Learning objectives

- Lap surgery has advantages for patients in terms of postop recovery, but poses challenges for anesthesia management perioperatively.
- An understanding of perioperative factors such as suppression of stress response, optimal fluid therapy, and multimodal pain management are essential for reducing morbidity and mortality in colorectal surgeries.
- Anesthesiologists can play an important role in improving the outcome of high-risk colorectal surgery by standardized perioperative care.

Introduction

Laproscopic colorectal (CR) surgery is commonly performed for colorectal malignancies, diverticular, and inflammatory bowel diseases. The advantages of laparoscopic colorectal surgery over open surgery are well known. Despite significant advances, such as laparoscopic techniques and multidisciplinary perioperative management, morbidity and mortality remain high and vary among institutions. An understanding of perioperative factors such as suppression of stress response, optimal fluid therapy, and multimodal pain management is essential for reducing morbidity and mortality in colorectal surgeries.

Preoperative assessment and optimization

For elective noncancer surgery, a detailed evaluation and treatment of medical problems should be performed prior to operations to improve outcome. However, in patients requiring cancer or urgent surgery (e.g. for obstruction or perforation), time may be limited. Use of scoring systems and assessment of functional capacity may help in identifying high-risk patients and predicting complications. History, clinical examination, review of monitored parameters, and laboratory investigations (e.g. arterial blood gas analysis and serum electrolytes) are vital to judge the severity of problems (e.g. fluid deficit) apart from routine laboratory investigations. During emergency surgery, the main goals are to identify deteriorating vital physiological end-organ functions and their causes, for example sepsis and hypovolemia.

Cardiac and respiratory diseases are commonly present among patients undergoing major CR surgery. General fitness of a patient is a better predictor, for outcome after surgery for colorectal cancer, than chronological age [1]. Cardiopulmonary exercise testing (CPET) has been suggested as an integrated objective measurement of functional reserve and is useful in predicting complications and outcome. The results of CPET have a high predictive value for patients at risk of developing cardiopulmonary complications in the postoperative period [2].

The Physiological and Operative Severity Score for the Enumeration of Mortality and Morbidity (POSSUM) and the Portsmouth-POSSUM (P-POSSUM) were developed in 1991 and 1996, respectively. The POSSUM-based scoring system predicts complications and outcome.

Preoperative preparation

To improve recovery after CR surgery, traditional clinical measures such as mechanical bowel preparation (MBP) and routine insertion of nasogastric tubes have been challenged [3]. Control of cardio-respiratory diseases, incentive spirometry, and chest physiotherapy should be started at earliest. Prevention of thrombo-embolic complications should be done by preoperative prophylactic doses of anticoagulants, intraoperative mechanical compression devices and stockings, and postoperative early mobilization [4]. Antimicrobial prophylaxis with aerobic and anaerobic coverage reduces surgical site infection significantly [5]. Hypoalbuminemia, anemia, and weight loss have been associated with increased postoperative complications such as infections [6], anastomotic complications, and impaired wound healing leading to increased length of hospital stay [7]. Several strategies to counteract the catabolic stress response have been suggested: shortening fasting periods, use of nutritional support and glycemic control [8], and laparoscopic techniques have all been shown to be beneficial.

Physiological changes occurring during laparoscopic surgery

Effect on respiratory system
The increased intra-abdominal pressure due to pneumopertioneum, along with a steep trendelenburg position, displaces the diaphragm cephalad. This will lead to reduction in lung volumes (tidal volume, minute volume, functional residual capacity) resulting in basal atelectasis and increased airway pressure. Restriction in diaphragmatic mobility promotes uneven distribution of ventilation, which results in ventilation-perfusion mismatch with hypoxemia and hypercarbia. Ventilatory impairment is more severe if there is associated airway and alveolar collapse, predisposing to postoperative chest infections. The end-tidal carbon dioxide ($ETCO_2$) is generally used by anesthesiologists as a noninvasive substitute for the arterial carbon dioxide level ($PaCO_2$). The $PaCO_2$ is generally higher than the $ETCO_2$ by a 5–10 mm Hg gradient during general anesthesia. Patients with preexisting cardiopulmonary disease were noted to have a significant increase in $PaCO_2$ and a decrease in pH after CO_2 insufflation, which are not reflected by comparable increases in $ETCO_2$ [9]. These patients also had inspiratory pressures that were significantly higher than baseline values after CO_2 insufflation. Low cardiac output (CO) increases dead space ventilation, which is reflected by a wider arterial-to-$ETCO_2$ gradient. Additional factors such as long duration of laparoscopy, intra-abdominal pressure (IAP) greater than 15 mm Hg, or subcutaneous emphysema can elevate $PaCO_2$. Radial artery cannulation for the purpose of frequent blood gas monitoring should also be considered in situations of intraoperative hypoxemia, profound elevation of $eTCO_2$, and high airway pressures.

Effect on cardiovascular system
Most of the cardiovascular changes occur due to creation of pneumo-peritoneum, patient position (steep trendelenburg and lithotomy), anesthesia, and hypercapnia. Creation of pneumo-peritoneum causes an increase in systemic vascular resistance, mean arterial pressure, and cardiac filling pressures. The increase in systemic vascular resistance may be due to an increased sympathetic output from CO_2 absorption and a neuro-endocrine response to pneumoperitoneum, and increase in systemic vascular resistance which may increase myocardial oxygen demand. Cardiopulmonary changes are proportional to the magnitude of intra-abdominal pressure attained during laparoscopy. Significant changes occur at an intra-abdominal pressure greater than 12–15 mm Hg.

Gas insufflation may cause arrhythmias including AV dissociation, nodal rhythm, sinus bradycardia, and asystole. Response is more pronounced at the beginning of insufflation probably due to a vagus-mediated reflex initiated by stretching of the peritoneum.

Gas embolus has been reported as a cause of cardiac arrest during laparoscopy. Alpha 2 agonist and beta-antagonist group of drugs like metoprolol, dexmedetomidine and clonidine, and sympathetic blockade with epidural local anesthetic agents can counteract the effect of increase in systemic vascular resistance (SVR).

Renal and metabolic effect
An intra-abdominal pressure greater than 15 mm Hg adversely affects renal function and urine output. Renal blood flow and glomerular filtration rate decrease because of increase in renal vascular resistance due to an increase in systemic vascular resistance.

An increase in intra-abdominal pressure above 15 mm Hg may produce lactic acidosis, probably due to a decrease in cardiac output and by impairing hepatic clearance of blood lactate. As with all surgeries, there is an associated stress response with elevated cortisol and circulating catecholamines.

Gastrointestinal effect
Pneumoperitoneum leads to an increase in intra-abdominal pressure as well as an increase in barrier pressure (barrier pressure = lower esophageal pressure – intragastric pressure). Therefore, previous risks of aspiration and regurgitation may have been overestimated and are now being reassessed.

Anesthetic techniques and intraoperative monitoring

Most anesthesiologists prefer general anesthesia with short-acting opioids and inhalational anaesthetic agents over sole regional anesthesia during laparoscopic colorectal surgery. Muscle relaxation with nondepolarizing agent allows controlled ventilation compensating for the various changes in oxygenation and ventilation. Concomitant neuraxial blockade with an epidural may be used with general anesthesia. Intraoperative epidural local anesthetic administration permits a decrease in the amounts of inhalational anesthetics, opioids, and muscle relaxants used. It may be beneficial to insert an epidural catheter if conversion to open surgery is likely.

It is well known that N_2O tends to diffuse into closed airspaces causing bowel distension. The combination of an orogastric tube and epidural anesthesia aids in bowel contraction and allows for better visualization [10].

Routine intraoperative monitors include standard five-lead electrocardiogram, systemic blood pressure with NIBP, pulse oximetry, capnography, temperature monitoring, and airway pressure monitoring. A urinary bladder catheter and nasogastric tubes are introduced to decompress the viscera, and avoid injury to the intra-abdominal contents during trocar insertion. Proper padding of pressure points should be done to avoid peripheral nerve injuries in prolonged surgeries in steep Trendelenburg and lithotomy positions.

The decision to place an invasive arterial monitor for advanced cardiac monitoring is reserved for cardiopulmonary compromised patients. Arterial blood gas measurement certainly allows more accurate monitoring of oxygenation and ventilation. Additional invasive monitoring with a pulmonary artery catheter or trans-oesophageal echocardiography may be considered in patients with severely compromised cardiopulmonary disease (American Society of Anesthesiologists class III–IV).

Maintaining perioperative normothermia reduces postoperative cardiac and coagulation complications, and should be standard care during colon surgery. Hypothermia causes several undesirable systemic changes, including an exaggerated stress response [11], and suppression of the immune function [12] in patients undergoing CR surgery. Active thermoregulation should be carried out both during open and laparoscopic CR surgery, as the reduced bowel exposure during the latter does not compensate for the marked effects of anesthesia on temperature regulation [13].

Goal-directed fluid therapy

Goal-directed hemodynamic management guided by SV or SVV (<15%) as endpoints reduces postoperative gastrointestinal complications. Fluids alone, or fluids and inotropes, are used to achieve defined end points. Flow, pressure, or volume-based goals have been used [14]. Interestingly, intraoperative or postoperative changes in central venous oxygen saturation (ScvO$_2$) have been found to predict complications. Intraoperative maintenance of ScvO$_2$ >73% may prevent complications [15].

During the perioperative period, fluid therapy and gastrointestinal function may complement or complicate each other. If fluid therapy is not optimal it may lead to hypovolemia or hypervolemia [16]; this in turn may cause gastrointestinal dysfunction (e.g. PONV or paralytic ileus). This further leads to fluid and electrolyte loss and metabolic problems. Liberal use of fluid during the perioperative period considering 'third space' loss, fluid loss due to mechanical bowel preparation, and replacement of preexisting deficit is an old philosophy. Restrictive fluid therapy and the use of vasopressors may raise concerns about systemic hypotension and reduced colon blood flow, respectively. It may compromise renal perfusion leading to renal failure. To achieve an optimal fluid balance, goal-directed (GD) crystalloids administration has been recommended [17].

Blood transfusion

Perioperative blood transfusion is also associated with increased colorectal cancer recurrence rates [18]. Allogenic blood transfusion is also an independent risk factor for developing postoperative infections most likely secondary to immunosuppression [19]. Intraoperative blood transfusion in colorectal surgery is associated with an increased length of stay and higher cost. Blood transfusions should be limited to strict indications only.

Recovery

Postoperatively, patients should be managed by multidisciplinary teams involving anesthesiologists, surgeons, nursing staff, nutritional experts, acute pain team, pharmacists, and physiotherapists in a high dependency unit (HDU). Early enteral nutrition has several advantages, such as improved anastomotic healing, improved calorie intake, a reduced incidence of infectious complications, reduced hyperglycemia, and insulin resistance [20]. Enteral nutrition is safe and more cost effective than parenteral nutrition (TPN), which requires a central line. It is also a care component of enhanced recovery.

Pain control

Pain relief in the postoperative period can be achieved by patient-controlled analgesia (PCA), wound infiltration, and transversus abdominis plane (TAP) block. Opioids have significant side effects on the gastrointestinal tract, such as nausea, vomiting, inhibition of gut motility, and constipation. In addition, NSAID and acetaminophen are commonly used to achieve multimodal analgesia. For laparoscopic CR surgery, there is no sufficient evidence for any specific postoperative analgesic method. Epidural analgesia may not offer the same benefits as in open surgery. However, epidurals may be indicated if patients have preoperative pulmonary morbidities and also if the procedure is converted to open surgery [21]. Laproscopy has its own postoperative advantages over open surgeries in terms of enhanced recovery and low analgesic requirements. Postoperative pain can be managed with intraperitonial instillation and trocar site injection of local anaesthetics (Bupivacaine 0.25%–0.125%, Ropivacaine 0.1%).

Morbidity and mortality

Colorectal surgery is a high-risk surgery and is associated with significant morbidity and mortality [22]. Predictive risk factors are mentioned in Table 9.1.

Important causes of in-hospital deaths were septic shock, terminal cancer, cardiac failure, broncho-pneumonia, acute respiratory distress, myocardial infarction, multiorgan failure, gastrointestinal hemorrhage, and stroke. The 30-day, in-hospital mortality during emergency surgery is three to four times higher in comparison to elective surgery. A wide variety of medical complications can occur after bowel surgery, with cardiovascular and pulmonary complications being the most frequent. Patients with renal failure have a significantly raised complication risk after bowel surgery, due to uremia and immunosuppression. Another frequent complication after abdominal surgery is postoperative delirium, with an incidence of 25%–35%, especially in the older patient population [23].

Summary

Laparoscopic surgery does present a unique challenge to anesthesiologist. The understanding of the physiological changes associated with increased abdominal pressure and positioning changes during surgery has improved over the years. Proper anesthetic management requires cooperation with the surgical team, as respiratory and cardiovascular parameters vary with each stage of surgery. Large volume fluid therapy may lead to gastrointestinal and systemic complications, therefore goal-directed fluid therapy is a standard of care. Postoperative issues such as nausea, vomiting, and ileus are more easily managed with preoperative planning. Anesthesiologists could play an important role to improve the outcome of high-risk colorectal surgery through vigilant perioperative care.

TABLE 9.1: Predictive Risk Factors for Postoperative Complications

Preoperative	Intraoperative	Postoperative
Age (<75)	Complexity of surgery	Sepsis
ASA Grade (>2)	Elective vs. emergency	Inadequate pain relief
MET equivalent <4	Cancer vs. noncancer surgery	Excess fluid administration
Anaemia, hypoalbuminemia significant weight loss	Right- vs. left-sided lesions	Medical complications
Chronic smoker	Intraoperative blood loss	Postoperative leaks
Morbid obesity	Intraoperative bowel injuries	
Presence of sepsis	Hypothermia	
	Excess fluid administration	

Key points

- Despite significant advances, such as laparoscopic techniques and multidisciplinary perioperative management, morbidity and mortality remain high and vary among different institutions.
- Preoperative assessment of patients for comorbidities and stratifying preoperative, intraoperative, and postoperative risk factors for complications are crucial for perioperative management and safe outcomes for the patient.
- Understanding of systemic physiological changes of laparoscopy plays a key role in managing anesthesia for lap colorectal surgery.
- CO_2 insufflation and steep positioning of patients during lap colorectal surgery impacts cardiorespiratory functions.
- Augmentation of physiology by pharmacological agents and ventilator strategies is important for a better postoperative outcome.
- Balance between over-transfusions and under-transfusions is critical for recovery of anastomosis in colorectal surgery, which can be achieved by adapting goal-directed fluid therapy perioperatively.
- It is well known that N_2O tends to diffuse into closed airspaces causing bowel distension. The combination of an orogastric tube and epidural anesthesia aids in bowel contraction and allows for better visualization.

References

1. Morris EJ, Taylor EF, Thomas JD et al. Thirty-day mortality after colorectal cancer surgery in England. *Gut* 2011;60:806–13.
2. Sjo OH, Larsen S, Lunde OC, Nesbakken A. Short term outcome after emergency and elective surgery for colon cancer. *Colorectal Dis* 2009;11:733–9.
3. Nelson R, Edwards S, Tse B. Prophylactic nasogastric decompression after abdominal surgery. *Cochrane Database Syst Rev* 2007; 2007(3):CD004929. doi:10.1002/14651858.CD004929.pub3.
4. Geerts WH, Bergqvist D, Pineo GF et al. Antithrombotic and thrombolytic therapy, 8 th ed. AACP guidelines: Prevention of venous thromboembolism. *Chest* 2008;133:381S–453.
5. Nelson RL, Glenny AM, Song F. Antimicrobial prophylaxis for colorectal surgery. *Cochrane Database Syst Rev* 2009;(1):CD001181. doi:10.1002/14651858.CD001181.pub3
6. Yamamoto T, Allan RN, Keighley MR. Risk factors for intra-abdominal sepsis after surgery in Crohn's disease. *Dis Colon Rectum* 2000;43:1141–5.
7. Garth AK, Newsome CM, Simmance N, Crowe TC. Nutritional status, nutrition practices and post-operative complications in patients with gastrointestinal cancer. *J Hum Nutr Diet* 2010;23:393–401.
8. Schricker T, Lattermann R. Strategies to attenuate catabolic stress response to surgery and improve perioperative outcomes. *Can J Anaesth* 2007;54:414–9.
9. Tramer M, Moore A, McQuay H. Omitting nitrous oxide from a propofol-based anesthetic does not affect the recovery of women undergoing outpatient gynecologic surgery. *Anes Thesiology* 2000;93:332–9.
10. Scheinin B, Lindgren L, Scheinin TM. Peroperative nitrous oxide delays bowel function after colonic surgery. *Br J Anaesth* 1990;64:154–8.
11. Frank SM, Higgins MS, Breslow MJ et al. The catecholamine, cortisol, and hemodynamic responses to mild perioperative hypothermia.A randomized clinical trial. *Anesthesiology* 1995;82:83–93.
12. Beilin B, Shavit Y, Razumovsky J, Wolloch Y, Zeidel A, Bessler H. Effects of mild perioperative hypothermia on cellular immune responses. *Anesthesiology* 1998;89:1133–40.
13. Danelli G, Berti M, Perotti V et al. Temperature control and recovery of bowel function after laparoscopic or laparotomic colorectal surgery in patients receiving combined epidural/general anesthesia and postoperative epidural analgesia. *AnesthAnalg* 2002;95:467–71.
14. Collaborative Study Group on Perioperative ScvO2 Monitoring: Multicentre study on peri- and postoperative central venous oxygen saturation in high-risk surgical patients. *Crit Care* 2006;10:R158.
15. Hiltebrand LB, Koepfli E, Kimberger O, Sigurdsson GH, Brandt S. Hypotension during fluid-restricted abdominal surgery: Effects of norepinephrine treatment on regional and microcirculatory blood flow in the intestinal tract. *Anesthesiology* 2011;114:557–64.
16. Giglio MT, Marucci M, Testini M, Brienza N. Goal-directed hemodynamic therapy and gastrointestinal complications in major surgery: A meta-analysis of randomized controlled trials. *Br J Anesth* 2009;103:837–46.
17. Amato A, Pescatori M. Perioperative blood transfusions for the recurrence of colorectal cancer. *Cochrane Database Syst Rev* 2006;1:CD005033.
18. Tartter PI. Blood transfusion and infectious complications following colorectal cancer surgery. *Br J Surg* 1998;75:789–92.
19. Carr CS, Ling KD, Boulos P, Singer M. Randomised trial of safety and efficacy of immediate postoperative enteral feeding in patients undergoing gastrointestinal resection. *BMJ* 1996;312:869–71.
20. Holte K, Andersen J, Jakobsen DH, Kehlet H. Cyclo-oxygenase 2 inhibitors and the risk of anastomotic leakage after fast-track colonic surgery. *Br J Surg* 2009;96:650–4.
21. Levy BF, Scott MJ, Fawcett W, Fry C, Rockall TA. Randomized clinical trial of epidural, spinal or patient-controlled analgesia for patients undergoing laparoscopic colorectal surgery. *Br J Surg* 2011;98:1068–78.
22. Janssen-Heijnen ML, Maas HA, Houterman S, Lemmens VE, Rutten HJ, Coebergh JW. Comorbidity in older surgical cancer patients: Influence on patient care and outcome. *Eur J Cancer* 2007;43:2179–93.
23. Morimoto Y, Yoshimura M, Utada K, Setoyama K, Matsumoto M, Sakabe T. Prediction of postoperative delirium after abdominal surgery in the elderly. *J Anesth* 2009;23:51–6.

Chapter 10

COMPLICATIONS IN LAPAROSCOPIC COLORECTAL SURGERY

Sanjiv Haribhakti and Shobhit Sengar

Contents

Learning objectives 48
Introduction and incidence 48
Classification of complications 48
Small bowel and duodenal injury... 49
Splenic injury.. 49
Pancreatic and gastric injury 49
Major vessel injury... 49
Surgical site infection... 49
Wound disruptions... 50
Early postoperative small bowel obstruction and postoperative ileus 50
Presacral bleeding.. 50
Ureteral injury... 50
Bladder injury 50
Urethral injury... 51
Urinary dysfunction... 51
Sexual dysfunction 51
Female infertility.. 52
Minor bleeding 52
Major bleeding 53
Anastomotic dehiscence and leaks 53
Chronic presacral sinus... 54
Strictures 54
Fistulas 54
Summary 54
Key points 54
Video... 55
References 55

Learning objectives

- Understand the mechanisms of various complications likely to occur in colorectal surgery, especially with reference to laparoscopic colorectal surgery.
- Learn about the incidence, etiology, risk factors, diagnosis, and management of these complications, with a special reference to prevention and early diagnosis.

Introduction and incidence

The safety of colorectal surgery has advanced dramatically over the last 50 years due to improvements in preoperative preparation, antibiotic prophylaxis, surgical techniques, and postoperative management. Despite these advances, colorectal surgery is associated with appreciable morbidity and mortality. Prospective studies [1,2] have shown that the rate of major morbidity ranged from 20% to 35%, and the 30-day mortality rate ranged from 2% to 8%. There does not appear to be a significant difference in 30-day mortality rate between malignant versus benign indications for surgery.

Independent preoperative risk factors associated with an increased risk of in-hospital complications include [1,2] age greater than 70 years, ASA physical status score – Grade III to V, emergency surgery, neurologic comorbidity, cardiorespiratory comorbidity, hypoalbuminemia, long duration of operative procedure, peritoneal contamination, and rectal excision. Additional independent preoperative risk factors associated with an increased risk of 30-day mortality include [1,2] loss of greater than 10% total body weight, age greater than 70 years, stage IV cancer (vs. earlier-stage cancer) and low surgeon case volume.

Classification of complications

A. Intra-abdominal injuries
   a. Small bowel and duodenal injury
   b. Splenic injury
   c. Pancreatic and gastric injury
   d. Major vessel injury
B. Wound complications
   a. Surgical site infection
   b. Wound disruptions
   c. Wound hernias
C. Early postoperative small bowel obstruction and postoperative ileus
D. Pelvic complications
   a. Presacral bleeding
   b. Ureteral injury
   c. Bladder injury
   d. Urethral injury

E. Genitourinary complications
   a. Urinary dysfunction
   b. Sexual dysfunction
   c. Female infertility
F. Anastomotic complications
   a. Minor bleeding
   b. Major bleeding
   c. Anastomotic dehiscence and leaks
   d. Chronic presacral sinus
   e. Strictures
G. Stoma-related complications – dealt in another chapter

Small bowel and duodenal injury

The incidence of small bowel injury during colorectal surgery is between 1% and 3% for open and laparoscopic techniques [3,4]. The risk of an inadvertent enterotomy increases with previous abdominal surgery, while injury to the duodenum is most likely to occur during right colon mobilization (Figure 10.1). Injury to the small bowel with the laparoscopic technique occurs in less than 1% of cases [5]. The therapeutic approach varies with the type and extent of injury. Veress needle injury to the small bowel rarely requires further intervention and can be managed conservatively. In contrast, a trocar injury to the small bowel requires primary operative repair, either laparoscopically or open. Full-thickness small bowel enterotomies are repaired in one or two layers. Serosal tears are repaired with seromuscular sutures. Technically, the most challenging repair is of an enterotomy of the duodenum. A primary repair should not compromise the duodenal lumen.

Splenic injury

The operative risk of splenic injury ranges from 0.4% to 8% for colonic procedures [6,7]. Injury occurs because of the close proximity of the colon to the spleen. During mobilization of the splenic flexure of the colon, excessive traction on the peritoneal attachments and omentum can lead to avulsion of a portion of the splenic capsule [8]. The risk of incidental splenic injuries is significantly greater for open compared to laparoscopic colorectal resection [9]. Other factors that increase the risk for iatrogenic splenic

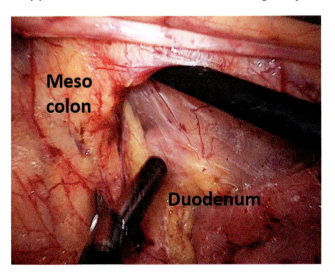

FIGURE 10.1 Relation of duodenum during right colonic mobilization.

injury include previous abdominal surgery, midline incision, obesity, and advanced age. Management of an intraoperative splenic injury includes splenic salvage (primary repair, splenorrhaphy) or splenectomy. Splenic salvage should be the first maneuver to control bleeding and a splenectomy reserved for cases when bleeding cannot be controlled by the previously described techniques. These patients who need an emergent splenectomy would need to be vaccinated for pneumococcal and H. influenza infections at the time of discharge.

Pancreatic and gastric injury

Injuries to the pancreas and stomach occur in less than 1% of colectomies, and are more likely to occur during a salvage splenectomy – or with dissection of dense adhesions, excessive use of electrocautery, and/or failure to develop an adequate plane [10]. Full-thickness gastric injuries are repaired in two layers, whereas serosal tears are repaired by seromuscular sutures only.

Major vessel injury

Major vessel injury during an open or laparoscopic colectomy is rare. Injuries can occur with traction on mesenteric vessels and splenic vessels during mobilization of the bowel with an open technique. The trocar can cause a fatal hemorrhage when inserted into the aorta or common iliac vessels; this occurs in less than 1% of laparoscopic case [5]. A vessel lacerated by a trocar usually requires immediate conversion to an open procedure for control of the bleeding vessel; however, there have been reports of successful laparoscopic management of major vascular injuries sustained during colectomy [11].

Surgical site infection

Colorectal operations are clean-contaminated procedures with an inherent risk of gross contamination of the peritoneal cavity and incision that can result in a surgical site infection (SSI) [12]. SSIs are classified as incisional or intra-abdominal (organ/space). The clinical criteria used to define a SSI include a purulent exudate draining from a surgical site, or a positive fluid culture obtained from a surgical site that was closed primarily.

The rate of SSIs following colorectal surgery varies in different reports from less than 1% to 20% [13]. In addition, superficial SSI may be more common in left compared to right colectomies (8% vs. 6%). This wide range depends upon the definition of SSI, time period for assessment of SSI, types of procedures, and inclusion of infections occurring after discharge [14]. In a prospective study of 59,365 patients who underwent colon resection, the overall infection rate was 13%; the rates of superficial, deep, and organ space infections were 8%, 1.4%, and 3.8%, respectively [15].

The risk factors for SSIs related to colorectal surgery [11,12] are perioperative blood transfusion, ASA grade 2 or 3, male gender, surgeons, types of operation, creation of an ostomy, contaminated wound, use of a drain, obesity, and long duration of operation.

A 'bundled' approach to SSI prevention has been shown to significantly decrease the rate of superficial SSIs (5.7% vs. 19.3%) and sepsis (2.4% vs. 8.5%) after colorectal surgery [16]. The preventive SSI bundle consists of existing evidence-based measures such as mechanical bowel preparation with oral antibiotics, antibiotic prophylaxis, and preparation of the surgical field with chlorhexidine, maintenance of euglycemia, and maintenance of normothermia during the perioperative period.

Management of an SSI depends upon the site of the infection. An intra-abdominal SSI can be treated by percutaneous catheter drainage or operative drainage.

Wound disruptions

Wound disruption occurs in 1.3% of colorectal resections, and it correlates with the mortality of patients [17]. Wound infection is the strongest predictor of wound disruption. Chronic steroid use, obesity, severe COPD, prolonged operation, non-elective admission, and serum albumin level are strongly associated with wound disruption. Utilization of the laparoscopic approach may decrease the risk of wound disruption when possible.

Early postoperative small bowel obstruction and postoperative ileus (see Video 17)

Small bowel obstruction (SBO) is the most frequent complication in the early postoperative period after colorectal surgery with a reported incidence ranging from 1.2% to 8.1% [18,19]. Inflammatory peritoneal adhesions account for the majority of cases. Early postoperative SBO, defined as occurring within the first 30 days following surgery, can be differentiated from a postoperative ileus on both clinical and radiographic grounds.

Immediate reoperation for early postoperative SBO should be avoided because of both the high rate of spontaneous resolution and the intense inflammatory response within the abdominal cavity in the perioperative period (from 10 days to 6 weeks). Indications for surgery should be limited to unresolved obstruction after prolonged nasogastric tube drainage, high-grade SBO, or suspected ischemic small bowel.

In contrast to the approach following open surgery, early small bowel obstruction following laparoscopic surgery usually requires early operative intervention. The cause of an SBO is more likely to be a peritoneal defect with herniation created by trocar placement or a peritoneal incision, not an inflammatory adhesion that generally results from an open procedure [20].

Presacral bleeding

Presacral bleeding results from injury to the presacral venous plexus, or to the internal iliac vessels or their branches [21]. The bleeding can be massive since the presacral complex contains large-caliber veins and produces high-pressure bleeding when disrupted. Intraoperative presacral bleeding occurs in approximately 4% to 7% [22,23]. Tumors fixed to the sacrum, preoperative radiation, previous pelvic surgery, a distal location of the tumor, and surgical maneuvers that violate the presacral fascia increase the risk of presacral bleeding [24]. Bleeding from the fragile presacral vessels can be life-threatening [17]. Morbidity and mortality is high when surgery is required to manage presacral bleeding [25].

Control of presacral bleeding is difficult because of the anatomy of the pelvis and the fragility of the venous plexus. Attempts to electrocauterize or suture ligate the vessels will lead to further vascular injury and increased bleeding. The initial management is to apply direct pressure over the bleeding site to achieve temporary control. This allows the anesthesia team time to resuscitate and replace volume loss, and prepare for possible additional blood loss.

Once the patient is stable, the most common technique after digital pressure to control the bleeding involves the application of sterile thumbtacks, or occluder pins, that are driven at right angles into the sacrum directly over the site of bleeding [26,27]. If occluder pins are not available, bone wax or bone cement is an effective alternative [28]. An epiploic flap and an omental flap have also been used to serve as plugs. If the above measures fail, pelvic bleeding may be controlled with tight pelvic packing with laparotomy pads. The abdomen is closed, and the laparotomy pads are removed 24 to 48 hours later, after patient stabilization in the intensive care unit [29].

Ureteral injury

The incidence of intraoperative ureteral injury with open or laparoscopic surgery ranges from 1% to 8% [30,31]. In a retrospective review of more than 2.1 million colorectal procedures identified from a U.S. nationwide database, the risk to ureters was 0.28% [17]. Ureteral injuries were independently associated with higher mortality ($p < 0.05$), morbidity ($p < 0.001$), and longer length of hospital stay ($p < 0.001$). Risk factors for injury included rectal cancer, adhesions, malnutrition, and performance of procedure in a teaching hospital. Protective factors included laparoscopic approach and right and transverse colectomies.

Identification of the ureters during pelvic and colorectal surgery is strongly advised to avoid injury. The ureters rest on the psoas muscle in the inferior medial course, and are crossed obliquely by the spermatic vessels and the genitofemoral nerve posteriorly (Figure 10.2). The ureter crosses the pelvic brim in front of or just lateral to the bifurcation of the common iliac artery. In colorectal surgery, injury to the ureter can occur during high ligation of the inferior mesenteric artery, mobilization of the upper mesorectum near the sacral promontory, dissection deep in the pelvis in the plane between the lower rectum, pelvic sidewall, and bladder base, and dissection of the most cephalad portion of the perineal dissection in an abdominoperineal resection.

The role of prophylactic ureteral catheterization is controversial. Although ureteral stents (catheters) facilitate intraoperative recognition of ureteral injuries, they do not appear to decrease the incidence of ureteral injury, and catheter placement is associated with a 1% risk of ureteral injury [32]. The authors use ureteral catheters in patients who have had severe diverticulitis or those undergoing reoperative pelvic surgery. Lighted ureteral stents (Figure 10.3) are useful for laparoscopic colectomies [33]. Only 20% to 30% of ureteral injuries are recognized during the operation [34]. Repair includes use of a stent or in cases of more extensive damage, advanced surgical repair.

Bladder injury

Bladder injuries are rare (<1%) during colorectal surgery. Bladder injury usually occurs when dissecting densely adherent rectosigmoid tumors or diverticular disease from the bladder wall.

Immediate repair is performed as a two-layer primary closure, and a Foley catheter is left in place for 7 to 10 days. A cystogram is performed prior to removing the catheter to assess for leaks. Injuries at the base of the bladder are technically more difficult to repair as the distal ureters are at risk for inadvertent suture ligature of the orifices. The repair is facilitated by making a cystotomy at the dome of the bladder and passing ureteral catheters in a retrograde fashion through the ureteral orifices. Injuries that are not recognized at the time of operation present with

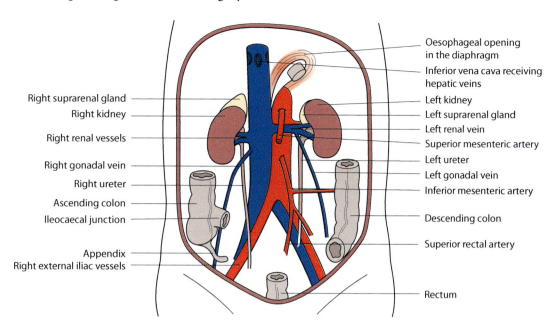

Right suprarenal gland
Right kidney
Right renal vessels
Right gonadal vein
Right ureter
Ascending colon
Ileocaecal junction
Appendix
Right external iliac vessels

Oesophageal opening in the diaphragm
Inferior vena cava receiving hepatic veins
Left kidney
Left suprarenal gland
Left renal vein
Superior mesenteric artery
Left ureter
Left gonadal vein
Inferior mesenteric artery
Descending colon
Superior rectal artery
Rectum

FIGURE 10.2   Surgical relations of ureter.

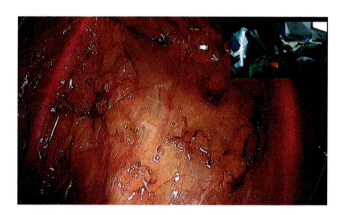

FIGURE 10.3   Lighted ureteric stents during laparoscopic colorectal surgeries.

urine peritonitis, or may result in the development of urinary tract fistulas. A primary repair is generally performed except in severe cases, when a temporary fecal or urinary diversion is performed [35].

Urethral injury

Iatrogenic injury to the urethra is rare (<1%) but can occur during the perineal portion of an abdominoperineal resection [36]. Urethral injuries have been reported as the most serious complication of transanal TME [37]. Intraoperative recognition of the injury usually occurs with visualization of the Foley catheter in the perineal defect. Primary repair of small injuries is preferred, with the urinary catheter left in place for four weeks to stent the repair.

In the postoperative period, injuries may present with urine draining from the perineal wound. A retrograde urethrogram may identify the level of injury. Management involves temporary urinary diversion (suprapubic catheterization) and delayed repair performed by an experienced urologist. Failure to diagnosis and repair a urethral injury may lead to strictures, incontinence, and erectile dysfunction.

Urinary dysfunction

The incidence of urinary dysfunction after proctocolectomy, primarily manifested as difficulty voiding, ranges between 30% and 60%, with the greatest risk following abdominoperineal resection [38]. Urinary dysfunction persisting beyond the early (30-day) postoperative period has been reported in 12% of patients [39]. For all low anterior or abdominoperineal resections, a Foley catheter remains in place for five days, or longer if symptomatic bladder dysfunction persists.

Urinary dysfunction is the result of one – or both of two factors: (i) anatomic changes in the pelvis, and autonomic nerve injury (Figure 10.4) leading to impairments in parasympathetic innervation to the detrusor muscle, and/or (ii) sympathetic innervation to the bladder neck, trigone, and urethra. Urodynamic studies may reveal a significant postoperative decrease in effective bladder capacity and increases in first sensation to void and residual urinary volume compared with the preoperative evaluation [40].

Autonomic sparing procedures can be effectively performed when dissecting the pelvis [41]. A prospective study of 20 patients undergoing a total mesorectal excision (TME) with an autonomic nerve preservation (ANP) technique and sphincter preservation found no significant difference between preoperative and postoperative mean residual volume after micturition [35].

Sexual dysfunction

Sexual dysfunction following rectal surgery is related to the extent of pelvic nerve dissection and occurs in both men and women. In men, damage to the sympathetic nerves during high ligation of the inferior mesenteric artery or posterior dissection at the sacral promontory can lead to retrograde ejaculation. In addition, damage to the parasympathetic plexus (nervi erigentes) during lateral and anterior dissection can lead to erectile dysfunction.

The pathophysiology of sexual dysfunction in women is likely multifactorial and includes damage to the parasympathetic nerves during deep pelvic dissection, as well as postoperative mechanical changes in the pelvis, which contribute to loss of

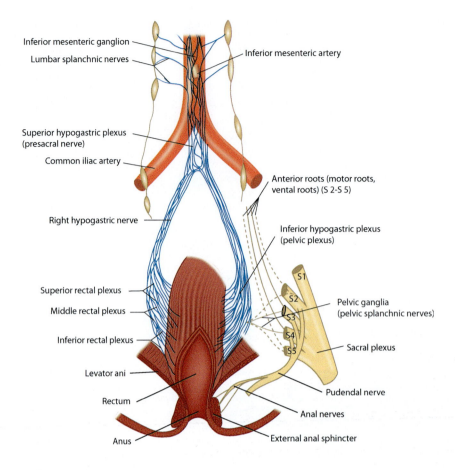

FIGURE 10.4   Anatomy of autonomic nerves.

sexual desire, vaginal dryness, altered orgasm, and dyspareunia. Sexual dysfunction is more difficult to diagnose in women, in part because the presence of incontinence often discourages women from engaging in sexual activity.

Sexual dysfunction is most common following rectal surgery for cancer because of the more extensive dissection required. Reported rates of sexual dysfunction in such patients range from 23% to 69% in men, and from 19% to 62% in women [42]. Here, the major risk factors for sexual dysfunction include advanced age, surgical technique (especially APR), and use of radiotherapy [43,44]. Sexual function can be preserved in patients undergoing rectal cancer surgery if nerve-sparing techniques are used. However, for patients with advanced rectal cancer (T3 or N+), combined modality treatment (including radiotherapy) is required. In those patients, the expected rate of sexual dysfunction can be much higher.

Female infertility

Female infertility is defined as one year of unprotected intercourse without conception in women of childbearing age. The infertility rate for women with inflammatory bowel disease prior to surgery is similar to that of the general population (less than 10%).

The rate of infertility following a restorative proctocolectomy is significantly increased, ranging in different studies from 26% to 48%, [45,46]. The cause of the increase in infertility is most likely mechanical, including fallopian tube occlusion and scarring, and not the disease process. A totally laparoscopic approach may reduce the risk of infertility in women undergoing ileal pouch anal anastomosis [47]. Women should be counselled preoperatively regarding the risk of infertility. If medically feasible, women with inflammatory bowel disease may choose to delay elective restorative proctectomy until their child bearing is complete.

Minor bleeding

Minor bleeding is defined as bleeding that does not require blood transfusion and/or intervention (endoscopic, angiographic, or surgical). It usually ceases within 24 hours. Minor anastomotic bleeding after hand-sewn or stapled anastomoses is common but rarely reported. It is usually manifested by the self-limited passage of dark blood with the patient's first few bowel movements. The risk of bleeding is increased in patients with a bleeding diathesis. Proposed techniques to reduce minor bleeding include [21] careful inspection of the staple line, especially for side-to-side and functional end-to-end anastomosis, inversion and inspection of the linear staple line prior to closure of the enterotomy through which a stapling instrument was passed has been advocated by the author; suture ligation, as opposed to electro-cauterization, of significantly bleeding points; utilization of the antimesenteric borders of each limb to construct the anastomosis, thereby avoiding inclusion of the mesentery into the staple line, and reinforcement of the anastomosis with an absorbable suture.

Major bleeding

Major bleeding is defined as one or more day of hemodynamic instability, need for blood transfusion or when emergency procedure is warranted (e.g. endoscopic, angiographic, surgical). The reported rate of major bleeding from an anastomosis following colorectal surgery ranges from 0.5% to 4.2% [48,49]. There is no significant association between the risk of bleeding and the technique used to perform the anastomosis (hand-sewn vs. stapled colocolic anastomoses) [52].

The management of patients with anastomotic bleeding should follow the same principles as the management of patients with lower gastrointestinal bleeding from other causes. Surgical intervention should be reserved for unstable patients, or those who fail conservative measures [51]. Initial management should be conservative with supportive care, including blood transfusions and correction of any underlying coagulopathy. Operative management should be considered early for patients with hemodynamic instability despite aggressive resuscitation. For persistent bleeding from a low anastomosis, a transanal operative approach is advocated. A proctoscopy is performed to evacuate clot, and bleeding points are suture ligated; for persistent bleeding from higher colorectal or ileocolic anastomoses, initial endoscopic management has been advocated.

Endoscopic management of bleeding includes isotonic saline washout, electrocoagulation, epinephrine injection, and application of hemostatic clips. For persistent bleeding from higher colorectal or ileocolic anastomoses, angiographic localization and control using intra-arterial vasopressin has been effective [50]. However, theoretically, there is a risk of ischemia and anastomotic dehiscence after angiography. Reoperation with resection of the bleeding anastomosis is necessary when endoscopic management is not successful.

Anastomotic dehiscence and leaks

The overall incidence of anastomotic dehiscence and subsequent leaks is 2% to 7% when performed by experienced surgeons [51,52]. The lowest leak rates are found with ileocolic anastomoses (1% to 3%), and the highest occur with coloanal anastomosis (10% to 20%).

Most anastomotic leaks usually become apparent between 5 and 7 days postoperatively. Late leaks often present insidiously with low-grade fever, prolonged ileus, and nonspecific symptoms attributable to other postoperative infectious complications. Small, contained leaks present later in the clinical course and may be difficult to distinguish from postoperative abscesses by radiologic imaging, making the diagnosis uncertain and underreported.

The clinical signs include pain, fever, tachycardia, peritonitis, feculent drainage, and purulent drainage. The radiographic signs include fluid collections and gas containing collections. The intraoperative findings include gross enteric spillage and anastomotic disruption.

Risk factors for a dehiscence and leak are classified according to the site of the anastomosis (extraperitoneal or intraperitoneal) [53].

Major risk factors for an extraperitoneal anastomotic leak include:

1. The distance of the anastomosis within 5 cm from the anal verge [54]
2. Anastomotic ischemia [55,56]
3. Male gender [57]
4. Obesity [58]

Major risk factors for an intraperitoneal anastomotic leak include:

1. ASA grade III to V [59]
2. Emergent surgery [59]
3. Prolonged operative time ≥ 4 hours [56]
4. Hand-sewn ileocolic anastomosis [59]

Controversial, inconclusive, or pertinent negative associations between the following variables and an anastomotic leak have been reported:

1. Neoadjuvant radiation therapy [60,61]
2. Drains [62,63]
3. Protective stoma [64–66]
4. Hand-sewn colorectal anastomosis [67,68]
5. Fibrin glue [69]
6. Laparoscopic procedure [70]
7. Mechanical bowel preparation
8. Nutrition [71–73]
9. Laparoscopic surgery [74]
10. Perioperative corticosteroids [75–77]
11. Nonsteroidal anti-inflammatory drugs (NSAIDs) [78–80]

Management of an anastomotic leak is dependent upon the patient's clinical condition, the nature of the leak, and, if an exploratory laparotomy is performed, the intraoperative findings. The following treatment options are available depending upon the clinical stability of the patient, radiographic findings, and feasibility of image-guided percutaneous drainage.

A subclinical leak, which is defined as a leak detected radiographically in patients with no clinical abdominal findings, can be managed expectantly.

For patients who present with localized peritonitis and low-grade sepsis, a diagnostic imaging workup is initiated. We perform a computed tomography (CT) scan with oral, intravenous, and rectal contrast. If a leak is present, the majority will be localized.

If a free intraperitoneal leak is demonstrated, the patient should be taken to the operating room for surgical management. If the patient is stable with small, contained abscesses (<3 cm), we recommend conservative management with broad-spectrum antibiotics and bowel rest. For larger abscesses (>3 cm), multiloculated collections, or multiple collections, an attempt at percutaneous drainage should be made. In those cases where image-guided drainage is not technically feasible, or where the patient's clinical condition deteriorates despite drainage, surgical intervention in the form of an exploratory laparotomy should be undertaken, as described in the following paragraph.

Patients who present with generalized peritonitis or high-grade sepsis with hypotension should be resuscitated and brought to the operating room for an exploratory laparotomy on an emergency basis. Surgical management is dependent upon the intraoperative findings. If an inoperable phlegmon is encountered, the safest approach is to place para-anastomotic drains and perform proximal temporary fecal diversion with either a loop ileostomy or colostomy.

For patients who have a major anastomotic defect (generally defined as >1 cm or greater than one-third the circumference of the anastomosis) [81], the options include resection of the anastomosis with the creation of an end stoma with/without mucus fistula, resection of the anastomosis with re-anastomosis and proximal diversion, or, rarely, exteriorization of both ends of the stoma.

In selected patients in whom the defect is minor and the tissue quality is adequate, one may consider primary repair of the anastomosis with drain placement and proximal diversion.

Management of patients with a pelvic abscess depends upon the patient's clinical condition, location of the abscess, and whether or not the abscess is in continuity with a leak. Consideration of proximal diversion is warranted in symptomatic patients. Determination of whether the abscess is contained or is in continuity with the leak can be made by performing a water-soluble contrast enema.

Patients with a contained abscess should be placed on intravenous antibiotics and undergo abscess drainage if the collection is larger than 3 cm. CT-guided drainage via a transabdominal, transvaginal, transanal, or transrectal route should be performed if technically feasible.

Anastomotic dehiscence and leaks are associated with an increased risk of mortality compared with patients without a leak (15.8% versus 2.5%), as well as a prolonged hospital stay, an increased rate of mortality, and an increase in cancer recurrence rates [82]. An anastomotic leak is associated with an increased risk for local recurrence for rectal and colon cancer [83].

Chronic presacral sinus

A chronic presacral sinus is an infrequent complication of a posterior leak in a coloanal or ileal pouch-anal anastomosis. A retrospective review of 100 consecutive cases of total mesorectal excision with proximal diverting ileostomy identified a para-anastomotic sinus in eight patients [84]. Spontaneous closure occurred in three patients, and a late malignant transformation developed in two.

Strictures

The incidence of an anastomotic stricture or stenosis after a colorectal anastomosis ranges from 0% to 30% [85,86]. This wide range is due at least in part to an imprecise definition of stricture. Studies have defined anastomotic stricture in terms of the inability to pass a proctoscope (12-mm diameter) [87,88] or a larger rigid sigmoidoscope (19-mm diameter) [83] through the stenosis. A clinically significant stricture typically presents with signs of a partial or complete bowel obstruction. The incidence of symptomatic strictures ranges from 4% to 10% [89]. An anastomotic stricture may be the result of tissue ischemia, inflammation, radiation, anastomotic leak, or recurrent disease [90]. Most patients with an anastomotic stricture do not require an intervention, most patients can be treated by endoscopic dilatation alone.

Malignant strictures: When the initial resection is performed for malignancy, it is imperative to rule out local recurrence. Malignant recurrence is reported to be rare in early strictures (up to 6 months), but the risk of local malignant recurrence increases with time. In the absence of distant metastatic disease, surgical resection of a malignant anastomotic stricture should be performed, with restoration of gastrointestinal continuity if technically feasible. In the presence of distant metastatic disease or unresectable locoregional disease, proximal fecal diversion may be warranted for palliation.

Benign strictures: Benign low colorectal, coloanal, and ileoanal strictures are usually effectively treated with repeated dilatation using an examining finger or rubber dilators. Higher colorectal, colocolic, or ileocolic strictures may be managed endoscopically. Endoscopic balloon dilatation is successful in 88% to 100% of benign cases. Endoscopic alternatives, employing the use of self-expanding metallic stents or endoscopic transanal resection of strictures, are effective in treating severe anastomotic strictures [91]. In refractory cases, surgical revision may be required, and, occasionally, permanent fecal diversion is warranted.

Fistulas

The risk of a fistula occurring after a colorectal, coloanal, or an ileocolic anastomosis ranges between 1% to 10% [92]. Rectourinary (rectovesical, rectourethral) fistulas following colorectal surgery are rare [93–96].

Stoma-related complications are dealt with in another chapter.

Summary

Postoperative complications are not uncommon after laparoscopic colorectal surgery. Thorough evaluation of the patient for the risks should be carried out, and optimization of the comorbidities of the patients should be done to reduce the risk of complications. Anastomotic complications, small bowel obstruction, wound-related complications, stoma-related problems, and intra-abdominal injuries to ureters and the autonomic nerves form the majority of the complications after colorectal surgery. There is some evidence to suggest that laparoscopy may reduce the risks of some of the complications, such as splenic injury and wound-related complications. Anastomotic leaks should be prevented by intraoperative technical factors and appropriate use of protective stomas, intraoperative leak tests, and transanal anastomotic tubes. Recent technology of near infrared (NIR) fluorescence imaging has been useful to identify ureters intraoperatively to avoid injuries in laparoscopic surgery, and to identify the vascularity of the anastomosis to reduce the risk of anastomotic leaks. NIR imaging should be employed wherever possible. Finally, early detection and appropriate management would ensure a good outcome. As with all complications, adequate counselling with the patients and relatives as well as documentation is of paramount importance to avoid any untoward consequences.

Key points

- Awareness of the high risk of postoperative complications in colorectal surgery.
- Preoperative optimization of patients with risk factors.
- Intraoperative maneuvers to prevent postoperative complications such as ureteric identification, automomic nerve preservation, use of leak tests, ICG and NIR fluorescence, use of stoma or trans-anastomotic drains and so forth to prevent complications.
- Postoperative close observation to detect complications early, such as anastomotic leak, and timely management can reduce the morbidity and mortality associated with these serious complications.

Video

VIDEO 17   https://youtu.be/2tud_dGBOaw

Laparoscopic Adhesiolysis for Intestinal Obstruction.

References

1. Alves A, Panis Y, Mathieu P et al. Postoperative mortality and morbidity in French patients undergoing colorectal surgery: Results of a prospective multicenter study. *Arch Surg.* 2005;140:278.
2. Ragg JL, Watters DA, Guest GD. Preoperative risk stratification for mortality and major morbidity in major colorectal surgery. *Dis Colon Rectum.* 2009;52:1296.
3. Rose J, Schneider C, Yildirim C et al. Complications in laparoscopic colorectal surgery: Results of a multicentre trial. *Tech Coloproctol.* 2004;8(Suppl 1):s25.
4. Franko J, O'Connell BG, Mehall JR et al. The influence of prior abdominal operations on conversion and complication rates in laparoscopic colorectal surgery. *JSLS.* 2006;10:169.
5. Lefor AT, Phillips EH. 52. Spleen. In: Norton JA, Barie PS, Bollinger RR, Chang AE, Lowry SF, Mulvihill SJ, Pass HI, Thompsons RW. (Eds.), *Surgery: Basic science and clinical evidence*, 2nd, Springer, 2008; 1111.
6. Holubar SD, Wang JK, Wolff BG et al. Splenic salvage after intraoperative splenic injury during colectomy. *Arch Surg.* 2009;144:1040.
7. Masoomi H, Carmichael JC, Mills S et al. Predictive factors of splenic injury in colorectal surgery: Data from the Nationwide Inpatient Sample, 2006–2008. *Arch Surg.* 2012;147:324.
8. Merchea A, Dozois EJ, Wang JK, Larson DW. Anatomic mechanisms for splenic injury during colorectal surgery. *Clin Anat.* 2012;25:212.
9. Isik O, Aytac E, Ashburn J et al. Does laparoscopy reduce splenic injuries during colorectal resections? An assessment from the ACS-NSQIP database. *Surg Endosc.* 2015;29:1039.
10. Ellison EC, Fabri PJ. Complications of splenectomy. Etiology, prevention, and management. *Surg Clin North Am.* 1983;63:1313.
11. Jafari MD, Pigazzi A. Techniques for laparoscopic repair of major intraoperative vascular injury: Case reports and review of literature. *Surg Endosc.* 2013;27:3021.
12. Platell C, Hall JC. The prevention of wound infection in patients undergoing colorectal surgery. *J Hosp Infect.* 2001;49:233.
13. Tang R, Chen HH, Wang YL et al. Risk factors for surgical site infection after elective resection of the colon and rectum: A single-center prospective study of 2,809 consecutive patients. *Ann Surg.* 2001;234:181.
14. Blumetti J, Luu M, Sarosi G et al. Surgical site infections after colorectal surgery: Do risk factors vary depending on the type of infection considered? *Surgery.* 2007;142:704.
15. Segal CG, Waller DK, Tilley B et al. An evaluation of differences in risk factors for individual types of surgical site infections after colon surgery. *Surgery.* 2014;156:1253.
16. Itani KM. Care Bundles and Prevention of Surgical Site Infection in Colorectal Surgery. *JAMA.* 2015;314:289.
17. Keenan JE, Speicher PJ, Thacker JK et al. The preventive surgical site infection bundle in colorectal surgery: An effective approach to surgical site infection reduction and health care cost savings. *JAMA Surg.* 2014;149:1045.
18. Moghadamyeghaneh Z, Hanna M, Carmichael J et al. Wound Disruption Following Colorectal Operations. *World J Surg Online. World J Surg.* 2015;39(12):2999–3007.
19. Quan SH, Stearns MW Jr. Early postoperative intestinal obstruction and postoperative intestinal ileus. *Dis Colon Rectum.* 1961;4:307.
20. Lee SY, Park KJ, Ryoo SB et al. Early postoperative small bowel obstruction is an independent risk factor for subsequent adhesive small bowel obstruction in patients undergoing open colectomy. *World J Surg.* 2014;38:3007.
21. Shin JY, Hong KH. Risk factors for early postoperative small-bowel obstruction after colectomy in colorectal cancer. *World J Surg.* 2008;32:2287.
22. Velasco JM, Vallina VL, Bonomo SR, Hieken TJ. Postlaparoscopic small bowel obstruction. Rethinking its management. *Surg Endosc.* 1998;12:1043.
23. Dietz, DW. Postoperative complications. In: Wolff BG, Fleshman JW, Beck DE, Pemberton JH, Wexner SD. (Eds.), *The ASCRS Textbook of Colon and Rectal Surgery*, New York: Springer Science +Business Media, LLC, 2007; 141.
24. Pollard CW, Nivatvongs S, Rojanasakul A, Ilstrup DM. Carcinoma of the rectum. Profiles of intraoperative and early postoperative complications. *Dis Colon Rectum.* 1994;37:866.
25. Zama N, Fazio VW, Jagelman DG et al. Efficacy of pelvic packing in maintaining hemostasis after rectal excision for cancer. *Dis Colon Rectum.* 1988;31:923.
26. Hammond KL, Margolin DA. Surgical hemorrhage, damage control, and the abdominal compartment syndrome. *Clin Colon Rectal Surg.* 2006;19:188.
27. McPartland KJ, Hyman NH. Damage control: What is its role in colorectal surgery? *Dis Colon Rectum.* 2003;46:981.
28. Patsner B, Orr JW Jr. Intractable venous sacral hemorrhage: Use of stainless steel thumbtacks to obtain hemostasis. *Am J Obstet Gynecol.* 1990;162:452.
29. Arnaud JP, Tuech JJ, Pessaux P. Management of presacral venous bleeding with the use of thumbtacks. *Dig Surg.* 2000;17:651.
30. Becker A, Koltun L, Shulman C, Sayfan J. Bone cement for control of massive presacral bleeding. *Colorectal Dis.* 2008;10:409.
31. Metzger PP. Modified packing technique for control of presacral pelvic bleeding. *Dis Colon Rectum.* 1988;31:981.
32. Redan JA, McCarus SD. Protect the ureters. *JSLS.* 2009;13:139.
33. Halabi WJ, Jafari MD, Nguyen VQ et al. Ureteral injuries in colorectal surgery: An analysis of trends, outcomes, and risk factors over a 10-year period in the United States. *Dis Colon Rectum.* 2014;57:179.
34. Bothwell WN, Bleicher RJ, Dent TL. Prophylactic ureteral catheterization in colon surgery. A five-year review. *Dis Colon Rectum.* 1994;37:330.
35. Nam YS, Wexner SD. Clinical value of prophylactic ureteral stent indwelling during laparoscopic colorectal surgery. *J Korean Med Sci.* 2002;17:633.
36. Selzman AA, Spirnak JP. Iatrogenic ureteral injuries: A 20-year experience in treating 165 injuries. *J Urol.* 1996;155:878.
37. Alperin M, Mantia-Smaldone G, Sagan ER. Conservative management of postoperatively diagnosed cystotomy. *Urology.* 2009;73:1163.e17.
38. Rosenstein DI, Alsikafi NF. Diagnosis and classification of urethral injuries. *Urol Clin North Am.* 2006;33:73.
39. Bjørn MX, Perdawood SK. Transanal total mesorectal excision – a systematic review. *Dan Med J.* 2015;62(7):A5105.
40. Banerjee AK. Sexual dysfunction after surgery for rectal cancer. *Lancet.* 1999;353:1900.
41. Havenga K, Enker WE, McDermott K et al. Male and female sexual and urinary function after total mesorectal excision with autonomic nerve preservation for carcinoma of the rectum. *J Am Coll Surg.* 1996;182:495.
42. Chang PL, Fan HA. Urodynamic studies before and/or after abdominoperineal resection of the rectum for carcinoma. *J Urol.* 1983;130:948.
43. Pocard M, Zinzindohoue F, Haab F et al. A prospective study of sexual and urinary function before and after total mesorectal excision with autonomic nerve preservation for rectal cancer. *Surgery.* 2002;131:368.
44. Ho VP, Lee Y, Stein SL, Temple LK. Sexual function after treatment for rectal cancer: A review. *Dis Colon Rectum.* 2011;54:113.
45. Lange MM, Marijnen CA, Maas CP et al. Risk factors for sexual dysfunction after rectal cancer treatment. *Eur J Cancer.* 2009;45:1578.
46. Maas CP, Moriya Y, Steup WH et al. A prospective study on radical and nerve-preserving surgery for rectal cancer in the Netherlands. *Eur J Surg Oncol.* 2000;26:751.
47. Olsen KO, Joelsson M, Laurberg S, Oresland T. Fertility after ileal pouch-anal anastomosis in women with ulcerative colitis. *Br J Surg.* 1999;86:493.

48. Ørding Olsen K, Juul S, Berndtsson I et al. Ulcerative colitis: Female fecundity before diagnosis, during disease, and after surgery compared with a population sample. *Gastroenterology.* 2002;122:15.

49. Bartels SA, D'Hoore A, Cuesta MA et al. Significantly increased pregnancy rates after laparoscopic restorative proctocolectomy: A cross-sectional study. *Ann Surg.* 2012;256:1045.

50. Cirocco WC, Golub RW. Endoscopic treatment of postoperative hemorrhage from a stapled colorectal anastomosis. *Am Surg.* 1995;61:460.

51. Malik AH, East JE, Buchanan GN, Kennedy RH. Endoscopic haemostasis of staple-line haemorrhage following colorectal resection. *Colorectal Dis.* 2008;10:616.

52. Atabek U, Pello MJ, Spence RK et al. Arterial vasopressin for control of bleeding from a stapled intestinal anastomosis. Report of two cases. *Dis Colon Rectum.* 1992;35:1180.

53. Kingham TP, Pachter HL. Colonic anastomotic leak: Risk factors, diagnosis, and treatment. *J Am Coll Surg.* 2009;208:269.

54. Hyman N, Manchester TL, Osler T et al. Anastomotic leaks after intestinal anastomosis: It's later than you think. *Ann Surg.* 2007;245:254.

55. Sciuto A, Merola G, De Palma GD et al. Predictive factors for anastomotic leakage after laparoscopic colorectal surgery. *World J Gastroenterol.* 2018 June 7;24(21):2247–60.

56. Platell C, Barwood N, Dorfmann G, Makin G. The incidence of anastomotic leaks in patients undergoing colorectal surgery. *Colorectal Dis.* 2007;9:71.

57. Konishi T, Watanabe T, Kishimoto J, Nagawa H. Risk factors for anastomotic leakage after surgery for colorectal cancer: Results of prospective surveillance. *J Am Coll Surg.* 2006;202:439.

58. Boyle NH, Manifold D, Jordan MH, Mason RC. Intraoperative assessment of colonic perfusion using scanning laser Doppler flowmetry during colonic resection. *J Am Coll Surg.* 2000;191:504.

59. Vignali A, Gianotti L, Braga M et al. Altered microperfusion at the rectal stump is predictive for rectal anastomotic leak. *Dis Colon Rectum.* 2000;43:76.

60. Choi HK, Law WL, Ho JW. Leakage after resection and intraperitoneal anastomosis for colorectal malignancy: Analysis of risk factors. *Dis Colon Rectum.* 2006;49:1719.

61. Choy PY, Bissett IP, Docherty JG et al. Stapled versus handsewn methods for ileocolic anastomoses. *Cochrane Database Syst Rev* 2011;(9):CD004320. doi:10.1002/14651858.CD004320.pub3.

62. Rullier E, Laurent C, Garrelon JL et al. Risk factors for anastomotic leakage after resection of rectal cancer. *Br J Surg.* 1998;85:355.

63. Vignali A, Fazio VW, Lavery IC et al. Factors associated with the occurrence of leaks in stapled rectal anastomoses: A review of 1,014 patients. *J Am Coll Surg.* 1997;185:105.

64. Merad F, Yahchouchi E, Hay JM et al. Prophylactic abdominal drainage after elective colonic resection and suprapromontory anastomosis: A multicenter study controlled by randomization. French Associations for Surgical Research. *Arch Surg.* 1998;133:309.

65. Gastinger I, Marusch F, Steinert R et al. Protective defunctioning stoma in low anterior resection for rectal carcinoma. *Br J Surg.* 2005;92:1137.

66. Hüser N, Michalski CW, Erkan M et al. Systematic review and meta-analysis of the role of defunctioning stoma in low rectal cancer surgery. *Ann Surg.* 2008;248:52.

67. Matthiessen P, Hallböök O, Rutegård J et al. Defunctioning stoma reduces symptomatic anastomotic leakage after low anterior resection of the rectum for cancer: A randomized multicenter trial. *Ann Surg.* 2007;246:207.

68. Docherty JG, McGregor JR, Akyol AM et al. Comparison of manually constructed and stapled anastomoses in colorectal surgery. West of Scotland and Highland Anastomosis Study Group. *Ann Surg.* 1995;221:176.

69. Kim HJ, Huh JW, Kim HR, Kim YJ. Oncologic impact of anastomotic leakage in rectal cancer surgery according to the use of fibrin glue: Case-control study using propensity score matching method. *Am J Surg.* 2014;207:840.

70. Neutzling CB, Lustosa SA, Proenca IM, da Silva EM, Matos D. Stapled versus handsewn methods for colorectal anastomosis surgery. *Cochrane Database Syst Rev.* 2012;(2):CD003144. doi:10.1002/14651858.CD003144.pub2.

71. Clinical Outcomes of Surgical Therapy Study Group, Nelson H, Sargent DJ, Wieand HS et al. A comparison of laparoscopically assisted and open colectomy for colon cancer. *N Engl J Med.* 2004;350:2050.

72. Guillou PJ, Quirke P, Thorpe H et al. Short-term endpoints of conventional versus laparoscopic-assisted surgery in patients with colorectal cancer (MRC CLASICC trial): Multicentre, randomised controlled trial. *Lancet.* 2005;365:1718.

73. Iancu C, Mocan LC, Todea-Iancu D et al. Host-related predictive factors for anastomotic leakage following large bowel resections for colorectal cancer. *J Gastrointestin Liver Dis.* 2008;17:299.

74. Mäkelä JT, Kiviniemi H, Laitinen S. Risk factors for anastomotic leakage after left-sided colorectal resection with rectal anastomosis. *Dis Colon Rectum.* 2003;46:653.

75. Wang Y, Wang H, Jiang J et al. Early decrease in postoperative serum albumin predicts severe complications in patients with colorectal cancer after curative laparoscopic surgery. *World J Surg Oncol.* 2018;16:192.

76. Zheng H, Wu Z, Wu Y et al. Laparoscopic surgery may decrease the risk of clinical anastomotic leakage and a nomogram to predict anastomotic leakage after anterior resection for rectal cancer. *Int J Colorect Dis. Published Online.* 2019;34(2):319328.

77. Eriksen TF, Lassen CB, Gögenur I. Treatment with corticosteroids and the risk of anastomotic leakage following lower gastrointestinal surgery: A literature survey. *Colorectal Dis.* 2014;16:O154.

78. Trésallet C, Royer B, Godiris-Petit G, Menegaux F. Effect of systemic corticosteroids on elective left-sided colorectal resection with colorectal anastomosis. *Am J Surg.* 2008;195:447.

79. Gorissen KJ, Benning D, Berghmans T et al. Risk of anastomotic leakage with non-steroidal anti-inflammatory drugs in colorectal surgery. *Br J Surg.* 2012;99:721.

80. Bhangu A, Singh P, Fitzgerald JE et al. Postoperative nonsteroidal anti-inflammatory drugs and risk of anastomotic leak: Meta-analysis of clinical and experimental studies. *World J Surg.* 2014;38:2247.

81. Hakkarainen TW, Steele SR, Bastaworous A et al. Nonsteroidal anti-inflammatory drugs and the risk for anastomotic failure: A report from Washington State's Surgical Care and Outcomes Assessment Program (SCOAP). *JAMA Surg.* 2015;150:223.

82. Smith SA, Roberts DJ, Lipson ME et al. Postoperative Nonsteroidal Anti-inflammatory Drug Use and Intestinal Anastomotic Dehiscence: A Systematic Review and Meta-Analysis. *Dis Colon Rectum.* 2016;59:1087.

83. Phitayakorn R, Delaney CP, Reynolds HL et al. Standardized algorithms for management of anastomotic leaks and related abdominal and pelvic abscesses after colorectal surgery. *World J Surg.* 2008;32:1147.

84. Walker KG, Bell SW, Rickard MJ et al. Anastomotic leakage is predictive of diminished survival after potentially curative resection for colorectal cancer. *Ann Surg.* 2004;240:255.

85. Mirnezami A, Mirnezami R, Chandrakumaran K et al. Increased local recurrence and reduced survival from colorectal cancer following anastomotic leak: Systematic review and meta-analysis. *Ann Surg.* 2011;253:890.

86. Arumainayagam N, Chadwick M, Roe A. The fate of anastomotic sinuses after total mesorectal excision for rectal cancer. *Colorectal Dis.* 2009;11:288.

87. Schlegel RD, Dehni N, Parc R et al. Results of reoperations in colorectal anastomotic strictures. *Dis Colon Rectum.* 2001;44:1464.

88. Shimada S, Matsuda M, Uno K et al. A new device for the treatment of coloproctostomic stricture after double stapling anastomoses. *Ann Surg.* 1996;224:603.

89. Luchtefeld MA, Milsom JW, Senagore A et al. Colorectal anastomotic stenosis. Results of a survey of the ASCRS membership. *Dis Colon Rectum.* 1989;32:733.

90. Suchan KL, Muldner A, Manegold BC. Endoscopic treatment of postoperative colorectal anastomotic strictures. *Surg Endosc.* 2003;17:1110.

91. Fingerhut A, Elhadad A, Hay JM et al. Infraperitoneal colorectal anastomosis: Hand-sewn versus circular staples. A controlled clinical trial. *French Associations for Surgical Research. Surgery.* 1994;116:484.

92. Corman ML. Carcinoma of the rectum. In: Corman ML (Ed.), *Colon and Rectal Surgery*, 5th ed, Philadelphia: Lippincott Williams & Wilkins, 2005; 1002.

93. Forshaw MJ, Maphosa G, Sankararajah D et al. Endoscopic alternatives in managing anastomotic strictures of the colon and rectum. *Tech Coloproctol.* 2006;10:21.

94. Goriainov V, Miles AJ. Anastomotic leak rate and outcome for laparoscopic intra-corporeal stapled anastomosis. *J Minim Access Surg.* 2010;6:6.

95. Muñoz M, Nelson H, Harrington J et al. Management of acquired rectourinary fistulas: Outcome according to cause. *Dis Colon Rectum.* 1998;41:1230.

96. Nunoo-Mensah JW, Kaiser AM, Wasserberg N et al. Management of acquired rectourinary fistulas: How often and when is permanent fecal or urinary diversion necessary? *Dis Colon Rectum.* 2008;51:1049.

Section III
Laparoscopy in Benign Colorectal Diseases

11 Laparoscopic Ileocecal Resection 59
12 Laparoscopic Appendectomy 62
13 Laparoscopic Sigmoid Colectomy for Diverticulitis 68
14 Laparoscopic Rectopexy for Rectal Prolapse... 75
15 Laparoscopic-Assisted Stomas and Stoma Reversal 85
16 Laparoscopic Restorative Proctocolectomy and Ileal Pouch Anal Anastomosis 90
17 Parastomal Hernias.. 109

Chapter 11

LAPAROSCOPIC ILEOCECAL RESECTION

Vismit Joshipura

Contents

Learning objectives 59
Introduction 59
Applied anatomy and physiology of the ileocecal area 59
Indications 60
Contraindications 60
Difference in resection between benign and malignant indications 60
Preoperative preparation 60
Results and consequences of resection 60
Summary 61
Key points 61
Video 61

Learning objectives

- Identify the terminal ileum, caecum in difficult anatomy
- Know the applied anatomy and physiology of the ileocecal area
- Know the benign conditions indicated for ileocecal resection
- Learn the preoperative planning and preparations for operation
- Understand the long-term consequences and physiological changes after ileocecal resection

Introduction

Among all resections of the luminal digestive tract, ileocecal resection needs some special mention because it involves resection and anastomosis of two different parts of the luminal digestive tract along with resection of a valve. Other examples of such resections are various gastrectomies followed by their reconstruction. There are no defined borders for ileocecal resection; however, loosely, any resection in the area in the vicinity of the ileocecal valve can be termed as ileocecal resection. This resection is sometimes loosely termed a right-quarter colectomy. The reconstructed ends are completely different in diameter, thickness, microbiological flora, vascularity, motility, and function.

Applied anatomy and physiology of the ileocecal area

The terminal ileum is smaller in diameter but has a thicker wall as compared to the cecum and ascending colon. Sometimes, it is very difficult to identify the terminal ileum. In such situation, a distinct 'fat pad' present exactly at the terminal ileum may serve as a constant landmark to identify the altered anatomy. Similarly, a distinct strip of taenia coli may help to identify the cecum and ascending colon in difficult terrain. The root of the appendix is exactly at the lower most point of the taenia coli.

The vasa recta of the terminal ileum are very crowded and smaller in diameter near the mesenteric border of the ileum, and

in benign conditions we do not require to resect all the way to the root of the mesentery; we can use energy sources to divide vascular supply close to the bowel. The ileocolic artery and vein are generally surrounded with a thick fat pad and lymph nodes, and one should be cautious in handling these vessels. The marginal artery of Drummond connects the ileocolic artery and the right colic artery (if present) and the right branch of middle colic artery, so we can safely divide the ileocolic artery without the risk of ischemia to ascending colon.

The appendix can be used as a handle to lift the cecum at the time of mobilization of the ascending colon. There is a distinct space between the posterior layer of the mesentery (and mesocolon) and the right Gerota's fascia, unless violated by inflammatory process. The right ureter and third part of duodenum are in close proximity to our area of dissection.

In females, the right ovary and the right fallopian tubes are to be kept in mind, as sometimes dense inflammatory conditions may pull right adnexal structures near the bowels.

Physiologically, the terminal ileum is an important area for absorption. It absorbs unused bile acids back, and it is the area of absorption of fat soluble vitamins (A, D, E and K) and vitamin B12. The ileocecal valve halts the stream of enteric contents a while for final nutrient absorption by the small intestine. This function is especially important in patients with compromised bowel lengths.

The cecum contains a far greater number of aerobic and anaerobic microbes compared to the terminal ileum, and ileocecal valve prevents reflux of the caecal contents – and in that manner microbes – to the terminal ileum.

Cecum is the most capacious and the most distensible part of the large intestine. It is a relatively thin-walled structure and the blood vessels supplying it runs parallel to the wall. This anatomical fact is important for surgeons because in cases of distal colonic obstruction, the brunt of the pressure comes on the thin-walled distensible cecum, closed at one end by the IC valve, and after a certain point of increasing pressure, the blood vessels in the stretched wall starts occluding and viability of the caecal wall comes under threat.

The cecum and the ascending colon is the area where most of the water and remaining bile salts are absorbed from the luminal contents. The capacity of this area to absorb water content is so great that the luminal contents in terminal ileum are exclusively liquid, while contents in the transverse colon are almost semi-solid. Microbiota of the cecum and ascending colon also produce short-chain fatty acids – nutrients to the mucosal cells of the colon.

As the terminal ileum is the most proximal part to the portion of the luminal digestive tract full of microbes, it has a special immunological mechanism, which is the reason the terminal ileum is a common site for Crohn's disease and tuberculosis.

Indications

Ileocecal resection is indicated in benign conditions for the following indications. However, laparoscopy is mostly used in non-emergency or semiemergency patients.

1. Tuberculosis
2. Crohn's disease
3. Nonspecific strictures
4. Acute mesenteric ischemia
5. Injury – blunt or sharp abdominal injury or iatrogenic injury, such as perforation or hemorrhage due to colonoscopy
6. Endometriosis involving the IC region
7. Bleeding from the cecum, not controllable by endoscopy
8. Caecal perforation or devitalization of the caecal wall due to typhilitis
9. Appendicular lump, where it does not seem possible to dissect the appendix safely
10. Benign or premalignant polyps not amenable for endoscopic treatment

Contraindications

Caecal volvulus (with or without ischemia) is the only benign indication in which formal right hemicolectomy, instead of ileocecal resection, is the treatment of choice.

Laparoscopy is mostly used as a diagnostic tool in emergency situations such as profound bleeding from a caecal pathology or perforation.

Difference in resection between benign and malignant indications

Resection for benign conditions do not warrant additional lengths of intestine for margin clearance, and no need to tackle vessels at their roots for lymph node clearance, unlike malignant conditions. However, in cases of suspected inflammatory bowel disease and tuberculosis, it is advisable to resect a couple of representative mesenteric lymph nodes along with the intestine for a better histopathological review. Similarly, grossly enlarged nodes with abscess formation should be resected in benign conditions as well.

Preoperative preparation

In preoperative planning and preparations for laparoscopic surgery, the history of previous abdominal and gynecological surgeries is especially noted due to possible adhesions and incisional hernias. Also, in patients with strictures, one can expect to deal with distended bowels. Special attention should be paid to fluid electrolytes and nutritional parameters while planning surgery in patients having a diseased ileocecal area, and deficiencies should

be rectified beforehand, if any. In cases of Crohn's disease, steroids and biologics should be stopped at least 4 to 6 weeks prior to the planned resection, especially if primary anastomosis is contemplated.

Preoperative imaging studies and endoscopies must be reviewed by the operating surgeon. Special attention should be paid to right ureter, iliac vessels, duodenum, and right adnexal structures in female patients.

Even if a primary anastomosis is planned, the possibility of stoma should be discussed with the patient, and a stoma therapist should mark the stoma. Thrombo-prophylaxis and/or mechanical devices for the prevention of deep venous thrombosis should be used.

Mechanical bowel preparation is generally not required for ileocecal resection. However, it is used for laparoscopic resections, as deflated bowel loops are easier to maneuver, and it is used for other rare situations when intra-operative colonoscopy is planned. Preoperative antibiotic prophylaxis should be third generation cephalosporin and metronidazole. Energy sources are very useful adjuncts in laparoscopic ileal resection because many smaller vessels are to be dealt with.

Complete laparoscopic resection with the use of staplers to divide the bowels and to anastomose them intra-corporeally is technically feasible, but to reduce cost, mobilization and vessel control can be done via laparoscopy, and then final resection and anastomosis can be done via a relatively smaller incision. Restoration of the bowel continuity is mostly established by side-to-side anastomosis because the diameters of both resected ends are different, and the orientations of the mesentery and mesocolon are more convenient with side-to-side anastomoses. In cases of Crohn's disease, side-to-side anastomosis has reduced incidences of anastomotic recurrence of the disease, as compared to end-to.end anastomosis. Either stapled or hand-sewn anastomosis can be performed. See Video 7.

Results and consequences of resection

Overall, the ileo-ascending anastomosis is considered one of the reliable anastomoses among various anastomoses performed in the digestive tract. However, the possibility of leak increases in cases of inflammatory bowel disease, amoebic typhilitis, and acute mesenteric ischemia. In cases of Crohn's disease, disease recurrence at the anastomotic site is fairly common, and rates for reoperation at 5 years and 10 years following an initial resection is close to 25% and 35%, respectively. Use of postoperative azathioprine or biologics is recommended to reduce the possibility of recurrence of Crohn's disease after surgery.

Long-term consequences and physiological changes should be kept in view in surgeries for benign disease. As mentioned earlier, the terminal ileum is a distinct and fairly important area for nutrient absorption, and its loss may lead to deficiency of fat soluble vitamins and vitamin B12. However, physiological adaptation of the remaining bowels generally compensates the loss after a certain period of time. Possibilities of gall stones increases in patients with an absent terminal ileum due to a disturbance in the bile acid pool. Oxalate urinary stones are formed more frequently in patients with a loss of the terminal ileum because the colon gets a greater quantity of free oxalate to absorb. Loss of the ileocecal valve and the initial part of colon may lead to diarrhea, or at least increased stool frequency, in some patients. Similarly, loss of the ileocecal valve allows the colonic flora to populate the distal small bowel, which may lead to possible disturbances in digestive function.

Summary

Ileocecal resection is a challenging surgery, as it involves resection and anastomosis of two different parts of the luminal digestive tract along with resection of a valve. The applied anatomy and physiology of the ileocecal area is to be kept in mind while planning a resection. Prior to resection, a thorough evaluation to identify the medical morbidities is imperative, so that the operative approach and involvement of multidisciplinary teams can be adjusted as necessary. Preoperative imaging studies and endoscopies must be reviewed by the operating surgeon. Overall, the ileo-ascending anastomosis is considered one of the reliable anastomoses among various anastomoses performed in the digestive tract. However, the possibility of leak increases in cases of inflammatory bowel disease, amoebic typhilitis, and acute mesenteric ischemia. Long-term consequences and physiological changes should be kept in view in surgeries for benign disease. Gall stones, oxalate urinary stones, diarrhea or at least increased stool frequency, or disturbances in digestive function may present consequently to ileocecal valve resection. Though ileocecal resection is a relatively easier surgery, its selection process, execution, and consequences require meticulous planning. Laparoscopy is a feasible option, with its inherent advantages of being minimally invasive. Laparoscopy-assisted resections balances cost and benefit in the Indian scenario as per our belief.

Key points

- In ileocecal resection, the reconstructed ends are completely different in diameter, thickness, microbiological flora, vascularity, motility, and function.
- With female patients, special attention must be paid when dissecting the right ureter, iliac vessels, duodenum, and right adnexal structures.
- Restoration of the bowel continuity is mostly established by ileocolic side-to-side anastomosis.
- Gall stones, oxalate urinary stones, diarrhea or increased stool frequency, and disturbances in digestive function are common sequelae to this surgery.

Video

VIDEO 7   https://youtu.be/8ScZFfWB0MU

Laparoscopic Ileocecal Resection.

Chapter 12

LAPAROSCOPIC APPENDECTOMY

Atul Shah and Rajat Srivastava

Contents

Learning objectives 62
Introduction 62
Indications 62
Absolute contraindications 62
Relative contraindications 62
Selection of patients 62
Preoperative preparation 62
OR setup 63
Operative steps 63
Postoperative course and recovery 66
Postoperative complications 66
SILS appendicectomy 66
Advantages of laparoscopic surgery 67
Disadvantages of laparoscopic surgery 67
Summary 67
Key points 67
Video 67
References 67

Learning objectives

- Know indications and contraindications of appendicectomy
- Know the operative principles and standardized steps of the procedure
- Know how to tackle the problems faced with in a difficult appendix with abscess, perforation, and acute or chronic cases
- Know postoperative care and complications

Introduction

Appendicectomy continues to be one of the most common surgical procedure in general surgery. The first description of a resection of the appendix was by Amyand in 1735, the procedure was performed on an 11-year boy suffering from an inguinal hernia containing an inflamed appendix [2]. An appendicectomy through a right iliac fossa incision was described by McBurney in 1894 [3].

In 1983, Kurt Semm [1], from the University of Kiel, performed the first successful laparoscopic appendicectomy. However, laparoscopic appendicectomy was not as widely accepted as laparoscopic cholecystectomy until 1991, because there were many different techniques described with varying results, and there was no uniformity in port placement and surgical technique.

Indications

Indications of laparoscopic appendicectomy are almost the same as for conventional appendicectomy, with advantages conferred by the use of laparoscopy in certain situations such as,

1. Appendicitis in obese patients, young women
2. Patients with confusing clinical pictures with RIF pain (Figure 12.1)
3. Right lower abdominal pain in women of childbearing age, to achieve better visualization of the pelvic organ
4. Perforated appendix with localized or generalized peritonitis

Absolute contraindications

1. Hemodynamic instability
2. Lack of surgical expertise

Relative contraindications

1. Restrictive cardiac or pulmonary comorbidity
2. Severe small bowel obstruction or ileus, malrotation with a perforated appendix

Selection of patients

Practically all patients from the pediatric to geriatric group can be included for laparoscopic appendicectomy, provided there is no restrictive comorbidity (Figure 12.1).

Preoperative preparation

Detailed history, physical exam, necessary blood investigations, and imaging modalities must be obtained for the patient.

The clinical presentation of acute appendicitis can vary from mild symptoms to signs of generalized peritonitis and sepsis. Hence, the value of individual clinical variables to determine the likelihood of acute appendicitis in a patient is low [4]. Thus, biochemical testing and imaging modalities have value in confirming appendicitis. The elevated C-reactive protein levels render the

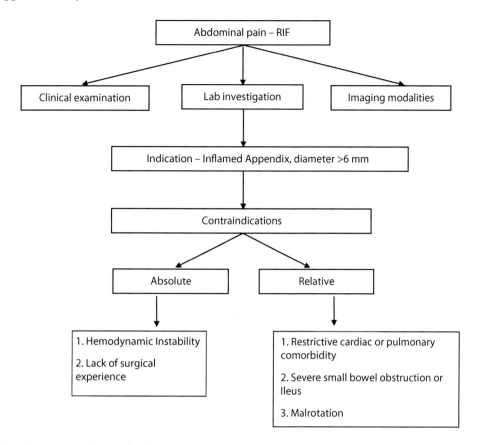

FIGURE 12.1 Flowchart approach to Right iliac Fossa pain.

highest diagnostic accuracy, followed by increased numbers of leucocytes with an area under the curve of 0.75 [95% CI 0.71–0.78] and 0.72 [95% CI 0.68–0.76], respectively [4].

Imaging studies in patients with a clinical suspicion of acute appendicitis can reduce the negative appendectomy rate, which has been reported to be as high as 15%. Counselling of patient about possibility of conversion to an open surgery. Preoperative dose of antibiotic.

  i. Ultrasonography, is noninvasive, avoids radiation, and is associated with a sensitivity rate between 71% and 94%, and a specificity rate between 81% and 98% [5]. Therefore, ultrasonography is reliable for confirming the presence of appendicitis, but is unreliable to exclude appendicitis.
 ii. Abdominal computed tomography (CT), has a sensitivity and specificity rates between 76%–100% and 83%–100%, respectively, and therefore, it is superior to ultrasonography [6].
iii. Magnetic resonance imaging (MRI) is used in pregnant patients and children with inconclusive findings at ultrasonography. A recent meta-analysis on MRI in 363 patients with appendicitis, yielded a sensitivity rate of 97%, a specificity rate of 95%, a positive likelihood ratio of 16.3 [95% CI 9.10–29.10], and a negative likelihood ratio of 0.09 [95% CI 0.04–0.20] [7].
    1. Counselling of patient about possibility of conversion to an open surgery.
    2. Preoperative dose of antibiotic.

Operative principles: The standard principles of laparoscopic appendicectomy are (Figure 12.2):

1. Access to the peritoneal cavity – entry and port placement
2. Identifying the pathology, diagnostic evaluation
3. Division of mesoappendix
4. Tackling the base of appendix
5. Specimen retrieval
6. Associated procedure if any
7. Lavage, drainage and port closure

OR setup

Standard OR setup with the patient in a supine position and a slight left lateral tilt with both arms by the side of the patient. Surgeon stands on the left side of the patient with cameraman next to surgeon towards the head end. The monitor is placed on the right side, opposite to the surgeon.

Operative steps (see Video 8)

1. *Peritoneal access and port placement:* The first entry for the pneumo-peritoneum is made through an infraumbilical incision, except in patients with peritonitis and small bowel obstruction, where an open entry or Palmer's point entry is preferred.

    Initial abdominal pressure is kept at 15 mm of Hg for the first port entry, and then the working pressure is usually 12 mm of Hg in adults and 10 mm of Hg in pediatric patients.

    After the first camera port, two other working ports are placed under direct vision (Figures 12.3 and 12.4).

    There are many different options of working ports as per the surgeon's preference, dexterity, and position of the appendix; the different options are:

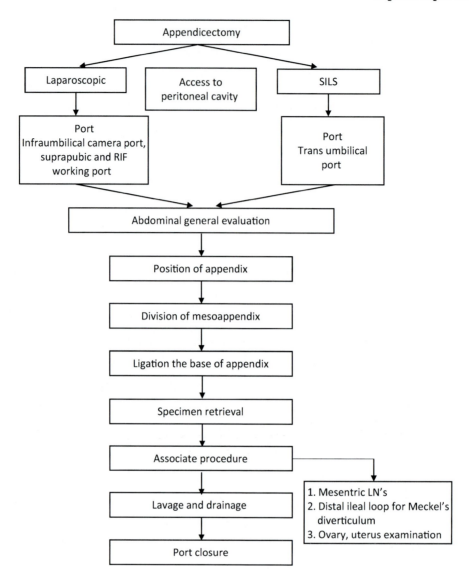

FIGURE 12.2   Flowchart steps of laparoscopic appendicectomy.

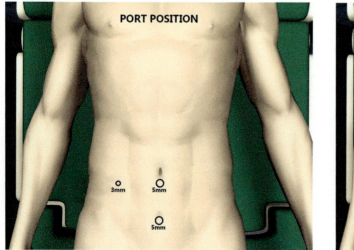

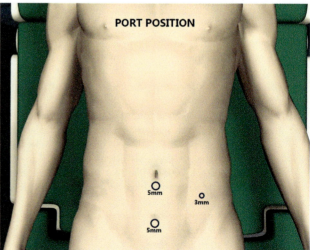

FIGURE 12.3   Standard port placement Infraumbilical right.   **FIGURE 12.4**   Standard port placement Infraumbilical left.

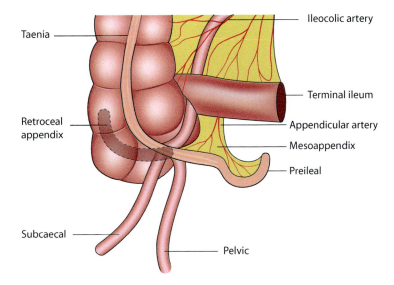

Taenia

Ileocolic artery

Retroceal appendix

Terminal ileum

Appendicular artery

Mesoappendix

Preileal

Subcaecal

Pelvic

FIGURE 12.5 Different positions of appendix.

i. Infraumbilical camera port, suprapubic, and RIF working port.
ii. Suprapubic camera port, infraumbilical, and RIF working port.
iii. Infraumbilical camera port and suprapubic, and LIF working port.
iv. SILS port position, single incision multiport, single incision SILS port.
v. Fouth port, which may be required for retraction of distended ileum and distal small bowel.

2. *Identifying the pathology and diagnostic evaluation*: As a standard practice, we need to evaluate the point of entry for any local injury, and then the whole abdominal cavity is inspected for any localized or generalized collection, the position of the omentum, the condition of the small bowel, and the location of tha caecum and appendix (Figure 12.5). Using two atraumatic instruments, the appendix can be located by gently lifting the caecum and tracing the tinea to the base of the appendix. Incision on the lateral and inferior peritoneal fold, with mobilization of the caecum may help to localize the retrocaecal appendix. In case of acute appendicitis, gentle omental separation or adhesiolysis may be needed to locate the appendix.

Patients with appendicular abscess, or dense adhesion, may require extensive adhesiolysis with a harmonic scalpel.

3. *Division of the mesoappendix*: The mesoappendix can be tackled in two ways:
i. Dissect at the root of the mesoappendix and coagulate the vessel at the base and keep the mesoappendix with the appendix (Figure 12.6).
ii. Dissect close to the appendix and leave the mesoappendix and bare the appendix completely up to the base (Figure 12.7).

Option for energy sources are:
i. Use of a bipolar (common).
ii. Use of a harmonic scalpel.
iii. Use of guarded monopolar coagulation – monopolar cautery should be used in short frequent bursts to avoid cecal injury.

iv. Use of a clip at the base after dissection.

In case of acute appendicitis with thick mesoappendix, we may have to coagulate and cut the mesoappendix sequentially in small fragments.

4. *Tackling the base of the appendix*: The base of the appendix is doubly ligated on patient side and one more single tie is used on specimen side.

The basic techniques:
i. *Staplers*: The first publications on the use in laparoscopic appendectomy were reported in 1990. It allows simultaneous sealing and division of both the mesoappendix and the appendix base. When the base of the appendix is very wide, we may have to use an EndoGIA 30 stapler close to the base on the caecum. It is both easy to apply and safe, even when the appendix base is inflamed and its diameter is too large. However, its advantage over other methods, in terms of reliability, has not been proven. The most

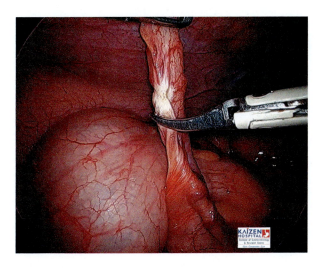

FIGURE 12.6 Dissect at the root of mesoappendix using bipolar cautery.

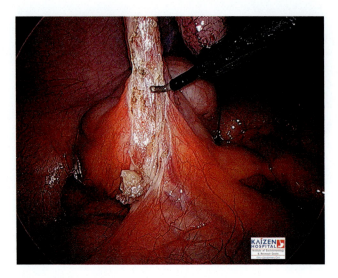

FIGURE 12.7   Dissect close to the appendix using hook.

important disadvantage is that it is more expensive than other methods [8].

  ii. *Endoloop*: Endoloop use has been proposed by several authors due to its safety in closing the appendix stump and its lower cost compared to staplers [9].

    I. Commercially available chromic catgut loop.

    II. Prepare a handmade endoloop with vicryl, using Roeder's knot and knot pusher [10] (Figure 12.8). The knot pusher is also available with the thread cutter in the same instrument.

  iii. *Extracorporeal knot*: Used with 90 cm long suture with extracorporeal knot tying and pushing with knot pusher.

  iv. *Intracorporeal knots*: Using vicryl suture two knots tied on the patient side and one on the specimen side, but has the disadvantage of prolonging the operation time [11].

    In special circumstances, one can use as well titanium clips, nonabsorbable polymer clips (Hem-o-lock clips), Ligasure, or division using bipolar cautery.

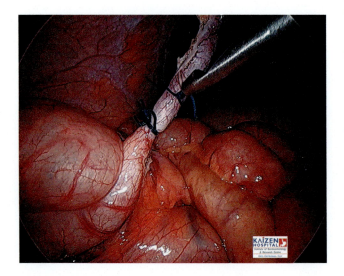

FIGURE 12.8   Roeder's knot and knot pusher.

Therefore, methods that are cheap and easy to apply should be considered as first choice.

  5. *Specimen retrieval*: Specimen is delivered using a retrieval bag to avoid wound contamination. Preferably the suprapubic port is converted to 10 mm for the retrieval.

  6. *Associated procedure*:

    i. In cases of diagnostic laparoscopy, where appendicular inflammation is not significant and mesenteric LNs are enlarged, we may take an lymph node (LN) biopsy.

    ii. Examination of the distal ileal loop for Meckel's diverticum should be carried out.

    iii. In female patients, pelvic organs should also be examined.

  7. *Lavage, drainage, closure*: After specimen retrieval, the abdominal cavity is inspected again for any bleeding or collection. A thorough peritoneal lavage is done. Usually, drains are not placed after an appendectomy, except in cases of friable appendicular stump, and risk of bleeding or leak. It is important to close the sheath of the 10 mm port site.

  8. *Special situation*:

    i. *Appendicular lump*: Careful blunt dissection is carried out to separate the omentum, small bowel, and colon to identify and dissect the appendix.

    ii. *Appendicular perforation*: Peritoneal lavage with large amounts of warm saline is needed. Then attention should be given to the base of the appendix and ligating the base.

    iii. *Retrograde appendectomy*: When the tip of the appendix is perforated and adherent to the omental mass omental mass or to the small bowel then the base then the base of the appendix can be dissected first, clipped, divided, and then the mesoappendix can be dissected close to the serosa of the appendix up to the tip.

    iv. *Necrotic appendicular base*: When the inflammation extends to the base and involves the caecum, then we may have to remove the part of the caecum either by endoGIA stapler, or by primary suturing.

    v. We may need extra ports for adhesiolysis.

Postoperative course and recovery

In uneventful cases the postoperative course is smooth and oral feeding is started within 6 to 8 hours.

In complicated cases, oral intake is delayed until bowel peristalsis returns. Intravenous antibiotics are given for 24 to 48 hours, which is then converted to oral antibiotic as per need.

Postoperative complications

Any complication associated with open surgery can also occur during laparoscopic surgery such as postoperative collection, stump blowout/leak, wound infection, and early or late intestinal obstruction. Appendicular stumpitis is also a known complication of appendectomies performed in acute cases, where there is a reasonable size stump left that gets infected and creates symptoms similar to acute appendicitis in patients with history of appendectomy.

SILS appendicectomy

SILS port technique is used, as first reported by Pelosi et al. [12], where the difficult ergonomics with the triangulation of the instruments and camera is avoided, by the use of special angulated instrument. Special angulated instrument can be used to overcome the issue.

The advantage is cosmetic as the total incision length is about 2.5 to 3 cm.

Advantages of laparoscopic surgery

1. Minimal invasive surgery with less pain, early recovery of bowel function, and fewer chances of wound infection.
2. Reduced incidence of wound infection and postoperative abscess formation with laparoscopic surgery.

Disadvantages of laparoscopic surgery

1. Increased chances of visceral and vessel injury with veress or trocar insertion in laparoscopic surgery.
2. Iatrogenic small bowel or colonic injury by instruments.
3. Thermal injury to the caecum or other small bowel loop due to nonpolar cautery current passing through the narrowed base, producing intense heat.

Summary

Laparoscopic appendectomy is the gold standard for the treatment of acute appendicitis. It allows for precise diagnosis, inspection of the abdominal cavity, including the bowel and pelvic organs, and tackling as well as difficult situations without extension or a change of incision. It imparts the advantages of minimal invasive access such as less pain, and early recovery and return to work.

Key points

- Laparoscopic appendectomy is the gold standard for the treatment of acute appendicitis with a standardized procedure.
- The role of imaging modalities and their accuracy in detecting doubtful cases of acute appendicitis.
- The advent of the SILS appendicectomy is equivocal to traditional laparoscopic appendicectomy.

Video

VIDEO 8   https://youtu.be/byZ44amV8HY

Laparoscopic Appendectomy.

References

1. Semm K. Endoscopic Appendectomy. *Endoscopy*. 1983 Mar;15(02):59–64.
2. Aly OE, Black DH, Rehman H, Ahmed I. Single incision laparoscopic appendicectomy versus conventional three-port laparoscopic appendicectomy: A systematic review and meta-analysis. *Int J Surg*. 2016 Nov;35:120–8.
3. Pearl RH, Hale DA, Molloy M, Schutt DC, Jaques DP. Pediatric appendectomy. *J Pediatr Surg*. 1995 Feb;30(2):173–81.
4. Andersson REB, Meta-analysis of the clinical and laboratory diagnosis of appendicitis. *Br J Surg*. 2004;91(1):28–37 doi:10.1002/bjs.4464
5. Carroll PJ, Gibson D, El-Faedy O et al. Surgeon-performed ultrasound at the bedside for the detection of appendicitis and gallstones: Systematic review and meta-analysis. *Am J Surg*. 2013 Jan;205(1):102–8.
6. Doria AS, Moineddin R, Kellenberger CJ et al. US or CT for Diagnosis of Appendicitis in Children and Adults? A Meta-Analysis. *Radiology*. 2006 Oct;241(1):83–94.
7. Barger RL, Nandalur KR. Diagnostic Performance of Magnetic Resonance Imaging in the Detection of Appendicitis in Adults. *Acad Radiol*. 2010 Oct;17(10):1211–6.
8. Rakić M, Jukić M, Pogorelić Z et al. Analysis of endoloops and endostaples for closing the appendiceal stump during laparoscopic appendectomy. *Surg Today*. 2014 Sep;44(9):1716–22.
9. Sahm M, Kube R, Schmidt S, Ritter C, Pross M, Lippert H. Current analysis of endoloops in appendiceal stump closure. *Surg Endosc*. 2011 Jan;25(1):124–9.
10. Yildiz F, Terzi A, Coban S, Zeybek N, Uzunkoy A. The handmade endoloop technique. A simple and cheap technique for laparoscopic appendectomy. *Saudi Med J*. 2009;30:224–7.
11. Kiudelis M, Ignatavicius P, Zviniene K, Grizas S. Analysis of intracorporeal knotting with invaginating suture versus endoloops in appendiceal stump closure. *Wideochir Inne Tech Malo Inwazyjne*. 2013;8:69–73.
12. Jawahar K, Sharanya R, Prakash S. Single-incision laparoscopic surgery versus conventional laparoscopic appendectomy. *Int Surg J*. 2018 Oct 26;5(11):3685.

Chapter 13

LAPAROSCOPIC SIGMOID COLECTOMY FOR DIVERTICULITIS

Paul Trinity Stephen and Rohin

Contents

Learning objectives 68
Introduction 68
Acute diverticulitis... 68
Diagnosis of acute diverticulitis... 69
Management of acute complicated diverticulitis 69
Choice of procedure... 69
Laparoscopic versus open approach 70
    Advantages of laparoscopy in an acute setting 70
    Disadvantages of laparoscopy in an acute setting... 71
    Prerequisites for laparoscopy in an acute setting 71
    Technical challenges in laparoscopy in the acute setting 71
Laparoscopic lavage in acute diverticulitis 71
    Literature review.. 71
    Patient positioning 71
    Port placement 71
    Operative steps 72
    Complications 72
    Conversion to laparoscopic colectomy.. 72
Laparoscopic sigmoid colectomy in acute diverticulitis 72
    Operative steps 73
    Complications 73
Summary 73
Key points 73
Video... 73
References 74

Learning objectives

- Diagnosis and staging of acute diverticulitis
- Management principles in acute complicated and uncomplicated diverticulitis
- Role of laparoscopy in acute diverticulitis – advantages, pitfalls and challenges
- Indications and technique for laparoscopic lavage in acute diverticulitis
- Role and technique of sigmoid colectomy in acute diverticulitis

Introduction

Colonic diverticulosis is common in the western world, with half the population being affected by the sixth decade of life, and two thirds by the ninth decade [1]. Indian studies show a much lower prevalence, even as low as 9.9% [2]. Most people with diverticular disease remain asymptomatic, and only 20%–25% develop clinical evidence of diverticulitis [3,4]. When diverticulitis does develop, it is mild or uncomplicated in most patients, and often resolves with nonoperative management [5,6]. A minority of patients develop complicated diverticulitis, characterized by a pericolic abscess, colonic perforation with purulent or fecal peritonitis, or a fistula. These patients are likely to require radiological intervention or surgery.

There are many options for surgical management of acute complicated diverticulitis. These include lavage and drainage, sigmoidectomy with end colostomy, or sigmoidectomy with colorectal anastomosis (with or without a proximal diverting stoma). All of these can be performed via the open or laparoscopic approach. Ideal surgical management of acute diverticulitis has been a widely debated topic, and depends on a number of disease and patient-related factors. There are multiple publications comparing various approaches, as well as multiple consensus statements available for management of acute diverticulitis, with detailed insights on the use of antibiotics, the role of radiological interventions, the role of laparoscopy as well as the need for resection, with or without a stoma [4,7–10].

In this chapter, we will focus on the surgical management of an acute attack of diverticulitis, with a special emphasis on laparoscopic approaches.

Acute diverticulitis

Acute diverticulitis develops in 20%–25% of patients with diverticular disease [3,4]. An acute episode may be uncomplicated or complicated. Complicated diverticulitis is defined as diverticulitis with a pericolic abscess, perforation with purulent or feculent peritonitis, or fistula formation.

A majority (85%) of patients developing diverticulitis will have acute uncomplicated diverticulitis [10]. These patients present

TABLE 13.1: The Hinchey Classification for Severity of Acute Complicated Diverticulitis

Hinchey Stage	Description
Stage 1	Pericolic abscess
Stage 2	Localized Pelvic or distant abscess
Stage 3	Generalized purulent peritonitis
Stage 4	Generalized feculent peritonitis

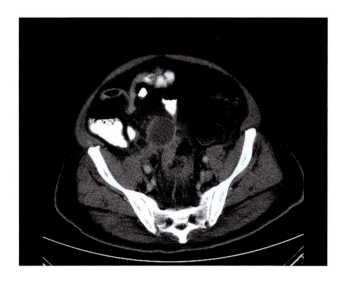

FIGURE 13.1 CT scan showing acutely inflamed and thickened sigmoid colon with diverticulae, and a pericolic abscess.

with abdominal pain in the left lower quadrant and change in bowel habits. They may have associated low-grade fever. Most of these patients will improve with nonoperative management, including antibiotics, bowel rest and a low fiber diet.

Patients with complicated diverticulitis may present with a localized phlegmon or generalized peritonitis. They have abdominal pain with associated high fever. Clinical examination may reveal tenderness in the left lower quadrant of the abdomen, or rebound tenderness and guarding in cases with generalized peritonitis. Extraperitoneal inflammation can present with back pain, as well as lower limb pain. Patient may also present with large bowel obstruction in cases with stricture, or recurrent urinary tract infection with or without fecaluria in cases with fistulation to the urinary bladder.

Complicated diverticular disease may be treated by radiological drainage, laparoscopy or laparotomy, with or without sigmoid resection, depending on the presentation. The Hinchey classification [11] (Table 13.1) is useful to classify and stage acute complicated diverticulitis, and aids in developing management strategies.

Diagnosis of acute diverticulitis

CT scanning is the imaging modality of choice for the diagnosis of acute diverticulitis. It has a sensitivity of up to 98% and an overall accuracy of 97% [12,13]. It gives information on the extent of disease, presence of pericolic collections, free air in the peritoneal cavity or the retroperitoneum, as well as generalized peritonitis (Figure 13.1). The CT scan therefore confirms the diagnosis, as well as stages the disease, aiding in formulating a management strategy. CT scans may also sometimes reveal unexpected findings such as a colonic neoplasm.

Colonoscopy is not usually performed in the acute setting. Patients with complicated diverticulitis should be evaluated with a colonoscopy after the acute episode has settled [4,10]. Other blood investigations such as total and differential leucocyte count, as well as C-reactive protein may help in assessing the severity of sepsis and inflammation.

Management of acute complicated diverticulitis

Acute uncomplicated diverticulitis is managed with antibiotics. In acute complicated diverticulitis, clinically stable patients with a pericolic abscess or phlegmon can be managed with radiology-guided drainage of the abscess along with antibiotics. Some small abscesses of <4 cm may be managed with antibiotics alone [14]. Most patients respond to this management, and surgery is rarely required. For patients not improving with drainage, or where drainage is technically not feasible, an operative intervention may be required. Patients with generalized peritonitis (purulent or feculent) will require surgical intervention.

Surgical options include a washout (lavage), with or without sigmoid colon resection. In cases where sigmoid resection is

performed, a decision has to be made on performing a Hartmann's procedure, or restoring bowel continuity. Both these procedures, lavage and resection, can be performed laparoscopically, in carefully selected individuals. Figure 13.2 outlines a flowchart for the management of acute complicated diverticulitis.

Choice of procedure

Patients with Hinchey 3 and 4 diverticulitis will usually require a surgical procedure. The options in such cases include a peritoneal lavage, or a sigmoid resection. In cases of sigmoid resection, one has to choose between performing a Hartmann's operation or a primary anastomosis with a covering stoma.

The choice of procedure depends on many factors. Patient factors include age, nutritional status, comorbidities, Hinchey stage as well as general hemodynamic stability of the patient. Other factors that dictate the choice of procedure include the infrastructure available, expertise of the surgical team as well as presence of high dependency or intensive care facilities.

A sigmoid resection is always preferred in patients with generalized feculent peritonitis. In individuals who are malnourished, chronically ill, have multiple comorbidities, are hemodynamically unstable, or have proximal obstruction, a Hartman's type resection is preferred. In the absence of all the above, an anastomosis may be considered [15]. We cover all such anastomosis with a proximal loop ileostomy. For patients undergoing a Hartman's type resection, it is important to realize that while reversal is technically possible, most individuals do not get their stoma reversed, in effect making this a permanent stoma. On the other hand, if a primary anastomosis is performed with a covering stoma, it is more likely to be reversed [16].

In patients with purulent peritonitis, in the presence of hemodynamic instability, a resection is preferred. In stable patients with purulent peritonitis, a peritoneal lavage may be considered as a therapeutic option. A lavage results in a shorter hospital stay and lower risk of stoma formation, with comparable morbidity and mortality [17–19]. Risk of recurrence following lavage is also low, favoring its use in select situations. Literature around this treatment option is covered later in the chapter. Figure 13.3 outlines some of the factors that help in decision-making in a patient with acute complicated diverticulitis.

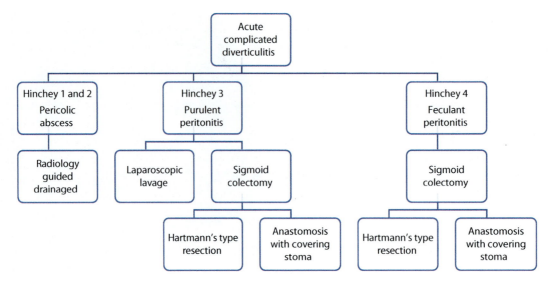

FIGURE 13.2   Algorithm for management of acute complicated diverticulitis.

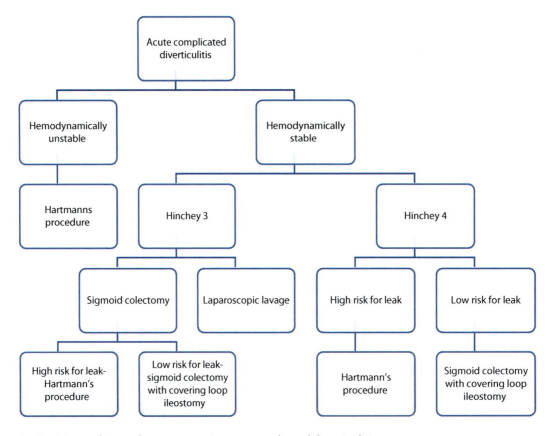

FIGURE 13.3   Decision-making and management in acute complicated diverticulitis.

Laparoscopic versus open approach

All the above procedures can be performed both open and laparoscopically. The decision to perform a laparoscopic or open approach depends on multiple factors.

Advantages of laparoscopy in an acute setting
Laparoscopy in the acute setting has many advantages including a smaller wound, less postoperative pain and earlier recovery.

Hospital stay has been shown to be shorter in the laparoscopic approach when compared to an open approach. In select cases, if only a lavage is performed, resection as well as stomas may be avoided. A recent meta-analysis revealed lower complication rates with laparoscopy compared to open sigmoid resection. However, patients undergoing open resection were sicker, and therefore this result needs to be interpreted with caution [20]. Laparoscopy can also be used as a diagnostic tool, leading to an early diagnosis.

Disadvantages of laparoscopy in an acute setting

Laparoscopy in the acute setting does have its pitfalls. In cases where a lavage is performed, the biggest worry is the danger of performing an inadequate operation. This often happens because of failure to drain all pus pockets. Patients undergoing laparoscopic lavage are at three times higher risk of having persistent peritonitis and abscesses, when compared to those having sigmoid resection [21].

With laparoscopic lavage, there is always the risk of missed cancer, which would have been detected if resection would have been carried out. It is therefore mandatory to perform a colonoscopy on such patients in about six weeks' time, once they have recovered [4,10].

The learning curve for laparoscopy in an acute setting is steep, and one must be comfortable with advanced laparoscopic colorectal procedures to perform these cases. As the tissues are more friable, there is a higher risk of visceral injuries.

Long-term data on outcomes of laparoscopy in the acute setting are not available, and the available data needs to be interpreted cautiously. Mild cases may be managed laparoscopically, and some of these may have been managed with medical management alone. The sicker patients tend to get managed with open surgery and therefore comparisons between the two may be biased. There is a need for well-conducted randomized controlled trials in this field.

Prerequisites for laparoscopy in an acute setting

Prior to undertaking any surgical procedure, the diagnosis of complicated diverticulitis should be confirmed with a CT scan. All required equipment such as a mobile table, Allen stirrups, and an antislip mattress should be available. These are essential as they allow the patient to be positioned in a steep Trendelenburg position, as well as allow access to the perineum, should it be required during the operation.

Prior experience of performing complex colorectal surgery, as well as other laparoscopic procedures is highly desirable. Intracorporeal suturing skills are a useful tool to have, should closure of a perforation in the colon be required.

Technical challenges in laparoscopy in the acute setting

Laparoscopy in an acutely inflamed setting, with possible purulent or feculent peritonitis, can be very challenging. Some of the technical challenges one may encounter are discussed below:

- Access to the peritoneal cavity to establish pneumoperitoneum may be difficult. In the presence of bowel distension, there is a high risk of bowel injury with any of the closed methods for creating pneumoperitoneum. We prefer an open Hassan's method at the umbilicus to create pneumoperitoneum in all such cases.
- These patients usually have some element of sepsis. Pneumoperitoneum may add to the cardiac stress, leading to some patients becoming unstable after the creation of pneumoperitoneum. In such cases, one must promptly convert to an open procedure.
- Vision is usually limited with presence of diffuse peritoneal contamination. The views are often suboptimal, with dilated bowel loops and little space in the peritoneal cavity. Ability to retract is also limited due to these circumstances. The tissues can be edematous and friable and are prone to damage and perforation. Both on and off camera injuries are possible, and one has to be very gentle during retraction and dissection.

- The planes may be blurred due to inflammation and edema, thereby posing a risk to visceral, neural, and vascular structures.
- Stapling in an acutely inflamed bowel may be difficult and prone to leakage. One must try and staple in the normal upper rectum, rather than the distal sigmoid colon. Use of a stapler with appropriate staple height is essential to minimize the risk of a distal stump blowout.
- Due to the presence of adhesions, there is a risk of an inadequate lavage. This will lead to failure of the patient to improve, with continuing sepsis and the need for further interventions.

Laparoscopic lavage in acute diverticulitis

Literature review

The concept of laparoscopic lavage and drainage has attracted the attention of many surgeons. Multiple case series have shown this to be an effective modality to treat purulent peritonitis, with shorter hospital stay, decreased stoma rates, and acceptable outcomes. The DILALA randomized controlled trial found shorter operative time and length of stay in patients undergoing laparoscopic lavage compared to sigmoid resection [22]. The SCANDIV trial again found comparable outcomes between the two groups, except that there were more missed cancers in the laparoscopic lavage group [23]. In another recent randomized controlled trial, the LADIES trial, the laparoscopic lavage arm was terminated early secondary to an increased rate of adverse events associated with surgical reintervention in the lavage arm [24]. Many meta-analysis have shown that laparoscopic lavage carries a higher risk or reintervention (percutaneous intervention or operative), but lower rate of stoma formation [17,18,21].

Looking at all the above literature, one can conclude that laparoscopic lavage has its limitations, and should be offered only to a highly select group of patients, while most patients should be offered resection.

Patient positioning

The patient is positioned in a modified lithotomy, or Lloyd Davies position, using Allen stirrups. Use of the Allen stirrups allows for repositioning of the legs, should access the perineum be necessary for intraoperative endoscopy or transanal stapling. The patient should be placed on a bean bag or an antislip mattress with the hip at the edge of the table. This prevents the patient from slipping during the steep Trendelenburg position. Both hands should be tucked in by the side of the patient to allow the surgeon and the assistants enough room.

The operation starts with the patient supine, however the patient can be placed in a steep Trendelenburg position with the left side elevated, if better access to the sigmoid colon is desired.

There is great variation in literature about the operative setup. We prefer to place the operative stack on the patient's left at the foot end. The surgeon and the camera holder stand on the patient's right, along with the scrub nurse, and the assistant stands on the patient's left (Figure 13.4).

Port placement

In the acute setting, we prefer an open Hassan's technique to establish pneumoperitoneum. This port can then be incorporated into the extraction site, should one be required. Other ports placed under vision include a 5 mm right iliac fossa port, a 10 mm right lumbar port (camera port), and a 5 mm left lumber port for retraction, mirroring the right lumbar port. In people with a small abdominal cavity, sometimes the umbilical port is too close

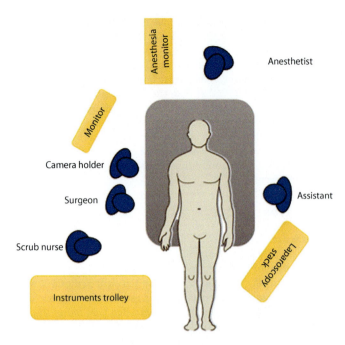

FIGURE 13.4 Theatre setup for a laparoscopic lavage/sigmoid resection.

to the sigmoid colon to allow easy manipulation. In these cases, we place a 5 mm port in the right upper quadrant to facilitate dissection. Our main working ports are the right iliac fossa port as well as the umbilical port, with the left lumbar port used for retraction. Figure 13.5 shows the usual port placement for the procedure.

Operative steps

The initial step is to perform a full abdominal survey to look at the extent of disease. In case of feculent peritonitis, one has to decide early if a conversion to open, or a change of plan to laparoscopic resection is warranted.

The abdominal cavity is thoroughly washed with warm saline, irrigated in all quadrants of the abdomen. Although there are reports of using antibiotics mixed in the saline, or betadine with the saline, we prefer warm normal saline without any additives for lavage. The amount of saline to be used is not standard, but lavage is carried out until the fluid sucked out is clear. All pockets

are opened into and pus drained. One has to be very gentle while breaking the adhesions as the bowel is usually friable and can be injured easily. The suction tip can be used gently to both wash as well as break adhesions, as most adhesions are acute and easily released. We avoid using any power source to break or dissect the adhesions. There may be some minimal bleeding from the raw areas as the adhesions are broken, which usually stops spontaneously. It is important to progress in a stepwise fashion (clockwise or anticlockwise) to wash out all quadrants of the abdomen, without missing any areas. The area of the sigmoid colon, including the pelvis is also washed thoroughly. If a large perforation is encountered, sigmoid resection must be undertaken.

Once lavage is complete, a drain is placed in the pelvis and the ports are removed under vision. Intravenous antibiotics should be continued and the patient monitored closely for signs of deterioration.

Complications

Incomplete lavage with residual pockets of pus is one of the most common causes of persisting symptoms [21]. Visceral and neurovascular injuries are common and one must be very gentle in handling tissues. If the patient fails to improve after lavage, or becomes septic again after an initial improvement, immediate CT scanning or laparotomy is warranted to look for the cause and address it. Delay in initiating this may lead to increased morbidity and mortality. A subset of these patients end up needing a sigmoid resection.

Conversion to laparoscopic colectomy

In patients with a large perforation, feculent peritonitis, or hemodynamic instability, a sigmoid colectomy is more appropriate rather than lavage alone. Suturing of a large perforation in an inflamed bowel is not advisable, and is likely to lead to further complications. Once the decision to perform a sigmoid colectomy is made, one must decide to perform the operation laparoscopically or open. In case of laparoscopic surgery, the steps are the same as described later in the chapter. Decision to anastomose or bring out an end stoma is again dictated by the various factors elucidated earlier.

Laparoscopic sigmoid colectomy in acute diverticulitis

The patient positioning and port placement remains the same as described for laparoscopic lavage. However, the right lower

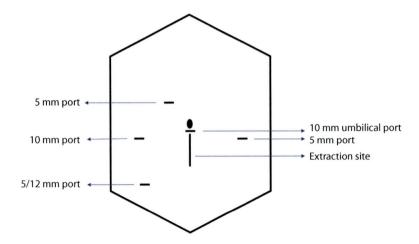

FIGURE 13.5 Port placement for laparoscopic lavage/sigmoid resection.

quadrant port is a 12 mm port rather than a 5 mm port, for introduction of a stapler for rectal transection. We prefer an infraumbilical midline extraction site for the specimen.

Once pneumoperitoneum is established, a full abdominal survey is performed. All quadrants of the abdomen are inspected in a stepwise fashion, to confirm the diagnosis and assess the extent of contamination. Following this, a systematic laparoscopic lavage must be performed, as described above. Once the lavage has been performed, one must set up for the sigmoid colectomy. The steps of the sigmoid colectomy are essentially same as for any other indication, with a few caveats:

- The tissues are edematous and friable, and identification of the ureter may be more difficult in such situations.
- Since this is essentially a benign process, a radical resection encompassing the entire mesentery, as well as high ligation of the vessel, is not required. We often perform low ligation of the vessel and just adequate excision of the mesentery.
- The distal resection must be in the upper rectum, making sure all diseased colon is removed. It is tempting to leave behind a sigmoid stump, or to bring the distal end as a mucous fistula, but this will leave behind residual disease, leading to further complications.

Operative steps

A steep Trendelenburg and left side up position helps in moving all the small bowel out of the pelvis. We prefer a medial to lateral approach. However, a lateral to medial approach may also be used.

The retraction on the sigmoid colon is important and both the operating and the assisting surgeon should provide retraction cephalad and anteriorly to expose the sigmoid mesentery. A peritoneal incision is made just above the sacral promontory to expose the avascular plane below the sigmoid mesentery. This plane, which hugs the sigmoid mesocolon and is superficial to the hypogastric nerves, ureter, and vascular structures is important to identify correctly. The pneumoperitoneum often opens up this plane once the peritoneal incision is made. This plane is then developed cephalad, caudad, and from medial to lateral, up to the lateral abdominal wall. The left ureter and the left gonadal vessels should be identified and preserved. If the ureter cannot be identified, the most likely explanation is that it has been mobilized with the mesocolon, and the plane of dissection is too deep.

The next step is to ligate the inferior mesenteric vessels. This need not be at the origin of the vessel because of the benign nature of the disease. We tend to perform a low ligation, leaving the left colic artery intact. The mesocolon is then further dissected off the retroperitoneal structures, until the left colon is adequately mobilized. If an anastomosis is planned, sometimes splenic flexure mobilization may be needed.

The upper rectum is mobilized next, and a point of transection is identified in the upper rectum. The lateral attachments of the sigmoid colon are now taken down to free the whole colon. Care must be taken at this point to safeguard the ureter. The mesorectum is divided at the point of distal transection and the upper rectum divided with an endoscopic stapler.

The proximal resection point is identified as a point of heathy colon and the colonic mesentery is divided until this point. The colon is then exteriorized.

We prefer an infraumbilical midline incision to deliver the specimen, and the proximal division is performed extracorporeally under vision, usually with a stapler. In cases where a stoma is planned, the proximal end is then placed back in the abdominal cavity and then delivered via a trephine at a premarked stoma site.

Laparoscopy is performed again, to look at the orientation of the stoma, and a drain is placed in the pelvis after further washout. The extraction site and other port sites are then closed.

In cases of primary anastomosis, the anvil of a circular stapler is placed in the proximal bowel and a purse string suture taken to secure it in place. Pneumoperitoneum is reestablished and a stapled colorectal anastomosis is performed. An air leak test is performed, followed by a wash and drain insertion. We routinely perform a covering loop ileostomy in these cases.

Complications

Some of the possible complications include a distal stump blowout, or missed pus pockets in the abdominal cavity. Off camera injuries also remain a real risk, especially in the presence of adhesion or edematous bowel. Ureteric injuries must be safeguarded against and ureteric stents may be used selectively. In cases of primary anastomosis, there is a chance for anastomotic leak, which may require relaparotomy, or dismantling the anastomosis with an end stoma.

Summary

Patients with Hinchey 3 and 4 acute diverticulitis need surgical intervention. The operation of choice in these patients is sigmoid resection. Decision to perform a Hartmann's procedure or a primary anastomosis depends on multiple factors and needs to be individualized for each patient. A laparoscopic approach for sigmoid colectomy is feasible and acceptable, and has some advantages over an open approach. It can, however, be technically challenging.

In a select group of patients with Hinchey 3 diverticulitis, who are clinically stable, a laparoscopic lavage may be offered. These patients have a shorter hospital stay and lower stoma rates; however, the incidence of reintervention and need for further continued treatment is higher in this group of patients. All patients managed with laparoscopic lavage must undergo a colonoscopy after recovery, in order to rule out a sigmoid cancer.

Key points

- CT scanning is the imaging modality of choice for the diagnosis of acute diverticulitis.
- Diverticulitis with a pericolic abscess, perforation with purulent or feculent peritonitis, or fistula formation is defined as complicated diverticulitis.
- The Hinchey classification is useful to classify and stage acute complicated diverticulitis, and plan management strategies.
- Patients with Hinchey 3 and 4 diverticulitis will usually require a surgical procedure.
- A sigmoid resection is always preferred in patients with generalized feculent peritonitis.
- In stable patients with purulent peritonitis, a peritoneal lavage may be considered as a therapeutic option.
- Laparoscopic approaches in the acute setting, although technically challenging, have some advantages over open surgery.

See Video 9.

Video

VIDEO 9   https://youtu.be/i-DXy-6VJTw

Laparoscopic Sigmoid Colectomy for Diverticulitis.

References

1. Buchs NC, Mortensen NJ, Ris F, Morel P, Gervaz P. Natural history of uncomplicated sigmoid diverticulitis. *World J Gastrointest Surg.* 2015;7:313–8.

2. Kamalesh NP, Prakash K, Pramil K, Zacharias P, Ramesh GN, Philip M. Prevalence and patterns of diverticulosis in patients undergoing colonoscopy in a southern Indian hospital. *Indian J Gastroenterol Off J Indian Soc Gastroenterol.* 2012;31:337–9.

3. Heise CP. Epidemiology and pathogenesis of diverticular disease. *J Gastrointest Surg Off J Soc Surg Aliment Tract.* 2008;12:1309–11.

4. Feingold D, Steele SR, Lee S, Kaiser A, Boushey R, Buie WD, Rafferty JF. Practice parameters for the treatment of sigmoid diverticulitis. *Dis Colon Rectum.* 2014;57:284–94.

5. Andersen JC, Bundgaard L, Elbrønd H, Laurberg S, Walker LR, Støvring J, Danish Surgical Society. Danish national guidelines for treatment of diverticular disease. *Dan Med J.* 2012;59:C4453.

6. Horesh N, Wasserberg N, Zbar AP, Gravetz A, Berger Y, Gutman M, Rosin D, Zmora O. Changing paradigms in the management of diverticulitis. *Int J Surg Lond Engl.* 2016;33(Pt A):146–50.

7. Deery SE, Hodin RA. Management of Diverticulitis in 2017. *J Gastrointest Surg Off J Soc Surg Aliment Tract.* 2017;21:1732–41.

8. Sartelli M, Catena F, Ansaloni L et al. WSES Guidelines for the management of acute left sided colonic diverticulitis in the emergency setting. *World J Emerg Surg WJES.* 2016;11:37.

9. Fozard JBJ, Armitage NC, Schofield JB, Jones OM, Association of Coloproctology of Great Britain and Ireland. ACPGBI position statement on elective resection for diverticulitis. *Colorectal Dis Off J Assoc Coloproctology G B Irel.* 2011;13(Suppl 3):1–11.

10. Stollman N, Smalley W, Hirano I, AGA Institute Clinical Guidelines Committee. American Gastroenterological Association Institute Guideline on the Management of Acute Diverticulitis. *Gastroenterology.* 2015;149:1944–9.

11. Hinchey EJ, Schaal PG, Richards GK. Treatment of perforated diverticular disease of the colon. *Adv Surg.* 1978;12:85–109.

12. Ambrosetti P. Acute diverticulitis of the left colon: Value of the initial CT and timing of elective colectomy. *J Gastrointest Surg Off J Soc Surg Aliment Tract.* 2008;12:1318–20.

13. Ambrosetti P, Becker C, Terrier F. Colonic diverticulitis: Impact of imaging on surgical management -- a prospective study of 542 patients. *Eur Radiol.* 2002;12:1145–9.

14. Siewert B, Tye G, Kruskal J, Sosna J, Opelka F, Raptopoulos V, Goldberg SN. Impact of CT-guided drainage in the treatment of diverticular abscesses: Size matters. *AJR Am J Roentgenol.* 2006;186:680–6.

15. Constantinides VA, Tekkis PP, Athanasiou T, Aziz O, Purkayastha S, Remzi FH, Fazio VW, Aydin N, Darzi A, Senapati A. Primary resection with anastomosis vs. Hartmann's procedure in nonelective surgery for acute colonic diverticulitis: A systematic review. *Dis Colon Rectum.* 2006;49:966–81.

16. Constantinides VA, Heriot A, Remzi F, Darzi A, Senapati A, Fazio VW, Tekkis PP. Operative strategies for diverticular peritonitis: A decision analysis between primary resection and anastomosis versus Hartmann's procedures. *Ann Surg.* 2007;245:94–103.

17. Marshall JR, Buchwald PL, Gandhi J, Schultz JK, Hider PN, Frizelle FA, Eglinton TW. Laparoscopic Lavage in the Management of Hinchey Grade III Diverticulitis: A Systematic Review. *Ann Surg.* 2017;265:670–6.

18. Cirocchi R, Di Saverio S, Weber DG, Taboła R, Abraha I, Randolph J, Arezzo A, Binda GA. Laparoscopic lavage versus surgical resection for acute diverticulitis with generalised peritonitis: A systematic review and meta-analysis. *Tech Coloproctology.* 2017;21:93–110.

19. Shaikh FM, Stewart PM, Walsh SR, Davies RJ. Laparoscopic peritoneal lavage or surgical resection for acute perforated sigmoid diverticulitis: A systematic review and meta-analysis. *Int J Surg Lond Engl.* 2017;38:130–7.

20. Cirocchi R, Fearnhead N, Vettoretto N, Cassini D, Popivanov G, Henry BM, Tomaszewski K, D'Andrea V, Davies J, Di Saverio S. The role of emergency laparoscopic colectomy for complicated sigmoid diverticulits: A systematic review and meta-analysis. *Surg J R Coll Surg Edinb Irel.* 2019;17:360–9.

21. Penna M, Markar SR, Mackenzie H, Hompes R, Cunningham C. Laparoscopic Lavage Versus Primary Resection for Acute Perforated Diverticulitis: Review and Meta-analysis. *Ann Surg.* 2018;267:252–8.

22. Angenete E, Thornell A, Burcharth J et al. Laparoscopic Lavage Is Feasible and Safe for the Treatment of Perforated Diverticulitis With Purulent Peritonitis: The First Results From the Randomized Controlled Trial DILALA. *Ann Surg.* 2016;263:117–22.

23. Schultz JK, Yaqub S, Wallon C et al. Laparoscopic Lavage vs Primary Resection for Acute Perforated Diverticulitis: The SCANDIV Randomized Clinical Trial. *JAMA.* 2015;314:1364–75.

24. Di Saverio S, Birindelli A, Catena F, Sartelli M, Segalini E, Masetti M, Jovine E. The Ladies Trial: Premature termination of the LOLA arm and increased adverse events incidence after laparoscopic lavage may be influenced by inter-hospital and inter-operator variability? Take-home messages from a center with laparoscopic colorectal expertise. *Int J Surg Lond Engl.* 2016;36:118–20.

Chapter 14

LAPAROSCOPIC RECTOPEXY FOR RECTAL PROLAPSE

Sanjiv Haribhakti and Jitender Singh Chauhan

Contents

Learning objectives 75
Introduction 75
Historical perspective 75
Types of rectal prolapse 76
Oxford rectal prolapse grading system (ORPG) 76
Indications for surgery 76
Goals of surgery 76
Surgical options 76
Selection of approach and controversies 77
Preoperative evaluation 77
Preoperative preparation 78
Operative principles for posterior suture/mesh/resection rectopexy 78
OR setup 78
Port placements 78
Operative steps of laparoscopic suture/resection rectopexy 79
Operative techniques 79
Postoperative care and early outcomes 80
Postoperative complications 80
Long-term functional results 81
Robotic rectopexy 82
Summary 82
Key points 82
Videos 83
References 83

Learning objectives

- Select the right patient for the right procedure by understanding structural deformities and functional issues along with the disease.
- Determine the best surgical approach for a given patient by his/her physical condition, age, and baseline bowel function, as well as the surgeon's experience and preference.
- Know the benefits and limitations of various abdominal and perineal procedures for rectal prolapse.
- Understand the operative principles and techniques of the various procedures.
- Review and analyze the current studies on long-term results of different procedures.
- Explore results of various surgical procedures in meta-analysis.

Introduction

Laparoscopic rectopexy (LR) has become the gold standard operation for rectal prolapse. Rectal prolapse has a multifactorial etiology, and also tends to affect multiple compartments. Commonly, it is associated with uterine or vault prolapse (middle compartment), and bladder or urethral prolapse (anterior compartment). There are several structural deformities along with the rectal prolapse, such as edematous peritoneal folds, deep pouch of Douglas, redundant sigmoid colon, and so forth which also needs to be addressed along with the rectal prolapse. Many patients have

functional issues such as chronic severe constipation antecedent to the prolapse, and many develop fecal incontinence (FI) after the prolapse, which also needs to be addressed while treating the prolapse. Thus, rectal prolapse surgery should take these factors into account before selecting the right patient for the right procedure.

Historical perspective

Suspension of the rectum to the sacrum has been performed for more than 100 years. In 1934, Carrasco [1] reported suturing the rectum to the sacrum, a concept resurrected by Cutait [2] in 1959. An anterior suspension of the rectum to the posterior vaginal wall with sutures was described by Lloyd-Davies [3] in 1949, whereas the term ventral rectopexy was introduced by Deucher [4] in 1960. An anterior suspension was also reported by Nigro [5], who in 1970 suspended the rectum to the pubis. An antero-posterior rectopexy was also suggested by Nicholls and Simson [6] in 1986. Nonetheless, for decades there has not been any Level 1 evidence to support that the addition of rectopexy to mobilization of the rectum would decrease recurrences [7]. A recent randomized control trial comparing rectopexy with no rectopexy in 252 patients concluded that rectopexy decreases recurrence rates at 5-year follow ups [8]. Laparoscopic rectopexy, first described in 1992 [9], has since emerged as the preferred approach to the surgical treatment of full-thickness rectal prolapse (FTRP).

Ventral mesh rectopexy (VR) is a well-established abdominal prolapse procedure for the management of rectal prolapse. The goals of the D'Hoore VR involve correcting the prolapsed rectum by suturing a mesh, or biological graft material, to the anterior rectum and suspending it to the anterior longitudinal ligament of the sacrum [10]. This technique avoids posterior rectal dissection and potential neurological injury, which may result in a new onset of constipation. Over the last decade, large patient series have shown that VR is effective at correcting rectal prolapse, improving bowel continence, and reducing symptoms of obstructed defecation [11].

Types of rectal prolapse

1. External (ERP) – Full thickness – Complete (Procidentia) or Partial mucosal
2. Internal (IRP) – Obstructed daefecation syndrome (ODS) – Intususception, mucosal

Oxford rectal prolapse grading system (ORPG)

- Grade 1 and 2 are recto-rectal intussusceptions [12] (Figure 14.1)
- Grade 3 and 4 are recto-anal intussusception rectal prolapses
- Grade 5 describes an external rectal prolapse

Indications for surgery

1. The presence of external rectal prolapse (ERP) is an indication for surgical repair because of the eventual progression of symptoms, weakening of the sphincter complex, and risk of bleeding and incarceration. Fecal incontinence and/or constipation associated with rectal procidentia are also indications of surgery.
2. For internal rectal prolapse (IRP), patients with grade 3 or 4 IRP (ORPG) with ODS negatively affecting quality of life, and resistant to conservative management are considered for surgery. Pain and bleeding due to a solitary rectal ulcer (SRUS) caused by an IRP is also an indication for surgery.

Contraindications (C/I) for rectopexy [13]. According to Dutch Guidelines 2017:

Absolute C/I:

1. Patient unable to tolerate general anesthesia for severe medical comorbidities
2. Pelvic floor dyssynergia with ODS

3. Pregnancy or active proctitis
4. Posterior suture rectopexy should not be used for treating patients with internal rectal prolapse due to its effects on constipation

Relative C/I:

1. Strong psychosomatic overlay in internal rectal prolapse
2. History of rectal radiotherapy or inflammatory bowel disease
3. Male patients with severe morbid obesity
4. Severe endometriosis
5. History of severe episode of diverticulitis
6. Severe adhesions after previous transabdominal surgery or after peritonitis

Goals of surgery

1. Cure the prolapse
2. Avoid complications such as bleeding and improve fecal incontinence
3. Treat constipation, prevent worsening of constipation
4. Treat other organ prolapse along with rectal prolapse
5. Prevent recurrence of prolapse

Surgical options

More than 300 different procedures to treat rectal prolapse syndromes have been described. Thus far, no technique has been shown to be superior. This was confirmed by an international survey in 2012, showing no uniformity of surgical procedure [14].

Abdominal Procedures – Laparoscopic, open, or robotic (Table 14.1) [15]:

1. Posterior suture rectopexy
2. Posterior mesh rectopexy (wells)
3. Sigmoid resection and rectopexy
4. Ventral mesh rectopexy
5. Rectal mobilization alone without rectopexy
6. Anterior sling rectopexy (ripsteins)

Perineal Procedures:

1. Rectosigoidectomy (Altemiers procedure)
2. Mucosal stripping and muscular plication (Delorme procedure)

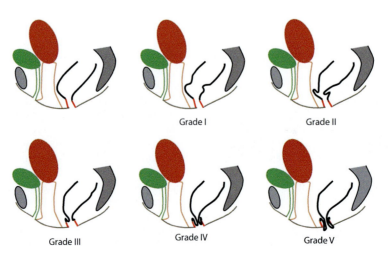

FIGURE 14.1 Oxford Rectal Prolapse Grade for grading of internal and external rectal prolapse.

TABLE 14.1: Abdominal Procedures for Pelvic Floor Disorders

Type of Procedure	Operation Technique
Suture rectopexy (Sudeck)	Complete rectal mobilization to level of levators Suture of rectum to presacral fascia
Anterior sling rectopexy (Ripstein)	Complete rectal mobilization to level of levators, circular wrapping of mesh around rectum, and attachment to the promontory
Lateral mesh rectopexy (Orr-Loygue)	Anterior and posterior complete rectal mobilization fixation by two lateral mesh strips to promontory
Ventral mesh rectopexy (D'Hoore)	Strictly anterior rectal dissection to level of levators Fixation of mesh strip on distal rectum and to promontory
Posterior mesh rectopexy (Wells)	Complete rectal mobilization to level of levators Semicircular mesh around rectum posterior, fixation to promontory
Resection rectopexy (Frykman-Goldberg)	Complete rectal mobilization to level of levators sigmoid resection and suture fixation of rectum to promontory
Rectal mobilization without rectopexy	Complete rectal mobilization to level of levators no fixation

3. Transanal procedures – STARR, contour STARR, double hemorrhoid stapling, transanal rectopexy, or transanal excision of nonhealing rectal SRUS

Selection of approach and controversies

The best surgical approach for a given patient is determined by his/her physical condition, age, and baseline bowel function, as well as the surgeon's experience and preference.

1. *Laparoscopic, open, or robotic*: Abdominal procedures for rectal procidentia can be performed with open or one of the minimally invasive techniques [16]. Although minimally invasive rectal procidentia repair is safe and effective, it has not been shown to be superior to open surgery in patient-important outcomes such as recurrence or postoperative bowel function. Thus, the operative approach should be determined by the surgeon; minimally invasive surgery is an option when the requisite expertise and equipment are available.

2. *Abdominal vs. perineal procedures*: Recurrence rates after an abdominal repair are generally lower than after a perineal repair. For those who are candidates (physically fit) for an abdominal procedure, we suggest an abdominal rather than a perineal repair. For patients who are not candidates (physically unfit) for an abdominal procedure, we use one of the perineal procedures to repair their rectal procidentia. In general, the perineal procedures are better tolerated than abdominal procedures, because they can be performed without general anesthesia and result in fewer complications and less pain. Additionally, perineal procedures are also preferred to abdominal procedures in the clinical settings [17], such as failed previous transabdominal repair, prior pelvic surgery, prior pelvic radiation therapy, and also in young males in order to minimize the risk of erectile dysfunction. There is little, if any, risk of damage to the hypogastric nerves with the perineal procedures.

3. *For perineal procedure*: Delorme or Altemiers procedures. For technical reasons, a perineal mucosal sleeve resection and muscular plication of the rectal procidentia (Delorme procedure) are typically performed for short-segment (<3 to 4 cm) rectal prolapses; a perineal rectosigmoidectomy (Altemeier procedure) is performed for rectal procidentias that are longer.

4. *Rectopexy vs. mobilization alone*: For patients undergoing an abdominal repair, we suggest performing a rectopexy rather than no rectopexy. In a randomized trial, patients who did not undergo a rectopexy had a higher recurrence rate than patients who underwent a rectopexy (8.6 versus 1.5%) [8].

5. *Suture rectopexy vs. mesh rectopexy*: The technique of rectopexy (suture vs. mesh) is determined by surgeon preference, as one technique has not been shown to be superior to other [18]. The author abandoned routine use of laparoscopic mesh rectopexy in favor of laparoscopic suture rectopexy since 2006, in order to avoid mesh-related morbidity, as results of efficacy and recurrences are equivalent. However, in patients with recurrence after suture rectopexy, a mesh rectopexy may be used.

6. *Suture rectopexy vs. resection rectopexy*: Sigmoid resection has been shown to reduce constipation in those who report this symptom preoperatively. Thus, for patients who have preexisting constipation, we suggest a sigmoid resection performed concomitantly with a rectopexy. Patients without baseline constipation should undergo a rectopexy without concomitant sigmoid resection.

7. *Posterior suture rectopexy vs. ventral mesh rectopexy*: Both are effective options in external rectal prolapse, and no head-to-head comparisons are available between the two. The author's choice is to use ventral mesh rectopexy for internal rectal prolapse and in those patients who have mild to moderate constipation, as this procedure improves constipation. For most patients with procidentia with mild constipation, the author's choice is lap posterior suture rectopexy, and in those with severe constipation, to add a lap resection to the rectopexy.

8. *Resection of redundant pouch of Douglas*: Douglas pouch removal was part of the original procedure and is probably one of the reasons why the recurrence rate is so low (around 3% in the long term) [19]. The rationale for that is based on the fact that in patients suffering from rectal prolapse, one of the anatomical abnormalities is the deep Douglas pouch.

9. *Rectal vs. Pelvic organ prolapse*: Concomitant pelvic organ prolapse (POP) can be present in up to one-third of patients who present with rectal prolapse. In patients who have a combined rectal/pelvic organ prolapse, an evaluation by a multidisciplinary team (i.e. surgeon, gynecologist, urologist) for a combined surgical repair procedure may be required, depending upon the symptoms and patient risk profile. One NSQIP study [20] of 3600 patients undergoing rectopexy along with sacro-colpopexy, demonstrates that the combined procedure adds 67 minutes to the operative time when compared to rectopexy alone, and did not increase hospital stay or 30-day complications.

Preoperative evaluation

1. Preoperative workup for GA including cardiopulmonary status evaluation.

2. *Sigmoido/colonoscopy*: Sigmoidoscopy helps to look for rectal ulcers, or SRUS, in young patients with bleeding. However, in elderly patients, colonoscopy may rule out other pathology (e.g. malignancy) which warrant specific treatment.

3. *Defecography*: Not useful in external rectal prolapse; nevertheless imaging is useful in patients for whom the prolapse cannot be reproduced on physical examination, or when symptoms are present suggestive of additional pelvic floor disorders [21,22]. Defecography, either via traditional fluoroscopy or dynamic magnetic resonance imaging (MRI), can reveal defects associated with rectal prolapse in up to 80% of patients with obstructive defecation symptoms [23].

4. *Anal manometry*: Anal manometry serves as a useful baseline assessment of sphincter function, as the internal anal sphincter muscle weakens from chronic dilation and can demonstrate low resting pressures. Manometry would objectively document sphincter pressures to help predict continence following repair and the potential need for postoperative biofeedback, although studies show it rarely changes the operative approach [24,25]. Paradoxical puborectalis contraction (PPC) can also be seen in patients with obstructed defecation syndrome (ODS). Pelvic floor dyssynergia is a contraindication for rectopexy.

5. *Transanal ultrasonography (US)*: Transperineal US is not indicated in external rectal prolapse and does not reliably predict internal rectal prolapse. Done by an expert in pelvic floor US, it can demonstrate pelvic floor descent on straining. 3D US can accurately perform sphincter mapping in patients with fecal incontinence.

6. *MR defecography*: Nowadays considered to be a gold standard investigation for pelvic floor descent. The landmarks to be seen are descent below the pubococcygeus (PC) line on rest, and straining. The H Line and M Line denotes the widening of the pelvic hiatus and pelvic descent, respectively. Depending on the level of descent, many studies have classified the severity of descent into mild, moderate, and severe.

7. *Colonic transit study*: It is performed for operative candidates who have a severe or longstanding history of constipation to determine if a sigmoid colectomy, or even total abdominal colectomy, is indicated to treat the constipation associated with the prolapse.

8. *Pelvic physiology studies*: Anorectal physiology studies, including electromyography (EMG) and pudendal nerve terminal motor latency (PNTML) testing, have been commonly used in patients with fecal incontinence secondary to obstetrical injuries, although their use in patients with procidentia with incontinence has been less extensively studied.

Preoperative preparation

It is similar to any laparoscopic colorectal procedure, including bowel preparation, DVT prophylaxis, and protocols for ERAS.

Operative principles for posterior suture/mesh/resection rectopexy

The techniques used for rectal mobilization (anterior vs. posterior) and rectopexy (suture vs. mesh), as well as the surgical approach (open, laparoscopic, or robotic) are not standardized and depend upon the surgeon's preference and expertise [26].

OR setup

OR setup is similar to laparoscopic rectal resection. If resection is definitely not planned, the patient is placed in a supine position.

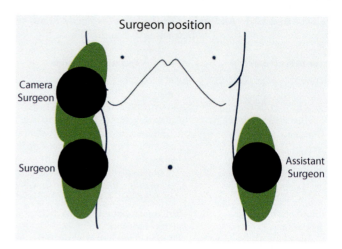

FIGURE 14.2 The operating surgeon and the camera surgeon stand on the right side of the patient, and the monitor is positioned on the left side of the patient, facing the surgeon.

After anesthesia, it is important to check in a left lateral position that the prolapse is completely reduced, or else it should be done before painting and draping. If there is any possibility that the sigmoid colon may need any resection, the patient is placed in a low lithotomy position similar to that for an anterior resection. The operating surgeon and the camera surgeon stand on the right side of the patient, and the monitor is positioned on the left side of the patient, facing the surgeon (Figure 14.2). The assistant surgeon stands on the left of the patient.

Port placements

Our preferred port placement is similar to the standard five port placement for laparoscopic colorectal surgery (Figure 14.3). The 10 mm 0-degree telescope port is at the umbilicus. The other four ports are all 5 mm ports. The variations in port placement would be to avoid one assistant port, or to use all 5 mm ports with 5 mm telescope in thin lean patients, where the needle can be inserted from the skin directly.

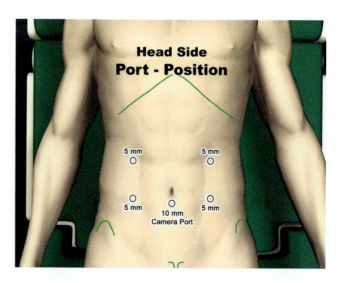

FIGURE 14.3 Port placement is similar to the standard 5 port placement for laparoscopic colorectal surgery.

Operative steps of laparoscopic suture/resection rectopexy

1. Complete posterior rectal mobilization
2. Limited lateral and anterior mobilization
3. Preservation of autonomic nerves
4. Hitching the rectum to the sacral promontory after traction
5. Sigmoid resection and rectopexy for severe constipation and redundant sigmoid

Operative techniques

Lap suture rectopexy (see Video 10): The first step of any abdominal procedure is to mobilize the rectum. Although surgeons differ in their techniques of rectal mobilization (posterior, anterior, or a combination of both), it is generally agreed that the lateral stalks of the rectum should be preserved during dissection because they contain nerves that innervate the rectum. Division of the lateral stalks during rectal mobilization may cause worsening or new-onset constipation postoperatively. However, preservation of the lateral stalks may increase the recurrence rate of rectal procidentia. The hypogastric nerves are preserved at the level of the sacral promontory and in the posterior dissection of rectum (Figure 14.4). In women, mobilize the rectum anteriorly to the level of the mid to upper-third of the vagina. In men, mobilize the rectum anteriorly for a few centimeters to allow for straightening of the rectum and additional scarring. After complete rectal mobilization, rectopexy is performed by affixing the pararectal tissue to the presacral fascia/sacral periosteum in the sacral promontory using nonabsorbable sutures or mesh. Place two nonabsorbable sutures (e.g. 00 Ethibond™ or Prolene™) in the presacral fascia/sacral periosteum approximately 1 cm apart in a horizontal mattress fashion (Figure 14.5a,b). To avoid accidental ligation of the blood supply, kinking of the bowel, or damage to the underlying nerves sutures should be placed only on one side of the rectal mesentery.

Lap Posterior Mesh Rectopexy (Wells): After complete rectal mobilization as described above, mesh rectopexy requires affixing a piece of mesh to the sacrum with sutures or tacks, and affixing the rectum to the mesh with sutures. Depending upon the

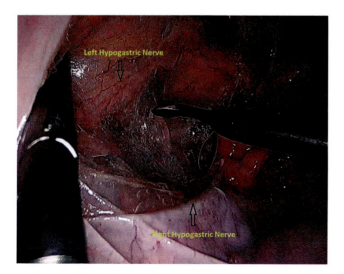

FIGURE 14.4 Hypogastric nerves are preserved at the level of the sacral promontory and in the posterior dissection of the rectum.

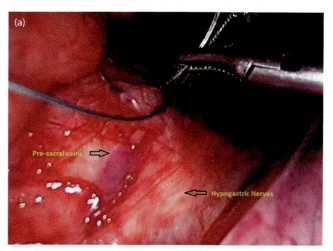

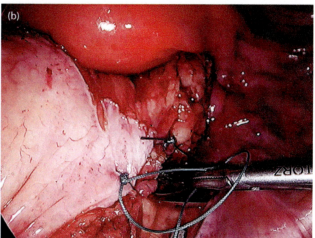

FIGURE 14.5 (a,b) Suture rectopexy, with presacral fascia/sacral periosteum in a horizontal mattress fashion.

technique used, the mesh can be placed posterior or anterior to the rectum. The posterior mesh rectopexy (Wells procedure) is similar to the anterior mesh rectopexy, except that the mesh is secured to the sacrum between the posterior rectum and sacral promontory.

Lap resection Rectopexy (see Video 12): If the sigmoid colon is redundant in a patient with preexisting constipation and a rectal procidentia, a sigmoid resection is typically performed with through rectopexy. The distal transection is at the level of the sacral promontory, after complete rectal mobilization and rectal traction (Figure 14.6). The proximal transection level is identified by selecting the location where there is no tension on the anastomosis and no residual redundant descending/sigmoid colon. In patients who undergo a sigmoid resection, rectopexy is typically performed after the sigmoid anastomosis for technical reasons (Figure 14.7).

LVMR (see Video 11): In a ventral rectopexy, the rectum is mobilized anteriorly, but not posterolaterally [27]. Following mobilization, the anterior wall of the rectum is sutured to a long strip of mesh that is affixed to the sacral promontory (Figure 14.8). Ventral mesh rectopexy is typically performed without a concomitant sigmoid resection. Both biologic and nonabsorbable meshes have been used [28]. Anterior mobilization of the distal rectum and mesh suspension performed during ventral mesh rectopexy can correct not only rectal procidentia but also rectoceles and internal rectal prolapse, and can be combined with

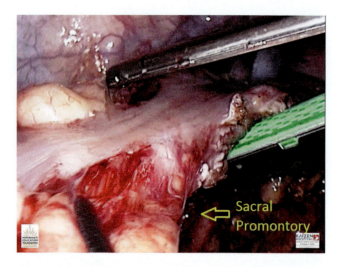

FIGURE 14.6 Distal transection at the level of the sacral promontory after complete rectal mobilization and rectal traction.

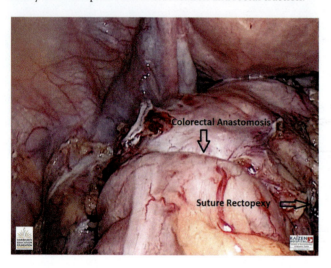

FIGURE 14.7 A rectopexy is typically performed after the sigmoid anastomosis – just distal to the anastomosis – in patients who undergo a sigmoid resection.

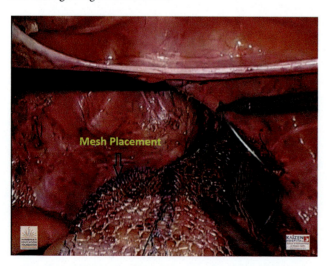

FIGURE 14.8 Following anterior mobilization, the anterior wall of the rectum is sutured to a long strip of mesh that is affixed to the sacral promontory.

vaginal prolapse procedures, such as sacrocolpopexy, in patients with multicompartment pelvic floor defects [29]. A ventral mesh rectopexy can be carried out laparoscopically, and has a low rate of postoperative constipation because of its avoidance of posterolateral rectal mobilization. A recent trial [30] concluded that ventral mesh rectopexy is an effective procedure for treating PFD, exhibiting a low rate of complications and an acceptable rate of recurrence.

Anterior sling rectopexy (Ripstein's): Anterior mesh rectopexy (Ripstein's procedure) incorporates an anteriorly based mesh sling for fixation of the rectum to the sacral hollow. The original Ripstein procedure was associated with a high complication rate because the mesh completely encircled the rectum anteriorly, causing obstruction or mesh erosion. A modified Ripstein procedure uses posterior fixation of the mesh to the sacrum with attachment of the ends of the mesh to the rectum laterally. Ripstein's operation is rarely performed today.

Postoperative care and early outcomes

The typical postoperative course includes early ambulation and initiation of enteral feeding after both perineal and abdominal repairs. Enhanced recovery protocols in colorectal surgery should be utilized to optimize postoperative care. Patients are encouraged to have oral liquids after 4–6 hours, and semisolid diet is advanced on 1–2 days. Patients are generally discharged home in 3–4 days. Few centers have performed these as day care surgeries.

For patients with a history of constipation, an aggressive bowel regimen is maintained for the first 1–2 weeks following surgery to avoid constipation and excessive straining that may lead to recurrence of rectal procidentia. Most patients will be able to return to normal activities, including work, in four weeks after surgery. Heavy lifting or straining of the abdominal and perineal muscles is to be avoided until the muscles are fully healed in approximately a few month's time.

Postoperative complications

1. *Recurrence*: Recurrence of complete rectal prolapse after rectal prolapse repair has been reported as high as 10%–20%. It is a relatively uncommon complication when rectopexy is performed, with reported rates of 0%–9% in laparoscopic rectopexy, compared with 0%–13% and 5%–20% in open rectopexy and perineal repairs, respectively [16,31,32]. There are very few reports on the ideal treatment for recurrence. Systematic review of the literature has failed to develop an algorithm for treatment of recurrent rectal prolapse [33]. Steele et al. reported significantly more re-recurrences following a perineal procedure, when compared with an abdominal surgery after reoperation for recurrent external rectal prolapse [34]. In one study, focused on laparoscopic ventral rectopexy for recurrent prolapse [35], the 5-year re-reccurence rates were 25% and 9.7% in recurrent and primary LVR, respectively. The authors concluded that patients with recurrent prolapse, especially if their initial procedure was a Delorme, should be counseled that they are at an increased risk for prolapse recurrence.

2. *Constipation*: Postoperative constipation after posterior mesh rectopexy stands around or even exceeds the 50% threshold, this being the case when the procedure is performed either via an open or laparoscopic approach [36,37]. Laparoscopic ventral rectopexy, however, appears to result in less constipation, with reported improvement rates of 72% [38].

3. *Urinary and sexual dysfunction*: A study [39] of 217 patients undergoing LVMR demonstrated that the number of sexually active patients decreased from 71% before surgery, to 54% at FU, while satisfaction rates remained relatively unchanged. In conclusion, the impact of LVR on the SF of patients seemed limited in this study.

4. *Mesh related complications*: The systematic review of Abed et al. [40] showed a mesh erosion rate of 10.3% (110 studies, range 0% to 29.7%) within 12 months after transvaginal pelvic organ prolapse repair, which has brought this important issue into the spotlight. In general, mesh complication rates of 0%–6.7%, along with mesh erosion contributing between 0% and 3.7% are described [41,42]. Erosion of the mesh, although rare, can result in significant morbidity and pose a surgical challenge during its management. A review [43] concluded that, though this rare complication is amenable to corrective surgery, its morbidity needs to be considered in the argument of mesh vs. sutured rectopexy.

5. Vertebral discitis is a rare but debilitating complication and is more frequently reported in recent studies [44].

Long-term functional results

The long-term results of different procedures are summarized in a table as below (Table 14.2):

Minimally invasive surgery (e.g. laparoscopic, laparoscopic-assisted, or robotic-assisted): It has the advantages of reduced postoperative pain, early return of bowel function, and shortened length of hospital stay. But also the disadvantages of longer operating times, more specialized technical skills and costly equipment, higher rates of intraoperative complications (e.g. bowel injury), and selective patient eligibility (e.g. lack of extensive intra-abdominal adhesions, tolerance of pneumoperitoneum) [45]. Robotic-assisted surgery combines the advantages of laparoscopic surgery (e.g. less postoperative pain, faster recovery) with those of open surgery (e.g. high-quality 3D vision, restoration of the eye-hand-target axis), but has as well the disadvantages of high costs, higher recurrence rates, and long procedure times [46–48].

Laparoscopic suture rectopexy (LSR): In a study evaluating long-term follow-up after LSR for 10 years [49], the authors concluded that LSR led to few complications, had an actuarial recurrence rate of 20%, improved continence and quality of life with no worsening of constipation at 10 years. The meta-analysis by Sajid et al. of 668 patients undergoing either laparoscopic rectopexy or open rectopexy showed no statistical difference in recurrence ($p = 0.51$), incontinence ($p = 0.57$), or constipation ($p = 0.82$) between the two groups [16]. This concurred with the subsequent meta-analysis carried out by Cadeddu et al. [50]. This meta-analysis summarized the results of published trials (Table 14.3).

Laparoscopic resection rectopexy (LRR): In a 20-year study from Germany, 264 patients underwent laparoscopic resection rectopexy for ODS [51]. The mortality rate was 0.75% (n = 2), the rate of complications requiring surgical re-intervention was 4.3% (n = 11), and the rate of minor complications was 19.8% (n = 51). Follow-up data were available for 161 patients with a mean follow-up of 58.2 months (±47.1 months). Long-term results showed that 79.5% of patients (n = 128) reported at least an improvement of symptoms.

Laparoscopic Ventral Mesh Rectopexy (LVMR): In a meta-analysis of 789 patients in 12 nonrandomized studies of LVMR, the pooled recurrence rate was 3.4% [11]. Complications occurred in 14% to 47% of patients. In all 12 studies, the fecal incontinence rate was lower after than before surgery, with a decrease of 45%. Constipation rates decreased after surgery in 24% of patients. A cohort of 245 consecutive patients analyzed by Formijne et al. demonstrated that there was a significant correlation to support the use of laparoscopic ventral rectopexy when considering the complications of constipation and incontinence [52]. They found that there was statistically significant data demonstrating a reduction in constipation ($p < 0.001$) and incontinence ($p < 0.001$) in their patient group. D'Hoore et al.'s work appears to support this with 28 out of 31 patients with incontinence experiencing a significant improvement in continence, and 16 out of 19 patients with constipation stating their symptoms had resolved [10]. In a nationwide study of 4304 patients from France [53] in age groups >70 years, the minor morbidity rate was <10%, whereas major complication

TABLE 14.2: Outcome of Laparoscopic Procedures for Pelvic Floor Disorders (Rickert et al. [15])

	Minor Complication	Major Complication	Mortality	Conversion	Incontinence	Constipation	Recurrence
LSR	0%–16%	2%–11%	0%	0%–5%	48%–82%(+)	11%(−)–70%(+)	2%–20%
LMR	0%–5%	0%–3%	0%	0%–3%	76%–92%(+)	38%(−)–36%(+)	1.3%–6%
LVR	0%–36%	0%–5%	0%–0.4%	0%–7.4%	70%–90%(+)	60%–80%(+)	0%–14%
LRR	11%–21%	0%–4%	0%–0.8%	0%–6%	62%–94%(+)	53%–80%(+)	0%–11%

TABLE 14.3: Summary of Results in Meta-Analysis (Cadeddu et al. [50])

Technique No. of Trials/Year	No. of Points	Continence Improved	Constipation Improved	Recurrence Range (%)	Follow up Months
Open Suture Rectopexy 6 trials, 1983–2009	287	15%–81%	30–83%	3%–9% (4%)	4–144
Open Mesh Rectopexy 15 trials, 1972–2000	1155	3%–78%	0%–69%	0%–9% (4%)	24–84
Lap Suture Rectopexy 7 trials, 1999–2007	180	0%–82%	0%–76%	0%–7% (2.5%)	24–67
Lap Mesh Rectopexy 13 trials, 1999–2008	607	10%–92%	19%–80%	0%–7% (2.6%)	18–106
Open Resection Rectopexy 7 trials, 1985–1999	393	11%–90%	18%–56%	0%–8% (4%)	17–98
Lap Resection Rectopexy 6 trials, 1998–2005	244	38%–100%	8%–76%	0%	12–36

rates were <1%. The mortality was 0.04%. The authors concluded that LVMR appears to be safe in select elderly patients.

VMR has, especially in Europe, emerged as the preferred treatment for full-thickness rectal prolapse to obtain the best postoperative functional results. The only randomized controlled double-blind trial to compare preoperative to postoperative changes in functional outcome, between LVMR and laparoscopic posterior sutured rectopexy (LPSR), was not able to show that VMR was superior to PSR in terms of functional outcome at one year for full-thickness rectal prolapse [54].

In a large cohort of 919 patients undergoing LVMR, 919 consecutive patients (869 women and 50 men) underwent LVR. A 10-year recurrence rate of 8.2% (95% confidence interval, 3.7–12.7) for external rectal prolapse repair was noted. Mesh-related complications were recorded in 18 patients (4.6%), of which mesh erosion to the vagina occurred in seven patients (1.3%). In five of these patients, LVR was combined with a perineotomy. The rates of both fecal incontinence and obstructed defecation decreased significantly ($p < 0.0001$) after LVR compared to the preoperative incidence (11.1% vs. 37.5% for incontinence and 15.6% vs. 54.0% for constipation) [55].

In a recent large meta-analysis of 17 studies comprising 1242 patients of a median age of 60 years, conversion to open surgery was required in 22 (1.8%) patients. The mean complication rate was 12.4%, and the mean rate of recurrence of full-thickness external rectal prolapse was 2.8%. The median follow-up duration was 23 months. Male patients ($p = 0.008$) and length of the mesh <20 cm were significantly associated with full-thickness recurrence of rectal prolapse. The rates of improvement in fecal incontinence and constipation after LVMR were 79.3% and 71%, respectively [56].

In a study [57] of LVR, 52 adult male patients with symptoms caused by external rectal prolapse underwent ventral rectopexy. A total of nine (17.3%) patients faced complications. There were two (3.8%) serious surgical complications during the 30-day period after surgery that necessitated reoperation. None of the complications were mesh-related. Recurrence of the prolapse was noticed in nine patients (17%), and postoperative mucosal anal prolapse symptoms persisted in 11 patients (21%). As a result, the reoperation rate was high. Altogether, 17 patients (33%) underwent reoperation during the follow-up period due to postoperative complications, or recurrent rectal or mucosal prolapse. They concluded that the ventral rectopexy technique should be modified or combined with other abdominal or perineal methods when treating male rectal prolapse patients. A word of caution for the widespread adoption of LVR has been sounded in another recent article, without high quality evidence [58].

In a study [59] comparing LRR and LVR for external rectal prolapse, both LRR and LVR seemed safe and suitable treatment strategies for external RP. Although there were more complications in the LRR cohort, this technique might offer better improvement in incontinence.

Robotic rectopexy

The robot enhances visualization and maneuverability to improve complex tasks in the deep pelvis, such as dissection and intracorporeal suturing [29]. Three recent studies, using synthetic mesh, discussed the complication rate following robotic ventral mesh rectopexy (RVMR) [60–62]. Robotic surgery showed a nonsignificant minimal advantage in terms of intra and postoperative complications compared to LVMR, as described in a meta-analysis of these three studies [63]. However, the studies were small and follow-up was short. A recent randomized trial [64] comparing laparoscopic and RVMR concluded that robot-assisted ventral mesh rectopexy

is more expensive than LVMR in the short-term, but incremental cost-effectiveness of RVMR may be acceptable at two and five years, suggesting this technique may offer value for the money. The current evidence [65] shows that LVMR and RVMR are safe procedures in terms of intraoperative, postoperative, and mesh-related complications. Both LVMR and RVMR generate an acceptable recurrence rate and satisfactory improvement of functional outcome, with only one small laparoscopic cohort reporting an overall nonsignificant deterioration with obstructed defecation after surgery [66]. There may be a trend towards a better outcome for obstructed defecation following RVMR as compared to LVMR, but the level of evidence is low [67]. LVMR and RVMR show similar good results for improvement of fecal incontinence. Based on the currently available data, no superiority for either technique can be determined.

Perineal procedures: The of two most commonly used perineal procedures are perineal rectosigmoidectomy (Altemeier procedure) and perineal mucosal stripping and muscle plication for rectal prolapse (Delorme procedure). In a randomized comparison involving 213 patients, the two perineal procedures achieved similar functional outcomes and recurrence rates [68].

Summary

Rectal prolapse is often a debilitating condition and surgery is necessary for adequate treatment. Deciding what surgical approach to offer is challenging [69], and this is made more so by the lack of clear guidelines and the evolution in the techniques available. The perineal approaches have historically been preferred for aged patients, or those with significant comorbid conditions, but abdominal procedures, with their improved durability and minimally invasive techniques, should be increasingly considered for most patients. Prior to treating a prolapse, a thorough evaluation – to identify slow transit constipation or other pelvic floor organ prolapse – is critical, so that the operative approach and involvement of multidisciplinary teams can be adjusted as necessary. Though technically challenging, laparoscopic ventral rectopexy is emerging as the procedure with good functional improvement, and acceptable recurrence and complications rates. Whether it is better performed with traditional multiport laparoscopy versus the robotic platform remains to be determined. Patients must be warned that not all disordered functions will improve with surgery. While fecal incontinence often improves, it may not totally resolve. Depending on the procedure performed, constipation may improve, remain the same, worsen, or in some cases, appear *de novo*. These steps can help ensure patient satisfaction and surgical success. The recent concerns about mesh erosion in LVMR point the authors of this review, in their clinical practice work, towards preferring a conventional posterior rectopexy with suture fixation to the sacrum for the treatment of full-thickness rectal prolapse [70]. For many patients with internal rectal prolapse and ODS, the authors do choose a LVMR, which has given good results.

Key points

- Rectal prolapse is a multifactorial and multicompartmental disease. It needs a thorough preoperative evaluation and multidisciplinary care in 25% of patients.
- Most patients with external prolapse need surgery. For patients with internal rectal prolapse abdominal rectopexy is increasingly becoming the procedure of choice, even among elderly patients.
- Minimally invasive options, such as laparoscopic and the robotic procedures, are increasingly being used and have given similar long-term results.

- Perineal operations are less commonly employed and are reserved for high-risk patients unable to tolerate GA.
- Laparoscopic suture rectopexy, laparoscopic resection rectopexy, and laparoscopic ventral mesh rectopexy have all shown good results in terms of low complications, low recurrence, and improvement in constipation and incontinence.

Videos

VIDEO 10   https://youtu.be/ypJvDAzUT9I

Laparoscopic Suture Rectopexy.

VIDEO 11   https://youtu.be/nt7I69C_uJ4

Laparoscopic Ventral Rectopexy.

VIDEO 12   https://youtu.be/3NHtvHMhEeY

Laparoscopic Resection Rectopexy.

References

1. Carrasco AB. *Contribution a l Etude du Prolapsus du Rectum.* Paris: Masson, 1934.
2. Cutait D. Sacro-promontory fixation of the rectum for complete rectal prolapse. *Proc R Soc Med.* 1959;52(Suppl):105.
3. Lloyd-Davies OV. Rectal prolapse: President's address. *JR Soc Med.* 1955;48:33–44.
4. Deucher F. Ventral rectopexy in the treatment of rectal prolapse. *Helv Chir Acta.* 1960;27:240–6.
5. Nigro ND. A sling operation for rectal prolapse. *Proc R Soc Med.* 1970;63(Suppl 1):106–7.
6. Nicholls RJ, Simson JN. Anteroposterior rectopexy in the treatment of solitary rectal ulcer syndrome without overt rectal prolapse. *Br J Surg.* 1986;73:222–4.
7. Bachoo P, Brazzelli M, Grant A. Surgery for complete rectal prolapse in adults. *Cochrane Database Syst Rev.* 2000:CD001758.
8. Karas JR, Uranues S, Altomare DF et al. No rectopexy versus rectopexy following rectal mobilization for full-thickness rectal prolapse: A randomized multicenter trial. *Dis Colon Rectum.* 2011;54:29–34.
9. Berman IR. Sutureless laparoscopic rectopexy for procidentia. Technique and implications. *Dis Colon Rectum.* 1992;35:689–93.
10. D'Hoore A, Cadoni R, Penninckx F. Long-term outcome of laparoscopic ventral rectopexy for total rectal prolapse. *Br J Surg.* 2004;91(11):1500–5.
11. Samaranayake CB, Luo C, Plank AW, Merrie AE, Plank LD, Bissett IP. Systematic review on ventral rectopexy for rectal prolapse and intussusception. *Color Dis.* 2010;12(6):504–12.
12. Wijffels NA, Collinson R, Cunningham C, Lindsey I. What is the natural history of internal rectal prolapse? *Color Dis.* 2010;12:822–30.
13. Van der Schans EM, Paulides TJ, Wijfels NA, Consten CJ. Management of patients with rectal prolapse: The 2017 Dutch guidelines. *Tech Coloproctol* 2018. https://doi.org/10.1007/s10151-018-1830-1.
14. Formijne Jonkers HA, Draaisma WA, Wexner SD, Broeders IA, Bemelman WA, Lindsey I, Consten EC. Evaluation and surgical treatment of rectal prolapse: An international survey. *Colorectal Dis.* 2013;15:115–9.
15. Rickert A, Kienle P. Laparoscopic surgery for rectal prolapse and pelvic floor disorders. *World J Gastrointest Endosc.* 2015 September 10;7(12):1045–54.
16. Sajid MS, Siddiqui MR, Baig MK. Open vs laparoscopic repair of full-thickness rectal prolapse: A re-meta-analysis. *Colorectal Dis.* 2010;12:515.
17. Mahmoud SA, Omar W, Abdel-Elah K, Farid M. Delorme's Procedure for Full-Thickness Rectal Prolapse; Does it Alter Anorectal Function. *Indian J Surg.* 2012;74:381.
18. Shin EJ. Surgical treatment of rectal prolapse. *J Korean Soc Coloproctol.* 2011;27(1):5–12.
19. Faucheron J-L, Trilling B, Girard E, Sage PY, Barbois S, Reche F. Anterior rectopexy for full-thickness rectal prolapse: Technical and functional results. *World J Gastroenterol.* 2015;21:5049–55.
20. Geltzeiler CB, Birnbaum BH, Silviera ML et al. Combined rectopexy and sacrocolpopexy is safe for correction of pelvic organ prolapse. *Int J Colorect Dis.* Pub online Aug 2018. https://doi.org/10.1007/s00384-018-3140-5.
21. Okamoto N, Maeda K, Kato R et al. Dynamic pelvic three-dimensional computed tomography for investigation of pelvic abnormalities in patients with rectocele and rectal prolapse. *J Gastroenterol.* 2006;41:802.
22. Hecht EM, Lee VS, Tanpitukpongse TP et al. MRI of pelvic floor dysfunction: Dynamic true fast imaging with steady-state precession versus HASTE. *AJR Am J Roentgenol.* 2008;191:352.
23. Mellgren A, Bremmer S, Johansson C et al. Defecography. Results of investigations in 2,816 patients. *Dis Colon Rectum.* 1994;37:1133.
24. Glasgow SC, Birnbaum EH, Kodner IJ et al. Preoperative anal manometry predicts continence after perineal proctectomy for rectal prolapse. *Dis Colon Rectum.* 2006;49:1052.
25. Woods R, Voyvodic F, Schloithe AC et al. Anal sphincter tears in patients with rectal prolapse and faecal incontinence. *Colorectal Dis.* 2003;5:544.
26. Felt-Bersma RJ, Tiersma ES, Cuesta MA. Rectal prolapse, rectal intussusception, rectocele, solitary rectal ulcer syndrome, and enterocele. *Gastroenterol Clin North Am.* 2008;37:645.
27. D'Hoore A, Penninckx F. Laparoscopic ventral recto(colpo)pexy for rectal prolapse: Surgical technique and outcome for 109 patients. *Surg Endosc.* 2006;20:1919.
28. Ogilvie JW Jr, Stevenson AR, Powar M. Case-matched series of a non-cross-linked biologic versus non-absorbable mesh in laparoscopic ventral rectopexy. *Int J Colorectal Dis.* 2014;29:1477.
29. Gurland B. Ventral mesh rectopexy: Is this the new standard for surgical treatment of pelvic organ prolapse? *Dis Colon Rectum.* 2014;57:1446.
30. Mäkelä-Kaikkonen JM, Rautio T, Kairaluoma M et al. Does Ventral Rectopexy Improve Pelvic Floor Function in the Long Term? *Dis Colon Rectum.* 2018;61:230–8.
31. Kairaluoma MV, Viljakka MT, Kellokumpu IH. Open vs.laparoscopic surgery for rectal prolapse: A case-controlled studyassessing short-term outcome. *Dis Colon Rectum.* 2003;46:353–60.
32. Rothenhoefer S, Herrle F, Herold A et al. DeloRes trial: Study protocol for a randomized trial comparing two standardizedsurgical approaches in rectal prolapse – Delorme's procedure versus resection rectopexy. *Trials.* 2012;13:155.
33. Hotouras A, Ribas Y, Zakeri S et al. A systematic review of the literature on the surgical management of recurrent rectal prolapse. *Color Dis.* 2015;17:657–64.
34. Steele SR, Goetz LH, Minami S, Madoff RD, Mellgren AF, Parker SC. Management of recurrent rectal prolapse: Surgical approach influences outcome. *Dis Colon Rectum.* 2006;49(4):440–5.
35. Gurland B, E Carvalho MEC, Ridgeway B, Paraiso MFR, Hull T, Zutshi M. Should we offer ventral rectopexy to patients with recurrent external rectal prolapse? *Int J Colorectal Dis.* 2017;32(11):1561–1567.
36. Benoist S, Taffinder N, Gould S, Chang A, Darzi A. Functional results two years after laparoscopic rectopexy. *Am J Surg.* 2001;182:168–73.
37. Aitola PT, Hiltunen K-M, Matikainen MJ. Functional results ofoperative treatment of rectal prolapse over an 11-year period: Emphasis on transabdominal approach. *Dis Colon Rectum.* 1999;42:655–60.

38. Boons P, Collinson R, Cunningham C, Lindsey I. Laparoscopic ventral rectopexy for external rectal prolapse improvesconstipation and avoids *de novo* constipation. *Color Dis.* 12:526–32.

39. Formijne Jonkers HA, Poierrié N, Draaisma WA et al. Impact of rectopexy on sexual function: A cohort analysis. *Int J Colorectal Dis. 2010*; June 2013. DOI 10.1007/s00384-013-1736-3.

40. Abed H, Rahn DD, Lowenstein L, Balk EM, Clemons JL, Rogers RG; Systematic Review Group of the Society of Gynecologic Surgeons. Incidence and management of graft erosion, wound granulation, and dyspareunia following vaginal prolapse repair with graft materials: A systematic review. *Int Urogynecol J.* 2011;22:789–98.

41. Smart NJ, Pathak S, Boorman P, Daniels IR. Synthetic or biological mesh use in laparoscopic ventral mesh rectopexy--a systematic review. *Colorectal Dis.* 2013;15:650–4.

42. Evans C, Stevenson AR, Sileri P, Mercer-Jones MA, Dixon AR, Cunningham C, Jones OM, Lindsey I. A Multicenter Collaboration to Assess the Safety of Laparoscopic Ventral Rectopexy. *Dis Colon Rectum.* 2015;58:799–807.

43. Patil NS, Saluja SS, Mishra PK et al. Intrarectal migration of mesh following Rectopexy: Case series and review of literature. *Int J Surg.* 2015;20:145–8.

44. Probst P, Knoll SN, Breitenstein S, Karrer U. Vertebral discitis after laparoscopic resection rectopexy: A rare differential diagnosis. *J Surg Case Rep.* 2014;2014(8).

45. Purkayastha S, Tekkis P, Athanasiou T et al. A comparison of open vs. laparoscopic abdominal rectopexy for full-thickness rectal prolapse: A meta-analysis. *Dis Colon Rectum.* 2005;48:1930.

46. Munz Y, Moorthy K, Kudchadkar R et al. Robotic assisted rectopexy. *Am J Surg.* 2004;187:88.

47. Heemskerk J, de Hoog DE, van Gemert WG et al. Robot-assisted vs. conventional laparoscopic rectopexy for rectal prolapse: A comparative study on costs and time. *Dis Colon Rectum.* 2007;50:1825.

48. de Hoog DE, Heemskerk J, Nieman FH et al. Recurrence and functional results after open versus conventional laparoscopic versus robot-assisted laparoscopic rectopexy for rectal prolapse: A case-control study. *Int J Colorectal Dis.* 2009;24:1201.

49. Foppa C. Martinek L, Arnaud JP, Bergamaschi R. Ten-year follow up after laparoscopic suture rectopexy for full-thickness rectal prolapse. *Colorect Dis.* 2014;16:809–14.

50. Cadeddu F, Sileri P, Grande M, De Luca E, Franceschilli L, Milito G. Focus on abdominal rectopexy for full-thickness rectal pro-lapse: A meta-analysis of the literature. *Tech Coloproctol.* 2012;16:37–53.

51. Laubert T, Kleemann M, Roblick UJ, Burk C, Hildebrand P, Lewejohann J, Schloricke E, Bruch HP. Obstructive defecation syndrome: 19 years of experience with laparoscopic resection Rectopexy. *Tech Coloproctol.* 2013;17:307–14.

52. Formijne Jonkers HA, Poierrie N, Draaisma WA, Broeders IAMJ, Consten ECJ. Laparoscopic ventral rectopexy for rectal prolapse and symptomatic rectocele: An analysis of 245 consecutive patients. *Color Dis.* 2013;15:695–9.

53. Gultekin FA, Wong MTC, Podevin J, Barussaud ML, Boutami M, Lehur PA, Meurette G. Safety of Laparoscopic Ventral Rectopexy in the Elderly: Results From a Nationwide *DatabaseDis Colon Rectum.* 2015;58:339–43.

54. Lundby L, Iversen LH, Buntzen S et al. Bowel function after laparoscopic posterior sutured rectopexy versus ventral mesh rectopexy for rectal prolapse: A double-blind, randomised single-centre study. *Lancet Gastroenterol Hepatol.* 2016. http://dx.doi.org/10.1016/S2468-1253(16)30085-1.

55. Consten ECJ, Iersel JJ, Verheijen PM et al. Long-term Outcome After Laparoscopic Ventral Mesh Rectopexy. An Observational Study of 919 Consecutive Patients. *Ann Surg.* 2015;262:742–8.

56. Emile SH, Elfeki H, Shalaby M et al. Outcome of laparoscopic ventral mesh rectopexy for full–thickness external rectal prolapse: A systematic review, meta–analysis, and meta–regression analysis of the predictors for recurrence. *Surg Endos.* Apr 2019;33:2444–55.

57. Rautio T, Kaikkonen JM, Vaarala M et al. Laparoscopic ventral rectopexy in male patients with external rectal prolapse is associated with a high reoperation rate. *Tech Coloproctol.* 2016;20:715–20.

58. Lundby L, Laurberg S. Laparoscopic ventral mesh rectopexy for obstructed defaecation syndrome: Time for a critical appraisal. *Colorectal Dis.* 2014;17, 102–3.

59. Formijne Jonkers HA, Maya A, Draaisma WA et al. Laparoscopic resection rectopexy versus laparoscopic ventral rectopexy for complete rectal prolapse. *Tech Coloproctol.* Feb 2014;18(7):641–6.

60. Wong MT, Meurette G, Rigaud J, Regenet N, Lehur PA. Robotic versus laparoscopic rectopexy for complex rectocele: A prospective comparison of short-term outcomes. *Dis Colon Rectum.* 2011;54:342–6.

61. Mäkelä-Kaikkonen J, Rautio T, Klintrup K et al. Robotic-assisted and laparoscopic ventral rectopexy in the treatment of rectal prolapse: A matched-pairs study of operative details and complications. *Tech Coloproctol.* 2014;18:151–5.

62. Mantoo S, Podevin J, Regenet N, Rigaud J, Lehur PA, Meurette G. Is robotic-assisted ventral mesh rectopexy superior to laparoscopic ventral mesh rectopexy in the management of obstructed defaecation? *Colorectal Dis.* 2013;15:e469–75.

63. Rondelli F, Bugiantella W, Villa F, Sanguinetti A, Boni M, Mariani E, Avenia N. Robot-assisted or conventional laparoscoic rectopexy for rectal prolapse? Systematic review and meta-analysis. *Int J Surg.* 2014;12(Suppl2):S153–9.

64. Kaikkonen JM, Rautio T, Ohinmaa A et al. Cost–analysis and quality of life after laparoscopic and robotic ventral mesh rectopexy for posterior compartment prolapse: A randomized trial. *Tech Coloproct,* publ online May 2019; 23:461–70.

65. Lersel JJ, Paulides TJC, Verheijen PM, Lumley JW, Broeders IA, Consten ECJ. Current status of laparoscopic and robotic ventral mesh rectopexy for external and internal rectal prolapse. *World J Gastroenterol,* 2016 June 7;22(21):4977–87.

66. van den Esschert JW, van Geloven AA, Vermulst N, Groenedijk AG, de Wit LT, Gerhards MF. Laparoscopic ventral rectopexy for obstructed defecation syndrome. *Surg Endosc.* 2008;22:2728–32.

67. Mäkelä-Kaikkonen J, Rautio T, Pääkkö E, Biancari F, Ohtonen P, Mäkelä J. Robot-assisted versus laparoscopic ventral rectopexy for external, internal rectal prolapse and enterocele: A randomised controlled trial. *Colorectal Dis.* 2016;18(10):1010–15

68. Senapati A, Gray RG, Middleton LJ et al. PROSPER: A randomised comparison of surgical treatments for rectal prolapse. *Colorectal Dis.* 2013;15:858.

69. Hrabe J, Gurland B. Optimizing Treatment for Rectal Prolapse. *Clin Colon Rectal Surg.* 2016;29:271–6.

70. Karagulle E, Yildirim E, Turk E, Akkaya D, Moray G. Mesh invasion of the rectum: An unusual late complication of rectal prolapse repair. *Int J Colorectal Dis.* 2006;21:724–7.

Chapter 15

LAPAROSCOPIC-ASSISTED STOMAS AND STOMA REVERSAL

Fazl Q Parray and Zamir A Shah

Contents

Learning objectives 85
Laparoscopic stoma formation. 86
Loop ileostomy 86
Loop stoma reversal 86
Colostomy 86
    Sigmoid colostomy 86
    Transverse colostomy. 87
    Sigmoid stoma reversal (Hartmann's reversal) 87
    Operative approach 87
    SILS stoma 88
Complications 88
Summary 88
Key points 88
Videos 88
References 88

Learning objectives

- Know about various indications for forming stomas such as an ileostomy or colostomy
- Become acquainted with technicalities of laparoscopic stoma formation
- Learn about the technicalities of laparoscopic stoma reversal

An ostomy is a purposeful anastomosis between a segment of the gastrointestinal tract and the skin of the anterior abdominal wall [1]. An ostomy can be created virtually anywhere along the gastrointestinal tract. For diversion of the fecal stream, the most common ostomies involve the distal small intestine (e.g. ileostomy) and large intestine (i.e. colostomy). Permanent or temporary fecal diversion is necessary for the surgical management of a wide variety of colorectal conditions. Permanent diversion is needed when diseases like carcinoma rectum involve the sphincter complex, or when the sphincter mechanism is badly damaged secondary to other nonmalignant diseases. Temporary or diverting stomas are needed in a variety of surgeries such as low anterior and ultralow resections, ileal pouch anal anastomosis, coloanal anastomosis, transanal transabdominal resections (TATA), transanal total mesorectal excisions (TaTME), complex ano-rectal fistulas, ano-rectal traumas, recto-vaginal fistulas, perineal floor reconstruction, perineal burn injuries, large bowel obstructions, and unresectable malignancies before down staging. These temporary or diverting stomas are constructed mainly with an aim to give healing time to a distal anastomosis and to prevent reconstructive procedures from a fecal infection.

Minimally invasive techniques have been applied with increasing frequency to intestinal surgical procedures. Although stoma creation and end stoma reversal have traditionally required formal laparotomy or a mini laparotomy, these procedures are well suited for a minimally invasive approach in the hands of an expert laparoscopic surgeon. A minimally invasive approach avoids a large abdominal incision and therefore minimizes postoperative pain, ileus, and wound complications. Other advantages may include a lesser use of postoperative narcotics, shorter hospital stays, and earlier initiation of other therapies such as chemotherapy or radiation therapy [2–4].

Over the last decade, laparoscopic stoma formation has gained wide acceptance as an alternative to open abdominal surgery [5–9]. When compared to open techniques, the laparoscopic approach carries several potential advantages including earlier return to bowel function, less pain, less morbidity, and shorter hospital stays [10,11]; however, at the cost of an increased operating time and an increased learning curve for the surgeon. The other big advantage of laparoscopy, which probably remains under emphasized, is that it is more evidence-based and all of the surgeon's assistants are also watching and contributing under the magnified view displayed on the screen – ensuring better teaching and learning of the whole team. LS creation not only minimizes surgical trauma but also allows the inspection of the intra-abdominal cavity, and if necessary, possible biopsies of any suspected lesions.

Laparoscopic ileostomy and colostomy is an effective treatment for several benign and malignant disorders. Laparoscopic multi-port stoma creation is considered safe and feasible having low morbidity, as well as ensuring better visualization and identification of bowel loops and the ileo-caecal and recto-sigmoid junction, except in some difficult cases with multiple surgeries and dense adhesions.

When feasible, laparoscopic ostomy formation is preferred to ostomy formation by laparotomy or mini laparotomy. Obesity and cardiopulmonary morbidity are no longer considered absolute contraindications to laparoscopy. In fact, if pneumoperitoneum can be safely established and maintained, these patients may fare better in the postoperative setting. There are no randomized trials comparing ostomy creation via traditional open surgical approaches versus minimally invasive approaches. However, multiple observational studies have documented the safety and favorable short-term outcomes of laparoscopic ostomy creation in comparison to surgery requiring a laparotomy [12–15].

Laparoscopic ostomies may also be easier to reverse [16]; probably for the reasons of less hand handling of gut, which subsequently may result in less postoperative adhesions, thus facilitating the ease of returning the gut to the peritoneal cavity.

The main technical principles for optimal stoma construction include proper stoma siting on the abdominal wall, adequate mobilization of the bowel, preservation of the blood supply, and eversion of the bowel wall during stoma maturation. Most laparoscopic techniques use two to three trocars, including one positioned through the premarked ostomy site. In our colorectal division at the Sher-i-Kashmir Institute of Medical Sciences, in Srinagar, we ensure (as a protocol) to have stoma sites marked preoperatively by our stoma therapists, which definitely ensures the proper stoma sitting and decreases the postoperative morbidity associated with them. Preoperative stoma marking, postoperative stoma care, and selection of appropriate stoma appliances by stoma therapists have proved significant factors in decreasing the morbidity and improving the overall quality of life in our stoma patients. Conversion to open surgery is uncommon, ranging from 0% to 16%, with more recent studies reporting rates in the single digits [17–19]. The rate of conversions will ultimately decrease in every setup, as soon as one negotiates the learning curve of laparoscopy.

Laparoscopic stoma formation

Laparoscopic stoma formation provides an improved anatomical view for stoma formation and abdominal exploration. Improved visualization offers a more accurate choice of bowel for stoma creation, especially in obese patients. The said, the procedure is carried out under general anesthesia in a supine position. The technique for laparoscopic stoma creation is not standardized, but certain general principles do apply.

Loop ileostomy

Preoperatively, the patient should be marked to ensure optimal trocar placement. Bowel preparation should be used to ensure easier bowel handling. Pneumoperitoneum can be established via an open or a closed technique at the umbilical port. Once the camera has been inserted through a 10 mm umbilical port, the surgeon determines where additional ports can be safely inserted; one more 10 mm port can be put at a four finger breadths down from the umbilical port but in the mid clavicular line, and one more 5 mm port can be made at a two finger breadths above the symphysis pubis. It is advantageous if one trocar can be placed through the marked stoma location for assistance in mobilization.

The patient is placed in a head-down and left-up position and try to identify the ileo–cecal junction. For an ileostomy, terminal ileal adhesions and mesenteric bands may need to be lysed. Go approximately 15 cm proximal to this junction towards the ileum and mark the distal side of the ileum with a double clip (D for distal, D for double). Put one more clip 6 cm proximal to the double clip to mark the proximal side. Try to catch the center of the ileum between the marked clips with the right-sided trocar and cut a two finger breadth parietal wall disc around the trocar, and deliver the marked ileal loop from this cut area. Remove laparoscopic instruments from the abdomen to avoid any inadvertent injury to bowel loops after loss of pneumoperitoneum. Rotate the marked loop to get the distal end proximally on stoma site and ensure that at least 6 cm of loop, or both markers, are above the skin level. Fix the everted loop at the 3 and 9 o'clock positions with an absorbable suture with fascia. Incise two-thirds of the circumference 1 cm away from the double clip mark to construct a mucous fistula, and then intussuscept the

proximal loop on the single clip side on itself in order to make a stoma pout. The mucous fistula site should be fixed to the skin with a 2 bite technique: one on the ileal edge and one on the skin. The stoma pout should be fixed to the skin with a 3 bite technique: one on the ileal edge, one on the ileal wall, and one on the skin edge to hold the pout eversion. The advantage of having the mucous fistula proximally and pout distally is that contents from the pout go easily in the stoma bag, rather than spilling in the mucous fistula. Clean the area nicely after completing the procedure – wipe it dry and apply a see-through stoma bag on the loop ileostomy. The advantage of a 'see-through bag' is that one can easily observe for any color changes, edema, or congestion of the stoma.

Loop stoma reversal (see Videos 5 and 6)

Stoma reversal should never be taken lightly. This surgery can invite more morbidity and even mortality in case the procedure is not planned properly. A proper evaluation should include:

- Exclusion of any recurrent or metastatic disease
- Ensuring that the distal anastomosis is not stenosed, which can be excluded through digital rectal examination or a cologram
- Ensuring that the rest of the gut distal to the stoma does not harbor any additional disease, which can be excluded by colonoscopy
- Ensure that the stoma closure is done at least 8 weeks after completion of adjuvant treatment, in order to encounter less adhesions and achieve a better immune status

Ideally loop stomas can be closed laparoscopically under general anesthesia. Patients are put in a supine position with a right up position. Disengage the loop, freshen the edges, push them inside the peritoneal cavity, close the stoma site using the umbilical port for the camera and two ports in the left mid-clavicular line at a four fingers breadths from each other. After pneumoperitoneum, identify the two ends and use an endo cartridge through the 12 mm port and perform side-to-side anastomosis. Then use one more endo cartridge to close the open ends transversely.

We do not find any specific advantage of this procedure laparoscopically. It is more time consuming, costlier, since the stoma opening is already present, even the cosmetic advantage is not much. We rather use a circular incision just on the mucocutaneous edge of the stoma, mobilize it all around until the peritoneal cavity, deliver the mobilized loops out, ensure that there are no injuries during adhesiolysis by leak test in both loops separately, then freshen the edges of the stoma without breaking the posterior wall and use interrupted 3–0 Vicryl for anastamosing the two ends of the ileum. After doing the leak test again, anastamosed bowel is returned to the peritoneal cavity. In case there is a need for resection, because of injury or perforation at the time of mobilization, then we perform resection of two ends to exclude injured parts, before anastomosis. We close the wound in layers, after putting in a subcutaneous drain. We mobilize subcutaneous tissue to facilitate the purse-string closure of the stoma site, which then produces a very small and acceptable scar after a few weeks.

Colostomy

Sigmoid colostomy

Patient should be placed in a supine position under general anesthesia. A 10 mm umbilical port is used for the camera. In the right mid clavicular line, use an upper 5 mm port situated at four finger breadths lateral and oblique to the umbilical port, then use a 10 mm port at 4 finger breadths below this port as a working port. On left side, use a premarked stoma site as one more port for holding and ultimately delivering the gut. Give a head down and left up position to the operation table. In case of a sigmoid stoma, the bowel is mobilized by incising the lateral peritoneal attachments. The proposed bowel for stoma is grasped with an Endo-Babcock. The skin and fascia are incised around the port site, and the loop of bowel delivered for stoma creation. The preference of the surgeon and the indication for stoma creation will dictate the need for a loop or end stoma. Ensure a good mobilization before the final delivery of the loop in order to avoid any traction on the stoma, which may lead to retraction or ischemia of the stoma.

In cases where a 'long Hartmann's stump' is left behind, the distal end may be tucked at the site of the actual stoma. This may be placed in either a subfascial or subcutaneous position. Eventual reversal should then require nothing more than a peristomal incision, rather than a full laparotomy.

In construction of a loop, or end colostomy, we do not need a pout-like ileostomy; rather, we need to fix the gut with fascia with two stitches in case of a temporary stoma, or four stitches in case of a permanent end stoma, then the circumferential margins are fixed all around flush to the skin. In case of a loop, there will be two openings, one for excreta and one as a mucous fistula; however, with an end stoma, there will be only one opening. At the end of procedure, clean the area and fix a stoma bag.

Most commonly, however, a Hartmann's colostomy is performed for rectosigmoid disease. Therefore, the rectal stump is left within the pelvis, and prevented from dropping into the lower pelvis by tacking the rectum to the promontory of the sacrum or the anterior abdominal wall using Prolene™ sutures. These sutures also assist in eventual laparoscopic identification of the staple line. In the case of resection for diverticular disease, care must be taken to resect the entire distal sigmoid colon. Leaving behind only the rectum simplifies the reversal, as further bowel resection will not be needed. It is also important not to dissect the presacral space unnecessarily during the initial colon resection. Any dissection will result in fibrosis of this plane, complicating Hartmann's reversal.

During bowel exteriorization and subsequent inspection of bowel orientation laparoscopically, the loss of pneumo-peritoneum may produce some difficulty. The trocar can be placed through the ostomy site and secured to the peritoneum. The peritoneum is subsequently incised and the stoma brought out without much difficulty.

When creating an ostomy laparoscopically, particular attention should be paid to avoid twisting of the exteriorized bowel (for a loop ostomy), or kinking of the mesentery (for an end ostomy). Marking proximal and distal ends and repeating peritoneal insufflation may be used to confirm the correct orientation of the bowel after it is passed through the fascia [20].

Transverse colostomy
The same principles can be applied except that besides the umbilical camera port, the other ports may be placed on two sides in the mid clavicular lines, taking care of the phenomenon of triangulation with the surgeon. The surgeon can position himself in between legs in lithotomy position with head up position.

Sigmoid stoma reversal (Hartmann's reversal)
At times, this continues to be a very demanding and difficult surgery. Always seek consent for reversal, and never forget to explain that in case of severe adhesions, or a frozen pelvis, one may not be able to reverse it. Too much adhesiolysis, or unnecessary heroics, at the time of reversal may invite more morbidity and even mortality.

The preoperative workup before planning a stoma closure should include a total colonic evaluation using a cologram/pouchogram or colonoscopy via the stoma and rectum to guide the surgical approach. The presence of any remaining distal sigmoid colon, the location of the Hartmann's stump, the length of residual descending colon, the height of the splenic flexure, as well as the presence of other colonic disease can be thus ascertained. In case of malignancy, proper evaluation for disease recurrence, progression or synchronicity should be ruled out before contemplating stoma reversal.

There are very few contraindications for a laparoscopic reversal. If none of the steps described above have been taken, the reversal process will be much more complicated, leading to a much higher rate of conversion. In addition, if diffuse purulent or feculent peritonitis was present at the index resection, one would expect dense adhesions.

Operative approach
The patient is subjected to general anesthesia and placed in a low lithotomy position. A 10 mm umbilical port is made for the camera, another 5 mm port is situated mid clavicular, obliquely up at four fingers breadths from the umbilicus, and a 10 mm port four fingers breadths down from this port. Position patient in head down and left up. Examine the abdominal cavity thoroughly in detail. Lyse adhesions if any, mobilize the left colon, identify and mobilize the rectal stump. Once satisfied that the anastomosis of the two ends can be achieved with ease and comfort, only then proceed for the stoma take down. Release it completely from surrounding parietal wall. Fix an anvil of circular stapler in this end with 2−0 Prolene™. The laparoscopic instruments and trocars should be out as you lose pneumoperitoneum at the time of take down, then push the stoma with the anvil inside the peritoneal cavity, and close the stoma opening. Reestablish pneumoperitoneum and the ports, use a grasper to hold the anvil in the proper orientation towards the rectum. Ask your assistant to come from the perineal side, and dilate the anal opening gently using two fingers and jelly. Push the circular stapler gently inside the rectum until you see from inside the stretched out end of the circular stapler in the rectum. Start opening the stapler until it penetrates the rectum and you can see the brown mark. Engage the anvil into the stapler until you hear a self-locking click. Then tell your assistant to start closing the circular stapler, taking care of the proper orientation of the stump, and ensuring that no other structure gets nipped between the two ends of the anastomosis. Close the circular stapler completely, until you see the green mark in the index window, then wait for 30 seconds until tissue edema is squeezed out, then disengage the lock and fire the stapler.

Hold it there for a minute or so to achieve hemostasis. Open the stapler circular knob by two turns, then bring out the stapler gradually with fishtail movements. Examine both the doughnuts for completeness. Push normal saline in the pelvis and perform a leak test by pushing 50 cc of air from the anal side and blocking the gut proximal to the anastomosis by a gentle push of the grasper. Ensure there is no leak, if there is some leakage then one may need to take some remedial measures such as putting a stitch, or a proximal diversion like a loop ileostomy. Use one of the port sites to push in a tube drain, which should be placed in the pelvis behind the anastomosis and fixed with skin. Clean the abdomen, deflate pneumoperitoneum and close the port sites, sealing them with dressings.

There are several adjuncts that may be of assistance during the laparoscopic dissection. If difficulty is encountered, a hand-assist device may be placed at the stoma site, as a bridge to converting to open surgery. In many cases, the vagina or bladder will become adhered to the rectal stump. Identification of the correct tissue planes may be enhanced by placing a dilator in the rectum or vagina, or filling the bladder with saline. Prior to anastomosis, if the original pathology was diverticular disease, any remaining sigmoid colon must be resected.

SILS stoma

Single-incision laparoscopic stoma creation is an effective technique that allows full intra-abdominal visualization and bowel mobilization, while reducing the need for additional skin incisions beyond that of the stoma site [21]. SILS stoma for transverse loop colostomy represents a feasible surgical procedure, allowing stoma creation at the ideal stoma sites marked preoperatively. Reductions in the number of port sites, and the avoidance of additional skin incisions, may result in improved cosmetic outcomes and quality of life for the patient [22]. SILS is a minimally invasive technique, suitable for patients in whom the stoma site was preoperatively decided [23].

Complications

The overall morbidity of laparoscopic stoma creation is low, but complications such as stoma or small bowel obstruction can be significant. Early postoperative blockage of the stoma or small bowel is often related to intraoperative events like twisting of the bowel as it is brought out through the abdominal wall, or maturing the wrong limb of the bowel in the case of an end stoma. Contributing factors leading to such complications include obesity, a redundant colon, or using the small bowel with its free mesentery that can easily twist. Several techniques are available to avoid twisting of the bowel, or maturing the wrong limb of the stoma. Intracorporeal marking of the proximal and distal limb of the bowel with clips or sutures of different colors can be helpful for proper identification of the bowel, once exteriorized. In the case of an end stoma, intracorporeal transection of the bowel and grasping the proximal end prior to creating the stoma trephine is another approach. Intra-abdominal inspection and visualization of the bowel with the camera can be performed after the stoma is matured, but this is not an option with the two-trocar technique. Although all these steps are effective, they do contribute to additional operative time, as in the case of intracorporeal suturing, or the added cost of a clip applier or stapler [24].

Summary

Laparoscopy has become one of the most acceptable and sought after surgical procedure for most abdominal surgeries because of less pain, earlier return to work, and better cosmesis. Even though gastrointestinal stomas are usually psychologically traumatic procedures, laparoscopies performed in good centers and trained hands have made them more acceptable compared to open stoma surgeries. The latter, because of large laparotomy scars, invariably make the results cosmetically more unsightly and predispose patients to more surgical site infections and longer hospital stays – making them more prone to adhesions and obstructions, which adds to the burden of a messy and mutilating surgery at the time of stoma reversal. This is usually avoided in laparoscopic stoma creation and stoma reversal. In addition to the advantages already mentioned, it also allows the surgeon a chance to have a look on the other abdominal viscera in order to rule out any metastatic disease.

Key points

- Laparoscopy allows the surgeon to visualize the whole gut with a magnified view.
- Laparoscopy orients the surgeon more optimally to identify the proper loop before delivering it outside.
- Laparoscopic stoma creation and reversal requires expert hands to make the procedure more patient friendly.

Videos

VIDEO 5   https://youtu.be/iaZh1qDX6Fs

Restoration of Loop Ileostomy – Part 1.

VIDEO 6   https://youtu.be/5_9yFGlfcTA

Restoration of Loop Ileostomy – Part 2.

References

1. Cataldo PA. Technical tips for stoma creation in the challenging patient. *Clin Colon Rectal Surg.* 2008;21:17–22.
2. Stephenson ER Jr, Ilahi O, Koltun WA. Stoma creation through the stoma site: A rapid, safe technique. *Dis Colon Rectum.*1997 ;40:112–5.
3. Young CJ, Eyers AA, Solomon MJ. Defunctioning of the anorectum: Historical controlled study of laparoscopic vs. open procedures. *Dis Colon Rectum.* 1998;41:190–4.
4. Anderson ID, Hill J, Vohra R, Schofield PF, Kiff ES. An improved means of faecal diversion: The trephine stoma. *Br J Surg.* 1992;79:1080–1.
5. Fuhrman GM, Ota DM. Laparoscopic intestinal stomas. *Dis Colon Rectum.* 1994;37:444–9.
6. Weiss UL, Jehle E, Becker HD, Buess GF, Starlinger M. Laparoscopic ileostomy. *Br J Surg.* 1995;82:1648.
7. Ludwig KA, Milsom JW, Garcia-Ruiz A, Fazio VW. Laparoscopic techniques for fecal diversion. *Dis Colon Rectum.* 1996;39:285–8.
8. Schwandner O, Schiedeck TH, Bruch HP. Stoma creation for fecal diversion: Is the laparoscopic technique appropriate? *Int J Colorectal Dis.* 1998;13:251–5.
9. Liu J, Bruch HP, Farke S, Nolde J, Schwandner O. Stoma formation for fecal diversion: A plea for the laparoscopic approach. *Tech Coloproctol.* 2005;9:9–14.
10. Lyerly HK, Mault JR. Laparoscopic ileostomy and colostomy. *Ann Surg.* 1994;219:317–22.
11. LoftJakobsen H, Harvald TB, Rosenberg J. No-trocar laparoscopic stoma creation. *Surg Laparosc Endosc Percutan Tech.* 2006;16:104–5.
12. Young CJ, Eyers AA, Solomon MJ. Defunctioning of the anorectum: Historical controlled study of laparoscopic vs open procedures. *Dis Colon Rectum.* 1998;41:190–4
13. Hollyoak MA, Lumley J, Stitz RW. Laparoscopic stoma formation for faecal diversion. *Br J Surg.* 1998;85:226–8.
14. Almqvist PM, Bohe M, Montgomery A. Laparoscopic creation of loop ileostomy and sigmoid colostomy. *Eur J Surg.* 1995;161:907–9.
15. Scheidbach H, Ptok H, Schubert D et al. Palliative stoma creation: Comparison of laparoscopic vs conventional procedures. *Langenbecks Arch Surg.* 2009;394:371–4.
16. Hiranyakas A, Rather A, da Silva G, Weiss EG, Wexner SD. Loop ileostomy closure after laparoscopic versus open surgery: Is there a difference? *Surg Endosc.* 2013;27:90–4.
17. Swain BT, Ellis CN Jr. Laparoscopy-assisted loop ileostomy: An acceptable option for temporary fecal diversion after anorectal surgery. *Dis Colon Rectum.* 2002;45:705–7.
18. Schwandner O, Schiedeck TH, Bruch HP. Stoma creation for fecal diversion: Is the laparoscopic technique appropriate? *Int J Colorectal Dis.* 1998;13:251–5.
19. Oliveira L, Reissman P, Nogueras J, Wexner SD. Laparoscopic creation of stomas. *Surg Endosc.* 1997;11:19–23.
20. Liu J, Bruch HP, Farke S, Nolde J, Schwandner O. Stoma formation for fecal diversion: A plea for the laparoscopic approach. *Tech Coloproctol.* 2005;9:9–14.

21. Miyoshi N, Fujino S, Ohue M et al. Standardized technique for single-incision laparoscopic-assisted stoma creation. *World J Gastrointest Endosc.* 2016;8(15):541–5.
22. Hasegawa J, Hirota HM, Kim S, Mikata J, Shimizu Y, Nezu R. Single-incision laparoscopic stoma creation: Experience with 31 consecutive cases. *Asian J Endosc Surg.* 2013(Aug);6(13):181–5.
23. Kengo H, Masanori K, Masahiro H et al. Laparoscopic versus Open stoma creation: A retrospective analysis. *J Anus Rectum Colon.* 2017;1(3):84–8.
24. Abbas MA, Tejirian T. Laparoscopic Stoma Formation. *JSLS.* 2008 Apr–Jun;12(2):159–61.

Chapter 16

LAPAROSCOPIC RESTORATIVE PROCTOCOLECTOMY AND ILEAL POUCH ANAL ANASTOMOSIS

Sanjiv Haribhakti and Rajat Srivastava

Contents

Learning objectives 90
Introduction 90
Goals of surgery 90
Surgical options 91
Selection of patients 91
Indications for RPC-IPAA 91
Contraindications for RPC-IPAA 91
Advantages of RPC-IPAA 92
Disadvantages of RPC-IPAA 92
Operative principles of laparoscopic assisted RPC-IPAA 92
Preoperative preparation 92
Operative steps 92
    OR setup 92
    Port placement philosophy 92
    Operative technique 93
Postoperative care and usual recovery 103
Postoperative complications – early and late 103
    Pouchitis 103
    Pouch failure 104
    Stricture 104
    Fecal incontinence 104
    Pouch dysplasia/cancer 105
    Sexual dysfunction 105
    Female infertility 105
    Anal transition zone inflammation 105
    Anal transitional zone dysplasia 105
Functional results of RPC-IPAA 105
Controversies 105
Authors' experience 106
Summary 106
Key points 106
Videos 106
References 107

Learning objectives

- To understand the goals of surgery
- To Know the surgical alternatives and appropriatey select patients for each options
- To learn the indications, contra-indications, advantages and disadvantages of RPC-IPAA
- To understand the operative princiles with special refernece to preoperative care, operative steps, postoperative care and complications
- To learn the prevention, mechanism and management of postoperative complications
- To be aware of the controversies of RPC-IPAA

Introduction

Restorative proctocolectomy (RPC) and ileal pouch anal anastomosis (IPAA) has become a standard procedure for surgical management of ulcerative colitis over the last 3–4 decades [1]. The results have been good to excellent in over 90% of patients, improving their quality of life [2]. This procedure has been successfully performed with the minimally invasive approach, minimizing the incision-related morbidity and optimizing the cosmesis in young patients [3]. There are several ways of performing a laparoscopic RPC-IPAA operation [4]. In this chapter, the author describes his standard method for performing this procedure for ulcerative colitis (UC).

Goals of surgery

1. Curing the disease by total proctocolectomy, as UC and familial adenomatous polyposis (FAP) are diseases restricted to the colon
2. Preventing complications of disease including acute complications, recurrent relapses, and risk of malignancy

3. Preventing risks of medical treatment including steroid complications, as well as complications of immunosuppressants and biologics
4. Improving quality of life
5. Alleviating the risk of malignancy

Surgical options

1. Restorative proctocolectomy and ileal pouch anal anastomosis (RPC-IPAA) is the first procedure of choice whenever feasible. A majority of patients with UC or FAP would be offered this procedure.
2. Total proctocolectomy and permanent ileostomy (TPC) is selected when patients have poor anal sphincter tone associated with incontinence; are unwilling to accept staged operations or long term functional results of RPC-IPAA; have severe colonic Crohn's disease; are medically unable to tolerate an extended operation (e.g. comorbidities, advanced age), have very low or ultra-low rectal cancer, not amenable to sphincter-sparing procedures [5].
3. Total colectomy (TC) and ileorectal anastomosis (IRA). In selected 5% of patients, who have rectal sparing ulcerative colitis, this option can be exercised with the understanding that they may be required to have rectum resection in the future if the disease recurs. This approach is indicated in clinical settings such as pregnancy, and acute fulminant colitis requiring emergent operative management. Other indications include extreme obesity, a narrow pelvis, and uncertainty of diagnosis, such as ulcerative colitis versus Crohn's disease [6–8]. This option is also useful for young female patients who have not yet completed their family, to prevent infertility after RPC-IPAA. Later, after their family is complete, they can undergo RPC-IPAA.
4. Total proctocolectomy and continent ileostomy (Koch), which is no longer an option today, as morbidity is much higher, and RPC-IPAA has produced better results.

Selection of patients

Mild to moderate disease can essentially be controlled with medical treatment. All patients who have severe disease, or who have repeated remissions and are young, should be counseled for possible surgical management. They should be explained in detail, the pros and cons of medical management versus surgical management. Patients should also be actively involved in the decision making, as well as the timing of surgery. Broadly, surgery should not be offered too early in the disease, neither should it be delayed when the patient becomes sick. In the natural history of the disease, which is quite unpredictable, when the disease becomes more active and more severe, and shows less response to medical treatment, needing more of immunosuppressants or steroids, one should start thinking and discussing surgical options [9–11]. The patient should ideally earn the surgery, when in a severe disease, he/she wants it as a one-time curative option.

Indications for RPC-IPAA

Elective indications: This is the most common setting for performing the operation. The broad indication is failure of medical management, which is poorly defined. Occasionally, in severe disease in young patients, the patient's preference for a one-time treatment is also a valid indication, provided the surgeon is experienced and can perform this procedure with acceptable morbidity and mortality. The main indications in elective setting include:

Definite indications:

1. Moderate or severe disease with repeated relapses affecting the quality of life
2. Moderate or severe intractable disease, causing malnutrition
3. Steroid dependent disease
4. Need for prolonged immunosuppressants or biologics
5. Steroid related toxicities
6. Diagnosis or suspicion of malignancy

Controversial indications:

7. Extracolonic complications
8. Pancolitis
9. Young patients
10. After acute severe colitis, once remission is achieved by steroids or biologics
11. Patient preference for a one-time treatment
12. Socio-economic reasons

Emergency: In an emergency, severe complications may require emergent or early surgery. The morbidity and mortality of these procedures are significantly higher than for the elective procedures.

1. Acute severe colitis, with no response to aggressive medical management, including steroids in 3–5 days
2. Acute severe colitis, failure of remission after biologics
3. Toxic megacolon
4. Severe lower GI bleeding
5. Colonic perforation

Contraindications for RPC-IPAA

Absolute contraindications:

1. The patient cannot tolerate a major surgery under GA or pneumoperitoneum due to severe cardiopulmonary disease.
2. *Inadequate sphincter function*: Should be assessed by a digital examination and squeeze in all patients before RPC-IPAA. Those patients who have an inadequate tone should undergo anorectal manometry and biofeedback to improve their tone. Patients with poor anal tone, or those who have incontinence should not be subjected to RPC-IPAA.
3. *Crohn's disease*: A biopsy of the colon and colonoscopic appearance should be assessed before surgery to rule out Crohn's disease. RPC-IPAA should not be performed in cases of suspected or proven Crohn's disease. In indeterminate colitis, we would prefer a 3-stage approach by doing a total colectomy and ileostomy, and decide for RPC-IPAA or ileorectal anastomosis for the next stage after the final biopsy is available.
4. Patients, especially the elderly, unwilling to accept the long-term functional results of RPC-IPAA – with a higher frequency of stool, 4 to 6 times in a day, occasional minor incontinence.

Relative contraindications:

1. *Morbid obesity*: This would cause difficulty in bringing the fatty mesentery down in spite of a lengthening procedure.
2. *Emergency surgery*: For acute severe colitis and its complications. Most surgeons would prefer a total colectomy and ileostomy rather than RPC-IPAA.

3. *Previous abdominal operations and adhesions*: It is a relative contraindication for the laparoscopic approach depending on the skill of the surgeon and the severity of adhesions.
4. Mild to moderate disease well controlled with medical management: Patients should not be subjected to the risks of RPC-IPAA.

Advantages of RPC-IPAA

1. *Cure for the disease*: Eliminates the colon, and cures the disease
2. Avoids the complications of disease such as repeated relapses, bleeding and severe acute complications
3. Avoids medical treatment and related morbidity and cost. Avoids the complications of repeated steroids, immuno-suppressants, and biologics
4. Preserves the sphincter
5. Significantly alleviates the risk of malignancy

Disadvantages of RPC-IPAA

1. Major procedure with significant morbidity and a small risk of mortality
2. Often needs two, or rarely, three stages
3. Functional results in the long term need to be accepted
4. Risk of pouchitis in the long term should be explained
5. One time cost of the procedure, and the use of staplers

Operative principles of laparoscopic assisted RPC-IPAA

1. Laparoscopic mobilization of the entire colon and rectum, including splenic and hepatic flexures
2. Ultralow rectal division on the pelvic floor just above the ATZ with a small rectal cuff
3. Minilaparotomy (periumbilical/pfannenstiel/stoma site) for specimen extraction or transanal specimen removal
4. Creation of 15 cm-long Ileal J-pouch by staple technique
5. Mobilization of DJ flexure and other maneuvers for tension free pouch anal anastomosis
6. Ileal J pouch anal anastomosis by circular stapled anastomosis, avoiding rotation and tension on the mesentery
7. Proximal diverting ileostomy, or transanal anastomotic drainage tubes
8. Stoma restoration 2–3 months later

Preoperative preparation

1. For general anaesthesia: Preoperative laboratory profile specifically including s. albumin; also, cardiopulmonary assessment for major surgery under GA
2. Evaluation for sepsis and malnutrition for severe disease and patients on immunosuppressants, steroids, or biologics
3. Mechanical bowel preparation and prophylactic antibiotics
4. DVT prophylaxis
5. ERAS protocols

Operative steps

OR setup

The patient is placed in a supine position in the operating room under general anesthesia, on a mechanized operating table that

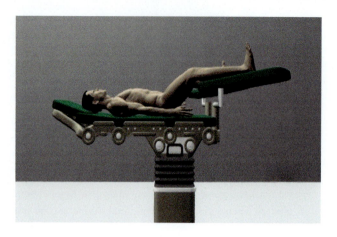

FIGURE 16.1 Patient position.

can go down low, up to 24 inches. The patient is placed in a lithotomy position with stirrups in such a way that the hip joint flexion is minimal and the thighs are almost in a straight line with the torso (Figure 16.1).

The OR Setup is arranged in such a way that the monitor faces the surgeon, just below eye level. It is advisable to have a large HD monitor for colorectal surgeries. Nowadays, as 4K or 3D camera systems are available, they have not been found to be superior to the currently used HD camera systems. An additional HD monitor is preferably placed opposite the assistant to give him/her an ergonomic view (Figure 16.2).

The surgeon stands opposite to the area of surgery, facing the disease. For left colonic or rectal resections, the surgeon is on the right side of the patient, and the camera surgeon is to the left of the surgeon, with the main monitor on the left side facing the surgeon (Figure 16.3). For right-sided colonic resections, the surgeon stands on the left side of the patient, with the camera surgeon on the left of the surgeon, or between the legs and the monitor is on the right side of the patient facing the surgeon (Figure 16.4). The assistant nurse is on the leg-end side of the table and for left resections, stands to the right of the patient, and for right resections stands to the left of the surgeon. All the laparoscopic cables and the camera cables come from the head-end side of the OR personnel.

Port placement philosophy

The port placement for all laparoscopic colorectal procedures is standardized. We use a five-port technique for lap RPC and IPAA. The standard five ports are placed in such a fashion that the 10 mm camera port is at the umbilicus, whereas all other four working ports are placed in the four quadrants of the abdomen (Figure 16.5). Occasionally, an additional sixth port is used in the epigastrium, or suprapubic location (Figure 16.6). The RIF port, which is the surgeon's right working port, is a 12 mm port (for stapled division of the low rectum) placed down low, at the level of the anterior superior iliac spine (ASIS), and is slightly lateral to the mid axillary line to get a good angle for rectal dissection and stapled low rectal division. The 5 mm port is in the right upper abdomen, which is the surgeon's left working port, and is slightly to the left of the midline. The two assistant 5 mm ports are at the mid axillary line, equidistant from the umbilicus and the ASIS for lower port, umbilicus and costal margin for the upper port. All the skin incisions for all ports, including the camera, should be such that the trocars fit snugly in the skin incision so they do not move during instrument exchanges, and do not come out accidentally. The sixth port in the suprapubic region is needed occasionally for uterine traction in females, or for vertical division of

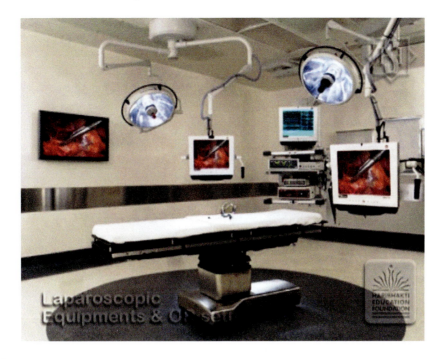

FIGURE 16.2 OR Setup.

the low rectum by stapler. The sixth port in the epigastrium is needed occasionally for splenic flexure mobilization from medial to lateral, using a supracolic approach.

We prefer to use a 10 mm straight viewing telescope for all colorectal resections, and have never switched to a 30-degree telescope. As the colon is freely mobile and viscous, through adequate traction most procedures – such as medial to lateral dissection, splenic flexure mobilization, and low rectal dissection – can easily be accomplished with a straight viewing telescope. The main reason for this preference is the wider view available and better orientation in the pelvis. Many surgeons are more comfortable

with a 30-degree telescope, and continue to use them. It is a matter of personal preference. The authors use a 30-degree telescope for all other laparoscopic procedures, including UGI, HPB, bariatric, and hernia surgeries, apart from colorectal procedures.

Operative technique

We adopt a standardized technique for lap RPC-IPAA, which we have standardized since 2006. We also published the first report of a single incision lap RPC-IPAA in 2015 [12]. There are several ways of doing this procedure; however, our standard method is described here in steps, as well as some variations:

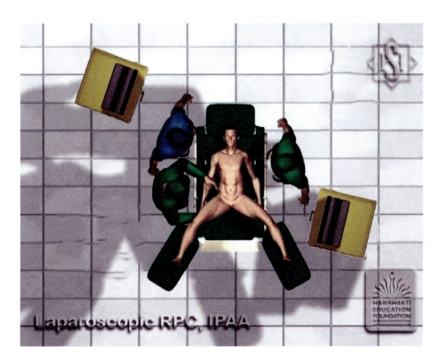

FIGURE 16.3 OR setup for left colonic or rectal resections, surgeon is on the right side of the patient.

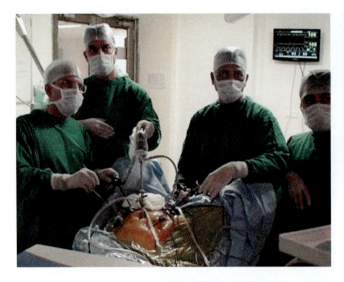

FIGURE 16.4 OR setup for right colonic resections, surgeon stands on the left side of the patient.

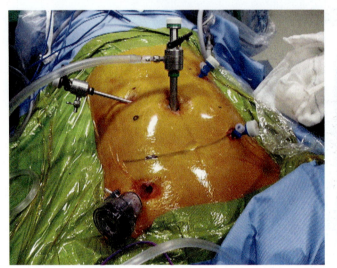

FIGURE 16.5 Standard 5 ports placement.

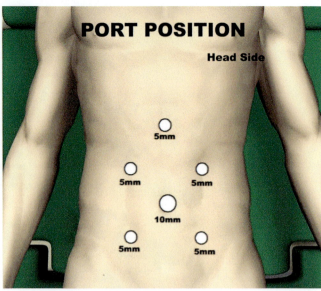

FIGURE 16.6 An additional 6th port is used in the epigastrium.

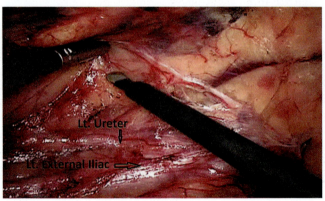

FIGURE 16.7 Medial to lateral dissection of left colon.

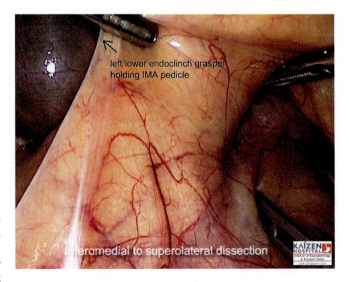

FIGURE 16.8 Left lower endoclinch grasper holds IMA pedicle and lifts pedicle to stretch the peritoneum.

1. *Left colon mobilization*: We first start with a left colonic mobilization. With the OR setup, and all ports inserted as explained above, initial assessment is performed. In a steep Trendelenburg position, the small bowel loops are retracted out of the pelvis with an atraumatic bowel grasper, and folded on themselves to see the DJ flexure clearly. The anesthetist is instructed to avoid nitrous oxide during the procedure to avoid bowel distension. We do not use epidural anesthesia for preventing bowel distension, as suggested by some authors.

   a. *Medial to lateral dissection*: The first step is to perform a medial to lateral dissection of the left colon, which essentially separates the mesocolic structures, such as IMA, from the retroperitoneal structures, such as the left ureter and left gonadal vein (Figure 16.7). The left lower endoclinch grasper holds the IMA pedicle and lifts the pedicle to stretch the peritoneum (Figure 16.8). The left upper endoclinch grasper holds the mesorectum at the rectosigmoid, and lifts it upwards to accentuate the peritoneal stretch (Figure 16.9). After visualization of the landmarks, such as the

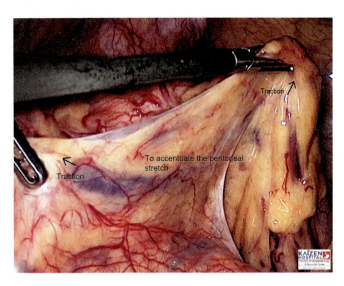

FIGURE 16.9 Left upper endoclinch grapser holds the meso-rectum at the rectosigmoid and lifts it upwards to accentuate the peritoneal stretch.

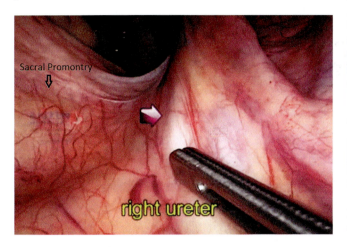

FIGURE 16.10 Visualization of the landmarks, sacral promontory, and right ureter.

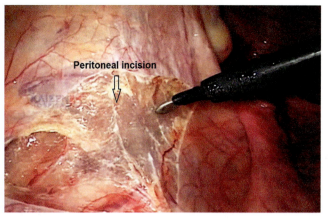

FIGURE 16.11 Peritoneal incision at the sacral promontory.

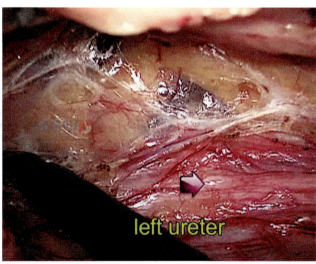

FIGURE 16.12 Identification of the left ureter, dissection proceeds in front of left ureter.

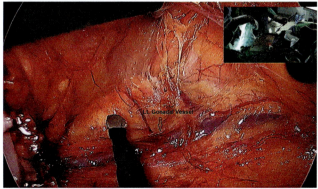

FIGURE 16.13 Identification of left gonadal vein, dissection proceeds in front of left gondal vein.

sacral promontory and the right ureter (Figure 16.10), a peritoneal incision is placed at the sacral promontory and extended cranially towards the root of IMA, and caudally towards the rectum (Figure 16.11). Medial to lateral dissection is done in the vascular areolar tissue plane accentuated by pneumoperitoneum. IMA and the mesocolic structures are dissected away from the retroperitoneal structures in the correct plane. The left ureter is always identified (Figure 16.12), and the dissection proceeds in front of the left ureter. Next, the left gonadal vein is identified (Figure 16.13), and the dissections proceeds in front of the left gonadal vein to reach up to the white line of Toldt, laterally (Figure 16.14).

b. *IMA ligation*: Now the IMA root is ligated with Hemolock™ clips (Figure 16.15) and divided distally. Further dissection demonstrates the inferior mesenteric vein(IMV), which is also ligated with Hemolock™ clips and divided (Figure 16.16).

c. *Splenic flexure mobilization*: The next step is to start the splenic flexure mobilization from medial to lateral in the infracolic tunnel behind the left mesocolon

(Figure 16.17). This dissection is extended in the avascular areolar tissue plane to separate the mesocolon from the left Gerota's fascia covering the left kidney, to reach up to the distal pancreas superiorly and splenic flexure and the descending colon laterally up to the white line of Toldt. The next step of splenic flexure mobilization involves medial to lateral dissection in

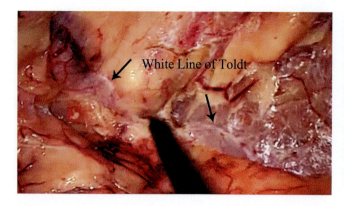

FIGURE 16.14 Dissection performed laterally till the white line of Toldt.

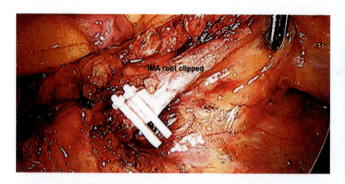

FIGURE 16.15 IMA root is ligated with hemolock clips and divided distally.

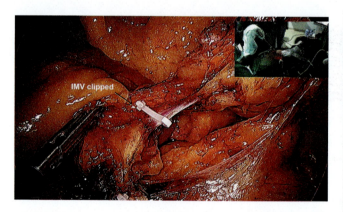

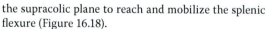

FIGURE 16.16 Inferior mesenteric vein (IMV), ligated with hemolock clips and divided.

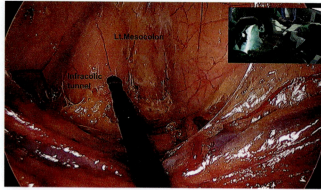

FIGURE 16.17 Splenic flexure mobilization from medial to lateral in the infracolic tunnel behind the left mesocolon.

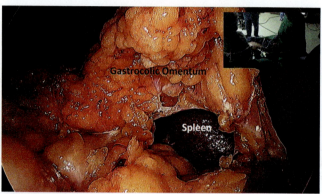

FIGURE 16.18 Splenic flexure mobilization involves medial to lateral dissection in supracolic plane.

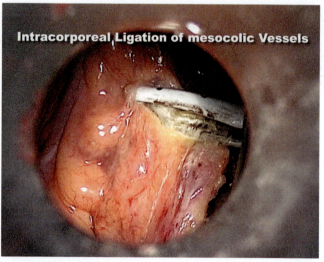

FIGURE 16.19 Left pericolic vessels, if divided intracorporeally.

the supracolic plane to reach and mobilize the splenic flexure (Figure 16.18).

   d. *Pericolonic vessels*: If the pericolic vessels are to be divided intracorporeally, it is done at this stage by lifting the mobilized left colon with both the assistant graspers (Figure 16.19), and dividing the pericolic vessels with Ligasure™ close to the colon, up to the distal transverse colon. This is an optional step, as with a periumbilical mini-laparotomy, the same step can be done extracorporeally.

   e. *Lateral colonic attachment*: Next, the lateral attachments of the left colon are divided starting from the sigmoid

colon (Figure 16.20). The two assistant graspers retract the left colon towards the right side, the lower one down on the floor and the upper one right and up. Once the peritoneum is divided, the previous plane of medial to lateral dissection is entered. The surgeon continues to divide the lateral attachments from the sigmoid (Figure 16.21a) to the descending colon and reaches to the splenic flexure (Figure 16.21b). The assistant grasper's traction

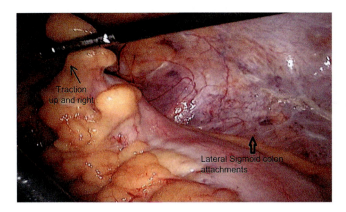

FIGURE 16.20 Lateral attachments of the sigmoid colon, divided by right-sided traction of the sigmoid colon.

needs to be changed as the dissection proceeds cranialy. Finally, the splenic flexure is completely mobilized from a lateral to medial approach, after detaching the gastrocolic omentum, and entering the lesser sac to visualize the posterior wall of the stomach (Figure 16.22a,b).

2. *Splenic flexure mobilization*: There are several ways and approaches to mobilize the splenic flexure, which is a very important step in left colorectal resections, especially lap RPC-IPAA and lap low anterior resection.
   a. *Infracolic – medial to lateral*: This approach has already been described above

b. *Supracolic – medial to lateral*: The gastrocolic omentum is detached from the distal transverse colon and proximal descending colon
c. *Lateral to medial*: As described above
d. *Top to down:* Final mobilization to check the complete mobilization

3. *Rectal mobilization*: The next step is to mobilize the rectum.
   a. *Right and posterior*: We start with the right and posterior mobilization of the rectum. With the upper assistant grasper pulling the rectum out and up (Figure 16.23), and the lower assistant grasper giving a countertraction, the surgeon dissects in the avascular plane with a monopolar spatula or hook. For the posterior mobilization, the assistant retracts the rectum anteriorly, and the surgeon dissects in the avascular holy plane, between the mesorectal fascia and presacral fascia, going down into the pelvis (Figure 16.24).
   b. *Left and posterior*: For dividing the left rectal attachments, the assistant retracts the rectum towards the right and the floor, with the upper grasper held at the rectosigmoid (Figure 16.25). The left attachments of the rectum are divided close to the rectum after identifying once again the left ureter.
   c. *Anterior peritoneum*: The anterior peritoneum is divided from the right to the left side after the assistant pulls the rectum with his upper grasper and gives and anterior countertraction with his lower grasper (Figure 16.26). In benign disease, as well as in most

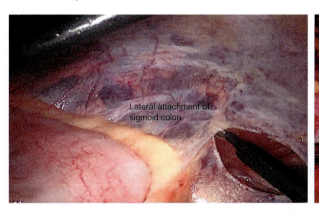
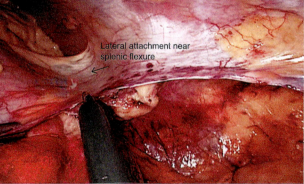

FIGURE 16.21 (a) Division of lateral attachments from the sigmoid colon. (b) Division of lateral attachments to reach until the splenic flexure.

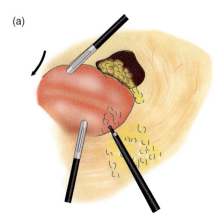
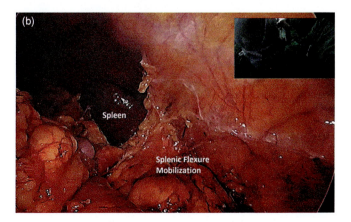

FIGURE 16.22 (a) Posterior mobilization of the splenic flexure from lateral to medial. (b) Complete mobilization of the splenic flexure.

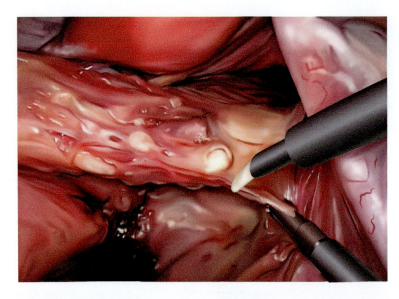

FIGURE 16.23   Right and posterior mobilization of the rectum, upper assistant grasper pulling the rectum out and up.

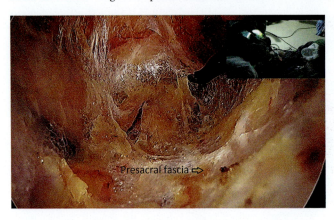

FIGURE 16.24   Posterior mobilization of the rectum in the avascular holy plane, between the mesorectal fascia and presacral fascia going down into the pelvis.

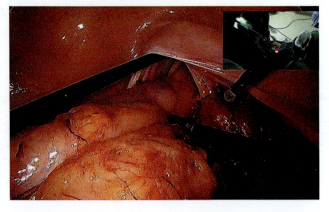

FIGURE 16.26   The anterior peritoneum is divided from right to the left side, after the assistant pulls the rectum with his upper grasper and gives anterior countertraction with his lower grasper.

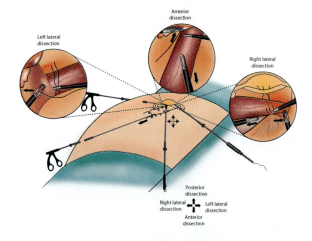

FIGURE 16.25   Left rectal lateral ligament division, the assistant retracts the rectum towards the right and the floor, with the upper grasper held at the rectosigmoid.

cases of malignancy, especially in males, the anterior dissection proceeds behind the Denonvillier's fascia to prevent injury to the autonomic nerves.

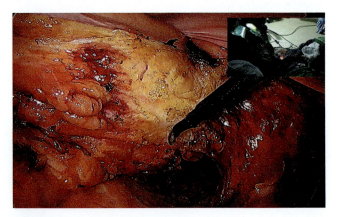

FIGURE 16.27   Right lateral ligaments are then divided close to the pelvic fascia one after the other.

d. *Lateral dissection*: Right and left lateral ligaments are then divided close to the pelvic fascia one after the other (Figures 16.27 and 16.28). The middle rectal vessels would need to be coagulated to prevent bleeding.

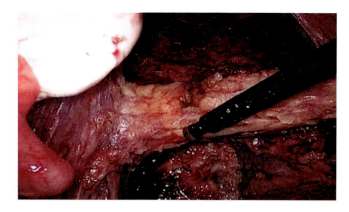

FIGURE 16.28 Left lateral ligaments are then divided close to the pelvic fascia one after the other.

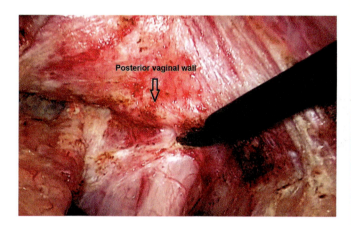

FIGURE 16.29 Anterior dissection is performed in females between the vagina and rectum.

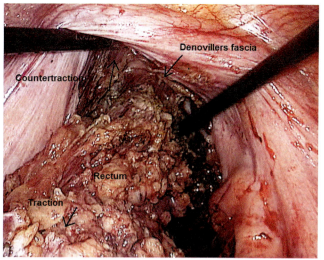

FIGURE 16.30 In males anterior dissection is behind the Denonvilier's fascia.

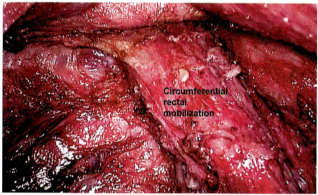

FIGURE 16.31 Circumferential dissection of the lowest portion of the rectum is done thoroughly before stapler division of the low rectum.

e. *Anterior dissection*: Further anterior dissection is performed in females between the vagina and the rectum to the lower most point, avoiding any injury to the vagina (Figure 16.29). In males, this dissection occurs behind the Denonvilier's fascia (Figure 16.30).

f. *Posterior dissection*: Finally, the complete posterior dissection is done.

g. Circumferential dissection of the lowest portion of the rectum is done thoroughly before the stapler division of low rectum (Figure 16.31).

4. *Low rectal division*: Is done with a roticulating stapler either 45 or 60 mm from the RIF port by pulling and stretching of the rectum by the assistant, initially to the left, for inserting the stapler in the lower rectum, and then to the right side, to see for correct application before firing (Figure 16.32a,b). A digital rectal examination should be done before firing the stapler to determine the level

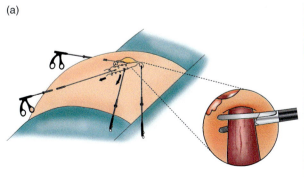

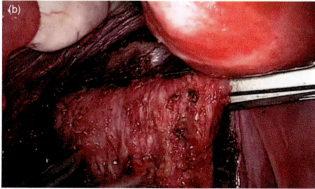

FIGURE 16.32 (a,b) Application of stapler in the lower rectum, and then to the right side to see for correct application before firing.

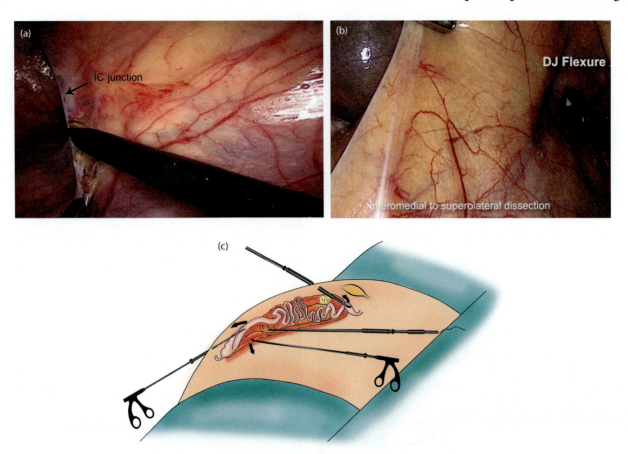

FIGURE 16.33   (a,b) The lower right grasper of the assistant holds and lifts the mesentery near the IC junction, and the upper right grapser holds and lifts the mesentery near the DJ flexure. (c) Complete view of the root of the mesentery elevated with both graspers in Chinese fan fashion.

of rectal division which should be 3–5 cm from the anal verge. A vaginal examination is optional in female patients when in doubt.

5. *Right colon mobilization*: For right colon mobilization, the entire surgical team shifts to the left of the patient, and the assistant to the right of the patient.

 a. *Inferomedial to superolateral*: In a steep Trendelenburg position, the small bowel loops are folded cranially by the surgeon with atraumatic bowel graspers. Next, the root of the mesentery is held up by the assistant for medial to lateral, or inferior to superior dissection of the right colon. The lower right grasper of the assistant holds and lifts the mesentery near the IC junction, and the upper right grasper holds and lifts the mesentery near the DJ flexure (Figure 16.33a,b). During this dissection, the second part of the duodenum is dissected away from the mesocolon medially, and laterally the Gerota's fascia is separated up to the hepatic flexure of the colon, in the avascular plane (Figure 16.34) up to the white line of Toldt.

 b. *Gastrocolic omentum*: Dissected away from the right colon close to the colon.

 c. *Pericolonic vessels*: If the pericolonic vessels are taken intracorporeally, then this step is now performed as in the left colon, starting from the transverse colon and going towards the ileocaecal region, remaining close to the colon using Ligasure™ (Figure 16.35).

 d. *Hepatic flexure mobilization*: For this step, the patient is placed in straight position, with a 20 degree Trendelenburg and right-side elevated. The gastrocolic omental is detached from the proximal transverse

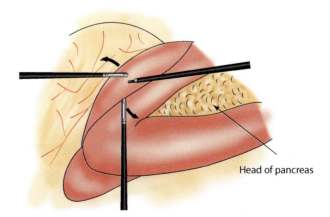

FIGURE 16.34   Second part of the duodenum is dissected away from the mesocolon medially and laterally, up to the hepatic flexure of the colon.

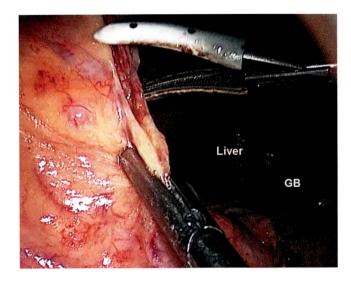

FIGURE 16.35 Right pericolonic vessels are taken intracorporeally, towards the ileocaecal region, remaining close to the colon using Ligasure.

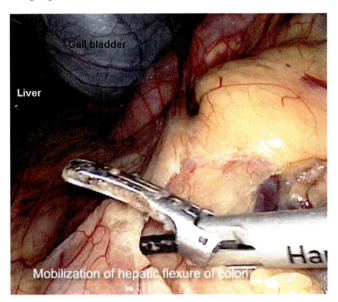

FIGURE 16.36 Hepatic flexure is mobilized from medial to lateral in the supracolic approach.

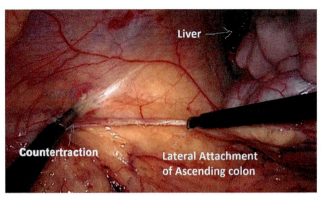

FIGURE 16.37 Lateral attachments of the right colon are divided to completely free the right colon.

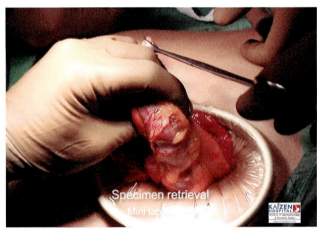

FIGURE 16.38 Specimen removed from the periumbilical mini-laparotomy wound.

colon. Next, the hepatic flexure is mobilized from medial to lateral in the supracolic approach (Figure 16.36), making sure the duodenum is visualized and is away from the dissection plane.

e. *Lateral attachments*: Finally, the lateral attachments of the right colon are divided to completely free the right colon (Figure 16.37).

6. *Minilaparotomy for specimen extraction*: A Pfannenstiel incision of approx. 6 to 7 cm is preferred for specimen extraction. Other options are periumbilical skirting (Figure 16.38), or a RIF muscle splitting at the stoma site. Alternate options are using a natural orifice, i.e. transanal/transvaginal route for specimen extraction.

a. *Small bowel assessment*: We first exteriorize the small bowel and examine for any unsuspected injuries. With the small bowel out of the abdomen, the entire

mobilized colon is exteriorized. The ileocaecal junction is divided as close to the IC junction as possible with a linear stapler (Figure 16.39). The staple line is invaginated by continuous sutures.

b. *Mobilization of the DJ flexure*: If this is not done intracorporeally, this step is now performed when all the small bowels are out of the abdomen. This will allow the ileal loop to reach the pelvic floor easily.

c. *Ileal J pouch creation*: Now a 15 cm ileal J pouch is created by folding the terminal ileum onto itself (Figure 16.40). The apex of the pouch is chosen at the area which easily comes below the pubic bone by stretching the pouch. Double firing of linear cutter stapler of 75/80 mm is performed to create the pouch. Haemostasis in the pouch staple line is secured. Now an anvil of no. 28/29 mm circular stapler is inserted into the apex of the pouch and the purse string closure is done (Figure 16.41).

d. *Stoma marking*: We prefer to perform a stoma marking and insert a no. 10 infant feeding tube around the bowel at the site of the proposed stoma, about 40–50 cm from the pouch. A marking is also done for the proximal and distal site by cauterization. Once this is done, the anvil is placed back in the abdomen. All the small bowels are once again exteriorized to make sure they do not internally herniate behind the mesentery.

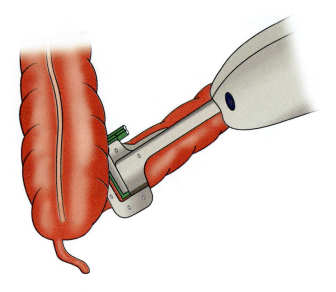

FIGURE 16.39 Ileocaecal junction is divided as close to the IC junction as possible with linear stapler.

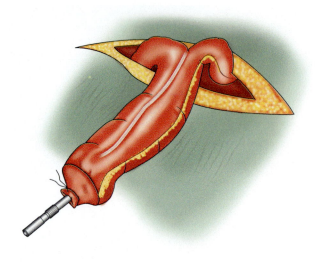

FIGURE 16.41 Anvil of circular stapler is inserted into the apex of pouch for doing ileo-anal anastomosis and purse-string closure.

7. *Re-creation of pneumoperitoneum*: There are several ways to recreate pneumoperitoneum.
   a. *Temporary closures can be performed by*:
      i. *Sutures/clips*: Towel clips can be used to avoid gas leakage.
      ii. *Handport device*: Frequently our choice is for the handport.
      iii. *Wound protector and glove* (Figures 16.42 and 16.43): Another economical and readily available method. A 10 mm trocar can be inserted through one of the fingers of the glove.
   b. *Final closure*: For a Pfannenstiel incision, where no trocars needs to be inserted, permanent closure can be performed for the fascia and the skin, and then pneumoperitoneum can be reestablished.
8. *Pouch anal anastomosis*: Now the pouch anal anastomosis is performed under telescopic vision (Figure 16.44).

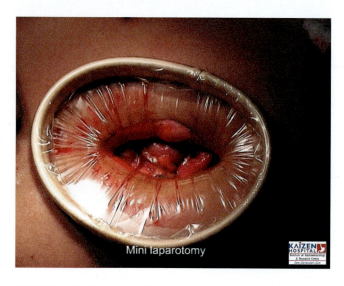

FIGURE 16.42 Wound protector to re-create pneumoperitoneum.

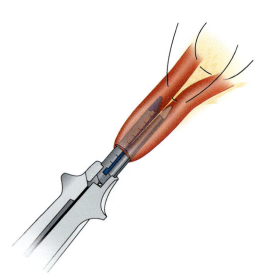
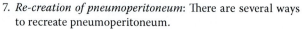

FIGURE 16.40 Two Linear cutter staplers used to create a 15-cm ileal J-pouch.

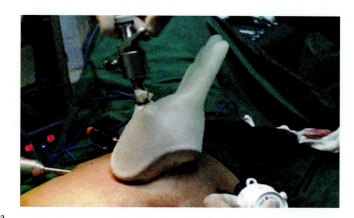

FIGURE 16.43 Glove port to re-create pneumoperitoneum.

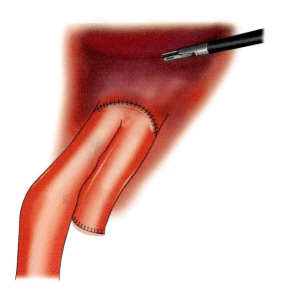

FIGURE 16.44 Pouch anal anastomosis is performed under telescopic vision.

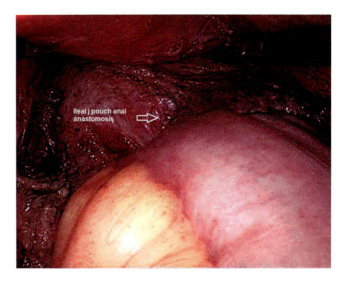

FIGURE 16.45 Leak test of pouch and pouch-anal anastomosis performed with saline irrigation in the pouch.

Again, the small bowel is retracted from the pelvis, suction and lavage is given in the pelvis, and pelvic haemostasis is achieved before the anastomosis, by inserting a gauze piece and using bipolar coagulation if there is any ooze. A circular stapler of no. 28/29 is used for the anastomosis. The lie and tension of the pouch is checked before the anastomosis to ascertain whether any pouch lengthening procedure needs to be performed. One surgeon comes to the perineum for the anastomosis. He gently does a digital examination and a gentle two finger dilatation of the anal canal for stapler insertion. The rectal cuff is small, and thus it is important that during stapler insertion there is no excess force used that could injure the rectal stump. Countertraction of the anal skin can be achieved by using three towel clips or Ellis forceps applied at 3, 7, and 11 o'clock on the anal skin – held by an assistant, while the surgeon gently inserts the stapler with rotating movements. This must be done under telescope vision and with adequate retraction of the pelvic structures, including the uterus in females and the bladder. Once the stapler is in the pouch, under vision the anastomosis is performed. One must make sure there is no rotation of the pouch mesentery, no tension on the anastomosis, and that there are no internal herniations of the small bowel. Before firing the stapler, make sure the vagina is not in the stapler by doing a vaginal examination, as a pouch vaginal fistula is one of the worst, but avoidable complications. Once the stapler is removed, the doughnuts are checked, hemostasis is checked, and a leak test is performed (Figure 16.45). A drain is kept in the pelvis and abdominal closure performed.

9. *Loop stoma/drain tube*: Most patients will have a diverting loop ileostomy, as they are on steroids or immunosuppressants, or have malnutrition. Some selected patients can have a one stage pouch with a transanastomotic drain tube in the pouch.

10. *Stoma closure*: Stoma closure is generally performed after 2–3 months, once the doses of steroids are tapered to a maintenance dose of 5 mg patients improve their nutrition.

Postoperative care and usual recovery

Postoperatively, once the stoma functions start, usually on the first or second day, liquids are started, which are increased to semisolids on the third or fourth POD, and then to a normal diet by the fifth to seventh day. Many patients need nutritional support as they are malnourished. A close watch is established for any symptoms of distension, nausea, or vomiting as postoperative intestinal obstruction is a common complication, needing bowel rest for a few days after which it usually settles, but occasionally needs a re-laparoscopy, or more rarely, a laparotomy for relief.

Postoperative complications – early and late

General complications of laparoscopic colorectal surgery are described in another chapter, whereas specific complications of RPC-IPAA are described here. For RPC-IPAA, the in-hospital and 30-day mortality rates are low (<1%); however, the overall morbidity rates approach 65% (Table 16.1) [13]. Early and late postoperative complications include bowel obstruction, anastomotic dehiscence, pelvic abscess, wound infection, urinary tract infection, anastomotic stenosis requiring mechanical dilatation, large enteric losses from an ileostomy, impotence, retrograde ejaculation, and dyspareunia [14,15]. Hemorrhage from the rectal stump is rare.

Acute and chronic complications can necessitate removal of the ileal reservoir and construction of a permanent ileostomy. For example, a retrospective review of 1005 patients undergoing an IPAA found that the pouch was removed in 15 of 858 patients (1.7%) with ulcerative colitis, and 19 of 147 patients (12.9%) with a diagnosis other than ulcerative colitis [16].

Pelvic sepsis is a common early complication of IPAA and occurs in 6% to 16% of patients [17]. Postoperative anastomotic leak with pelvic sepsis is associated with poor pouch function. A controlled septic condition does not preclude salvage surgery. Furthermore, excision of the pouch is associated with a high risk of complications, particularly delayed perineal wound healing [18,19].

Pouchitis

Pouchitis is an inflammatory condition of the ileal pouch reservoir of an ileal pouch-anal anastomosis. Among patients who have

TABLE 16.1: Proposed Classification of Complications of RPC IPAA [13,14]

Surgical and mechanical	Anastomotic leaks
	Pelvic sepsis and abscess
	Pouch sinuses
	Pouch fistulae
	Strictures
	Afferent limb syndrome and efferent limb syndrome
	Infertility and sexual dysfunction
	Portal vein thrombi
	Pouch prolapse, twisted pouch bleeding, sphincter injury, or dysfunction
Inflammatory and infectious	Pouchitis
	Cuffitis
	CD of the pouch
	Proximal small-bowel bacterial overgrowth
	Inflammatory polyps
Functional	Irritable pouch syndrome
	Anismus
	Pseudo-obstruction
Dysplastic and neoplastic	Dysplasia or cancer of the pouch
	Dysplasia or cancer of the anastomosis
Systemic and metabolic	Anemia
	Bone loss
	Vitamin B-12 deficiency

TABLE 16.2: Diagnostic Algorithm of Ileal Pouch Disorders

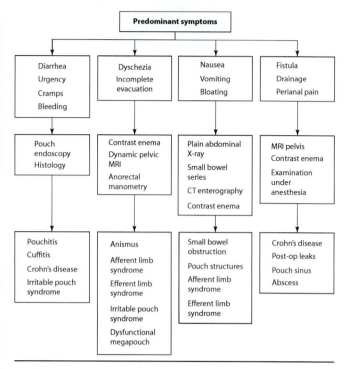

undergone IPAA, the reported incidence of pouchitis ranges from 23% to 59% [20]. Patients who have undergone an IPAA for UC have a higher incidence of pouchitis as compared to patients with FAP. The pathogenesis of pouchitis is unclear, but it is hypothesized to result from an abnormal immune response to altered luminal and/or mucosal bacteria in genetically susceptible hosts. The pathogenesis is multifactorial and genetic factors, changes in gut microbiota, and abnormal mucosal immunity play an important role. Pouchitis is not an isolated disease entity, it likely represents a disease spectrum ranging from acute antibiotic-responsive pouchitis to chronic antibiotic-refractory pouchitis (CARP). Several other pouch disorders have been recognized, such as the irritable pouch syndrome and anismus (anorectal dysfunction) (Table 16.2) [14].

Patients with pouchitis typically have a wide range of clinical presentations, ranging from increased stool frequency, urgency, abdominal cramps, pelvic pressure, tenesmus, and night-time fecal seepage to incontinence.

On pouchoscopy, pouchitis is characterized by the presence of diffuse erythema, friability, granularity, exudates, erosions, and/or ulcerations [22]. On histology, pouchitis is characterized by acute inflammation with neutrophil infiltration, crypt abscess, and mucosal ulceration, often superimposed on a background of chronic changes including villous atrophy, crypt distortion or hyperplasia, pyloric gland metaplasia, and chronic inflammatory cell infiltration [23]. Differential diagnosis includes Cuffitis, Crohn's disease, and surgery-associated mechanical complications such as anastomotic sinus or leak, decreased pouch compliance, diversion pouchitis, and irritable pouch syndrome (IPS).

The majority of patients with acute pouchitis respond well to a short course of antibiotics. Approximately 40% of patients with acute pouchitis will have a single episode of pouchitis, and 60% will have at least one recurrence. Prevention of recurrence is possible with a long course of probiotics rather than antibiotics. Mesalamine or steroids are rarely necessary.

Pouch failure

The pouch failure rate in a large series is estimated at 1.7% for ulcerative colitis versus 13.8 for Crohn's disease. The factors that increased the risk of pouch failure, using a multivariable regression analysis for ulcerative colitis [24], are hand-sewn versus stapled anastomosis, Crohn's disease diagnosis versus mucosal ulcerative colitis, and indeterminate colitis and diagnosis of diabetes versus no diabetes. Crohn's disease involving the ileal pouch is generally associated with a high failure rate and pouch-related fistulas [25]. The complications associated with failure are extensive, and the options for reconstructive surgery in patients with Crohn's disease should be questioned [26]. On the other hand, in a series of 204 patients with Crohn's disease who underwent primary IPAA, the overall 10-year pouch retention was 71% [27]. Pouch retention rates were higher and functional results were most favorable when the diagnosis of Crohn's disease was established preoperatively, or immediately following surgery (85% to 87% 10-year pouch retention). Outcomes in patients with delayed diagnosis fared worse, but half of them still retained their pouch at 10 years.

In addition, excessive weight gain is a risk factor for pouch failure. In a multivariate analysis of 846 patients undergoing a restorative proctocolectomy with nine months of observation, patients experiencing weight gain were significantly more likely to develop pouch failure compared with patients without weight gain (18.4 vs. 12.3%, HR 1.69%, 95% CI 1.01–2.84, p = 0.048) [28].

Stricture

Anal canal stricture has been reported in up to 11% of patients [29]. Nonfibrotic strictures generally respond well to transanal or endoscopic dilation [30], while fibrotic strictures require reoperation.

Fecal incontinence

In the same systematic review cited above [31], mild and severe fecal incontinence during the day was reported in 17% and 3.7%

of patients, respectively. The corresponding rates during the night were 13.1% and 4.5%. Urge incontinence during the day was reported in 7.3% of patients.

Overall, the rate of complete bowel continence that can be achieved after ileal pouch-anal anastomosis (IPAA) varies between 53% and 76% depending upon studies. Those patients who are continent have, on average, six stools a day, with more than 75% having at least one bowel movement at night [32,13].

Pouch dysplasia/cancer
About 1% of patients develop dysplasia or carcinoma after surgery, which occurs in the retained rectum, anal transitional zone, or ileal pouch, depending upon the procedure performed [34,35]. Thus, regular (at least yearly) endoscopic surveillance is mandatory for early detection of dysplasia, and pouch excision may be required in cases of carcinoma [36] Recommended screening strategies for patients with ulcerative colitis are discussed elsewhere.

Sexual dysfunction
IPAA has been associated with a small risk of sexual dysfunction and the risk is greatest in patients who require reoperative pelvic surgery. Postoperative impotence and retrograde ejaculation has been observed in approximately 1.5% and 4% of men, respectively. Transient dyspareunia occurs in about 7% of women, although coital frequency and the ability to experience orgasm remain unchanged [37,38].

Female infertility
Female fertility is significantly decreased after open IPAA, although successful pregnancies do occur regularly [39].

Patients who have had an IPAA procedure should not be discouraged from childbearing because of the pouch. Pregnancy and delivery are safe in patients with IPAA. Patients may experience a transient increase in stool frequency or incontinence during pregnancy, both of which resolve after delivery [40].

It remains controversial whether vaginal or cesarean delivery is better for women with a pelvic pouch. Vaginal delivery has the potential of disrupting the anal sphincter, nevertheless the mode of delivery should be dictated primarily by obstetric considerations [40].

Anal transition zone inflammation
Acute and chronic inflammation is common following an IPAA for patients with ulcerative colitis. In a retrospective review of 225 patients with a stapled IPAA, acute inflammation at the anal transition zone (ATZ) was identified in 4.6% of patients, chronic inflammation in 84.9%, and normal mucosa in 10.5%; no patient had evidence of dysplasia [42]. The presence of inflammation at the ATZ, however, does not negatively affect functional outcomes or quality of life.

Anal transitional zone dysplasia
ATZ dysplasia after stapled IPAA is infrequent and is usually self-limiting. ATZ preservation did not lead to the development of cancer with a minimum of 10 years of follow-up. Long-term surveillance is recommended to monitor dysplasia. If repeat biopsy confirms persistent dysplasia, we perform a mucosectomy with perineal pouch advancement and a neo-ileal pouch-anal anastomosis [43].

Unusual complications – A number of unusual late complications have been described, including [44–46] superior mesenteric artery syndrome, solitary ileal ulcer, traumatic ileal ulcer perforation, fibroid polyps, mucosal prolapse with outlet obstruction, puborectal spasm, sacral osteomyelitis, volvulus, and pharmacobezoar.

Functional results of RPC-IPAA
After surgery, the quality of life and defecatory and bowel function plateau at approximately one year and remain constant, with more than 90% of patients satisfied with the outcome of the operation and quality of life [47]. Long-term functional results and quality of life are best illustrated by a 30-year retrospective study of patients who underwent RPC-IPAA for chronic ulcerative colitis. At 30 years, 93% of patients maintained a functional pouch, although stool frequencies increased slightly (5.7 to 6.2 during day; 1.5 to 2.1 at night) compared with at one year. The cumulative probability of pouchitis, stricture, obstruction, and fistula were 80%, 57%, 44%, and 16%, respectively. Quality-of-life scores remained stable over the 30 years [1]. Two large studies looked at health-related quality of life (HRQoL) after pouch failure [2]. Overall, patients with a failed pouch reported significantly worse physical function, social functioning, energy level, and physical role function compared with the group with a functioning pouch.

Controversies
1. *Laparoscopic versus open approach*: Based upon observational studies, the complication rates and functional outcomes of the laparoscopic total proctocolectomy are similar to that of the open approach; however, patient acceptance, body image, cosmesis, and quality of life are better with the laparoscopic approach [3,4];
2. *One vs. two vs. three stage pouch*: The benefit of using a diverting loop ileostomy to reduce the risk of an anastomotic leak or dehiscence has not been clearly established [48]; however, we selectively use this approach to minimize the risk of a leak, dehiscence, or pelvic sepsis [49,50];

Staged approach to IPAA: Following proctocolectomy, an ileal pouch-anal anastomosis (IPAA) can be performed in stages as follows:

One-stage IPAA: An ileal pouch is made and anastomosed to the anus. The operation is completed in a single stage.

Two-stage IPAA: The same ileal pouch anal anastomosis is made, but is protected by a loop ileostomy from the fecal stream. The loop ileostomy is subsequently reversed in a second operation. Although there is no evidence that a loop ileostomy protects against serious complications such as anastomotic leak [51], many surgeons still routinely perform IPAA in two stages.

Three-stage IPAA: The first stage of a three-stage IPAA is a total abdominal colectomy and ileostomy. This is followed by a completion proctectomy with an IPAA and loop ileostomy as the second stage operation. Finally, the loop ileostomy is reversed as the third stage.

Three-stage IPAA was routinely performed in patients treated with antitumor-necrosis-factor (anti-TNF) agents (e.g. infliximab) due to concerns over infection [52]. However, contemporary studies and a meta-analysis found no advantage to the three-stage IPAA in such patients [50].

Patients should be advised that a permanent ileostomy will be required if an IPAA is not technically possible. In a large series of 1789 patients undergoing proctocolectomy, IPAA was attempted but abandoned intraoperatively in 4.1% [53] of patients. An ileostomy may also be required if the pouch fails postoperatively due to anastomotic complications, infection, fistulization, development of Crohn's disease, disease recurrence, or poor function.

3. *J vs. W vs. S Pouch*: The J-pouch is the preferred ileal reservoir because of the efficiency of construction and optimal functional results. Alternatives to the J-pouch configuration for the ileal reservoir include three- and four-limbed pouches, such as an S or W pouch. These alternative configurations are rarely performed due to complexity of construction [36].

4. *Stapled vs .hand sewn pouch*: The best data comparing the two anastomotic techniques came from a nonrandomized, prospective study of 3382 patients undergoing IPAA. Compared with a stapled anastomosis, a hand-sewn anastomosis was associated with a higher frequency of anastomotic stricture, septic complication, bowel obstruction, and pouch failure. Patients who had the hand-sewn anastomosis reported more incontinence, seepage, and pad usage, as well as dietary, social, and work restrictions [41].

5. *Mucosectomy vs. no mucosectomy*: A stapled IPAA, which requires a small amount of rectal tissue to be spared for the anastomosis, preserves the ATZ in the rectal cuff [47] and is performed only in patients with no evidence of ATZ dysplasia of any grade, and no polyps at the dentate line.

We perform a transanal mucosectomy, which removes all rectal mucosa, and a hand-sewn IPAA for inflammatory bowel disease (IBD) patients with biopsy-proven dysplasia, regardless of the degree or location [21,33,42], and as well for familial polyposis (FAP) patients with polyps involving the dentate line.

Authors' experience

From January 2000 to September 2019, from the author's prospectively maintained database, a total of 170 patients with ulcerative colitis underwent surgery. 56 cases were excluded from the study (14 – total proctocolectomies with end ileostomy, 7 – emergency open IPAA, 35 – elective open IPAA). 114 (67%) patients who underwent elective laparoscopic IPAA were included in the study. The mean age was 36.2 years. Out of 114 patients, 109 underwent a two-stage procedure. The mean operating time was 281 min. Conversion to open surgery occurred in 6 (5.2%) patients. Postoperative morbidity and mortality occurred in 37 (32.4%) and 2 (1.8%) patients, respectively. The median length of stay was 13.3 (6–33) days. Major immediate postoperative complications were intestinal obstruction 22 (19.2%), anastomotic leak 6 (5.2%), and pouch haemorrhage 4 (3.5%). Long-term functional outcomes revealed a 24-hr frequency of stool of 5.7 per day (3–15), a daytime average of 4 per day, and a nocturnal average of 1.7 per day. Long-term complications were pouchitis 20 (17.5%) and fecal incontinence (2.6%; major: none, minor: 3).

Summary

Restorative proctocolectomy (RPC) and ileal pouch anal anastomosis (IPAA) has become a standard procedure for surgical management of ulcerative colitis over the last 3–4 decades. This surgery becomes necessary in 10%–30% of patients within one decade after diagnosis of UC. RPC-IPAA is a curative and continence-preserving procedure that avoids the long-term risks

of medical treatment, and has made surgical management a more attractive option. The quality of life and the defecatory and bowel function plateau at approximately one year and remain constant, with more than 90% of patients satisfied with the outcome of the operation and quality of life. Long-term functional results and quality of life are best illustrated by a 30-year retrospective study of patients who underwent RPC-IPAA for chronic ulcerative colitis which showed that 93% of patients maintained a functional pouch, although stool frequencies increased slightly (5.7 to 6.2 during day; 1.5 to 2.1 at night) compared to at one year. In the natural history of the disease, which is quite unpredictable, when the disease becomes more active, more severe, and shows less response to medical treatment, requiring more immunosuppressant or steroids, one should start thinking and discussing surgical options. The patient should ideally earn the surgery, when in a severe disease, he/she wants it as a one-time curative option.

Key points

- RPC-IPAA is the surgical treatment option for patients who have failed medical management for ulcerative colitis.
- RPC-IPAA is a curative and continence-preserving procedure and by avoiding long-term risks of medical treatment, this procedure has made surgical management a more attractive option.
- The J-pouch is the preferred ileal reservoir because of the efficiency of construction and optimal functional results.
- Stapled anastomosis is better than hand sewn anastomosis, having decreased complication rates; however, we perform a hand-sewn IPAA with a transanal mucosectomy, which removes all rectal mucosa, for IBD patients with biopsy-proven dysplasia, regardless of the degree or location, and as well for FAP patients with polyps involving the dentate line.
- This procedure has been successfully performed with the minimally invasive approach, minimizing the incision-related morbidity and optimizing the cosmesis in young patients. It has minimal postoperative morbidity and favorable results, showing that 90% of patients have a good quality of life.
- The patient should ideally earn the surgery, when in a severe disease, he/she wants it as a one-time curative option.

Videos

VIDEO 13   https://youtu.be/c1xDI6HsXgg

Laparoscopic Restorative Proctocolectomy and Ileal Pouch for Ulcerative Colitis – Part 1.

VIDEO 14   https://youtu.be/Jil7wJnMwHA

Laparoscopic Restorative Proctocolectomy and Ileal Pouch for Ulcerative Colitis – Part 2.

References

1. Lightner AL, Mathis KL, Dozois EJ et al. Results at Up to 30 Years After Ileal Pouch-Anal Anastomosis for Chronic Ulcerative Colitis. *Inflamm Bowel Dis.* 2017;23:781.
2. Lepistö A, Luukkonen P, Järvinen HJ. Cumulative failure rate of ileal pouch-anal anastomosis and quality of life after failure. *Dis Colon Rectum.* 2002;45:1289.
3. Fichera A, Silvestri MT, Hurst RD et al. Laparoscopic restorative proctocolectomy with ileal pouch anal anastomosis: A comparative observational study on long-term functional results. *J Gastrointest Surg.* 2009;13:526.
4. Dunker MS, Bemelman WA, Slors JF et al. Functional outcome, quality of life, body image, and cosmesis in patients after laparoscopic-assisted and conventional restorative proctocolectomy: A comparative study. *Dis Colon Rectum.* 2001;44:1800.
5. The American Society of Colon and Rectal Surgeons. Wexner SD, Rosen L, Lowry A et al. Practice parameters for the treatment of mucosal ulcerative colitis--supporting documentation. The Standards Practice Task Force. *Dis Colon Rectum.* 1997 Nov;40(11):1277–85.
6. Hurst RD, Finco C, Rubin M, Michelassi F. Prospective analysis of perioperative morbidity in one hundred consecutive colectomies for ulcerative colitis. *Surgery.* 1995;118:748.
7. Daperno M, Sostegni R, Rocca R. Lower gastrointestinal bleeding in Crohn's disease: How (un-)common is it and how to tackle it? *Dig Liver Dis.* 2012;44:721.
8. Dayan B, Turner D. Role of surgery in severe ulcerative colitis in the era of medical rescue therapy. *World J Gastroenterol.* 2012;18:3833.
9. Wexner SD, Rosen L, Lowry A et al. Practice parameters for the treatment of mucosal ulcerative colitis--supporting documentation. The Standards Practice Task Force. The American Society of Colon and Rectal Surgeons. *Dis Colon Rectum.* 1997;40:1277.
10. Martel P, Majery N, Savigny B et al. Mesenteric lengthening in ileoanal pouch anastomosis for ulcerative colitis: Is high division of the superior mesenteric pedicle a safe procedure? *Dis Colon Rectum.* 1998;41:862.
11. Radice E, Nelson H, Devine RM et al. Ileal pouch-anal anastomosis in patients with colorectal cancer: Long-term functional and oncologic outcomes. *Dis Colon Rectum.* 1998;41:11.
12. Haribhakti S, Madnani M, Mistry J, Soni H, Shah A, Patel K. Laparoscopic restorative proctocolectomy ileal pouch anal anastomosis: How I do it?. *J Min Access Surg.* 2015;11(3):218.
13. Michelassi F, Lee J, Rubin M et al. Long-term functional results after ileal pouch anal restorative proctocolectomy for ulcerative colitis: A prospective observational study. *Ann Surg.* 2003;238:433.
14. Shen B, Remzi FH, Lavery IC et al. A proposed classification of ileal pouch disorders and associated complications after restorative proctocolectomy. *Clin Gastroenterol Hepatol.* 2008;6:145.
15. Farouk R, Pemberton JH, Wolff BG et al. Functional outcomes after ileal pouch-anal anastomosis for chronic ulcerative colitis. *Ann Surg.* 2000;231:919.
16. Fazio VW, Ziv Y, Church JM et al. Ileal pouch-anal anastomoses complications and function in 1005 patients. *Ann Surg.* 1995;222:120.
17. Farouk R, Dozois RR, Pemberton JH, Larson D. Incidence and subsequent impact of pelvic abscess after ileal pouch-anal anastomosis for chronic ulcerative colitis. *Dis Colon Rectum.* 1998;41:1239.
18. Karoui M, Cohen R, Nicholls J. Results of surgical removal of the pouch after failed restorative proctocolectomy. *Dis Colon Rectum.* 2004;47:869.
19. Prudhomme M, Dehni N, Dozois RR et al. Causes and outcomes of pouch excision after restorative proctocolectomy. *Br J Surg.* 2006;93:82.
20. Lohmuller JL, Pemberton JH, Dozois RR et al. Pouchitis and extraintestinal manifestations of inflammatory bowel disease after ileal pouch-anal anastomosis. *Ann Surg.* 1990;211:622.
21. Holder-Murray J, Fichera A. Anal transition zone in the surgical management of ulcerative colitis. *World J Gastroenterol.* 2009;15:769.
22. Shen B, Achkar JP, Lashner BA et al. Endoscopic and histologic evaluation together with symptom assessment are required to diagnose pouchitis. *Gastroenterology.* 2001;121:261.
23. Moskowitz RL, Shepherd NA, Nicholls RJ. An assessment of inflammation in the reservoir after restorative proctocolectomy with ileoanal ileal reservoir. *Int J Colorectal Dis.* 1986;1:167.
24. Manilich E, Remzi FH, Fazio VW et al. Prognostic modeling of preoperative risk factors of pouch failure. *Dis Colon Rectum.* 2012;55:393.
25. Reese GE, Lovegrove RE, Tilney HS et al. The effect of Crohn's disease on outcomes after restorative proctocolectomy. *Dis Colon Rectum.* 2007;50:239.
26. Tekkis PP, Heriot AG, Smith O et al. Long-term outcomes of restorative proctocolectomy for Crohn's disease and indeterminate colitis. *Colorectal Dis.* 2005;7:218.
27. Melton GB, Fazio VW, Kiran RP et al. Long-term outcomes with ileal pouch-anal anastomosis and Crohn's disease: Pouch retention and implications of delayed diagnosis. *Ann Surg.* 2008;248:608.
28. Wu XR, Zhu H, Kiran RP et al. Excessive weight gain is associated with an increased risk for pouch failure in patients with restorative proctocolectomy. *Inflamm Bowel Dis.* 2013;19:2173.
29. Prudhomme M, Dozois RR, Godlewski G et al. Anal canal strictures after ileal pouch-anal anastomosis. *Dis Colon Rectum.* 2003;46:20.
30. Shen B, Lian L, Kiran RP et al. Efficacy and safety of endoscopic treatment of ileal pouch strictures. *Inflamm Bowel Dis.* 2011;17:2527.
31. Hueting WE, Buskens E, van der Tweel I et al. Results and complications after ileal pouch anal anastomosis: A meta-analysis of 43 observational studies comprising 9,317 patients. *Dig Surg.* 2005;22:69.
32. Hahnloser D, Pemberton JH, Wolff BG et al. Results at up to 20 years after ileal pouch-anal anastomosis for chronic ulcerative colitis. *Br J Surg.* 2007;94:333.
33. Silvestri MT, Hurst RD, Rubin MA et al. Chronic inflammatory changes in the anal transition zone after stapled ileal pouch-anal anastomosis: Is mucosectomy a superior alternative? *Surgery.* 2008;144:533.
34. Kariv R, Remzi FH, Lian L et al. Preoperative colorectal neoplasia increases risk for pouch neoplasia in patients with restorative proctocolectomy. *Gastroenterology.* 2010;139:806.
35. Banasiewicz T, Marciniak R, Paszkowski J et al. Pouchitis may increase the risk of dysplasia after restorative proctocolectomy in patients with ulcerative colitis. *Colorectal Dis.* 2012;14:92.
36. Sagar PM, Pemberton JH. Intraoperative, postoperative and reoperative problems with ileoanal pouches. *Br J Surg.* 2012;99:454.
37. Wax JR, Pinette MG, Cartin A, Blackstone J. Female reproductive health after ileal pouch anal anastomosis for ulcerative colitis. *Obstet Gynecol Surv.* 2003;58:270.
38. Cornish JA, Tan E, Teare J et al. The effect of restorative proctocolectomy on sexual function, urinary function, fertility, pregnancy and delivery: A systematic review. *Dis Colon Rectum.* 2007;50:1128.
39. Hahnloser D, Pemberton JH, Wolff BG et al. Pregnancy and delivery before and after ileal pouch-anal anastomosis for inflammatory bowel disease: Immediate and long-term consequences and outcomes. *Dis Colon Rectum.* 2004;47:1127.
40. Bharadwaj S, Philpott JR, Barber MD et al. Women's health issues after ileal pouch surgery. *Inflamm Bowel Dis.* 2014;20:2470.
41. Kirat HT, Remzi FH, Kiran RP, Fazio VW. Comparison of outcomes after hand-sewn versus stapled ileal pouch-anal anastomosis in 3,109 patients. *Surgery* 2009; 146:723.
42. Fichera A, Ragauskaite L, Silvestri MT et al. Preservation of the anal transition zone in ulcerative colitis. Long-term effects on defecatory function. *J Gastrointest Surg.* 2007;11:1647.
43. Remzi FH, Fazio VW, Delaney CP et al. Dysplasia of the anal transitional zone after ileal pouch-anal anastomosis: Results of prospective evaluation after a minimum of ten years. *Dis Colon Rectum.* 2003;46:6.

44. Taylor WE, Wolff BG, Pemberton JH, Yaszemski MJ. Sacral osteo-myelitis after ileal pouch-anal anastomosis: Report of four cases. *Dis Colon Rectum.* 2006;49:913.

45. Jain A, Abbas MA, Sekhon HK, Rayhanabad JA. Volvulus of an ileal J-pouch. *Inflamm Bowel Dis.* 2010;16:3.

46. Mmeje C, Bouchard A, Heppell J. Image of the month. Pharmacobezoar: A rare complication after ileal pouch-anal anastomosis for ulcerative colitis. *Clin Gastroenterol Hepatol.* 2010;8:A28.

47. Litzendorf ME, Stucchi AF, Wishnia S, et al. Completion muco-sectomy for retained rectal mucosa following restorative proc-tocolectomy with double-stapled ileal pouch-anal anastomosis. *J Gastrointest Surg* 2010; 14:562.

48. Gorfine SR, Gelernt IM, Bauer JJ et al. Restorative proctocolec-tomy without diverting ileostomy. *Dis Colon Rectum.* 1995;38:188.

49. Lovegrove RE, Constantinides VA, Heriot AG et al. A comparison of hand-sewn versus stapled ileal pouch anal anastomosis (IPAA) following proctocolectomy: A meta-analysis of 4183 patients. *Ann Surg.* 2006;244:18.

50. Hicks CW, Hodin RA, Bordeianou L. Possible overuse of 3-stage procedures for active ulcerative colitis. *JAMA Surg.* 2013;148:658.

51. Remzi FH, Fazio VW, Gorgun E et al. The outcome after restor-ative proctocolectomy with or without defunctioning ileostomy. *Dis Colon Rectum.* 2006;49:470.

52. Schluender SJ, Ippoliti A, Dubinsky M et al. Does infliximab influ-ence surgical morbidity of ileal pouch-anal anastomosis in patients with ulcerative colitis? *Dis Colon Rectum.* 2007;50:1747.

53. Browning SM, Nivatvongs S. Intraoperative abandonment of ileal pouch to anal anastomosis--the Mayo Clinic experience. *J Am Coll Surg.* 1998;186:441.

Chapter 17

PARASTOMAL HERNIAS

Arun Prasad and Sanjiv Haribhakti

Contents

Learning objectives 109
Introduction 109
Incidence of PH. 109
History of laparoscopy in stomal surgery. 109
Classification of PH 110
Risk factors. 110
Diagnosis of PH. 110
Indications and contraindications for surgery 110
Surgery for PH. 110
Prevention of parastomal hernia 111
    Transrectus or pararectus 111
    Size of the trephine. 111
    Extraperitoneal approach 111
    Role of prophylactic mesh. 111
Techniques of repair. 112
Onlay mesh repair 112
Intraperitoneal mesh repair 112
Laparoscopic versus open repair 113
Recurrence. 113
Recurrent PH repair. 113
Robotic PH repair. 113
Summary 114
Key points 114
Videos 114
References 114

Learning objectives

- Classify PH to improve the ability to compare different studies and their results
- Study risk factors for the development of PH
- Understand indications and contraindications for surgery
- Learn techniques for prevention of PH
- Determine the best surgical approach for a given patient
- Know the benefits and limitations of various operations for reducing PH recurrence
- Understand the operative principles and techniques of the various procedures
- Review and analyze the current studies on long-term results of different procedures
- Explore results of various surgical procedures in meta-analyses

Introduction

The most common long-term complication following stoma creation is parastomal hernia (PH), which according to some authors is practically unavoidable [1]. They are uncommon in the early postoperative period (0%–3%), but the incidence of PH increases with time, ranging from 14.1% to 40% [2]. As a general rule, reinforcing the abdominal wall with a prosthetic mesh is the treatment of choice, with a low rate of complications and relapses over a long period of time.

Incidence of PH

Based on data available from the literature globally, the incidence of hernia relative to the respective type of stoma can be summarized as follows:

- End colostomy: 4%–48% (mean: 15%)
- Loop colostomy: 0%–30% (mean: 4.0%)
- End ileostomy: 2%–28% (mean: 7%)
- Loop ileostomy: 0%–6% (mean: 1%)

A separate clinical problem is the incidence of PH recurrence following corrective surgery. Depending on the selected reconstructive technique, the results can be summarized as follows:

- After surgery with stoma transposition: 0%–76% (mean: 24%)
- After mesh plasty: 0%–33% (mean: 3%)
- Simple tissue plasty: 46%–100% (mean: 65%)

History of laparoscopy in stomal surgery

The first use of laparoscopy in stoma surgery was in 1991, in a procedure performed by Lange while conducting a loop colostomy. Since then, the number of stomata aided by laparoscopy has been on a steady increase, including the development of minimally invasive methods such as laparoscopic procedures involving only a single incision – SILS [3]. No randomized studies are available [4]. Laparoscopic techniques are becoming popular for PH surgery. However, the recurrence percentages are similar (8%–56%) to results for open plasty [5]. Unfortunately, the reports lack randomized studies and most papers pertain to a relatively small number of patients [6]. Moreover, hernia recurrence may occur not only at the location of the newly formed stoma but, according to the quoted authors, there is also a 1%–32% risk of recurrence at the location of the removed stoma [7].

Classification of PH

There are many classifications for PH (Table 17.1). Szczepkowski's classification is most commonly used. In 2014, the European Hernia Society (EHS) published a new classification based on Szczepkowski's classification to improve the ability to compare different studies and their results, which could result in developing new evidence-based therapeutic guidelines. The EHS grid for classification of PH is given in Table 17.2.

Risk factors

In terms of patient-dependent factors, the significant parameters are [8]: age >60 years (some authors mention 67 years as the age limit), obesity with body mass index (BMI) >30 kg/m2, waist circumference >100 cm, diabetes, smoking, systemic and local infection, hard physical labor, ASA classification >II, low tensile strength of abdominal wall, chronic cough and/or chronic obstructive pulmonary disease (COPD), steroid therapy, eating or immune disorders and collagen metabolism disorders, Crohn's disease, cancer, and ischemia.

It is believed that among surgical factors contributing to the increased incidence of PH, the most important include urgency of surgery, stoma type, preoperative marking of the stoma location, prior PH surgery, surgeon's experience and qualifications, referral

TABLE 17.1: Classification for PH

Moreno-Matias (2009) and Seo (2011)	Szczepkowski (2011)
0-CT image normal, peritoneum follows the wall of the bowel forming the stoma, with no formation of a scar	I-isolated, small PH
Ia-bowel forming the colostomy with a sac of under 5 cm	II-small PH with coexisting midline incisional hernia without any significant front abdominal wall deformity
Ib-bowel forming the colostomy with a scar of over 5 cm	III-isolated, large PH with front abdominal wall deformity
II-sac containing omentum	IV-large PH with coexisting midline incisional hernia, with front abdominal wall deformity
III-sac containing an intestinal loop rather than the bowel forming the stoma	

TABLE 17.2: EHS Grid for Classification of PH

EHS Parastomal Hernia Classification		Small ≤5 cm	Large >5 cm
Concomitant Incisional hernia?	No	I	III
	Yes	II	IV
		P ☐	R ☐

Note: **P** stands for primary hernia, **R** stands for recurrent hernia and ☐ is check-box for tick mark.

level of the healthcare institution, type of suture and mesh, stoma creation technique, and the size of the stoma orifice in integuments above 3 cm (the accepted optimum is 2/3 of the intestine width) [9].

A somewhat less evident correlation between the incidence of hernia and the use of the following surgical techniques can also be inferred from the literature; however, the literature review and meta-analysis did not confirm their prognostic significance: position of the stoma relative to the rectus muscle, placing of the fixing sutures to the fascia, and closing the lateral extraintestinal space forming the stoma [10].

Diagnosis of PH

In the vast majority of cases, the only clinical symptom is a deformity of the abdominal wall around the stoma, which is the basis for the diagnosis. Some hernias can be overlooked due to the patient's obesity, or difficulty in performing a physical examination due to severe pain during palpation. This is also the case when there are contracted scars on the abdominal skin or coexisting hernias along the laparotomy incision line, and in cases of neurogenic abdominal muscle relaxation. In this respect, diagnostic imaging techniques such as ultrasound or CT may prove useful [7,12].

Indications and contraindications for surgery

Surgery should be avoided in asymptomatic patients due to the inherent risks and high incidence of recurrence. Surgical repair is indicated for patients who develop acute PH complications and for those with chronic symptoms that impair quality of life.

Absolute indications are incarceration, strangulation, obstruction, parastomal fistula, perforation, and stomal ischemia. Relative indications are history of incarceration, recurrent obstruction, difficulty in maintaining the collection device, hernia-related pain, erosion of the surrounding skin, inability to accept the stoma aesthetically, and other concomitant complications such as stenosis or prolapse.

Absolute contraindications for elective surgery is terminal malignant disease. Relative contraindications for elective surgery are unresectable or metastatic cancer, serious comorbidity, and scheduled temporary stoma closure.

Surgery for PH

There are a number of methods that can be employed in corrective surgery depending on the approach route, possible transposition of the stoma, the use of mesh reinforcement, or the use of minimally invasive techniques. Open techniques without prosthetic implantation can be divided into: those without stoma transposition and those with stoma transposition [13].

Surgical options for correcting a PH are local primary repair, relocation, and repair with mesh. Local primary repair does not require a laparotomy and dissection can be minimal. The fascial defect around the stoma is plicated, and is technically easy. The results, however, are disappointing, with recurrence rates ranging from 46%–100% [14,15], limiting its clinical applicability. Ideally, it should only have a role in those patients where a larger complex surgical repair is considered high risk, or in cases where mesh repair is strongly undesirable. Relocation of the stoma can be performed through a formal laparotomy, or by way of a local peristomal incision. The rate of recurrence at the relocated site remains problematic, ranging from 24%–40% [16,17]. In fact, the recurrence rate at the new site should be expected to be at least as high as that after the initial stoma creation. A second repair with relocation is associated with an even higher expected chance of recurrence (71%) [18]. Relocating the stoma to the same side of the abdominal wall further increases the likelihood of a recurrence (80%–86%). Overall, the data are limited comparing direct repair to relocation. In the short term, it seems that relocation offers a better outcome [19]. However, with longer postoperative follow-up, the re-recurrence rates appear to be disappointingly high, regardless of whether direct repair or relocation was performed.

Prevention of parastomal hernia

Transrectus or pararectus
No clear consensus exists regarding the ideal location of trephination through the abdominal wall musculature. Studies have suggested that the course through the rectus abdominis is favorable [20]. Others have found no correlation of the position of the stoma in relation to the rectus abdominis, and the rates of PH [21]. Although not clearly protective against PH, a stoma positioned through the rectus abdominis is advocated due to any lack of disadvantage and belief in superior appliance fit [22].

Size of the trephine
The size of the trephination is also a matter of some debate. As a general guideline, an aperture of two finger breadths is an acceptable size. Martin and Foster suggested the trephine will expand with time and application of tangential intra-abdominal forces. Their recommendations were more precise: 2 cm for ileostomies and 1.5 cm for colostomies [8]. Several investigators have used mechanical devices to assure accurate and reproducible aperture sizes [24–26]; however, whether such devices are truly superior to conventional methods is not proven. It is best to avoid dogmatic adherence to strict sizes, but rather to use a guided approach in which the smallest aperture is fashioned to a size that allows passage of the bowel without vascular compromise.

Extraperitoneal approach
Goligher initially described the extraperitoneal stoma in 1958, and remained a strong proponent of the technique [27]. Early findings indicated a decreased incidence of hernia formation through the use of the extraperitoneal course [28]. Recent reports have supported these findings and have demonstrated a statistically significant reduction in hernia rates [29,30]. However, prospective randomized studies are still lacking, and the role of the extraperitoneal stoma as a preventive measure remains unclear [30].

Role of prophylactic mesh
Due to the high rate of PH formation postoperatively, it is not surprising that the use of mesh as a prophylactic measure has been advocated by some. Prevention of PH using mesh during the initial operation was first described in 1986 [31]. Since this early study, many advances in hernia repair have been made, namely the development of large-pore lightweight synthetic and biologic meshes. One of the primary concerns of mesh repair in PH is the insertion of a foreign body into a potentially contaminated field. Mesh infection rates, in the setting of PH repair, range from 0% to 13% [32,33]. Steele et al. in a large study regarding mesh infection in PH repairs, reported on 58 patients, showed that even with the bowel in direct contact with mesh and exposed to a clean contaminated field, the wound infection, fistula, and mesh erosion rates remained low at 3%, 3%, and 2%, respectively. The authors concluded that the utilization of mesh for PH repair is safe in a clean contaminated field [34]. In another prospective trial, 25 patients undergoing elective colorectal surgery had creation of a permanent colostomy with concomitant placement of synthetic mesh. The authors estimated the procedure added 10–15 minutes to the surgery total time. Follow-up was 12 months with two PH. Mesh erosion through the skin without infection or abscess occurred in two patients; these were treated locally without explantation [35]. In a multicenter prospective study, 20 patients underwent abdominoperineal excision and colostomy with mesh reinforcement. With a median follow-up of 24 months, the PH rate was 5% and no infectious complications occurred [36]. Figel et al. have reported on the feasibility and safety of biologic mesh for prophylaxis as well [37]. Recent meta-analyses have shown favorable results in support of using mesh in a prophylactic manner [38,39]. Data from randomized studies, however, remain sparse. Serra-Aracil et al. conducted a trial on prophylactic implantation of lightweight, large-pore partially biodegradable mesh, which included a control group with no mesh. The implantation was estimated to add no more than 20 minutes to the total operative time. Mesh implantation was associated with a statistically significant reduction of PH occurrences (14.8 vs. 40.7%) [40]. In another prospective randomized study, 27 patients were randomized to either sublay mesh implantation with colostomy, or a conventional colostomy creation only. At 12-month follow-up, the clinical trial arm demonstrated no PH, while the control arm demonstrated eight hernias (p = 0.003) [41]. A 5-year follow-up of the original study continues to support the effectiveness of the use of prophylactic mesh [42]. Although important issues still remain, such as the choice of the mesh type and the technique of placement, these randomized studies suggest the safety and effectiveness of the use of prophylactic mesh in reducing the risk of PH formation. Furthermore, the surgical techniques have been well described in the literature, are relatively easily incorporated into the primary operation (adding 10–20 minutes to operative time), and appear to be well tolerated by patients. Cost-effectiveness of prevention has also been put forth as a potential advantage [37].

A systematic review and systematic meta-analysis have shown that prophylactic mesh placement is safe and effectively reduces the risk of PH after end [43] and loop [39] stomas. In the former meta-analysis for end stoma by Wang et al., six RCTs containing 309 patients were included. PH occurred in 24.4% (38 of 156) of patients with mesh and 50.3% (77 of 153) of patients without mesh. Stoma-related morbidity was similar between mesh group and non-mesh group. Another systematic review and meta-analysis looked at the cost effectiveness of this approach. In this study [45], eleven RCTs were included. Four hundred fifty-three patients were randomized to mesh, with 454 controls. Significant reductions were seen in the number of hernias detected clinically, and on computed tomography scan. Reductions persisted for synthetic and composite meshes. Operative time was similar, with zero incidence of mesh infection/fistulation, and fewer peristomal complications. Synthetic mesh demonstrated a favorable cost profile, with composite approximately cost neutral, and biological incurring net costs. They concluded that reinforcing elective stomas with mesh (primarily synthetic) reduces subsequent PSH rates, complications, repairs, and saves money.

In a Cochrane database review 2018, 10 RCTs involving a total of 844 participants, the incidence of PH was 22 per 100 participants receiving prophylactic mesh compared to 41 per 100 participants having a standard ostomy formation. There were no differences in the need for reoperation, operative time, postoperative length of hospital stay, or stoma-related infections. They found a low quality of evidence due to the large heterogeneity of cases, meshes, as well as high variability in follow-up duration and technique of parastomal herniation detection.

Techniques of repair

Techniques with prosthetic reinforcement can be divided into open techniques, laparoscopic techniques, and robotic techniques [46].

Depending on the method and layer wherein the prosthetic is implanted, the currently employed surgical techniques can be classified as follows: superficial mesh (onlay technique), preperitoneal mesh (sublay technique), and intraperitoneal mesh (inlay technique).

Onlay mesh repair

Onlay mesh repair is performed by making an incision in the abdominal wall, typically in the midline, well away from the stoma. In some situations, a lateral incision may be appropriate. A subcutaneous dissection along the rectus and oblique fascia is performed circumferentially around the stoma. The contents of the hernia are reduced into the abdomen, and the abdominal wall defect is closed using a tension-free mesh repair. While all of the series describing this technique are small, nonrandomized, and lack long-term follow-up, these reports describe low perioperative complication rates but recurrence rates ranging from 0% to 20%. Undermining the skin around the stoma also risks ischemic injury to the skin, which can result in significant management problems with the stoma appliance. The use of closed suction drains overlying the mesh appears to reduce complications resulting from seroma collections [47]; however, this needs to be balanced against the possible risk of mesh infection, which is higher for this technique than for intraperitoneal placement of mesh.

Intraperitoneal mesh repair

There have been three primary ways described for intraperitoneal mesh repair, the 'Sugarbaker' technique, the 'key-hole' technique, and the 'Sandwich repair'. The Sugarbaker technique was first described in 1985. A laparotomy was performed, and after the hernia was reduced, the sac resected, and the stoma trephine reduced to an appropriate size (just enough to admit the surgeon's finger), the ostomy opening is covered with an intraperitoneally placed prosthetic mesh that is sutured to the fascia. The bowel is lateralized and secured between the mesh and the peritoneum,

thereby lateralizing the forces which press the bowel ventrally onto the abdominal wall, shifting them from pushing up toward the defect and causing these forces to press ventrally against an intact abdominal wall (Figure 17.1). In the seminal paper describing this technique, there were six recurrent and one primary PHs repaired, with no recurrences reported with a 5-year follow-up [48]. In another slightly larger study, 20 open PH repairs with the Sugarbaker technique, using a mesh with an overlap of at least 5 cm, were reviewed retrospectively. There was a 15% recurrence rate with a mean follow-up of 42 months. Complications of the procedure included bowel obstruction secondary to dense adhesions, wound infection, seroma formation, and pain at the site of transfascial sutures [49]. Initial use of this technique may cause anxiety due to the sharp angle created in the large bowel conduit. Surgeons should be reassured that with appropriate technique, this will not result in obstruction. If biologic mesh is used, eventually native tissue ingrowth results in, essentially, an extraperitoneal-type colostomy. In general, this approach is not used for small bowel stomas.

The intraperitoneal approach aims to avoid local direct access to the stoma, which theoretically reduces the risk of infection by treating the hernia intra-abdominally. One of the variations was described by Sugarbaker, wherein the mesh is not only sutured around the hernia orifice, but also forms a bridge over the extracted colon, giving the effect of peritonization [48] (Figure 17.1).

The other primary option for surgical repair is the 'key-hole' technique. In the keyhole technique, a cut-out of mesh is made to circumferentially surround the ostomy and cover the entire hernia defect [51,52]. One of the tricks of this technique is to not make the keyhole too small so as to cause a bowel obstruction, but not to make it so large as to increase the risk of herniation (Figure 17.2). Hansson et al. found that the laparoscopic keyhole technique had higher rates of recurrence than laparoscopic Sugarbaker repairs, 34.6 versus 11.6%, respectively. It appears that using a solid piece of mesh rather than a cut piece of mesh provides a lower recurrence rate as well as shorter operative times.

The sandwich technique has also been described for laparoscopic repairs. This is a combination of both the keyhole and Sugarbaker techniques, using a piece of mesh in the intraperitoneal position as in the keyhole technique and then lateralizing the bowel and covering this with another piece of mesh using the Sugarbaker

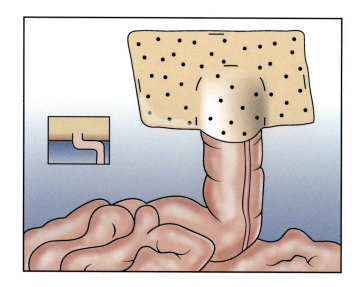

FIGURE 17.1   Sugarbaker repair.

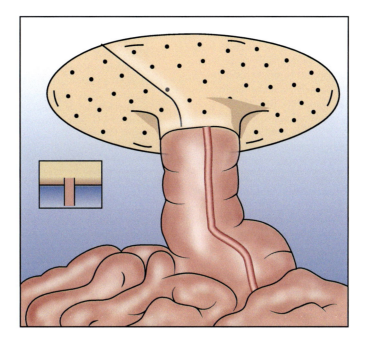

FIGURE 17.2   Keyhole repair.

technique. This technique does result in an area of mesh overlapping with mesh, which is generally avoided. There is only one study looking at this technique, performed by Berger and colleagues, that includes 42 patients with only a 2.1% rate of hernia recurrence [53]. This technique, although only studied in a small group of people, did have the lowest recurrence rate for laparoscopic repairs.

Laparoscopic versus open repair (see Videos 15 and 16)

There are multiple theoretical advantages to the use of laparoscopy when treating PH. First, it avoids another large incision and potential hernia site in the abdominal wound and allows faster postoperative recovery. It also provides a better view of the defect, allowing a more precise repair and reinforcement with mesh and greater overlap of the defect [11]. Unfortunately, there have been variable levels of success reported in the literature. Most studies demonstrate low infection rates (0%–5%) and conversion to an open procedure is infrequent. In Hansson and colleagues' review, they looked at 363 laparoscopic repairs and found a conversion to open rate of 3.6% [23]. The most common reasons for conversion include inadvertent enterotomy and dense adhesions [44,50].

In an overall comparison made between open and laparoscopic cases using NSQIP data from 2005 to 2011, it was determined the laparoscopic approach was associated with better short-term results than open surgery, includeing a 3-day reduction in length of hospital stay, a shorter operative time, a 58% reduction in morbidity, and a 65% reduction in the odds of a superficial skin infection [44].

Recurrence

The various types of PH repair are associated with a wide range of recurrence rates due to variations of the definition of a PH recurrence, either radiographic, clinical, or symptomatic; type of stoma; size of hernia defect; indications for a repair; and length of time of follow-up. Recurrence rates for primary suture repair are high, ranging from 30% to 76%. In a systematic review, primary suture repair significantly increased the risk for recurrent hernia compared to mesh repair [23]. There were no significant differences between open and laparoscopic hernia repair for recurrence; the open Sugarbaker technique had significantly fewer recurrences compared with the keyhole technique, but this was not the case for the laparoscopic approach. The following recurrence rates were noted:

- Primary suture repair: 69.4%
- Onlay mesh: 17.2%
- Sublay mesh: 6.9%
- Open, intraperitoneal mesh
  - Sugarbaker: 15%
  - Keyhole: 7.2%
- Laparoscopic mesh
  - Sugarbaker: 11.6%
  - Keyhole: 11.6%
  - Sandwich: 2.1%

Recurrent PH repair

Recurrent PH presents many challenges for repair. Recurrent repair is best performed if there was no mesh previously used. If mesh was used as an onlay or sublay and the hernia recurred, one option is to perform a Sugarbaker repair. If all else fails, relocating the stoma to the other side of the abdomen and using prophylactic mesh during creation of the new stoma is the next best option.

Robotic PH repair

There are a few case reports and video vignettes of parastomal hernioplasty done by the robotic assistance. Both the Sugarbaker type and retrorectus repair with or without transverses abdomonis release (TAR) have been described. A novel retrorectus Sugarbaker type of repair has also been performed (personal communication – Eric Pauli and Arun Prasad).

Summary

PH is a highly prevalent problem. In reality, almost every stoma will ultimately result in some degree of PH, if followed long enough. The complications of hernia range from asymptomatic to potentially life-threatening. The traditional paradigm of direct repair and stoma re-siting has largely been abandoned due to unacceptable recurrence rates at the initial site, as well as at the new site. The sublay or intra-abdominal approach offers the lowest recurrence rate, and is our recommendation. The decision whether to approach the surgery laparoscopically or open is based on the surgeon's level of experience and comfort. Finally, due to the known likely development of PH in the majority of cases, we recommend prophylactic parastomal reinforcement at the time of permanent stoma creation. Given the increased use of laparoscopy at the time of many colectomies, as well as the ease of placement, we favor a sublay or intraperitoneal technique in these cases.

Key points

- The most common long-term complication following stoma creation is PH, the incidence increases with time, ranging from 14.1% to 40%.
- Surgery should be avoided in asymptomatic patients due to the inherent risks and high incidence of recurrence.
- Surgical repair is indicated for patients who develop acute PH complications and for those with chronic symptoms that impair quality of life.
- Surgical options for correcting a PH are local primary repair, relocation, and repair with mesh.
- Out of all the methods used to prevent PH, prophylactic mesh repair appears to be most useful and successful in selected patients.
- Depending on the method and layer wherein the prosthetic is implanted, the currently employed surgical techniques can be classified as follows: superficial mesh (onlay technique), preperitoneal mesh (sublay technique), and intraperitoneal mesh (inlay technique).
- Techniques with prosthetic reinforcement can be divided into open techniques, laparoscopic techniques, and robotic techniques.
- The various types of PH repair are associated with a wide range of recurrence rates due to variations of the definition of a PH recurrence ranging from 2% (with sandwich repair) to 69% (with primary suture repair).

Videos

VIDEO 15   https://youtu.be/NJLZPlHjuhg

Lap Sugarbaker Hernioplasty for Parastomal Hernias.

VIDEO 16   https://youtu.be/kMTEJRvmRAw

Robotic Parastomal Hernioplasty for Parastomal Hernias.

References

1. Goligher JC. *Surgery of the Anus, Rectum and Colon.* 5th ed. Bailliere Tindall, 1985; 703–5.
2. Robertson I, Leung E, Hughes D et al. Prospective analysis of stoma-related complications. *Colorectal Dis* 2005;7(3):279–85.
3. Hasegawa J, Hirota M, Kim HM et al. Single-incision laparoscopic stoma creation: Experience with 31 consecutive cases. *Asian J Endosc Surg* 2013;6:181–5.
4. Carne PWG, Frye JNR, Robertson GM, Frizelle FA. Parastomal hernia following minimally invasive stoma formation. *ANZ J Surg* 2003;73:843–5.
5. Israelsson LA. Preventing and treating parastomal hernia. *World J Surg* 2005;29:1086–9.
6. Hansson BME, De Hingh IHJT, Bleichrodt RP. Laparoscopic parastomal hernia repair is feasible and safe: Early results of a prospective clinical study including 55 consecutive patients. *Surg Endosc Other Interv Tech* 2007;21:989–93.
7. Cingi A, Solmaz A, Attaallah W, Aslan A, Aktan AO. Enterostomy closure site hernias: A clinical and ultrasonographic evaluation. *Hernia* 2008;12:401–5.
8. Martin L, Foster G. Parastomal hernia. *Ann R CollSurg Engl* 1996;78:81–4.
9. Carne PWG, Robertson GM, Frizelle FA. Parastomal hernia. *Br J Surg* 2003;90:784–93.
10. Black P. Managing physical postoperative stoma complications. *Br J Nurs* 2009;18:4–10.
11. Hansson BM, Bleichrodt RP, de Hingh IH. Laparoscopic parastomal hernia repair using a keyhole technique results in a high recurrence rate. *Surg Endosc* 2009;23(7):1456–9.
12. Cingi A, Cakir T, Sever A, Aktan AO. Enterostomy site hernias: A clinical and computerized tomographic evaluation. *Dis Colon Rectum* 2006;49:1559–63.
13. Pilgrim CHC, McIntyre R, Bailey M. Prospective audit of parastomal hernia: Prevalence and associated comorbidities. *Dis Colon Rectum* 2010;53:71–6.
14. Williams JG, Etherington R, Hayward MW, Hughes LE. Para-ileostomy hernia: A clinical and radiological study. *Br J Surg* 1990;77(12):1355–7.
15. Allen-Mersh TG, Thomson JP. Surgical treatment of colostomy complications. *Br J Surg* 1988;75(5):416–8.
16. Rieger N, Moore J, Hewett P, Lee S, Stephens J. Parastomal hernia repair. *Colorectal Dis* 2004;6(3):203–5.
17. Riansuwan W, Hull TL, Millan MM, Hammel JP. Surgery of recurrent parastomal hernia: Direct repair or relocation? *Colo-rectal Dis* 2010;12(7):681–6.
18. Rubin MS, Schoetz DJ Jr, Matthews JB. Parastomal hernia. Is stoma relocation superior to fascial repair? *Arch Surg* 1994;129(4):413–8, discussion 418–419.
19. Cheung MT, Chia NH, Chiu WY. Surgical treatment of parastomal hernia complicating sigmoid colostomies. *Dis Colon Rectum* 2001;44(2):266–70.
20. Sjödahl R, Anderberg B, Bolin T. Parastomal hernia in relation to site of the abdominal stoma. *Br J Surg* 1988;75(4):339–41.
21. Ortiz H, Sara MJ, Armendariz P, de Miguel M, Marti J, Chocarro C. Does the frequency of paracolostomy hernias depend on the position of the colostomy in the abdominal wall? *Int J Colorectal Dis* 1994;9(2):65–7.
22. Israelsson LA. Parastomal hernias. *Surg Clin North Am* 2008;88(1):113–25, ixix.
23. Hansson BM, Slater NJ, van der Velden AS et al. Surgical techniques for parastomal hernia repair: A systematic reviewof the literature. *Ann Surg* 2012;255(4):685–95.
24. Resnick S. New method of bowel stoma formation. *Am J Surg* 1986;152(5):545–8.
25. Koltun L, Benyamin N, Sayfan J. Abdominal stoma fashioned by a used circular stapler. *Dig Surg* 2000;17(2):118–9.
26. Wang J, Dou Z, Wang T, Liu D, Wang L. Circular stapler-assisted extraperitoneal colostomy. *Dig Surg* 2010;27(6):521–4.
27. Goligher JC. Extraperitoneal colostomy or ileostomy. *Br J Surg* 1958;46(196):97–103.

28. Whittaker M, Goligher JC. A comparison of the results of extraperitoneal and intraperitoneal techniques for construction of terminal iliac colostomies. *Dis Colon Rectum* 1976;19(4):342–4.

29. Hamada M, Ozaki K, Muraoka G, Kawakita N, Nishioka Y. Permanent end-sigmoid colostomy through the extraperitoneal route prevents parastomal hernia after laparoscopic abdominoperineal resection. *Dis Colon Rectum* 2012;55(9):963–9.

30. Lian L, Wu XR, He XS et al. Extraperitoneal vs. intraperitoneal route for permanent colostomy: A meta-analysis of 1,071 patients. *Int J Colorectal Dis* 2012;27(1):59–64.

31. Bayer I, Kyzer S, Chaimoff C. A new approach to primary strengthening of colostomy with Marlex mesh to prevent paracolostomy hernia. *Surg Gynecol Obstet* 1986;163(6):579–80.

32. Lüning TH, Spillenaar-Bilgen EJ. Parastomal hernia: Complications of extra-peritoneal onlay mesh placement. *Hernia* 2009;13(5):487–90.

33. Longman RJ, Thomson WH. Mesh repair of parastomal hernias – a safety modification. *Colorectal Dis* 2005;7(3):292–4.

34. Steele SR, Lee P, Martin MJ, Mullenix PS, Sullivan ES. Is parastomal hernia repair with polypropylenemesh safe? *AmJ Surg* 2003;185(5):436–40.

35. Gögenur I, Mortensen J, Harvald T, Rosenberg J, Fischer A. Prevention of parastomal hernia by placement of a polypropylene mesh at the primary operation. *Dis Colon Rectum* 2006; 49(8):1131–5.

36. Hauters P, Cardin JL, Lepere M, Valverde A, Cossa JP, Auvray S. Prevention of parastomal hernia by intraperitoneal onlay mesh reinforcement at the time of stoma formation. *Hernia* 2012; 16(6):655–60.

37. Figel NA, Rostas JW, Ellis CN. Outcomes using a bioprosthetic mesh at the time of permanent stoma creation in preventing a parastomal hernia: A value analysis. *AmJ Surg* 2012;203(3):323–6, discussion 326.

38. Tam KW, Wei PL, Kuo LJ, Wu CH. Systematic reviewof the use of a mesh to prevent parastomal hernia. *World J Surg* 2010;34(11):2723–9.

39. Wijeyekoon SP, Gurusamy K, El-Gendy K, Chan CL. Prevention of parastomal herniationwith biologic/composite prosthetic mesh: A systematic review and meta-analysis of randomized controlled trials. *J Am Coll Surg* 2010;211(5):637–45.

40. Serra-Aracil X, Bombardo-Junca J, Moreno-Matias J et al. Randomized, controlled, prospective trial of the use of a mesh to prevent parastomal hernia. *Ann Surg* 2009;249(4):583–7.

41. Jänes A, Cengiz Y, Israelsson LA. Randomized clinical trial of the use of a prosthetic mesh to prevent parastomal hernia. *Br J Surg* 2004;91(3):280–2.

42. Jänes A, Cengiz Y, Israelsson LA. Preventing parastomal hernia with a prosthetic mesh: A 5-year follow-up of a randomized study. *World J Surg* 2009;33(1):118–21, discussion 122–123.

43. Wang S, Wang W, Zhu B, Song G, Jiang C. Efficacy of Prophylactic Mesh in End-Colostomy Construction: A Systematic Review and Meta-analysis of Randomized Controlled Trials. *World J Surg* 2016;40:2528–36.

44. Halabi WJ, Jafari MD, Carmichael JC et al. Laparoscopic versus open repair of parastomal hernias: An ACS-NSQIP analysis of short-term outcomes. *Surg Endosc* 2013;27(11):4067–72.

45. Findlay JM, Wood CP, Cunningham C. Prophylactic mesh reinforcement of stomas: A cost–efectiveness meta–analysis of randomised controlled trials. *Tech Coloproctol* 2018;22:265–70.

46. Tadeo-Ruiz G, Picazo-Yeste JS, Moreno-Sanz C, Herrero-Bogajo ML. Parastomal hernias: Background, current status and future prospects. *Cir Esp* 2010;87:339–49.

47. Kasperk R, Klinge U, Schumpelick V. The repair of large parastomal hernias using a midline approach and a prosthetic mesh in the sublay position. *Am J Surg* 2000;179(3):186.

48. Sugarbaker PH. Peritoneal approach to prosthetic mesh repair of paraostomy hernias. *Ann Surg* 1985;201(3):344–6.

49. Stelzner S, Hellmich G, Ludwig K. Repair of paracolostomy hernias with a prosthetic mesh in the intraperitoneal onlay position: Modified Sugarbaker technique. *Dis Colon Rectum* 2004;47(2):185–91.

50. Asif A, Ruiz M, Yetasook A et al. Laparoscopic modified Sugarbaker technique results in superior recurrence rate. *Surg Endosc* 2012;26(12):3430–4.

51. Van Sprundel TC, Gerritsen van der Hoop A. Modified technique forparastomal hernia repair in patients with intractable stomacareproblems. *Colorectal Dis* 2005;7(5):445–9.

52. Hofstetter WL, Vukasin P, Ortega AE, Anthone G, Beart RW Jr. New technique for mesh repair of paracolostomy hernias. *Dis Colon Rectum* 1998;41(8):1054–5.

53. Berger D, Bientzle M. Polyvinylidene fluoride: A suitable mesh material for laparoscopic incisional and parastomal hernia repair! A prospective, observational study with 344 patients. *Hernia* 2009;13(2):167–72.

Section IV
Laparoscopy Colorectal Cancer Surgery

18 Laparoscopic versus Open Colorectal Resection: An Evidence-Based Review 117
19 Laparoscopic Right Hemicolectomy for Right Colon Cancer 123
20 Laparoscopic Transverse Colectomy for Transverse Colon Cancer 128
21 Laparoscopic Hemicolectomy for Left Colon Cancer 131
22 Laparoscopic Anterior Resection and Total Mesorectal Excision for
   Rectosigmoid Cancer 139
23 Techniques for Laparoscopic Low Anterior Resection, Ultra Low Anterior
   Resection, and Inter Sphincteric Resection (ISR) 146
24 Laparoscopic Conventional Abdominoperineal (CAPE) and Extra-Levator
   Abdominoperineal Resection (ELAPE) 154
25 Laparoscopic Subtotal/Total/Proctocolectomy 160
26 Laparoscopic Management of T4 Tumor and Pelvic Exenteration for Locally
   Advanced Tumors 165
27 Laparoscopic Surgery in Obstructed and Recurrent Tumors 172
28 Resection for Colorectal Liver Metastasis 179
29 Specimen Retrieval after Laparoscopic Colectomy and NOSE 185

Chapter 18

LAPAROSCOPIC VERSUS OPEN COLORECTAL RESECTION: AN EVIDENCE-BASED REVIEW

Anish Nagpal

Contents

Learning objectives 117
Introduction 117
Historical perspectives of laparoscopic colorectal surgery.............................. 117
Filling the gap between open and laparoscopic surgery 118
    Laparoscopic-assisted techniques 118
    Hand-assisted techniques 118
Evidence for quality of life after laparoscopic colorectal cancer resection 118
Rectal cancer 119
    Efficacy of minimal invasive surgery for rectal malignancy 119
    Locally advanced rectal disease 120
        Indications for extended lymphadenectomy in rectal cancer................... 120
Future of laparoscopic colorectal surgery 120
Summary 121
Key points 121
References 121

Learning objectives

- Review the current scenario of laparoscopic colorectal surgery
- Evidence-based review of literature
- Learn practical guidelines

Introduction

The advances of laparoscopic surgery during the last three decades have been one of the major revolutions in the field of surgery. Since the application of laparoscopic surgery, minimally invasive techniques are being utilized in all aspects of gastrointestinal and urologic surgeries. Still, the acceptance of laparoscopic surgery in cancer care was resisted mainly due to its oncologic concerns and the substantial learning curve it presents for surgeons. In spite of all the technical difficulties and debatable early oncologic parameters, laparoscopic surgery persisted, and eventually favorable long-term outcomes data on its oncological parameters provided the major breakthrough. Over the past ten years, laparoscopic surgery has been increasingly applied to the resection of cancers. Level 1 evidence is now available, providing strong support for similar oncological outcomes between laparoscopic surgery and open surgery for colon cancers. The future of laparoscopic colorectal surgery will be based on prognostic factors of success, potentially limiting approaches that do not add to patient outcomes.

Historical perspectives of laparoscopic colorectal surgery

The first laparoscopic-assisted colectomy was reported by Jacobs et al. [1] According to Jacobs, laparoscopic-assisted colonic surgery was considered an evolving procedure, but he was confident that in time it had the potential to be as popular as laparoscopic cholecystectomy. The successful application of laparoscopic surgery to gallbladder disease and acute appendicitis encouraged Jacobs [1] to develop this technology further in an attempt to manage other pathologic disorders of the gastrointestinal (GI) tract, and therefore, he initiated a pilot program for laparoscopic colonic surgery. Twenty patients with ages ranging from 43 to 88 years (mean age 57 years) underwent laparoscope-assisted colon resection. Eighty percent of patients were able to tolerate a liquid diet on the first postoperative day, and 70% were discharged within 96 hr – eating a regular diet and having normal bowel movements.

Compared with routine laparoscopic procedures like cholecystectomy, appendectomy, or Nissen fundoplication, laparoscopic colorectal surgery is more challenging as it often involves more than one abdominal quadrant. Further, it requires determination of the correct target segment to be removed, safe identification and transection of named vascular structures, mobilization and resection of the bowel, and specimen retrieval and creation of an anastomosis. An early report, by Frederik J. Berends, raised concerns about high rates of port site recurrences of up to 21%, which led to the decreased use of laparoscopy for malignant disease [2]. Fortunately, the issue was investigated further in a number of reports whereby a port site recurrence rate closer to 1% was noted, which appeared to be in a similar range as wound implants after open surgery for colorectal cancer [3–6]. These were retrospective findings, but later a number of prospective randomized trials were undertaken (Table 18.1) to investigate the impact of laparoscopic surgery on oncological outcomes [7–12].

In the United States, a well-designed prospective randomized multicenter trial was conducted under the umbrella of the National Cancer Institute to document noninferiority of the laparoscopic approach when compared to open surgery [10,11]. Other trials were initiated in other parts of the world, most notably in Spain, the United Kingdom, and Hong Kong [8,9,12]. While the larger picture remained in evolution, all studies including several meta-analyses came to similar conclusions that laparoscopic

TABLE 18.1: **Important Breakthrough Trials**

Trial	Place	Type of Trial	Patients Enrolled	End points	Interpretation
Colon cancer laparoscopic or open resection study group (COLOR) trial [7]	Canada	PRT	627 patients lap 621 open	The primary endpoint was cancer-free survival 3 years after surgery.	Laparoscopic surgery can be used for safe and radical resection of cancer in the right, left, and sigmoid colon.
(MRC CLASICC) trial [8]	London	PRT	452 patients randomized to laparoscopic surgery (lap) compared with the 230 randomized to open procedure (open)	This study presents the short-term (3 month) cost analysis undertaken on a subset of patients entered into the CLASICC trial.	The short-term cost analysis for the CLASICC trial indicates that the costs of either laparoscopic or open procedure were similar, lap surgery costing marginally more on average than open surgery.
Laparoscopic resection of rectosigmoid carcinoma: prospective randomized trial [9]	Hong Kong		403 patients with rectosigmoid carcinoma were randomized to receive either laparoscopic assisted (n = 203) or conventional open (n = 200) resection of the tumor	Survival and disease-free interval were the main endpoints.	Laparoscopic resection of rectosigmoid carcinoma does not jeopardize survival and disease control of patients. The justification for adoption of the laparoscopic technique would depend on the perceived value of its effectiveness in improving short-term postoperative outcomes.
Clinical outcomes of surgical therapy study group [10] COST trial	USA	PRT	872 patients with adenocarcinoma of the colon to undergo open or laparoscopically assisted colectomy	The primary end point was the time to tumor recurrence.	In this multi-institutional study, the rates of recurrent cancer were similar after laparoscopically assisted colectomy and open colectomy, suggesting that the laparoscopic approach is an acceptable alternative to open surgery for colon cancer.
Barcelona trial lap-assisted vs. open colectomy [12]		RCT Single center	219		Improved perioperative outcomes and hospital stay in lap group. Survival benefit in stage III disease for lap group.

Abbreviations: PRT: Prospective Randomized Trial; RCT: Randomized Control Trial.

colectomy in skilled hands was associated with shorter postoperative recovery at the price of longer operative times; however, most notably it was safe and at least oncologically equivalent to the standard of open surgery [13–15]. However, a steep learning curve was acknowledged throughout the literature, and at least 20–50 laparoscopic cases were considered the minimum to achieve basic proficiency with the technique. Along those lines, the professional societies ASCRS, ACS, and SAGES supported the use of laparoscopy for cancer performed by appropriately trained surgeons who are engaged in training protocols.

Filling the gap between open and laparoscopic surgery

Several variations – such as the laparoscopic-assisted or the hand-assisted techniques – have been developed to bridge the gap between conventional open surgery and minimally invasive approaches.

Laparoscopic-assisted techniques
'Laparoscopic-assisted' is a broad term utilized variably for laparoscopic mobilization of the left colon and division of the inferior mesenteric pedicle for anterior resection, with subsequent rectal dissection being performed open via a low midline or Pfannenstiel incision, avoiding a high midline wound which would potentially be more painful and reduce cosmesis.

Hand-assisted techniques
A hybrid technique is the hand-assisted approach, which attempts to provide the advantages of laparoscopic surgery while

reducing the technical difficulties and increased operative time. It can be particularly useful for surgeons, who are relatively new to laparoscopic surgery, as a useful adjunct to becoming proficient in fully laparoscopic colorectal surgery. This technique involves the insertion of a hand port into the abdominal wall that allows the surgeons' hand to enter the abdominal cavity to assist in the operation, while maintaining a pneumoperitoneum and therefore continued visualization of the abdominal contents with the laparoscope. Although data comparing hand-assisted and laparoscopic colorectal surgery is limited in comparison to that comparing laparoscopic and open procedures, a Cochrane review of randomized controlled trials concluded that there was a significant decrease in conversion rates in the hand-assisted group, although there was no difference in complications or operating times [16].

Evidence for quality of life after laparoscopic colorectal cancer resection

Although the concern regarding port site metastases had been addressed by the turn of the century, and uptake of laparoscopic colorectal surgery began to increase as a niche interest, a lack of long-term data evaluating oncological outcomes – following cancer resection – prevented its use as a mainstream technique in the majority of units. At this time, data from large multicenter randomized controlled trials across the world have been published and suggest that short-term outcomes were at least equivalent to open surgery and may have some advantages on perioperative outcomes.

After colorectal surgery for malignancy, many patients experience a combination of physical and emotional problems for a long period of time. Symptoms such as fatigue, pain and disturbed bowel function, as well as problems in social and role functioning inevitably affect the patients' well-being. Assessment of self-reported quality of life is therefore increasingly important in clinical trials, and when considering the higher costs for laparoscopy and its cost-effectiveness. In addition, in cancer trials, it has been shown that assessing quality of life can contribute to improved treatment [17]. In 2010, Bartels SAL and Vlug MS published a systematic review of all available randomized controlled trials involving 2263 patients addressing the quality of life after laparoscopic and open colorectal surgery [18]. When patients were surveyed on their quality of life following both forms of surgery, using validated questionnaires, the authors concluded that: 'based on presently available high-level evidence, this systematic review showed no clinically relevant differences in postoperative quality of life between laparoscopic and open colorectal surgery' (Table 18.2).

Rectal cancer

Rectal cancer is managed in a multimodal fashion, with surgery continuing to be the mainstay of treatment. The use of laparoscopic treatment of rectal cancer has been limited, and is tempered by the relative complexity of the operation and questionable benefits in short-term postoperative and pathologic outcomes.

Efficacy of minimal invasive surgery for rectal malignancy

Total mesorectal excision (TME) has become the surgical treatment of choice for rectal cancer, because adopting the principles of TME achieves very low local recurrence rates. The adoption of the TME principles along with the estimation of the circumferential resection margin on the nonperitonealized surface of the resected rectal specimen are the most important predictors of local recurrence. Many have demonstrated that these principles can be followed with the MIS approach. While there are aspects of these principles that are easily accomplished with the MIS approach (high ligation, distal margin, and anastomosis), the integrity of the circumferential resection margin has been a concern in some studies [8,23,24].

One of the earliest surgical trials to encompass the role of laparoscopy in rectal cancer was the MRC CLASICC trial out of the United Kingdom [8]. This study was mainly carried out for evaluating the role of laparoscopy in colorectal cancer disease, and the subset of patients with rectal disease was limited. However, the rectal cancer patients treated with an MIS approach did have an increase in the rate of the circumferential resection margin (CRM) positivity, but this did not reflect in an increase in the local recurrence rate.

Other studies, like the COREAN and COLOR II trials, were both performed in a randomized fashion and neither found differences in the circumferential margin [26,27]. These studies went on to examine local recurrence rates and found no differences over relatively short time frames. In addition to these randomized controlled trials, many institutional series have been performed and have found no differences in recurrence rates. Both the COREAN [26] and COLOR II trial [27] compared laparoscopic to open rectal cancer resections and showed no difference in the quality of the oncologic resection, complication rates, and long-term survival outcomes. However, both trials had limitations such as a nonobese population, involvement limited to three tertiary centers with experienced surgeons, and a low complete mesorectal excision rate (73%) in the COREAN trial. Similarly, the COLOR II trial used neoadjuvant therapy in stage I patients, had a low rate of pathologic complete response (pCR), a high rate for CRM involvement for tumors located in the low rectum (22%) in the open group, and a high permanent stoma rate (29%) in the laparoscopic group. Since these two trials, two well-done major RCTs have been published on this topic: the ALaCaRT trial [24] and the ACOSOG-Z6051 trial [23], which are highlighted in Table 18.3.

Both trials failed to show noninferiority of the laparoscopic approach compared with open surgery for pathologic outcomes. In all four trials, the laparoscopic group had significantly longer operative time, less blood loss, and quicker return of bowel function, while two trials demonstrated a shorter hospital stay. In summary, the available RCT data do not support the use of laparoscopic resection in patients with rectal cancer at this time.

Surgery for rectal cancer remains fraught with complications. A minimally invasive approach is safe and effective and appears to improve short-term outcomes. While long-term oncologic outcome from some studies is pending, many have found no

TABLE 18.2: Summary of Key Papers on Laparoscopic Resection for Colorectal Cancer

Trial	Year of Publication	Type of Study	Numbers of Patients	Key Findings
Barcelona trial [12] Lap-assisted vs. open colectomy	2002	RCT Single center		Improved perioperative outcomes and hospital stay in lap group. Survival benefit in stage III disease for lap group
COST study [10] Lap vs. open colectomy	2004	RCT Multicenter	872	Longer operating time but quicker recovery for lap. No difference in morbidity, mortality, recurrence or survival
COLOR trial [19] Lap vs. open colectomy	2009	RCT Multicenter	1248	Supported findings of COST study
CLASICC trial [18,21] Lap vs. open colon and rectal cancers	2005, 2010 (5 yr follow-up)	RCT Multicenter	794 (2:1 lap:open)	Equivalent perioperative and oncological outcomes, 29% conversion rate. Higher CRM involvement for rectal cancers with lap
Abraham et al. [22] Short-term outcomes of lap vs. open	2004	Meta-analysis of RCTs	2521 12 RCTs	Longer operative times, less morbidity and quicker recovery for lap. Mortality and oncological outcomes equivalent
Cochrane review [20] Short-term outcomes after lap	2005	Systematic review		Less morbidity and quicker recovery for lap
Cochrane review [15] Long-term results after lap	2008	Systematic review		Equivalent oncological outcomes for lap vs. open

Abbreviations: lap: laparoscopic; RCT: Randomized control trial; CRM: circumferential resection margin.

TABLE 18.3: Trials Comparing Laparoscopic and Open Surgery for Rectal Cancer Patients

Trial	No of Patients	Primary Endpoint	Negative CRM	Clear Distal Margin	Complete or Near- Complete TME	Other
Kang et al. (2010) [36]	340	3-y DFS rate	97.1% lap vs. 95.9% open	100% lap vs. 100% open	91.8% lap vs. 88% open	3-y LR, DFS, OS: Similar Conversion rate: 1.5%
Van der Pas et al. (2013) [37]	1044	3-y LR rate	90% lap vs. 90% open	100% lap vs. 100% open	97% lap vs. 98% open	3-y LR, DFS, OS: Similar Conversion rate: 17%
Stevenson et al. (2015) [24]	475	Complete TME, CRM ≥ 1 MM Distal margin ≥ 1 mm	93% lap vs. 97% open	98% lap vs. 98% open	97% lap vs. 99% open	Conversion rate: 9%
Fleshman et al. (2015) [23]	248	Composite of CRM >1 mm, negative distal margin and completeness of TME	87.9% lap vs. 92% open	99% lap vs. 99% open	92% lap vs. 95% open	Conversion rate: 11.3%

Abbreviations: CRM: circumferential margin; DFS: disease-free survival rate; lap: laparoscopic; LR: local recurrence rate; OR time: operative time; OS: overall survival rate; TME: total mesorectal excision.

differences in local recurrence or disease-free survival. While there are clear positives to a minimally invasive operation, oncologic outcomes must be the top priority.

Therefore, the approach to the treatment of rectal cancer should be based on the experience of the surgeon. For those who feel comfortable with a minimally invasive approach, the platform of choice is dictated by their own experience.

Locally advanced rectal disease

Indications for extended lymphadenectomy in rectal cancer

Neoadjuvant chemoradiation therapy (CRT), followed by total mesorectal excision (TME) represents the standard of care for the treatment of locally advanced extraperitoneal rectal cancer [30,31]. However, metastases in the lateral pelvic lymph nodes (LPLN) occur in up to 25% of these patients [32,33], and LPLN involvement is associated with high rates of local recurrence and poor oncologic outcomes after neoadjuvant CRT and TME [34]. To lower the risk of local recurrence and improve long-term survival, TME with LPLN dissection and extended lymphadenectomy (EL) beyond the planes of TME has been widely adopted in Japan, even in the absence of enlarged LPLNs. However, the value of this strategy is still debated in Western countries for several reasons.

First, even though TME with EL appears to reduce the rate of local recurrence, it does not prevent the occurrence of tumor relapse in the lateral pelvis [35]. Second, LPLN metastases are considered distant metastases in Western literature. Third, with neoadjuvant CRT the radiation field include tumor and peri-rectal nodes.

Fourth, early perioperative outcomes are poorer after EL than for rectal surgery performed within the planes of the TME: EL is associated with longer operative time and greater intraoperative blood losses. Quality of life and both sexual and urinary functions are poorer than those reported after TME alone [25,28,29]. Hence, the real benefits from the minimally invasive approach in these patients remain unproven, and there have been very few retrospective studies comparing laparoscopic and open EL.

In conclusion, based on the current evidence, EL should be considered within a tailored multidisciplinary strategy in rectal cancer patients with enlarged LPLNs before neoadjuvant CRT, and the postoperative morbidity and the oncologic benefits should be balanced out. However, the results of large RCTs are needed to shed light on unanswered questions, including the role of a laparoscopic approach and induction preoperative chemotherapy on the outcomes of this complex patient population. These RCT results would also provide the opportunity to better select patients that would benefit from EL.

Future of laparoscopic colorectal surgery

A number of new approaches have been researched and are evolving. Robotic surgery has already evolved and is aggressively marketed even though it has the limitations of cost, bulkiness, and lack of tactile feedback. Single-port laparoscopic surgery and/ or natural orifice transluminal endoscopic surgery (NOTES) was once perceived to be the ultimate goal of minimally invasive surgery. The latter – as a result of a concerning incidence of complications in experimental settings – has not gotten beyond pilot settings. Transanal endoscopic microsurgery (TEMS), or transanal minimally invasive surgery (TAMIS) for colorectal diseases, has achieved convincing results for benign rectal lesions that are not amenable to colonoscopic removal, or too high for conventional transanal excisions. When it comes to the role in malignant disease, however, concerns exceed the ones for laparoscopic surgery for cancer insofar as local excision of rectal cancers has always been associated with unjustifiably high local recurrence rates. Laparoscopically-assisted colonoscopic polypectomies (endoscopic-laparoscopic resections) is a combination of two procedures and has been suggested for larger colon lesions similar to TEMS/TAMIS for rectal lesions. However, the difference is that typically a laparoscopic segmental colon resection is much less problematic than a rectal resection. Hence, it remains doubtful what – if any – parameter would define superiority of outcome compared to a laparoscopic resection in the first place. Furthermore, one should caution that the probability of harboring a malignancy within a polyp is equivalent to the size of the lesion. Manipulating such a malignancy to the point of transmural dissection would not only be a primarily insufficient oncological resection, but furthermore carry the risk of turning a curable tumor into a noncurable one if cancer cells are spilled into the peritoneal cavity.

Last but not least, at the present time, appropriate surgical tumor management is defined by the tissue specimen being retrieved. Gross and microscopic pathology are core elements of tumor staging, and are relevant prognostic and predictive factors for treatment planning of a multimodality management. A new form of surgery combining the use of surgery and real-time image guidance has gained popularity in the field of surgical research. Cybernetic surgery is a combination of augmented skills, such as augmented reality and computer generated realistic 3D environments with real image guidance. The main goal is to increase the safety and accuracy of surgical procedures. Also, the use of near-infrared fluorescence (NIF) provides an expansion for the application of laparoscopic and robotic surgery. NIF can be used to assess blood supply and sentinel lymph node mapping in both colorectal and gastroesophageal surgeries. Intraoperative indocyanine green (ICG) use can help in identifying the vascular and biliary anatomy, assessing organ and tissue perfusion, mapping lymph nodes, and real-time identification of lesions. In trying to predict future research, human and artificial intelligence may be considered one of the main target areas in new surgical platforms.

Summary

Laparoscopic surgery has been a major revolution in surgery and clearly has become a core technique in colorectal surgery. The fine tuning of its applications remains in evolution. At times of economic constraints, institutions should resist jumping on every single trend, but should employ the wisdom of controlled research to define true progress that results in measurable value for the patient. In the United Kingdom and United States, the National Institute of Clinical Excellence and the Society of American Gastrointestinal and Endoscopic Surgeons, respectively, now support laparoscopic resection for colorectal cancer performed by suitably experienced surgeons.

In conclusion, laparoscopic surgery for colorectal disease has moved from being an experimental procedure performed by a small number of pioneers in the early 1990s, to today being firmly established in the mainstream around the world. This has occurred despite the fact that laparoscopic surgery – during the initial stage of the learning curve – is more expensive and requires a longer operating time than the equivalent open colorectal procedure. Large-scale international multicenter randomized trial data has established that laparoscopic colorectal surgery is safe, both in terms of short-term perioperative outcomes and long-term oncological efficacy. We are now into the robotic era, which is perhaps the next stage of minimally invasive colorectal procedures.

Key points

- Surgery remains the mainstay of curative treatment for both colon and rectal cancers.
- Colon cancer outcomes have improved with the use of laparoscopic techniques, enhanced recovery pathways, and adjuvant chemotherapy.

- Multimodality management of rectal cancer continues to evolve, with total mesorectal excision being the cornerstone.
- Oncologic results from recent studies do support the use of laparoscopic resection in patients with rectal cancer.
- For locally advanced extraperitoneal rectal cancer, TME with LPLN dissection and extended lymphadenectomy (EL) is suggested, but awaits clinical trials. However, the role of laparoscopy in EL is doubtful.

References

1. Jacobs M, Verdeja JC, Goldstein HS. Minimally invasive colon resection (laparoscopic colectomy). *Surg Laparos Endosc Percut Tech* 1991;1:144–50.
2. Berends FJ, Kazemier G, Bonjer HJ, Lange JF. Subcutaneous metastases after laparoscopic colectomy. *Lancet* 1994;344:58.
3. Reilly WT, Nelson H, Schroeder G, Wieand HS, Bolton J, O'Connell MJ. Wound recurrence following conventional treatment of colorectal cancer. A rare but perhaps underestimated problem. *Dis Colon Rectum* 1996;39:200–7.
4. Hughes ES, McDermott FT, Polglase AL, Johnson WR. Tumor recurrence in the abdominal wall scar tissue after large-bowel cancer surgery. *Dis Colon Rectum* 1983;26:571–2.
5. Fleshman JW, Nelson H, Peters WR et al. Early results of laparoscopic surgery for colorectal cancer. Retrospective analysis of 372 patients treated by Clinical Outcomes of Surgical Therapy (COST) study group. *Dis Colon Rectum* 1996;39:S53–8.
6. Allardyce RA. Is the port site really at risk? Biology, mechanisms and prevention: A critical view. *Aust N Z J Surg* 1999;69:479–85.
7. Veldkamp R, Kuhry E, Hop WC et al. Colon cancer laparoscopic or open resection study group (COLOR) laparoscopic surgery versus open surgery for colon cancer: Short-term outcomes of a randomised trial. *Lancet Oncol* 2005;6:477–84.
8. Guillou PJ, Quirke P, Thorpe H, Walker J, Jayne DG, Smith AMH, Heath RM, Brown JM. Short-term endpoints of conventional versus laparoscopic-assisted surgery in patients with colorectal cancer (MRC CLASICC trial): Multicentre, randomised controlled trial. *Lancet* 2005;365:1718–26.
9. Leung KL, Kwok SP, Lam SC, Lee JF, Yiu RY, Ng SS, Lai PB, Lau WY. Laparoscopic resection of rectosigmoid carcinoma: Prospective randomised trial. *Lancet* 2004;363:1187–92.
10. Clinical Outcomes of Surgical Therapy Study Group. A comparison of laparoscopically assisted and open colectomy for colon cancer. *N Engl J Med* 2004;350:2050–9.
11. Weeks JC, Nelson H, Gelber S, Sargent D, Schroeder G. Short-term quality-of-life outcomes following laparoscopic-assisted colectomy vs open colectomy for colon cancer: A randomized trial. *JAMA* 2002;287:321–8.
12. Lacy AM, García-Valdecasas JC, Delgado S, Castells A, Taurá P, Piqué JM, Visa J. Laparoscopy-assisted colectomy versus open colectomy for treatment of non-metastatic colon cancer: A randomised trial. *Lancet* 2002;359:2224–9.
13. Bonjer HJ, Hop WC, Nelson H et al. Laparoscopically assisted vs open colectomy for colon cancer: A meta-analysis. *Arch Surg* 2007;142:298–303.
14. Jackson TD, Kaplan GG, Arena G, Page JH, Rogers SO. Laparoscopic versus open resection for colorectal cancer: A metaanalysis of oncologic outcomes. *J Am Coll Surg.* 2007;204:439–46.
15. Kuhry E, Schwenk WF, Gaupset R, Romild U, Bonjer HJ. Long-term results of laparoscopic colorectal cancer resection. *Cochrane Database Syst Rev* 2008;2008(2):CD003432. doi:10.1002/14651858. CD003432.pub2.
16. Moloo H, Haggar F, Coyle D, Hutton B, Duhaime S, Mamazza J, Poulin EC, Boushey RP, Grimshaw J. Hand assisted laparoscopic surgery versus conventional laparoscopy for colorectal surgery. *Cochrane Database Syst Rev* 2010;(10):CD006585.

17. Gujral S, Avery KN, Blazeby JM. Quality of life after surgery for colorectal cancer: Clinical implications of results from randomised trials. *Support Care Cancer* 2008;16:127–32.

18. Bartels SA, Vlug MS, Ubbink DT, Bemelman WA. Quality of life after laparoscopic and open colorectal surgery: A systematic review. *World J Gastroenterol* 2010;16:5035–41.

19. Buunen M, Veldkamp R, Hop WC et al. Survival after laparoscopic surgery versus open surgery for colon cancer: Long-term outcome of a randomised clinical trial. *Lancet Oncol* 2009;10:44–52.

20. Schwenk W, Haase O, Neudecker J, Müller JM. Short term benefits for laparoscopic colorectal resection. *Cochrane Database Syst Rev* 2005;(3):CD003145.

21. Jayne DG, Thorpe HC, Copeland J, Quirke P, Brown JM, Guillou PJ. Five-year follow-up of the medical research council CLASICC trial of laparoscopically assisted versus open surgery for colorectal cancer. *Br J Surg* 2010;97:1638–45.

22. Abraham NS, Young JM, Solomon MJ. Meta-analysis of short-term outcomes after laparoscopic resection for colorectal cancer. *Br J Surg* 2004;91:1111–24.

23. Fleshman J, Branda M, Sargent DJ et al. Effect of Laparoscopic-Assisted resection vs open resection of stage II or III rectal cancer on pathologic outcomes: The ACOSOG Z6051 randomized clinical trial. *JAMA* 2015;314(13):1346–55.

24. Stevenson AR, Solomon MJ, Lumley JW et al. Effect of Laparoscopic-Assisted resection vs open resection on pathological outcomes in rectal cancer: The Ala CaRT randomized clinical trial. *JAMA* 2015;314(13):1356–63.

25. Fujita S, Akasu T, Mizusawa J et al. Postoperative morbidity and mortality after mesorectal excision with and without lateral lymph node dissection for clinical stage II or stage III lower rectal cancer (JCOG0212): Results from a multicentre, randomised controlled, non-inferiority trial. *Lancet Oncol* 2012;13(6):616–21.

26. Jeong SY, Park JW, Nam BH et al. Open versus laparoscopic surgery for mid-rectal or low-rectal cancer after neoadjuvant chemoradiotherapy (COREAN trial): Survival outcomes of an open-label, non-inferiority, randomised controlled trial. *Lancet Oncol* 2014;15(7):767–74.

27. Bonjer HJ, Deijen CL, Abis GA et al. A randomized trial of laparoscopic versus open surgery for rectal cancer. *N Engl JMed* 2015;372(14):1324–32.

28. Georgiou P, Tan E, Gouvas N et al. Extended lymphadenectomy versus conventional surgery for rectal cancer: Ameta-analysis. *Lancet Oncol* 2009;10(11):1053–62.

29. Valentini V, Aristei C, Glimelius B et al. Multidisciplinary rectal cancer management: 2nd European Rectal Cancer Consensus Conference (EURECACC2). *Radiother Oncol* 2009;92(2):148–63.

30. Swedish Rectal Cancer T. Cedermark B, Dahlberg M, Glimelius B et al. Improved survival with preoperative radiotherapy in resectable rectal cancer. *N Engl J Med* 1997;336(14):980–7.

31. MacFarlane JK, Ryall RD, Heald RJ. Mesorectal excision for rectal cancer. *Lancet* 1993;341(8843):457–60.

32. Fujita S, Yamamoto S, Akasu T, Moriya Y. Lateral pelvic lymph node dissection for advanced lower rectal cancer. *Br J Surg* 2003;90(12):1580–5.

33. Ueno M, Oya M, Azekura K, Yamaguchi T, Muto T. Incidence and prognostic significance of lateral lymph node metastasis in patients with advanced low rectal cancer. *Br J Surg* 2005;92(6):756–63.

34. Hida J, Yasutomi M, Fujimoto K, Maruyama T, Okuno K, Shindo K. Does lateral lymph node dissection improve survival in rectal carcinoma? Examination of node metastases by the clearing method. *J Am Coll Surg* 1997;184(5):475–80.

35. Fujita S, Mizusawa J, Kanemitsu Y et al. Mesorectal excision with or without lateral lymph node dissection for clinical stage II/III lower rectal cancer (JCOG0212): A multicenter, randomized controlled, noninferiority trial. *Ann Surg* 2017;266(2):201–7.

36. Kang SB, Park JW, Jeong SY et al. Open versus laparoscopic surgery for mid or low rectal cancer after neoadjuvant chemoradiotherapy (COREAN trial): Short-term outcomes of an open-label randomised controlled trial. *Lancet Oncol.* 2010;11(7):637–45. doi:10.1016/S1470-2045(10)70131-5

37. van der Pas MH, Haglind E, Cuesta MA et al. Laparoscopic versus open surgery for rectal cancer (COLOR II): short-term outcomes of a randomised, phase 3 trial. *Lancet Oncol.* 2013;14(3):210–18. doi:10.1016/S1470-2045(13)70016-0

Chapter 19

LAPAROSCOPIC RIGHT HEMICOLECTOMY FOR RIGHT COLON CANCER

Harshad Soni and Jitender Singh Chauhan

Contents

Learning objectives 123
Introduction 123
Definition 123
Indications 123
Preoperative work up 123
Operative technique 123
    Positioning and port placement 123
Operative steps 124
Postoperative care 126
Role of SILS (single incision laparoscopic surgery) 126
Summary 126
Key points 127
Videos 127
References 127

Learning objectives

- Operating room set up for performing laparoscopic right hemicolectomy
- Port placement and equipment usage during surgery
- Standardized step-by-step approach to laparoscopic right hemicolectomy surgery
- Indication of surgery and pre- and postoperative care of patients planned for laparoscopic right hemicolectomy

Introduction

Colorectal cancer is the second most common cause of cancer in Western countries. In recent years, there has been a paradigm shift towards a minimally invasive approach, even for cases of malignancies. Laparoscopic right hemicolectomy yields all the benefits of laparoscopy and helps in radical removal of tumors along with lymph nodes.

Definition

Right hemicolectomy includes removal of the terminal ileum, cecum, ascending colon, hepatic flexure, and proximal parts of the transverse colon. In case of malignant lesion, it is mandatory to excise out the mesentery of terminal ileum and mesocolon of the right colon along with pericolic, paracolic and draining lymph nodes reaching up to the root of the major blood vessels (ileocolic, right colic and middle colic).

Indications

Common indication is a malignant lesion involving the cecum and the ascending colon. Apart from malignancy, the procedure is indicated for tuberculosis of the right colon, stricturing lesions of the right colon in Crohn's disease, or any other pathology compromising the functions of the right colon.

Extended right hemicolectomy is commonly performed for malignant disease of the hepatic flexure and the proximal transverse colon. When the dissection extends up to the mid-transverse region, then the right branch of the middle colic vessels is also dissected up to the root of the mesocolon along with all lymph nodes [1].

Preoperative work up

It is very important to perform a complete workup to allow the previous localization of the lesion by means of ultrasonography, computed tomography (CT) scan with contrast, and colonoscopy-guided biopsy. A baseline biochemical profile including complete blood count, carcino embryonic antigen (CEA), preoperative electrocardiogram, and chest radiograph must be performed as needed. Pulmonary function tests for patients with compromised respiratory function, and additional tests according to the patient's specific problems, are also indicated. CT scan of the abdomen for liver secondaries and chest X-ray/CT scan of the thorax for pulmonary metastasis are also required. The patient must be evaluated for cardiac morbidity and diabetes for better perioperative outcome. DVT prophylaxis should be given 12 hr prior to surgery and preoperative prophylactic antibiotics should be given at the induction of anesthesia.

Operative technique (see Videos 18 and 19)

Positioning and port placement

The patient is placed in a supine position with right-sided elevation of the body (similar to laparoscopic RPC IPAA, except 5 mm port in RIF) [2] (Figure 19.1). The patient must be fastened with sticking tape or broad straps to the operating table. The surgeon and camera surgeon stand on the left side of the abdomen, and the assistant surgeon stands on the right side of the patient. The laparoscopic trolley along with the monitor is positioned on the right side of the patient – opposite to the surgeon's position. An additional monitor is required for the assistant on the left side of

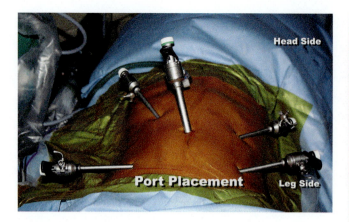

FIGURE 19.1   Port position in right hemicolectomy.

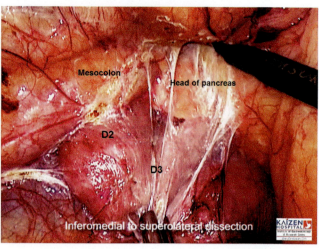

FIGURE 19.3   The second part of the duodenum is dissected away from the mesocolon medially, up to the hepatic flexure.

the patient. Next, ports are placed after achieving pneumoperitoneum with a veress needle. For the 10 mm infraumbilical camera port, the skin incision is vertical for possible extension for specimen extraction. Two 5 mm working ports for the assistant surgeon are placed on the left side of the abdomen, an upper 5 mm port in the mid-clavicular line between the left costal margin and the umbilicus, and the lower 5 mm port in the left iliac fossa in mid-clavicular line. Two assistant 5 mm ports are located on the right side of the abdomen in the midclavicular line, the upper port at right hypochondrium between the right subcostal to umbilicus and the lower port at right iliac fossa between right ASIS to umbilicus. A 10 mm zero-degree telescope is used. Commonly used surgical instruments are bowel graspers, atraumatic graspers, scissor, Maryland™ dissector, hook cautery, spatula cautery, suction cannula, right angle dissector, and so on. Ultrasonic energy and vessel sealer instruments are used according to need during the dissection.

Operative steps

a. *Inferomedial to superolateral:* In a steep Trendelenburg position, the small bowel loops are folded cranially by the surgeon with atraumatic bowel graspers. Next, the root of the mesentery is held up by the assistant for medial

to lateral, or inferior to superior dissection of the right colon. The lower right grasper of the assistant holds and lifts the mesentery near the IC junction (Figure 19.2a), and the upper right grasper holds and lifts the mesentery near the DJ flexure (Figure 19.2b). During this dissection, the second part of the duodenum is dissected away from the mesocolon medially (Figure 19.3) and laterally; the Gerota's fascia is separated up to the hepatic flexure of the colon, in the avascular plane up to the white line of Toldt.

b. *Major vascular pedicles:* The major three vessels are identified at the root of the mesocolon during laparoscopic right hemicolectomy. Inferomedial to superolateral dissection helps to reach up to origin of the vessels. The ileocolic artery and vein (Figures 19.4 and 19.5a,b), and right branch of the middle colic artery and vein are clipped and divided. The right colic vein present in 12%–15% of patients (Figure 19.6a), is also divided near its origin. For the tumor at the hepatic flexure, the middle colic artery is also dissected near its origin, clipped and divided to perform an extended right hemicolectomy (Figure 19.6b,c).

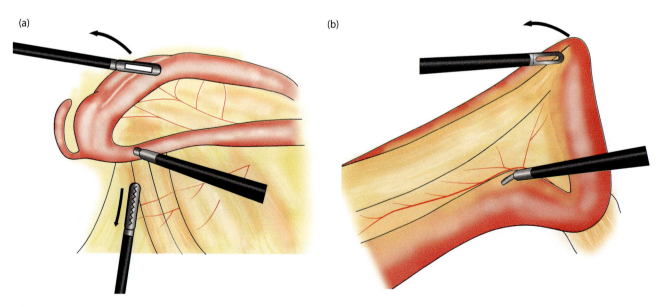

FIGURE 19.2   (a) Lower right grasper of the assistant holds and lifts the mesentery near the IC junction. (b) The upper right grasper holds and lifts the mesentery near the DJ flexure.

c. The gastrocolic omentum is kept along with the right colon (Figure 19.7).

d. *Hepatic flexure mobilization:* For this step, the patient is placed in straight position, with a 20° Trendelenburg and right-side mild elevation. The hepatic flexure is mobilized from medial to lateral in the supracolic approach, making sure the duodenum is visualized and is away from the dissection plane (Figure 19.8).

e. *Lateral attachments:* Finally the lateral attachments of the right colon are divided to completely free the right colon and terminal ileum (Figure 19.9).

f. At this point, specimen extraction is carried out using a peri-umbilical mini laparotomy, according to the lesion (approx. 5–7 cm). The specimen is removed after application of a wound protector (Figure 19.10). The terminal

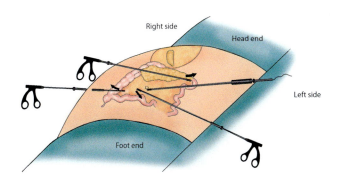

FIGURE 19.4 Ileocolic pedicle is demonstrated by adequate traction of both assistant graspers.

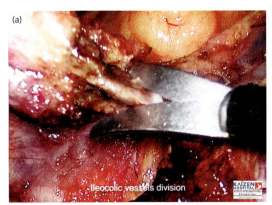
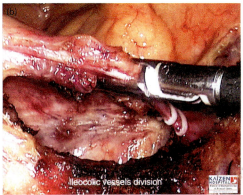

FIGURE 19.5 (a) Ileocolic artery is clipped and divided at its origin. (b) Ileocolic vein is clipped and divided at its origin.

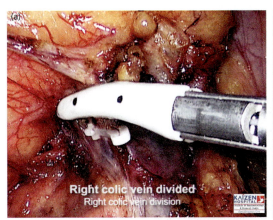
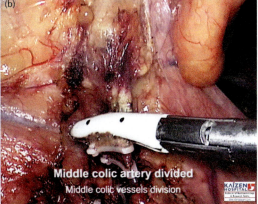
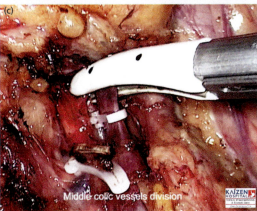

FIGURE 19.6 (a) Right colic vein (12%) is clipped and divided. (b) Middle colic artery is clipped and divided. (c) Middle colic vein is clipped and divided.

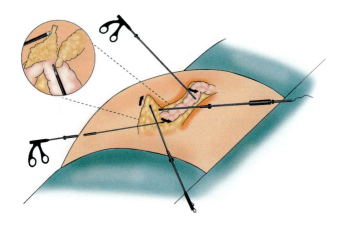

FIGURE 19.7   Right colon gastrocolic omentum is divided.

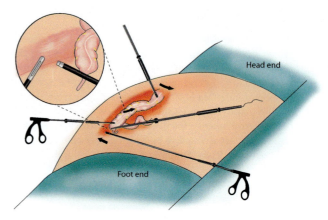

FIGURE 19.9   The lateral attachments of the right colon are finally divided to completely free the right colon and terminal ileum.

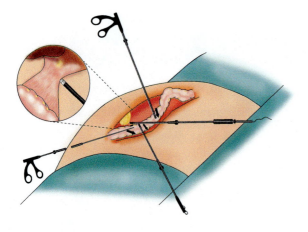

FIGURE 19.8   Hepatic flexure is mobilized from medial to lateral in the supracolic approach.

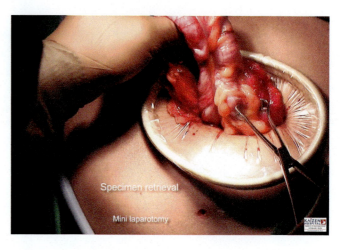

FIGURE 19.10   Specimen is removed after application of wound protector.

ileum and mid transverse colon are divided along with the mesocolon, and the ileo-transverse anastomosis is performed either hand sewn or with staplers. The mesentery and mesocolon are sutured to prevent future space for internal herniation. Thereafter, the bowel is delivered back in the peritoneal cavity, preventing any internal rotation. The mini laparotomy wound is closed with nonabsorbable suture.

Postoperative care

Postoperatively, the patient follows the ERAS protocol for colonic surgery. The Ryle's tube and Foley's catheter are removed according to patient's mobility, and the decrease in aspirated contents from the stomach. Antibiotics and analgesics are continued along with supportive IV fluids. DVT prophylaxis is stopped after five days of surgery. Mini laparotomy wound care should be taken to prevent wound sepsis.

The role of robotics in laparoscopic right hemicolectomy is explained in the chapter on robotics in laparoscopic colorectal surgery.

Role of SILS (single incision laparoscopic surgery)

With the use of rotaculator laparoscopic instruments, as well as SILS ports, this surgery can be performed with utmost efficiency. Saang Woo Lim et al. [3] have compared their 44 SILS right hemicolectomies with conventional multiport laparoscopic right hemicolectomy and concluded that it is a feasible and noninferior treatment option for colonic cancer, having similar results and a longer operating time. One can also use a hybrid technique by adding an additional port at the future abdominal drain site, and then perform the surgery.

Summary

Laparoscopic right hemicolectomy, for malignant and nonmalignant lesion of the ileo-cecal and right colonic lesions, is feasible with sound laparoscopic skills, teamwork, and good perioperative care. Standardized surgical steps for laparoscopic right hemicolectomy result in less operative complications with decreased chances of conversion to open surgery. SILS right hemicolectomy is a noninferior approach for right-sided colonic cancer.

Key points

- Laparoscopic right colonic mobilization needs thorough anatomical knowledge of retroperitoneal organs.
- Inferomedial to superolateral dissection is performed safeguarding ureters, nerves, and vessels.
- Specimen extraction is done with a peri-umbilical mini laparotomy.
- SILS is a feasible and noninferior treatment option for colonic cancer when compared to conventional multiport lap surgery, demonstrating similar results, but a longer operating time.

Videos

VIDEO 18   https://youtu.be/NWiIW2-oc2g

Laparoscopic Extended Right Hemicolectomy for Right Colon Cancer – Part 1.

VIDEO 19   https://youtu.be/ONkPRjNTZ2c

Laparoscopic Extended Right Hemicolectomy for Right Colon Cancer – Part 2.

References

1. Deo SV, Puntambekar SP. Laparoscopic right radical hemicolectomy. *J Minim Access Surg* 2012;8(1):21–4.
2. Haribhakti SP, Madnani MA, Mistry JH, Patel KS, Shah AJ, Soni HN. Laparoscopic restorative proctocolectomy ileal pouch anal anastomosis: How I do it? *J Minim Access Surg* July-September 2015;11(3):218–22.
3. Lim SW, Kim HR, Kim YJ. Single incision laparoscopic colectomy for colorectal cancer: Comparison with conventional laparoscopic colectomy. *Ann Surg Treat Res* 2014 Sep;87(3):131–8.

Chapter 20

LAPAROSCOPIC TRANSVERSE COLECTOMY FOR TRANSVERSE COLON CANCER

Prajesh Bhuta

Contents

Learning objectives 128
Introduction 128
Anatomy. 128
Evidence of laparoscopic resection 128
Preoperation preparation 128
Steps of laparoscopic transverse colectomy. 129
    Port placement 129
    Greater omentum dissection 129
    Ligation of the middle colic vein and artery 129
    Mobilization of the mesocolon. 129
    Delivery of the colon 129
Summary 130
Key points 130
References 130

Learning objectives

- To understand the anatomy of the vascular and lymphatic drainage of the right colon in relation to an extended right/transverse colectomy.
- To learn the steps of laparoscopic transverse colectomy.

Introduction

Transverse colon tumors have always remained an enigma as far as treatment options are concerned, as surgeons have different options and preferences for its surgical management. Carcinoma of the transverse colon accounts for 10% of all colorectal cancers. These tumors remain undetected until complications occur in 30%–50% of cases [3]. The commonest complications are perforation, fistulization, and obstruction. They are also more prone to involve other organs like the stomach and pancreas depending on the location [1,3]. These are present as T4 lesions in 20%–40% of cases, and the prognosis is much worse than colon cancer in other areas [2,3]. They also present a challenge in differential diagnosis between neighboring tumors, and also in benign diseases like Crohn's and tuberculosis. They can present as colonic strictures where preoperative diagnosis is sometimes not easy. The CT scan remains the gold standard for staging and deciding the surgical extent of resection for transverse colon tumors.

Anatomy

It is very important to understand the anatomy of the transverse colon for laparoscopic surgery, as the surgery is based on the site of tumor on the colon, lymphatic drainage, venous anatomy, and arterial supply. The middle colic artery is the main vessel which has to be sacrificed, and the anatomy around its origin is important for high ligation of the vessel. Vascular anatomical patterns (Figure 20.1) were classified according to whether the first jejunal vein ran behind (type A 79%), or in front of the superior mesenteric artery (type B). Type B is divided into B1 (10.5%) or B2 (10.5%), depending on whether the middle colic artery originated

cephalad or caudal to the vein. Also in 17% the middle colic vein drains into the inferior mesenteric vein, and in 8% the middle colic drains into the first jejunal vein.

Evidence of laparoscopic resection

There have been multiple trials over the last 10 years confirming the equivalence of laparoscopic versus open resection. There is also the benefit of faster recovery and less pain in laparoscopic surgeries [4–9]. The central location of transverse colon tumors poses difficult surgical choices for lymph node dissection, extent of resection, and reestablishment of intestinal continuity [10,12]. The type of surgery and the extent of lymphadenectomy are mainly based on tumor location. The tumor in the transverse colon can be divided into right and left transverse colon tumors, based on the location and the extent of lymph nodes along the marginal artery in the middle colic artery [10,12]. These groups of patients still present with disparities when selecting them for an aggressive or an extended approach. Lymph node metastasis has been reported to be confined to the middle colic artery if the tumor is on the left side of the transverse colon; however, metastases are detected along the right colic artery in 17% of patients with tumors on the right side of the middle colic artery [11]. Current studies have revealed that if there were no metastatic lymph nodes along the ileocolic artery, it would seem acceptable to undergo less aggressive surgery, with ileocaecal valve preservation, in transverse colon tumor patients [10,12]. The surgical options are selective transverse colectomy, right-extended hemicolectomy for right-sided tumors. and left-extended hemi-colectomy for left-sided transverse colon tumors. In many studies, transverse colectomy has shown to have similar outcomes, nevertheless most surgeons still prefer right- or left-extended colectomy for transverse colon tumors [13–16].

Preoperation preparation

Staging with CT scan is important not only to assess operability, but also to obtain an idea of the anatomy of the middle colic

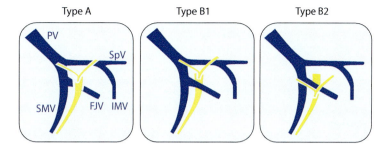

FIGURE 20.1 Vascular anatomical patterns.

artery and the jejunal veins. In case of small tumors, we need to tattoo the site preoperatively for localization, as sometimes it is difficult to assess the site of the tumor in laparoscopic surgery as transverse colon can be quite redundant. The patient's BMI and previous surgeries may necessitate changes in port placement and extraction.

Steps of laparoscopic transverse colectomy

1. Port placement
2. Greater omentum mobilization
3. First jejunal vein preservation
4. Middle colic artery and vein ligation
5. Mobilization of mesocolon
6. Delivery of the colon
7. Resection with end-to-end anastomosis

Port placement (Figure 20.2)
Generally, a five port technique is used as we need to access the splenic and hepatic flexure for adequate mobilization of the transverse colon. The ports should not be too far away from the umbilicus, especially among patients with a high BMI. Two screens are generally required as the surgeon will stand on the left side of the patient for right-sided dissection, but will have to switch sides for the splenic flexure mobilization.

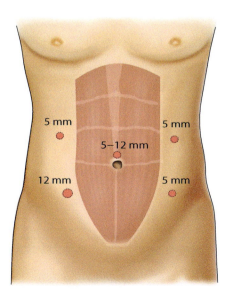

FIGURE 20.2 Port placement.

Greater omentum dissection
The first step is dissection of the omentum from the colon. If the surgeon decides to remove the omentum with the specimen, the omentum can be divided along the greater curvature of the stomach. Dissection of the omentum can be performed with the hook cautery, or an advanced bipolar device. We prefer not to address the MCV pedicle until the vascular control of the MCV can be obtained from the caudal and a ventral approach. This is very important as the bleeding, while attempting to divide the MCV, can be challenging to control. The dissection of the omentum allows access to control bleeding from the ventral aspect, if required.

Ligation of the middle colic vein and artery
There are various techniques to identify and divide the middle colic trunk.

1. One can identify the superior mesenteric artery and continue the medial dissection until the MCV is identified.
2. Use a window approach.
3. One can hold two ends of the transverse colon and lift them. The middle colic trunk can then be identified and the vascular pedicle divided just distal to the inferior aspect of the pancreas, but before it bifurcates, to allow for a complete lymphadenectomy.

Care must be taken to identify the first jejunal vein before ligation and preserved, as various anomalies can be present as described before. Excessive traction should be avoided at all cost.

Mobilization of the mesocolon
The mesocolon is mobilized by creating the plane between the stomach and the transverse colon, so as to mobilize the hepatic flexure. The colon is mobilized in the plane above Gerota's fascia. Occasionally, an accessory right colic vein can be encountered while mobilizing the hepatic flexure. It can be dealt with by harmonic scalpel or ligated. If sufficient mobilization is not achieved, the splenic flexure can be mobilized as well.

Delivery of the colon
A small periumbilical or supraumbilical incision is made. A wound protector usually aids with exposure. The colon is usually divided with a stapler. The anastomosis is usually constructed in an isoperistaltic fashion, as opposed to the typical antiperistaltic anastomosis. One can perform an end-to-end anastomosis with the stapler by making a colotomy in the proximal bowel, and using an endoluminal stapler followed by suture of the colotomy. It can also be performed with a hand sewn end-to-end anastomosis.

Summary

Laparoscopic transverse colectomy requires extensive surgical skills, and the surgeon should first gain experience in other colon surgeries before attempting this procedure. The type of procedure should be decided based on the patient's condition and the experience the surgeon has in each of the approaches mentioned.

Key points

- Staging with CT scan is important not only to assess operability, but also to obtain an idea of the anatomy of the middle colic artery and the jejunal veins.
- Middle colic artery is the main vessel, which has to be sacrificed, and the anatomy around its origin is important for high ligation of the vessel.

References

1. Kelley WE Jr, Brown PW, Lawrence W Jr, Terz JJ. Penetrating, obstructing, and perforating carcinomas of the colon and rectum. *Arch Surg* 1981 Apr;116(4):381–4.
2. Dutton JW, Hreno A, Hampson LG. Mortality and prognosis of obstructing carcinoma of the large bowel. *Am J Surg* 1976 Jan;131(1):36–41.
3. Lê P, Mehtari L, Billey C. [Carcinoma of the transverse colon]. *J Chir (Paris)* 2006 Sep-Oct;143(5):285–93.
4. Colon cancer laparoscopic or open resection study group. Kelley WE Jr, Brown PW, Lawrence W Jr et al. Survival after laparoscopic surgery versus open surgery for colon cancer: Long-term outcome of a randomised clinical trial. *Lancet Oncol* 2009;10:44–52. [Crossref] [PubMed]
5. Jayne DG, Thorpe HC, Copeland J et al. Five-year follow-up of the medical research council CLASICC trial of laparoscopically assisted versus open surgery for colorectal cancer. *Br J Surg* 2010;97:1638–45. [Crossref] [PubMed]
6. McKay GD, Morgan MJ, Wong SK et al. Improved short-term outcomes of laparoscopic versus open resection for colon and rectal cancer in an area health service: A multicenter study. *Dis Colon Rectum* 2012;55:42–50. [Crossref] [PubMed]
7. Hazebroek EJ. Color Study Group. COLOR: A randomized clinical trial comparing laparoscopic and open resection for colon cancer. *Surg Endosc* 2002;16:949–53. [Crossref] [PubMed]
8. Fleshman J, Sargent DJ, Green E et al. Laparoscopic colectomy for cancer is not inferior to open surgery based on 5-year data from the COST Study Group trial. *Ann Surg* 2007;246:655–62; discussion 662–4. [Crossref] [PubMed]
9. Zeng WG, Liu MJ, Zhou ZX et al. Outcome of laparoscopic versus open resection for transverse colon cancer. *J Gastrointest Surg* 2015;19:1869–74. [Crossref] [PubMed]
10. Kim HJ, Lee IK, Lee YS et al. A comparative study on the short-term clinicopathologic outcomes of laparoscopic surgery versus conventional open surgery for transverse colon cancer. *Surg Endosc* 2009;23:1812–7. [Crossref] [PubMed]
11. Zmora O, Bar-Dayan A, Khaikin M et al. Laparoscopic colectomy for transverse colon carcinoma. *Tech Coloproctol* 2010;14:25–30. [Crossref] [PubMed]
12. Lee YS, Lee IK, Kang WK et al. Surgical and pathological outcomes of laparoscopic surgery for transverse colon cancer. *Int J Colorectal Dis* 2008;23:669–73. [Crossref] [PubMed]
13. Chong CS, Huh JW, Oh BY et al. Operative method for transverse colon carcinoma: Transverse colectomy versus extended colectomy. *Dis Colon Rectum* 2016;59:630–9. [Crossref] [PubMed]
14. Akiyoshi T, Kuroyanagi H, Fujimoto Y et al. Short-term outcomes of laparoscopic colectomy for transverse colon cancer. *J Gastrointest Surg* 2010;14:818–23. [Crossref] [PubMed]
15. Fernández-Cebrián JM, Gil Yonte P, Jiminez-Toscano M et al. Laparoscopic colectomy for transverse colon carcinoma: A surgical challenge but oncologically feasible. *Colorectal Dis* 2013;15:e79–83. [Crossref] [PubMed]
16. Matsuda T, Iwasaki T, Hirata K et al. Optimal surgery for Mid-Transverse colon cancer: Laparoscopic extended right hemicolectomy versus laparoscopic transverse colectomy. *World J Surg* 2018;42:3398–404. [Crossref] [PubMed]

Chapter 21

LAPAROSCOPIC HEMICOLECTOMY FOR LEFT COLON CANCER

Ashwin deSouza and Shankar Malpangudi

Contents

Learning objectives 131
Introduction 131
Vascular anatomy of the left colon 131
Lymphatic drainage of the left colon... 132
Complete mesocolic excision (CME) 132
Resection templates for left colon cancer 133
Laparoscopic left hemicolectomy: Surgical technique 134
Surgical steps... 134
Summary 137
Key points 137
Video... 137
References 137

Learning objectives

- Understand the vascular anatomy of the left colon, including the variation in arterial supply, venous drainage, and their significance in surgical resection templates for left colon cancer.
- Understand the lymphatic drainage of the colon and the levels of lymph node involvement by malignant cell dissemination.
- Appreciate the unique anatomy of the splenic flexure with respect to its role as the watershed between the superior and inferior mesenteric arterial systems.
- Understand the principles of complete mesocolic excision for colon cancer, its technique and outcomes, as compared to conventional colectomy.
- Be aware of the various resection templates for cancer of the left colon and their oncological outcomes.
- Be able to tailor the surgical approach depending on the location of the tumor, the vascular anatomy of the colon, and the clinical presentation of the patient.
- Understand the principles and technique of laparoscopic left colon resection.

Introduction

A radical colectomy for cancer involves the resection of the tumor along with its supplying vascular pedicles at their origin, thereby resecting all the regional nodes and intervening lymphatics en masse. The template for radical colectomy has been defined depending on the location of the tumor in the colon. These templates are based on the vascular pedicles that are ligated for each tumor location, and not on the length and anatomical location of the bowel segment resected.

The resection template for a right hemicolectomy is fairly straightforward, and subsequent bowel continuity is always established by an ileocolic anastomosis. Depending on the location of the lesion in the right colon, the only factor that needs to be modified is whether or not the middle colic pedicle is ligated at its origin. Two standard templates have therefore evolved for right colon cancer, namely, the right and right extended hemicolectomy.

For tumors in the left colon however, surgical options are less clearly defined. Anatomically, the left colon extends from the left half of the transverse colon to the rectosigmoid junction at the sacral promontory. Upon resecting this entire segment of large bowel, the surgeon is left with the cut end of the transverse colon in the epigastrium to anastomose to the rectum at the sacral promontory. Though this is possible with the adoption of elaborate transmesenteric and/or right colon rotational maneuvers [1], the procedure is technically challenging. This has led surgeons and clinicians to question the oncological necessity of such an extensive resection for all lesions in the left colon. Detailed study of the vascular anatomy and the lymphatic drainage of the left colon has formed the basis of less extensive, but perhaps equally radical, resections from an oncological standpoint.

This chapter deals with the various templates for left colon resection and their oncological outcomes, and elaborates as well on the surgical technique of laparoscopic radical left hemicolectomy.

Vascular anatomy of the left colon

The left colon receives its arterial supply both from the superior and inferior mesenteric arteries (IMA). The left branch of the middle colic, which arises from the superior mesenteric artery (SMA), supplies the left half of the transverse colon. The rest of the left colon and rectum receives arterial supply from the inferior mesenteric artery through the left colic artery, sigmoid branches, and the superior rectal artery (Figure 21.1). The middle colic artery may be absent in 2%–22% of patients [2–5]. In these cases, the transverse colon gets its supply from anastomotic channels originating from the right colic artery [6].

The left colic artery is the first lateral branch of the inferior mesenteric artery, which divides into an ascending branch that courses towards the splenic flexure and a descending branch, which goes towards the sigmoid colon. Latarjet described two variations for the origin of the left colic artery [7]. These are important to note as they become relevant in the nodal dissection at the root of the IMA. Type 1, or a spread-out origin is one where the left colic artery has a separate origin several centimeters away from the origin of the IMA. The sigmoid vessels originate from

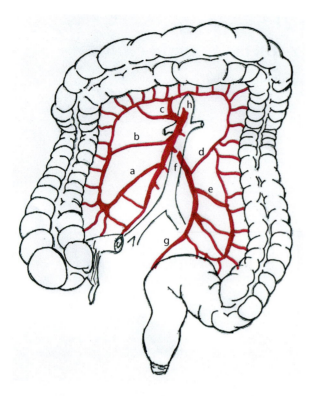

FIGURE 21.1 Arterial supply of the colon. (a) Ileocolic (b) Right colic (c) Middle colic. (d) Left Colic (e) First sigmoid (f) Inferior mesenteric artery (g) Superior rectal artery (h) Superior mesenteric artery.

the IMA a further few centimeters distal to the left colic artery origin. Type 2, or fan-shaped origin is one where the left colic and sigmoid branches share a common origin from the IMA, arising in a fan-shaped manner (Figure 21.2).

The marginal artery of Drummond is a continuous anastomotic channel that is fed by the terminal branches of the named vessels of the colon. Although there may be disagreement regarding the presence of direct communicating vessels between the superior and inferior mesenteric arteries, the presence of the marginal artery is largely undisputed [2,5,8–10].

The arc of Riolan, also known as the mesenteric meandering artery, the artery of Moskowitz, or by 11 other such synonyms [6], is an arterial communication between the middle colic and left colic arteries, thereby forming an important anastomotic channel between the superior and inferior mesenteric arteries. A recent publication [6] casts doubt on the presence of this artery, which according to the author represents the ascending branch of the left colic artery. Additional, more central communications between the superior and inferior mesenteric arteries are rare and have been described only in 0%–18% of patients [2–5,8,11,12].

The splenic flexure represents the watershed between the superior and inferior mesenteric artery supply. However, as reported by Griffith, the majority of blood supply to the splenic flexure is carried by the left colic artery, with only 11% of cases receiving blood supply from the left branch of the middle colic [2]. Although there exist a number of variations in the arterial supply to the left colon, some sort of anastomotic connection between the superior and inferior mesenteric arterial systems around the splenic flexure is present in nearly every individual.

The venous drainage of the left colon follows the arteries, ultimately forming the inferior mesenteric vein (IMV) that runs just

lateral to the duodenojejunal flexure to terminate into the splenic vein. In some patients, there may be a prominent splenic flexure vein that joins the IMV at or near its termination in the splenic vein [13]. Identifying and preserving this vein may help in the venous drainage of the residual colon after ligation of the IMV.

Lymphatic drainage of the left colon

As is the rule in all other organs of the gastrointestinal tract, the lymphatic drainage of the colon follows its arterial supply to the root nodes (or level 3 nodes) at the origin of the named vascular pedicles. Unique to the left colon is the splenic flexure, which forms a watershed between the superior and inferior mesenteric artery systems. There has been considerable debate regarding the preferred pathway for lymphatic drainage from malignant lesions at the splenic flexure. This is of importance when defining the nodal dissection template for splenic flexure lesions, in order to be considered oncologically adequate.

Vasey et al. evaluated the patterns of lymphatic drainage of the normal splenic flexure in 30 patients using laparoscopic scintigraphic mapping [14]. This study established a dominant lymphatic drainage towards the left colic artery in >95% of patients. The authors did notice a small volume of tracer flow to the left branch of middle colic in a significant number of patients. However, counts at the root of the middle colic and IMA were very low and did not show increase over time. This study supports the oncological adequacy of the left segmental colectomy for splenic flexure lesions, where the left branch of middle colic and the left colic pedicles are ligated.

Watanabe et al. evaluated the direction of lymphatic flow with real-time indocyanine green fluorescence following a peritumoral injection in 31 patients with colon cancer at the splenic flexure and node negative on preoperative imaging [15]. The authors found flow along the left accessory aberrant colic artery in the 12 cases where it was present, and in 61.3% of cases at the root of the inferior mesenteric vein. No case demonstrated flow in both directions, that is towards the left branch of middle colic and towards the left colic artery.

In a retrospective comparison between right extended and left hemicolectomy for splenic flexure lesions, deAngelis et al. failed to detect any nodal metastasis along the branches of the superior mesenteric artery, or at the root of the middle colic pedicle in any patient in this series [16]. However, nodal metastasis along the ileocolic pedicle [17], and along branches of the superior mesenteric artery, have been reported in about 10% of cases [18]. This may be on account of variations in vascular anatomy, or due to rerouting of lymphatic drainage in the setting of lymphatic blockage secondary to heavy nodal disease burden, as seen in locally advanced cancer at other sites [19].

Complete mesocolic excision (CME)

The surgical approach for rectal resection witnessed a paradigm shift in 1979 with the introduction of total mesorectal excision [20]. Adopting this technique of resecting the rectum by sharp dissection, and maintaining an intact mesorectal fascial envelope was associated with dramatic decreases in local recurrence and an improvement in survival [20,21]. Hohenberger et al. proposed a similar approach for radical colectomy which involved mobilization of the colon along the embryological fascial planes, maintaining an intact mesocolic fascia, ensuring a complete lymphadenectomy of all the nodal tissue, and dividing the supplying vessels at their origin [22]. Adopting this technique, the

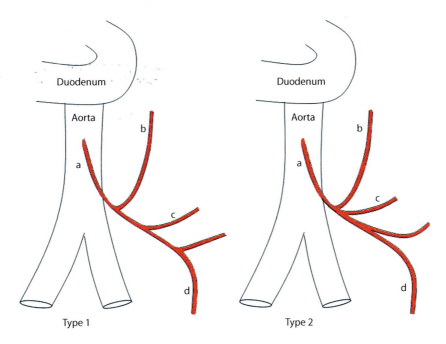

FIGURE 21.2 Inferior mesenteric artery branching – Latarjet classification (7). (a) Inferior mesenteric artery (b) Left colic artery (c) First sigmoid artery (d) Superior rectal artery.

Erlangen group was able to show a decrease in local recurrence rates and an improvement in cancer-related survival [22].

Lymphatic spread in colon cancer first occurs to the pericolic lymph nodes that lie along the marginal vessel. Subsequent spread occurs to the nodes along the supplying vascular pedicles. The longitudinal nodal spread would determine the length of colon, both proximal and distal to the tumor that would need to be resected to remove all involved nodes. In their initial paper, the Erlangen group pointed out that lateral spread in the pericolic nodes usually does not occur for more than 8 cm from the primary tumor [23,24], thus making a 10 cm margin on either side an appropriate length of resection. However, there is no consensus on the length of colon to be resected. Japanese recommendations stipulate resection of 10 cm of bowel proximal and distal to the lesion [25], while just 5–7 cm is recommended in the United States [26].

Through an elegant study involving systematic lymph node dissection of 662 radical colectomy specimens, Yamaoka et al. [25] determined that the pattern of lymph node spread changes with increase in T stage. No patient with a T1 lesion had lymph node metastasis in the nodes at the root of the vascular pedicle. Whereas this was present in 2%, 2.3%, and 3.7% in patients with T2, T3, and T4 tumors, respectively. Twenty-five specimens (3.7%) had positive lymph nodes in the colonic segment between 5 and 10 cm either proximal or distal to the primary tumor. Only one specimen (0.2%) demonstrated lymph node spread in the colonic segment beyond 10 cm from the primary tumor. This was in a T4 lesion. Based on these findings the authors conclude that CME is indicated in all patients with ≥T2 lesions (in view of the spread to the root nodes) and resection of 10 cm of bowel both proximal and distal to the primary tumor is necessary to resect all involved epicolic nodes [25].

Since the initial report from the Erlangen group in 2008, there have been a number of publications on the use of CME for radical colectomy for colon cancer [27]. When compared with conventional colectomy, CME has been associated with a better disease-free survival [28] and lower local recurrence rate [29]. CME can be performed laparoscopically [30–33] and is not associated with an increased morbidity [29]. The only drawback seems to be an increased operative time and isolated reports of increased vessel injury [34]. The oncological rationale of the approach has been endorsed in an international consensus statement [35], though it is not yet recommended as a standard of care for all colonic resections for cancer. Many centers, including our own have adopted CME for colon cancer, and as additional data becomes available, it is very likely that CME will be established as a standard of care for elective radical colectomy.

Resection templates for left colon cancer

The extent of any radical colectomy is defined on the basis of the location of the primary tumor. However, it would scarcely be considered appropriate to resect the entire left colon, that is from the middle of the transverse colon to the rectosigmoid junction at the sacral promontory, for lesions at all locations within this colonic segment. Lesions at the apex of the sigmoid colon may be resected with a sigmoid colectomy, dividing only the sigmoid vessels and preserving both the superior rectal and left colic arteries. Lesions in the descending limb of the sigmoid colon may require a high anterior resection where the IMA is divided either at the root or after the origin of the left colic artery. For lesions in the distal descending or proximal sigmoid colon, it may be more appropriate to include the left colic pedicle (along with the sigmoid vessels) in the resection template due to the more proximal location of the tumor. The superior rectal artery may be preserved for tumors at this location as the entire rectum is retained. The problem arises for splenic flexure lesions where there is a lack of consensus on the extent of resection.

The splenic flexure is defined as the portion of the large intestine from the distal third of the transverse colon to the proximal 10 cm of the descending colon [36]. As this region represents the watershed of arterial supply between the superior and inferior mesenteric arterial systems, various resection templates have been proposed, namely, extended right hemicolectomy, left segmental colectomy, and left hemicolectomy. The extended right hemicolectomy (ERH) removes the entire ascending colon, transverse colon, and an appropriate length of descending colon to achieve the desired distal margin (of 10 cm) from the tumor. The ileocolic, right colic, middle colic, and left colic pedicles are divided during this procedure [16,37]. The left segment colectomy (LSC) aims to resect the primary lesion at the splenic flexure with 10 cm of uninvolved large bowel on either side. The left branch of middle colic and the left colic arteries are ligated for this resection. Both the origin of the middle colic and the main IMA are preserved during a left segmental colectomy [38–40]. A formal left hemicolectomy (LH) includes the entire left colon, that is the distal transverse to the rectosigmoid junction and requires division of the left branch of middle colic and the main IMA pedicle at its origin. In patients with a redundant transverse colon, intestinal continuity can be restored with a colo-colic anastomosis between the transverse colon and the rectum [16,41]. However, if the bowel ends do not come together without tension, either a transmesenteric approach – or some sort of right colon rotation, for example Deloyer's procedure – is usually required [1].

To date, there is no consensus as to the most appropriate procedure for splenic flexure lesions. A number of studies have compared the short and long-term outcomes of ERH to either LH or LSC for splenic flexure lesions [16,42–48]. None of these studies have demonstrated any oncological superiority of one procedure over the other, making all three approaches oncologically adequate templates for splenic flexure lesions. The results of a recent survey among French surgeons showed that the left segmental colectomy was the preferred procedure of choice, which was adopted by 70% of the surgeons surveyed [49]. In the emergency setting, for an obstructing lesion at the splenic flexure, the extended right hemicolectomy may be the procedure of choice [43]. This is because the obstructed portion of the colon is removed and an ileocolic anastomosis is fashioned, which may be a more secure option vis-à-vis a colo-colic anastomosis in an obstructed system.

However, that being said, there are a few case reports of metastatic lymph nodes along the ileocolic pedicle in patients with splenic flexure lesions [17]. As discussed in the section of lymphatic drainage in this chapter, this may be on account of the redistribution of lymphatic spread in the presence of heavy lymph node burden, or due to the presence of variations in arterial anatomy. These 'distant' lymph nodes may be involved in up to 10% of patients, and are more commonly seen in patients with metastatic disease where a colectomy is being performed with curative intent [18]. Although the three surgical approaches for splenic flexure lesions – ERH, LH, and LSC – seem to be oncologically equivalent for splenic flexure lesions, it may be more appropriate to adopt the extended right hemicolectomy for obstructing lesions, for patients with variations in vascular anatomy, for example, for those who have an absent middle colic artery, for tumors with heavy nodal disease burden as visualized on preoperative imaging and in the setting of colectomy with curative intent in the presence of metastatic disease.

Laparoscopic left hemicolectomy: Surgical technique (see Video 31)

The use of laparoscopy in radical colectomy for colon cancer is well supported by evidence from multiple randomized controlled trials [50]. Complete mesocolic excision is safe and feasible via the laparoscopic approach [30–33]. A number of reports have confirmed the safety, feasibility, and acceptability of the oncological results of a laparoscopic approach for left colon resection [51,52]. Although laparoscopy for a left hemicolectomy can be considered as a standard of care, it does represent one of the more technically challenging colonic resections performed laparoscopically.

This is on account of the variations in vascular anatomy of the pedicles involved, and the variable position of the splenic flexure. At no point should there be a compromise in the oncological adequacy of the resection – just to be able to complete the procedure laparoscopically.

This section briefly describes the surgical technique of a laparoscopic segmental colectomy for a splenic flexure lesion. Please refer to Video 31 for this chapter.

a. *Patient position:* The patient is placed in a lithotomy position with less than 10° of flexion at the hip. A small sand bag is placed below the sacrum to elevate the pelvis and keep the lumbar spine flat. The arms are placed by the side and the patient is secured to the operation table with some sort of padded strapping, with care to ensure that all pressure points are adequately protected. We use padded supports for both shoulders and strapping across the patient's chest. Before draping the patient, the table is moved into a Trendelenberg, reverse Trendelenberg, and right and left lateral tilt positions to ensure that the patient is secure and that all lines, tubes, and catheters are not at risk of getting dislodged during subsequent intraoperative patient positioning.
b. *Operation theater layout:* The operation theater layout is as shown in Figure 21.3, with the operating surgeon standing on the patient's right, the cameraman to the surgeon's left and the second assistant diametrically across them. It is very useful to have two monitors at either side of the foot end of the table, so that all operating surgeons have access to good vision of the laparoscopic field with comfortable ergonomics.
c. *Port positions:* The port position is as shown in Figure 21.4. In patients with a high riding splenic flexure, or in obese individuals, it may be beneficial to have an additional 5 mm port in the right hypochondrium, as shown in the figure. This greatly increases laparoscopic access to the upper abdomen and shortens operative time, without any increase in morbidity.

Surgical steps

i. *Laparoscopic access and exposure:* Pneumoperitoneum is created either with the open Hassan technique or by using the Veress needle. The 12 mm port for the camera is then inserted in the supraumbilical position and a staging laparoscopy is performed to rule out the presence of metastatic disease. All quadrants of the abdomen should be surveyed, especially the right and left subdiaphragmatic recesses which are often overlooked. The remaining ports are then inserted and the greater omentum reflected below the left lobe of the liver. This helps to create a surgical working space for the subsequent positioning of the small bowel. The patient is then placed in a steep Trendelenberg position with a right tilt and the small bowel positioned in the right upper quadrant. This exposes the entire left colon.
ii. *Inferior mesenteric vein dissection:* The procedure is begun by first dissecting the inferior mesenteric vein. The peritoneal attachments around the duodeno-jejunal flexure (DJ) are then taken down with the help of cold scissors to expose the root of the inferior mesenteric vein at the lower border of the pancreas. It is preferable to avoid using an energy device to release the attachments of the DJ flexure as working from the right, the instrument arches over the

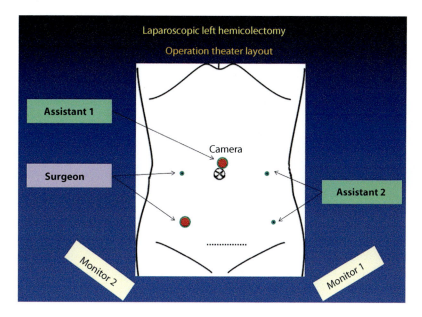

FIGURE 21.3   Laparoscopic left hemicolectomy – operation theater layout.

DJ flexure, risking lateral thermal injury to the bowel wall. The inferior mesenteric vein (IMV) is then held up by the assistant and the peritoneum incised just posterior to it to open up the retroperitoneal avascular place which is developed posterior to the vein in a medial to lateral fashion (Figure 21.5). The plane of dissection lies just posterior to the vein and care must be taken not to dissect in a deeper plane. The left gonadal vessels should be identified at this point and the plane maintained anterior to them, or one might inadvertently dissect posterior to the gonadal vein and risk injury to the left renal vein (Figure 21.5). The IMV is then clipped and divided.

iii. *Inferior mesenteric artery dissection:* The rectosigmoid is then held up by the assistant and the peritoneum on the right leaf of the rectal mesentery is incised just posterior to the inferior mesenteric artery (IMA) at the level of the sacral promontory. Medial to lateral dissection is then

performed, posterior to the IMA to visualize the inferior portion of the left gonadal vessels and the left ureter as they cross the pelvic brim. Nodal dissection is then completed at the root of the IMA to identify the left colic artery and IMV (Figure 21.6). The left colic artery is then divided at its origin from the IMA, and the lower end of the IMV clipped and divided at the level of the first sigmoid artery.

iv. *Splenic flexure mobilization:* With the vascular pedicles divided, the medial to lateral mobilization of the left colon is completed laterally to the abdominal wall and superiorly to the lower border of the pancreas. The transverse mesocolon is then held up by the assistant and the mesocolon lifted off the anterior surface of the pancreas. As this dissection proceeds towards the upper border of the pancreas one enters the lesser sac. The attachments of the transverse mesocolon to the lower border of the pancreas are then taken down with the harmonic scalpel moving towards the

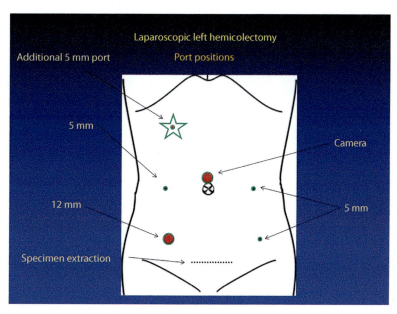

FIGURE 21.4   Laparoscopic left hemicolectomy – port position.

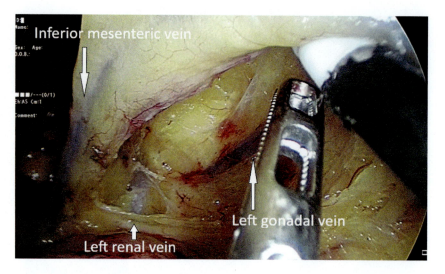

FIGURE 21.5   Development of the plane posterior to the inferior mesenteric vein.

splenic flexure. A gauze piece can be placed here to mark this location. The lateral attachments of the left colon are then taken down by sharp dissection beginning in the left iliac fossa and moving towards the splenic flexure. The omentum is then taken off the distal transverse colon and the final attachments of the colon at the bend of the splenic flexure are taken down to completely mobilize the left colon. For tumors at the splenic flexure, mobilization of the upper rectum is usually not necessary. The point of proximal and distal specimen transection, 10 cm away from the tumor is identified and the mesentery divided at this level with the help of an energy device.

v. *Anastomosis – intra vs. extra corporeal:* We prefer an end-to-end, hand sewn, extracorporeal anastomosis after exteriorizing the specimen through a Pfannenstiel incision. The classical Pfannenstiel incision splits and does not divide the rectus muscle, and is probably associated with the lowest rates of incisional hernia [53]. Alternatively, an intracorporeal side-to-side anastomosis can be fashioned using a linear laparoscopic stapler. The intra-corporeal anastomosis is no doubt feasible and could be associated with less pain and a faster return of bowel function [54]. However, this is technically more demanding and more time consuming.

vi. *Closure of mesenteric defect:* After a segmental left colectomy, one is left with a mesenteric defect that extends from the left half of the transverse colon to the sigmoid colon. It is technically very difficult to close this defect but fortunately this usually does not lead to any complications if left as is. However, we do restore pneumoperitoneum after the bowel is reposited and the Pfannenstiel incision closed, in order to ensure that the first loops of jejunum are placed anterior to the left colon which has been extensively mobilized. With this maneuver, we have not had any instance of postop internal herniation following laparoscopic left hemicolectomy. Symptomatic internal herniation, requiring surgical intervention, has been reported after laparoscopic left colectomy [55,56], though the incidence is only about 1% [56]. Considering all laparoscopic colectomies, the incidence of internal herniation is still lower, at about 0.65%, though the highest incidence is reported after laparoscopic left colectomy [57]. In view of the rarity of this complication, routine

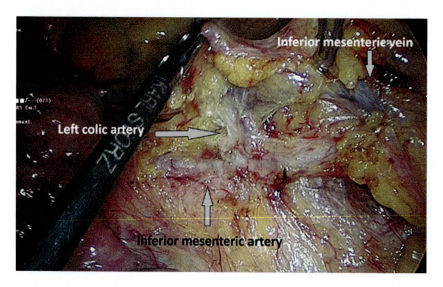

FIGURE 21.5   Nodal dissection at the inferior mesenteric artery.

closure of the mesenteric defect is not advocated after a laparoscopic left colectomy, though it may be considered in high risk individuals, on a case-to-case basis.

Summary

The left colon is unique as it receives its blood supply from both the superior and inferior mesenteric arterial systems. The left branch of the middle colic from the SMA and the left colic, and the sigmoid branches from the IMA are the vascular pedicles supplying the left colon. A number of variations in vascular anatomy have been defined and it is important for the surgeon to be aware of them.

The splenic flexure represents the watershed between the superior and inferior mesenteric arterial systems though in a majority of cases, the left colic artery serves as the dominant arterial supply and the preferred pathway for lymphatic drainage. In the presence of variations in vascular anatomy and in patients with heavy nodal disease burden, nonregional lymph nodes may also be involved with disease spread.

Complete mesocolic excision involves dissection of the colon in the embryological mesocolic plane, nodal dissection and ligation of the supplying vessels at their origin, and resection of 10 cm of bowel both proximal and distal to the primary tumor. Though this approach has not yet been established as standard of care for colonic resections for cancer, it does have a sound oncological basis and could probably lead to better survival rates.

Left hemicolectomy, extended right hemicolectomy, and segmental left colectomy have all been suggested as acceptable templates for radical colectomy for splenic flexure lesions. While the oncological outcomes of all three approaches are largely equivalent, there are some situations – for example obstructing lesions, limited metastatic disease etc. – where one approach could fare better that the other. The use of laparoscopy in radical colectomy for colon cancer is well supported by evidence from multiple randomized controlled trials. Complete mesocolic excision is also safe and feasible via the laparoscopic approach. However, laparoscopic radical colectomy with complete mesocolic excision is technically challenging, and each surgeon will have his or her unique learning curve.

Key points

- The left colon receives blood supply both from the superior and inferior mesenteric arteries.
- The left colic artery serves as the dominant pathway for blood supply and lymphatic drainage for lesions at the splenic flexure in the majority of cases.
- Though a number of variations in vascular anatomy of the left colon have been described, there usually exists some sort of anastomotic channel between the SMA and IMA at or around the splenic flexure.
- Patterns of lymphatic drainage and nodal involvement may differ in the presence of variations of the arterial anatomy, and in the setting of heavy nodal involvement of the pericolic and intermediate nodes.
- Complete mesocolic excision involves dissection of the colon in the embryological mesocolic plane, division of the vascular pedicles at their origin, and resection of at least 10 cm of bowel on either side of the tumor.
- CME has a sound oncological basis and could be associated with superior outcomes in terms of disease-free and overall survival.

- Extended right hemicolectomy, left hemicolectomy, and left segmental colectomy are oncologically equivalent resection templates for malignant lesions at the splenic flexure.
- Extended right hemicolectomy/subtotal colectomy may be preferred in the setting of emergency resection for obstructing splenic flexure tumors, radical resection with curative intent in the setting of metastatic disease, and in the presence of variations in the arterial supply of the left colon.
- Laparoscopy for radical left colectomy is an accepted standard of care with both extracorporeal and intracorporeal anastomosis as feasible options.

Video

VIDEO 31   https://youtu.be/5yczQJqytLI

Laparoscopic Left Segmental Colectomy.

References

1. Chen YC, Fingerhut A, Shen MY et al. Colorectal anastomosis after laparoscopic extended left colectomy: Techniques and outcome [published online ahead of print, 2020 Feb 14]. *Colorectal Dis.* 2020;10.1111/codi.15018. doi:10.1111/codi.15018
2. Griffiths JD. Surgical anatomy of the blood supply of the distal colon. *Ann R Coll Surg Engl* 1956 Oct;19(4):241–56.
3. Garćia-Ruiz A, Milsom JW, Ludwig KA, Marchesa P. Right colonic arterial anatomy. Implications for laparoscopic surgery. *Dis Colon Rectum* 1996 Aug;39(8):906–11.
4. Michels NA, Siddharth P, Kornblith PL, Parke WW. The variant blood supply to the descending colon, rectosigmoid and rectum based on 400 dissections. Its importance in regional resections: A review of medical literature. *Dis Colon Rectum* 1965 Aug;8:251–78.
5. Bertelli L, Lorenzini L, Bertelli E. The arterial vascularization of the large intestine. Anatomical and radiological study. *Surg Radiol Anat SRA* 1996;18(Suppl 1):A1–6, S1–59.
6. Lange JF, Komen N, Akkerman G et al. Riolan's arch: Confusing, misnomer, and obsolete. A literature survey of the connection(s) between the superior and inferior mesenteric arteries. *Am J Surg* 2007 Jun;193(6):742–8.
7. Latarjet A. *Traite' d'anatomie humaine Tome quatrie' me: Appareil de la digestion.* Paris: G Doin & Cie, 1949.
8. VanDamme JP. Behavioral anatomy of the abdominal arteries. *Surg Clin North Am* 1993 Aug;73(4):699–725.
9. Peters JH, Kronson JW, Katz M, De Meester TR. Arterial anatomic considerations in colon interposition for esophageal replacement. *Arch Surg Chic Ill.* 1960 1995 Aug;130(8):858–62; discussion 862–863.
10. Ventemiglia R, Khalil KG, Frazier OH, Mountain CF. The role of preoperative mesenteric arteriography in colon interposition. *J Thorac Cardiovasc Surg* 1977 Jul;74(1):98–104.
11. Cheng B, Chen K, Gao S, Tu Z. Colon interposition. *Recent Results Cancer Res.* 2000;155:151–60.
12. Stearns MW. Benign and malignant neoplasms of colon and rectum. Diagnosis and management. *Surg Clin North Am.* 1978 Jun;58(3):605–18.
13. Murono K, Miyake H, Hojo D et al. Vascular anatomy of the splenic flexure, focusing on the accessory middle colic artery and vein. *Colorectal Dis* 2020;22(4):392–98..
14. Vasey CE, Rajaratnam S, O'Grady G, Hulme-Moir M. Lymphatic drainage of the splenic flexure defined by intraoperative scintigraphic mapping. *Dis Colon Rectum* 2018 Apr;61(4):441–6.
15. Watanabe J, Ota M, Suwa Y, Ishibe A, Masui H, Nagahori K. Evaluation of lymph flow patterns in splenic flexural colon cancers using laparoscopic real-time indocyanine green fluorescence imaging. *Int J Colorectal Dis* 2017 Feb;32(2):201–7.

138   **Laparoscopic Colorectal Surgery**

16. de'Angelis N, Hain E, Disabato M et al. Laparoscopic extended right colectomy versus laparoscopic left colectomy for carcinoma of the splenic flexure: A matched case–control study. *Int J Colorectal Dis* 2016 Mar;31(3):623–30.

17. Sadler GP, Gupta R, Foster ME. Carcinoma of the splenic flexure--a case for extended right hemicolectomy? *Postgrad Med J* 1992 Jun;68(800):487.

18. Manceau G, Mori A, Bardier A et al. Lymph node metastases in splenic flexure colon cancer: Is subtotal colectomy warranted?: MANCEAU et al. *J Surg Oncol* 2018 Nov;118(6):1027–33.

19. Leijte JAP, van der Ploeg IMC, Valdés Olmos RA, Nieweg OE, Horenblas S. Visualization of tumor blockage and rerouting of lymphatic drainage in penile cancer patients by use of SPECT/CT. *J Nucl Med off Publ Soc Nucl Med* 2009 Mar;50(3):364–7.

20. Heald RJ, Ryall RD. Recurrence and survival after total mesorectal excision for rectal cancer. *Lancet Lond Engl* 1986 Jun 28;1(8496):1479–82.

21. Wibe A, Møller B, Norstein J et al. A national strategic change in treatment policy for rectal cancer--implementation of total mesorectal excision as routine treatment in Norway. A national audit. *Dis Colon Rectum* 2002 Jul;45(7):857–66.

22. Hohenberger W, Weber K, Matzel K, Papadopoulos T, Merkel S. Standardized surgery for colonic cancer: Complete mesocolic excision and central ligation - technical notes and outcome. *Colorectal Dis* 2009 May;11(4):354–64.

23. Toyota S, Ohta H, Anazawa S. Rationale for extent of lymph node dissection for right colon cancer. *Dis Colon Rectum* 1995 Jul;38(7):705–11.

24. Goligher JC. Rationale for extent of lymph node dissection for right colon cancer. In: *Surgery of the Anus, Rectum and Colon, Bailliere Tindall* (ed.),. 5th ed. London, 1984; 445.

25. Yamaoka Y, Kinugasa Y, Shiomi A et al. The distribution of lymph node metastases and their size in colon cancer. *Langenbecks Arch Surg* 2017 Dec;402(8):1213–21.

26. Vogel JD, Eskicioglu C, Weiser MR, Feingold DL, Steele SR. The American society of colon and rectal surgeons clinical practice guidelines for the treatment of colon cancer. *Dis Colon Rectum* 2017 Oct;60(10):999–1017.

27. Gouvas N, Agalianos C, Papaparaskeva K, Perrakis A, Hohenberger W, Xynos E. Surgery along the embryological planes for colon cancer: A systematic review of complete mesocolic excision. *Int J Colorectal Dis* 2016 Sep;31(9):1577–94.

28. Bertelsen CA, Neuenschwander AU, Jansen JE et al. Disease-free survival after complete mesocolic excision compared with conventional colon cancer surgery: A retrospective, population-based study. *Lancet Oncol* 2015 Feb;16(2):161–8.

29. Bertelsen CA, Neuenschwander AU, Jansen JE et al. 5-year outcome after complete mesocolic excision for right-sided colon cancer: A population-based cohort study. *Lancet Oncol* 2019 Nov;20(11):1556–65.

30. Athanasiou CD, Markides GA, Kotb A, Jia X, Gonsalves S, Miskovic D. Open compared with laparoscopic complete mesocolic excision with central lymphadenectomy for colon cancer: A systematic review and meta-analysis. *Colorectal Dis* 2016 Jul;18(7):O224–35.

31. Ehrlich A, Kairaluoma M, Böhm J, Vasala K, Kautiainen H, Kellokumpu I. Laparoscopic wide mesocolic excision and central vascular ligation for carcinoma of the colon. *Scand J Surg* 2016 Dec;105(4):228–34.

32. Feng H, Zhao X, Zhang Z et al. Laparoscopic complete mesocolic excision for stage II/III left-sided colon cancers: A prospective study and comparison with D3 lymph node dissection. *J Laparoendosc Adv Surg Tech* 2016 Aug;26(8):606–13.

33. Bracale U, Merola G, Pignata G et al. Laparoscopic resection with complete mesocolic excision for splenic flexure cancer: Long-term follow-up data from a multicenter retrospective study. *Surg Endosc* 2020;34(7):2954–62;

34. Freund MR, Edden Y, Reissman P, Dagan A. Iatrogenic superior mesenteric vein injury: The perils of high ligation. *Int J Colorectal Dis* 2016 Sep;31(9):1649–51.

35. Søndenaa K, Quirke P, Hohenberger W et al. The rationale behind complete mesocolic excision (CME) and a central vascular ligation for colon cancer in open and laparoscopic surgery : Proceedings of a consensus conference. *Int J Colorectal Dis* 2014 Apr;29(4):419–28.

36. Steffen C, Bokey EL, Chapuis PH. Carcinoma of the splenic flexure. *Dis Colon Rectum*. 1987 Nov;30(11):872–4.

37. Odermatt M, Siddiqi N, Johns R et al. Short- and long-term outcomes for patients with splenic flexure tumours treated by left versus extended right colectomy are comparable: A retrospective analysis. *Surg Today* 2014 Nov;44(11):2045–51.

38. Nakagoe T, Sawai T, Tsuji T et al. Surgical treatment and subsequent outcome of patients with carcinoma of the splenic flexure. *Surg Today* 2001;31(3):204–9.

39. Ceccarelli G, Biancafarina A, Patriti A et al. Laparoscopic resection with intracorporeal anastomosis for colon carcinoma located in the splenic flexure. *Surg Endosc* 2010 Jul;24(7):1784–8.

40. Pisani Ceretti A, Maroni N, Sacchi M et al. Laparoscopic colonic resection for splenic flexure cancer: Our experience. *BMC Gastroenterol* 2015 Jul 7;15:76.

41. Fiscon V, Portale G, Migliorini G, Frigo F. Splenic flexure colon cancers: Minimally invasive treatment. *Updat Surg* 2015 Mar;67(1):55–9.

42. Martínez-Pérez A, Brunetti F, Vitali GC, Abdalla S, Ris F, de'Angelis N. Surgical treatment of colon cancer of the splenic flexure: A systematic review and meta-analysis. *Surg Laparosc Endosc Percutan Tech* 2017 Oct;27(5):318–27.

43. Binda GA, Amato A, Alberton G et al. Surgical treatment of a colon neoplasm of the splenic flexure: A multicentric study of short-term outcomes. *Colorectal Dis* 2020 Feb;22(2):146–53.

44. Gravante G, Elshaer M, Parker R et al. Extended right hemicolectomy and left hemicolectomy for colorectal cancers between the distal transverse and proximal descending colon. *Ann R Coll Surg Engl* 2016 May;98(5):303–7.

45. Kim CW, Shin US, Yu CS, Kim JC. Clinicopathologic characteristics, surgical treatment and outcomes for splenic flexure colon cancer. *Cancer Res Treat* 2010;42(2):69.

46. Beisani M, Vallribera F, García A et al. Subtotal colectomy versus left hemicolectomy for the elective treatment of splenic flexure colonic neoplasia. *Am J Surg* 2018 Aug;216(2):251–4.

47. Rega D, Pace U, Scala D et al. Treatment of splenic flexure colon cancer: A comparison of three different surgical procedures: Experience of a high volume cancer center. *Sci Rep* 2019 Dec;9(1):10953.

48. The SFC Study Group. de'Angelis N, Martínez-Pérez A, Winter DC et al. Extended right colectomy, left colectomy, or segmental left colectomy for splenic flexure carcinomas: A European multicenter propensity score matching analysis. *Surg Endosc* 2020 Feb 18 [cited 2020 Feb 23]; Available from: http://link.springer.com/10.1007/s00464-020-07431-9

49. Manceau G, Benoist S, Panis Y et al. Elective surgery for tumours of the splenic flexure: A French inter-group (AFC, SFCD, FRENCH, GRECCAR) survey. *Tech Coloproctology* 2020 Feb;24(2):191–8.

50. Bonjer HJ, Hop WCJ, Nelson H et al. Laparoscopically assisted vs open colectomy for colon cancer: A meta-analysis. *Arch Surg Chic Ill 1960.* 2007 Mar;142(3):298–303.

51. Dewulf M, Kalmar A, Vandenberk B et al. Complete mesocolic excision does not increase short-term complications in laparoscopic left-sided colectomies: A comparative retrospective single-center study. *Langenbecks Arch Surg* 2019 Aug;404(5):557–64.

52. Mori S, Kita Y, Baba K et al. Laparoscopic complete mesocolic excision via mesofascial separation for left-sided colon cancer. *Surg Today* 2018 Mar;48(3):274–81.

53. DeSouza A, Domajnko B, Park J, Marecik S, Prasad L, Abcarian H. Incisional hernia, midline versus low transverse incision: What is the ideal incision for specimen extraction and hand-assisted laparoscopy? *Surg Endosc* 2011 Apr;25(4):1031–6.

54. Milone M, Angelini P, Berardi G et al. Intracorporeal versus extracorporeal anastomosis after laparoscopic left colectomy for splenic flexure cancer: Results from a multi-institutional audit on 181 consecutive patients. *Surg Endosc* 2018 Aug;32(8):3467–73.

55. Daskalaki A, Kaimasidis G, Xenaki S, Athanasakis E, Chalkiadakis G. Internal-mesocolic hernia after laparoscopic left colectomy report of case with late manifestation. *Int J Surg Case Rep* 2015;6:88–91.

56. Sim WH, Wong KY. Mesenteric defect after laparoscopic left hemicolectomy: To close or not to close? *Int J Colorectal Dis* 2016 Jul;31(7):1389–91.

57. Toh JWT, Lim R, Keshava A, Rickard MJFX. The risk of internal hernia or volvulus after laparoscopic colorectal surgery: A systematic review. *Colorectal Dis* 2016 Dec;18(12):1133–41.

Chapter 22

LAPAROSCOPIC ANTERIOR RESECTION AND TOTAL MESORECTAL EXCISION FOR RECTOSIGMOID CANCER

Avanish Saklani, S Barath Raj Kumar, and Sanket Bankar

Contents

Learning objectives 139
Introduction 139
Preoperative patient preparation. 139
Operating room: Patient position and draping with placement of equipment and team 140
    Position of the patient 140
    Position of the surgeon and equipment 140
Initiating the procedure: Port placement and laparoscopic instrumentation 140
    Port placement 140
    Instruments required 140
Performing the procedure. 140
    Medial to lateral dissection: Inferior mesenteric vein ligation 140
    Medial to lateral dissection: Mesocolic dissection 141
    Ligation of inferior mesenteric artery. 142
    Enter the lesser sac 142
    Haray maneuver and posterior pelvic dissection 142
    Lateral peritoneal dissection and mobilization of splenic flexure 143
    Back to pelvic dissection (anterior and lateral dissection) 143
    Distal rectal transection and anastomosis of the rectum 143
    Extracorporeal procedure. 144
    Summary 144
Key points 144
Videos. 144
References 145

Learning objectives

- Preoperative patient preparation
- Operating room – patient position and draping with placement of equipment and team
- Initiating the procedure – port placement and laparoscopic instrumentation
- Performing the procedure
- Knowing the relevant anatomy and physiology

Introduction

In India, the age standardized incidence rate of rectal cancer in men is 8.3 per 100,000 and 5.0 per 100,000 among women. The mortality rate is 3.3 per 10,000. The immutable metrics in the surgical treatment of rectal cancer are tumor biology and stage at presentation. Operative technique is the major area where the outcome of the disease can be improved. A meticulous dissection of the 'correct tissue in the correct plane' is fundamental in reducing the oncological and physiological complications. A few trials (COLOR II, COREAN, ACOSOG, and AlaCaRT) [1–4] have shown that the resection range and degree of lymph node dissection is nearly identical in laparotomy. A meta-analysis of 14 randomized trials showed similar rates of circumferential and distal margin involvement, mean numbers of lymph nodes retrieved, and mean distances to radial and distal margins [5]. Intermediate-term follow-up local recurrence and overall survival rates were also similar, while the long term results are pending. With earlier postoperative recovery, laparoscopy is a viable approach in rectal surgery [6].

> **Before starting the procedure, know this:**
>
> - Aim of oncological surgery is to distinguish between parts to be resected and parts to be preserved.
> - Most important 'instrument' in oncological surgery is good traction and countertraction.
> - Prevent oncological and physiological complications: No tumour should be left behind, no neural structures unintentionally cut.

Preoperative patient preparation

In patients undergoing elective rectal surgery, we give them a mechanical bowel preparation with polyethylene glycol when there is no obstruction. In patients with obstructive features, a phosphate enema would suffice. We keep a close monitor on the hydration status and electrolytes of the patients undergoing mechanical bowel prep.

Thromboprophylaxis is typically administered as subcutaneous injections of low-molecular-weight heparin the evening before along with compression stockings.

Operating room: Patient position and draping with placement of equipment and team

Position of the patient
The patient will be in a 30-degree Trendelenburg position with legs in low lithotomy, using Allen yellowfins stirrups. The knees are flexed without hip flexion (a modification of Lloyd-Davies position – see Figure 22.1). A 15-degree tilt towards the right is given. Gel bolster is placed and adjusted below the sacrum. Shoulder pads and strapping of the patient is performed at the level of chest so as to prevent the patient from slipping.

Position of the surgeon and equipment
The surgeon positions himself on the right side of the patient while the first assistant is on the left. The second assistant will be beside the surgeon to his left. The monitors are placed on the foot end of the patient on either side.

> **Respiratory physiology alterations due to position**
>
> Significant changes occur in airway pressure, airway resistance, and compliance.
>
> Careful monitoring of the respiratory variables is required as to prevent potential negative respiratory effects.
>
> The functional residual capacity is reduced because of pelvic and abdominal organs moving towards the diaphragm and causing compression of the lungs. To counter this, airway resistance is increased so as to maintain tidal volume.

Instrument	
Ports	5 – Three 12 mm and two 5 mm cannulae
Scope 30 degree	1
Bowel grasper	4 (Curved and straight)
Monopolar spatula	1
Needle holder	1
Alexis wound retractor	1
Glove port	1
Energy device	Harmonic Scalpel (Ethicon Endosurgery, Cincinnati, OH). or Ligasure (Valleylab)

Initiating the procedure: Port placement and laparoscopic instrumentation (see Video 20)

Port placement
We use 5 ports, which are placed as follows: a 12 mm camera port is placed at supraumbilical position (using a visiport trocar). Two more 12 mm ports and two 5 mm ports are placed in hypochondrium and iliac regions as shown in the Figure 22.2. The pneumoperitoneum is maintained at 10–12 mm Hg.

Instruments required
The staplers used are:

1. Endoscopic linear cutter: Echelon 60 mm Green
2. Circular EEA stapler

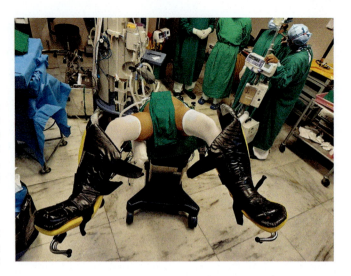

FIGURE 22.1 Patient Position. Modified Lloyd-Davies position with a right tilt.

Performing the procedure

After the preliminary step of thorough examination, the first point of order will be to obtain a good exposure to the rectum. The greater omentum is pulled up and tucked in below the liver. As a fallout, the transverse colon gets flipped up partially. Now run the small bowel loops using two bowel graspers, and place them in the right upper quadrant. This exposes the duodenum and the inferior mesenteric vein (IMV) (Figure 22.3). Placing a gauze here will prevent any downward movement of the duodenum and small bowel due to peristalsis.

> **Surgical anatomy**
>
> - Fascia is a term applied to any connective tissue layer covering organs that are large enough to be visible to the unaided eye.
> - Dissection of fascia between the colon/rectum and the neural system creates two other fascia – the pericolic fascia/rectal fascia propria (mesorectum) and the prehypogastric nerve fascia.
> - Never cut adipose tissue unintentionally – adipose tissue always encase vascular/neural bundles. Hence, cut adipose tissue only intentionally when you divide the vascular/neural branches to the rectum.

Identify the tumor. If there is difficulty in its identification, use a rigid sigmoidoscope to determine the tumor's extent and its lower limit.

Medial to lateral dissection: Inferior mesenteric vein ligation
We perform ligation of the IMV as the first step. This is contrary to the predominant teaching of ligating the inferior mesenteric artery (IMA) first. We have observed that the conversion rates (to open surgery) and the blood loss is less when ligating the IMV first. A randomized control trial also found similar findings with no change in operative time [8]. Start the dissection

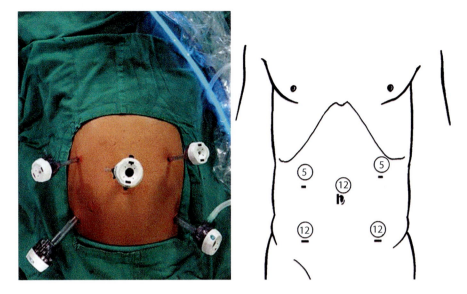

FIGURE 22.2   Showing port placements.

by releasing the fascia tethering the duodenum close to the IMV. Aid the assistant in holding the lower grasper near the superior rectal pedicle and the upper grasper more cephalad. Start by incising the peritoneum dorsal to the IMV, continuing the dissection superior to the IMA. Continue the medial to lateral dissection. As the predominant autonomic nerves are situated caudal to the IMA, dissection can be proceeded without injuring the nerves (Figure 22.4). On reaching close to the lower border of the pancreas, care must be taken not to injure the arc of Riolan (meandering mesenteric artery). The IMV is now ligated and resected below the pancreas.

Medial to lateral dissection: Mesocolic dissection

Position the assistant's grasper: the upper grasper holds the superior rectal pedicle and the lower grasper holds the mesocolon of the rectosigmoid, just above the level of the sacral promontory.

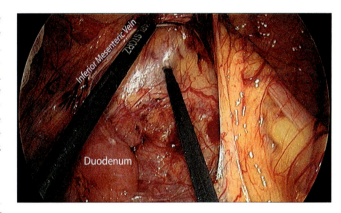

FIGURE 22.4   Delineating the IMV before its ligation.

The graspers need to be pulled ventrally and laterally. This forms a 'curtain' of mesocolon.

The incision starts on the peritoneum of the mesocolon at the level of the sacral promontory (Figure 22.5). Ask the assistant to temporarily relax his traction and make a horizontal cut on the peritoneum from the promontory to the root of the IMA. Once done, the assistant can apply the traction again – the horizontal line will tent up to form a mildly convex arch. This would be the line of dissection. Once the cut is made, the gas enters the

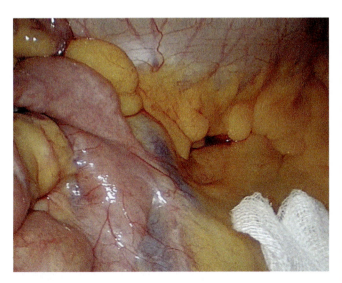

FIGURE 22.3   Exposure of duodenum and IMV after placing the small bowel in the right upper quadrant.

Camera position

The second assistant holds the camera in a manner such that the ureter runs horizontally form left to right. This is called the 'Retroperitoneal view'. This view will be maintained throughout the medial to lateral dissection, until the pelvic phase begins when the camera then switches on to the 'Pelvic view' – a cranio-caudal view centered around the sacral hollow.

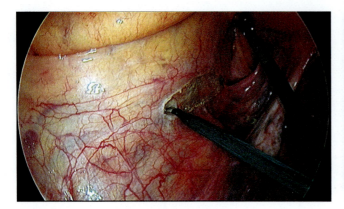

FIGURE 22.5   Medial to lateral dissection posterior to IMA.

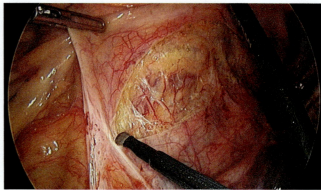

FIGURE 22.6   Medial to lateral dissection close to IMA.

fascial fibers and creates a 'foamy aerated' appearance. This aids in further dissection to a great extent. Hold the lower edge of the incised peritoneum and give countertraction with your left hand. Always dissect the fascial fibers and never the adipose tissue.

Progress with the dissection of fascia. Use the left-hand grasper and insert it below the IMA and anchor it upwards. This will add on to the traction. With the right hand, give downward strokes using a harmonic scalpel during the dissection so as to push down the neural structures. Keep in mind that fascia exists both ventral and dorsal to the autonomic nerves. Always stay on the ventral aspect of the nerve bundle. Another easier guide to dissection is to go close to the undersurface of the IMA – 'When in doubt, hug the IMA' (Figure 22.6).

Continuing in this plane, between the white line of Toldt and Gertota's fascia will be bloodless and will drop down all the retroperitoneal tissues (including the left ureter). This amounts to preventing any retroperitoneal organ injury and preserving the pelvic autonomic nerves (Figure 22.7).

> **Surgical anatomy**
>
> Lymphatic supply of the large bowel parallels its arterial supply. The large bowel lymphatics reside in the submucosa. The hierarchy of lymph nodes is as follows:
>
> The most proximal lymph nodes close to the bowel wall are the epicolic nodes. The paracolic lymph nodes are located along the marginal vessels. Intermediate nodes are found along the major vessels and subsequently drain to the principal nodes, which are at the origin of the IMA. Paraaortic nodes are the final point of drainage.

Ligation of inferior mesenteric artery

Once the medial to lateral dissection is complete up to the IMA, it is time to ligate the IMA. We prefer a high ligation of the IMA. This would remove all the regional nodes up to the principal nodes en bloc with the specimen. The mesocolon is held on both sides of the IMA. This would form a 'seagull' insignia (Figure 22.8). The root of the IMA is cleared of lymphatic tissue and is ligated with haemolock clips and cut.

Enter the lesser sac

The ligated end of the IMA and the superior edge of the peritoneum caudally will now be held by the assistant. Complete the medial to lateral dissection. The final step will be to enter the lesser sac. This can be achieved by incising the fascia superficial

to the pancreas. This step will be complimented by the lateral dissection of the colon and splenic flexure takedown later on.

> **Surgical anatomy**
>
> The superior hypogastric plexus is situated on the vertebral bodies anterior to the bifurcation of the aorta. Damage to this nerve plexus has been associated with erectile dysfunction in males.
>
> The pelvic splanchnic nerves, which are responsible for urinary continence and erectile function at vertebral levels S2–S4, track anteriorly and laterally to join the inferior hypogastric plexus anteriorly. This union occurs lower than the level of the origin of the IMA, and it is unlikely that these nerves are damaged outright in high ligation.
>
> Operatively, these nerves are more likely to be damaged during rectal mobilization in the pelvis, and this would occur in either high or low ligation. Hence, pelvic dissection is much more important in safeguarding the nerves.

Haray maneuver and posterior pelvic dissection

Having completed the medial to lateral dissection, we move on to the pelvis dissection. The first step will be performing a maneuver which will connect the abdominal and pelvic dissection. With the left-hand grasper giving traction on the mesocolon, use the open grasper in the right hand to straddle the sigmoid colon and give a sustained upward tug – this opens up the plane to pelvic dissection (Figure 22.9).

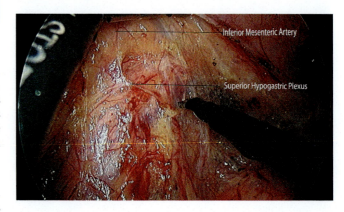

FIGURE 22.7   Medial to lateral dissection – preserving the autonomic nerves.

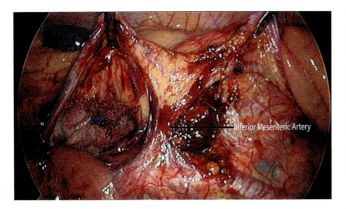

FIGURE 22.8 Seagull sign.

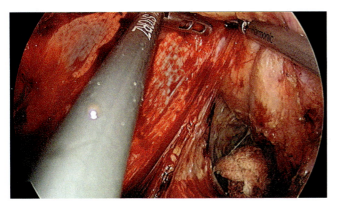

FIGURE 22.9 Haray maneuver.

The second assistant now changes the camera to a pelvic view. The posterior pelvic dissection is a continuity of the dissection of the sigmoid colon. A U-shaped dissection is followed posterior to the rectum following the same plane ventral to the neural structures – the rectal fascia propria (mesorectum) is hence formed. This initiates the total mesorectal excision posteriorly [7]. Any dissection, henceforth, will only be sharp. The reason being that any blunt dissection or push will catastrophically cause a breach in the mesorectum, and hence result in a positive circumferential resection margin.

The dissection is continued in to the concavity of the sacrum until an adequate distal rectal margin is reached, sparing the sphincter complex (Figure 22.10). Use an opened grasper or a bunched gauze in the left hand and give traction to the rectum. Alternatively, the assistant can use a fan retractor to give better visualization of the region. In case of a high rectal/rectosigmoid growth, 5 cm of mesorectal excision below the distal tumor margin is sufficient.

Lateral peritoneal dissection and mobilization of splenic flexure

With much of the hard work performed during the medial to lateral dissection, its fruits are now borne when performing the lateral peritoneal dissection. The assistant can relax during this dissection, albeit for a short period. The flimsy lateral peritoneal attachment of the colon is cut and circumferential dissection is completed until the splenic flexure is reached. Downwards traction is now given to the mobilized colon, and splenic flexure mobilization is complete.

Surgical anatomy

Denonvillier's fascia is the retroprostatic fascia that forms when the fascia connecting the rectum and prostate is cut. The Rectal fascia propria (mesorectum) is formed concomitantly.

Back to pelvic dissection (anterior and lateral dissection)

The posterior pelvic dissection is then continued laterally. The assistant pulls up the redundant colon upwards and to the side opposite to the laterality of dissection (upwards and to the right in left lateral dissection, and vice versa). The right and the left hypogastric nerves will be seen running laterally, which are preserved. The middle rectal vessel will then be encountered, which is then cauterized using the harmonic scalpel. An anterior peritoneal cut is then made on the rectovesical/rectouterine pouch close to the rectum (Figure 22.11). The assistant can now give traction ventrally over the bladder/uterus. The plane of dissection will be posterior to the Denonvillier's fascia in males and rectovaginal fascia in females. In males, once the seminal vesicles and the prostate is identified, dissection is carried out maintaining the intact mesorectum .

Distal rectal transection and anastomosis of the rectum

To aid in transection of the rectum, sling the rectum with a cotton tape (Figure 22.12). Use a needle holder to step up over the point of sling – this can be used to maneuver towards the right or the left when the endo stapler needs to be positioned. An Echelon 60 mm Green stapler is used for distal transection (Figure 22.13).

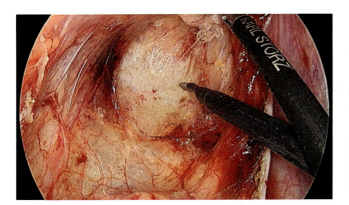

FIGURE 22.10 Posterior pelvic dissection.

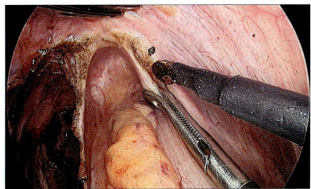

FIGURE 22.11 Anterior pelvic dissection.

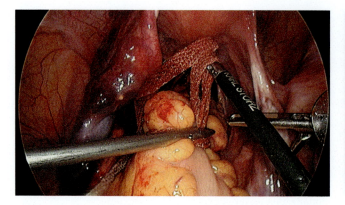

FIGURE 22.12 Slinging of rectum.

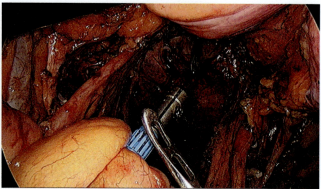

FIGURE 22.14 End-to-end anastomosis.

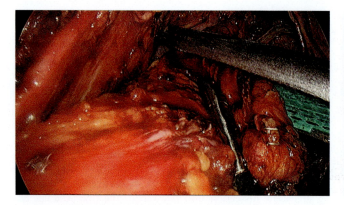

FIGURE 22.13 Firing of endoscopic linear cutter.

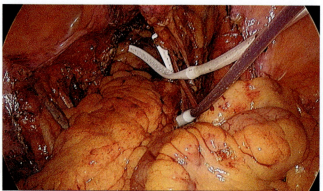

FIGURE 22.15 Placement of drains.

Rectal transection will require a few of staplers so as to get a near horizontal line of transection. Once transection is complete, the proximal end of the transected bowel is held on using a grasper with a ratchet and brought near the left iliac fossa port. Distal rectal wash is given and kept ready for anastomosis.

Extracorporeal procedure

The left iliac fossa port is then removed and the horizontal incision is increased so as to accommodate a medium sized Alexis wound retractor. The specimen is then delivered out, and proximal transection performed after obtaining adequate margins.

The proximal stapler line of the descending colon is opened and purse string sutures taken with 1 Prolene. The anvil of the EEA stapler is placed and the purse string tightened. The bowel is taken inside. A glove port is placed over the wound retractor so as to maintain the pneumoperitoneum. Lie of the mesocolon is checked and the stapler is introduced per rectally. End-to-end anastomosis is done (Figure 22.14).

We prefer placing two Jackson-Pratt drains anterior and posterior to the rectal anastomosis (Figure 22.15).

A defunctioning ileostomy is performed for all patients in whom the anastomosis is below the pelvic peritoneal reflection, and in those who have received neoadjuvant treatment.

Summary

TME is the standard of care in removing perirectal tissue when performing surgery of the rectum for an oncological cause. Rectal cancer surgery can be performed using either an open or minimally invasive approach. No one approach has been shown to be superior to the other. With the current emphasis on enhanced

recovery after surgery (ERAS), laparoscopic rectal surgery will complement the early recovery of the patient.

Key points

- A meticulous dissection of the 'correct tissue in the correct plane', is fundamental in reducing the oncological and physiological complications.
- We perform IMV ligation first, contrary to IMA ligation, and have observed that the conversion rates (to open surgery) and blood loss both diminish when ligating the IMV first.

See Videos 24 and 25.

Videos

VIDEO 20 https://youtu.be/sKko9cJIgTc

Laparoscopic Anterior Resection and TME for Rectosigmoid Cancer.

VIDEO 24 https://youtu.be/89rF20WnaxE

Anterior Resection and TME – Part 1.

VIDEO 25 https://youtu.be/OtAK6hTJwYU

Anterior Resection and TME – Part 2.

References

1. van der Pas MH, Haglind E, Cuesta MA et al. Laparoscopic versus open surgery for rectal cancer (COLOR II): Short-term outcomes of a randomised, phase 3 trial. *Lancet Oncol.* 2013;14(3):210–18. doi:10.1016/S1470-2045(13)70016-0

2. Jeong SY, Park JW, Nam BH et al. Open versus laparoscopic surgery for mid-rectal or low-rectal cancer after neoadjuvant chemoradiotherapy (COREAN trial): Survival outcomes of an open-label, non-inferiority, randomised controlled trial [published correction appears in Lancet Oncol. 2016 Jul;17 (7):e270]. *Lancet Oncol.* 2014;15(7):767–74. doi:10.1016/S1470-2045(14)70205-0

3. Fleshman J, Branda M, Sargent DJ et al. Effect of Laparoscopic-Assisted Resection vs Open Resection of Stage II or III Rectal Cancer on Pathologic Outcomes: The ACOSOG Z6051 randomized clinical trial. *JAMA* 2015;314(13):1346–55. doi:10.1001/jama.2015.10529

4. Stevenson ARL, Solomon MJ, Lumley JW et al. Effect of Laparoscopic-Assisted Resection vs Open Resection on Pathological Outcomes in Rectal Cancer: The ALaCaRT randomized clinical trial. *JAMA* 2015;314(13):1356–63. doi:10.1001/jama.2015.12009

5. Martínez-Pérez A, Carra MC, Brunetti F et al. Pathologic Outcomes of Laparoscopic vs Open Mesorectal Excision for Rectal Cancer: A Systematic Review and Meta-analysis. *JAMA Surg.* Published Online April 01, 2017;152(4):e165665. doi:10.1001/jamasurg.2016.5665

6. Yamada T, Okabayashi K, Hasegawa H et al. Meta-analysis of the risk of small bowel obstruction following open or laparoscopic colorectal surgery. *Br J Surg.* 2016;103(5):493–503. doi:10.1002/bjs.10105

7. Heald B. Autonomic nerve preservation in rectal cancer surgery -- the forgotten part of the TME message a practical 'workshop' description for surgeons. *Acta Chir Iugosl* 2008;55(3):11–6.

8. Planellas P, Salvador H, Farrés R et al. A randomized clinical trial comparing the initial vascular approach to the inferior mesenteric vein versus the inferior mesenteric artery in laparoscopic surgery of rectal cancer and sigmoid colon cancer. *Surg Endosc* 2019;33(4):1310–8. doi:10.1007/s00464-018-6551-z

Chapter 23

TECHNIQUES FOR LAPAROSCOPIC LOW ANTERIOR RESECTION, ULTRA LOW ANTERIOR RESECTION, AND INTER SPHINCTERIC RESECTION (ISR)

S Rajapandian, R Parthasarathy, Raghavendra Gupta, Sunil Kumar Nayak, and C Palanivelu

Contents

Learning objectives 146
Introduction 146
Indications... 146
Contraindications.. 147
Laparoscopic total mesorectal excision 147
   Preoperative preparation... 147
   Theater setup: Patient position.. 147
   Ports position.. 147
   Technique... 147
      Exploration of peritoneal cavity.. 147
      Division of the inferior mesenteric pedicle (medial to lateral approach) 147
      Medial to lateral mobilization of descending colon, splenic flexure, and transverse colon........ 148
      Mobilization of lateral attachments of rectosigmoid and descending colon 148
      Splenic flexure and transverse colon mobilization 148
      Pelvic dissection 148
      Posterior mobilization 148
      Medial and lateral mobilization 148
      Anterior mobilization... 148
      Distal occlusion 149
      Rectal transection 149
      Specimen removal... 149
      Anastomosis.. 149
      Assessment of anastomosis.. 150
   Intersphincteric resection... 150
   Diversion ileostomy 151
   Postoperative care.. 151
Postoperative follow-up... 151
Discussion 151
Summary 152
Key points 153
Videos.. 153
References 153

Learning objectives

In this chapter, we will be discussing the indications, preoperative evaluation, and technique of laparoscopic low anterior resection, ULAR, and ISR with intraoperative illustrative images.

- Know the indications and contraindications of each procedure
- Understand the structural anatomy which is important to perform the surgery
- Know the steps of the surgical procedure, and the added advantage of the laparoscopy

Introduction

Colorectal cancer is the third most common cancer in the world, and stands sixth in India [1]. Surgical management of rectal cancer has undergone a significant change during the past three decades, and the new concept of total mesorectal excision (TME) is now considered the golden standard for management of rectal cancer.

Although surgery remains the cornerstone of treatment for rectal cancer, multimodality therapy along with chemotherapy and radiotherapy has resulted in decreased local recurrence, increased colostomy-free survival, and increased overall survival rates.

Indications

1. Resectable carcinoma of rectum (T1-T3, N0-N2 lesions), i.e., stage I to III
2. Large benign rectal polyp (not amenable for endoscopic resection)
3. As part of other colonic resection procedures in palliation of ulcerative colitis and Crohn's disease
4. T4 lesions after NACRT

Contraindications

1. Tumor invasion into the sphincter complex, pelvic side wall, bladder, or prostate
2. Faecal incontinence
3. Unresectable M1 disease with minimal symptoms due to rectal tumor
4. Severe cardiopulmonary disease contraindicating laparoscopic surgery

> *Total-ISR is defined as complete internal anal sphincter (IAS) removal at the intersphincteric groove (ISG).*
>
> *Subtotal-ISR is IAS removal between the dentate line (DL) and ISG and involves two-thirds removal of the IAS.*
>
> *Partial-ISR is defined as IAS removal at the DL and involves one-third removal of the upper part of the IAS.*

(In our institute, we prefer partial ISR and are not performing total ISR due to poor postoperative quality of life.)

Laparoscopic total mesorectal excision

Preoperative preparation

All patients should undergo the following: Digital rectal examination, colonoscopy, CECT abdomen and chest, MRI pelvis or endoscopic ultrasound (EUS), and serum CEA apart from routine blood tests and LFTs (use of preoperative sigmoidoscopy should be preferably done by the operating surgeon to precisely identify the lower margin). Also, a routine preanesthetic checkup, cardiac evaluation, and pulmonary function evaluation should be done.

In patients planned for ISR, anal manometry should be done to assess anal function, resting pressures, and squeeze pressures, apart from DRE.

Patient to be kept nil by mouth from prior midnight except for medications. We always give tab Erythromycin (1gm + Tab. Rifagut 400 mg – oral antibiotic prophylaxis) the day before the surgery, along with bowel preparation with polyethylene glycol.

DVT prophylaxis: Compression stockings and low molecular weight heparin the night before surgery. Preoperative antibiotics: Injectable Ceftriaxone/Inj. Cefazolin 1g+Inj.metronidazole 500 mg 1 hr before incision.

Theater setup: Patient position (see Videos 21 and 22)

The patient is placed in a modified lithotomy position with the legs secured to the operating table with velcro or safety straps.

Anal sphincter involvement is further assessed and the distal rectum is washed with betadine saline solution to reduce the potential for tumor shedding. Ureteral stents are considered selectively in large, bulky, upper tumors, or inflammatory lesions.

Ports position (Figure 23.1)

1. The pneumoperitoneum is created by Verres needle through the midline and a right para umbilical 10 mm port is introduced for the camera.
2. Initially, a 5 mm, and then later a 12 mm port is inserted in right lower quadrant 2–3 cm medial and superior to the ASIS.
3. A 5 mm port is inserted in right lumbar region, in between the camera port and 2nd port.
4. A 5 mm left upper quadrant port inserted for retraction and splenic flexure mobilization.
5. A 5 mm suprapubic port is inserted in the midline for bladder/uterus retraction (optional).
6. A 5 mm port is inserted in left lower quadrant (optional).

Technique
Exploration of peritoneal cavity

The peritoneal cavity is thoroughly assessed for distant metastasis on the liver, peritoneal surface, and small bowel. Assessment of the pelvis follows the upper abdomen and adhesions, if any, due to previous surgeries are lysed. Any ascitic fluid noted should be sent for HPE/Cytology.

Division of the inferior mesenteric pedicle (medial to lateral approach)

The sacral promontory is identified and the peritoneum over it is incised on the medial aspect of the mesosigmoid, and continued up to the DJ flexure. A window is made between the mesocolon over the inferior mesenteric artery and Toldt's fascia, extended up

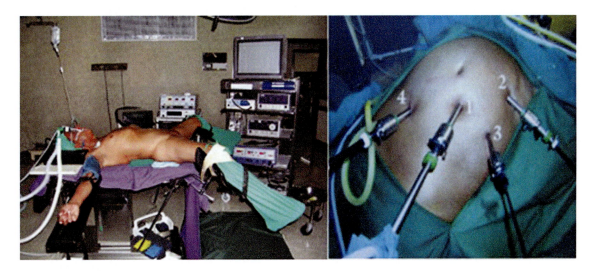

FIGURE 23.1 Port position.

to the level of the duodenojejunal flexure. The origin of the inferior mesenteric pedicle is identified and the pedicle skeletonized.

The IMA (high ligation) is divided proximal to the left colic artery (Figure 23.2). Then the IMV (Figure 23.3) is identified in a similar fashion between the duodenum and the IMA, and divided at the inferior side of the pancreas, usually well above the IMA ligation.

Medial to lateral mobilization of descending colon, splenic flexure, and transverse colon

The plane of dissection is continued from the medial to lateral aspect, proceeding towards the lateral parietal wall between the mesocolon and Toldt's fascia.

Identification of the lower border of pancreas is the limit of the cranial dissection. Subsequently, the lateral peritoneal attachment is incised from the sigmoid to the level of splenic flexure.

Mobilization of lateral attachments of rectosigmoid and descending colon

The dissection now continues up along the white line of Toldt, towards the splenic flexure. In this way, the lateral and any remaining posterior attachments are freed, making the left colon and sigmoid a midline structure.

Splenic flexure and transverse colon mobilization

The splenic flexure and the left colon should be mobilized in all cases of sphincter saving mesorectal excision, to achieve tension

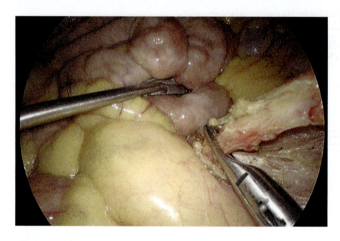

FIGURE 23.2   IMA ligation.

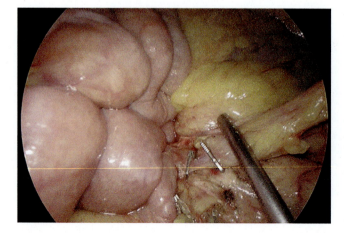

FIGURE 23.3   IMV ligation.

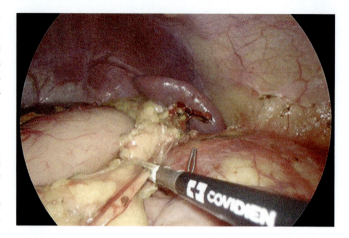

FIGURE 23.4   Splenic flexure mobilization.

free anastomosis (Figure 23.4). Division of the splenocolic and retro colic ligaments releases the splenic flexure. The gastrocolic portion of the greater omentum on its left end and the attachment of the transverse mesocolon to the inferior border of the pancreas are released separately. The marginal vessels of the colon are protected by keeping the level of division at the inferior border of the pancreas.

The descending colon, splenic flexure, and the distal transverse colon are completely mobilized at the end of this phase. This helps to obtain an adequate length of proximal colonic segment for tension-free anastomosis at the level of the pelvic floor.

Pelvic dissection

Pelvic dissection starts with the identification of the avascular plane of Heald. The peritoneum overlying the sacral promontory is incised and is continued distally along the right side of the rectum into the pelvis.

At this point of dissection, the pelvic autonomic plexus (or superior hypogastric plexus), and the left and right hypogastric nerves emerge sagitally below the level of the bifurcation of the aorta. The peritoneal incision is made on the left side of the rectum and is continued distally into the pelvis. Both the incisions are joined down to the anterior reflections in a U-shaped manner (recto vesical fold in males and rectovaginal fold in females).

Posterior mobilization

The posterior dissection is then continued down into the pelvis just above the fascia propria as low as possible, as this helps in subsequent lateral and anterior dissection. The posterior aspect of the mesorectum can be identified and dissection continues in this avascular plane towards the pelvic floor. Rectosacral fibers are divided at the level S4 to enter the pelvic floor, which straightens the rectum from the sacrum's curvature. The levators are now cleared on both sides. The division of the midline raphe completes the posterior dissection. With this approach, the rectum is lengthened to 4–5 cm.

Medial and lateral mobilization

The peritoneum is divided on the right side of the rectum reaching anteriorly. Similarly, the left side peritoneum is divided to reach anteriorly. At the distal limit of the recto uterine or recto vesicular pouch, the medial peritoneal incision is carried anterior to the rectum and left to right peritoneal incisions are connected.

Anterior mobilization

The dissection is started in the midline. Below the level of peritoneal reflection there is little tissue that covers the lower anterior

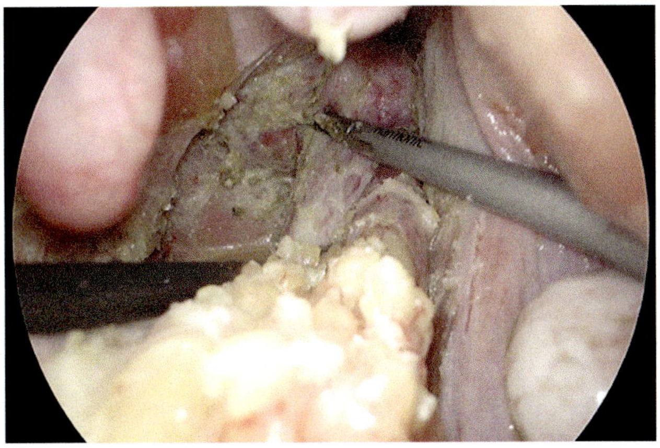

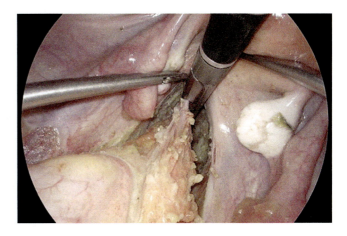

FIGURE 23.5 View after TME in ULAR.

FIGURE 23.7 Rectal transection using linear staplers.

rectum. During the anterior mobilization, care must be taken to avoid injuring the cavernous nerves (periprostatic plexus) while dissecting the anterior part to the Denioviillers fascia close to the seminal vesicles in males, and vaginal wall in females. The dissection is pursued by alternating lateral, anterior, and posterior dissection down to the pelvic floor until circumferential mobilization of the bowel is accomplished (Figure 23.5). The longitudinal muscle of the rectum and the levator ani should be clearly visualized at the end of the dissection.

After complete mobilization, the distal limit of the tumor and clearance below can be assessed by digital examination or sigmoidoscopy. At the end of dissection, the entire mesorectum is excised up to the level of the levator ani. The stapler has to be applied only after complete denudation.

Distal occlusion

The distal resection line, 2–5 cm distal to the tumor is precisely identified using sigmoidoscopy (Figure 23.6) or by rectal examination. Once the distal resection line has been freed from the mesorectum, a right-angle bowel clamp or stapler is applied to occlude the lumen distal to the growth.

Rectal transection

The mesorectum is dissected to at least 2–3 cm below the distal level of the tumor.

The rectum is transected at a level just below the occluding stapler line with 1 or 2 applications of the 60 mm linear endostapler

that has been passed through the right-lower-quadrant trocar, as perpendicularly to the bowel as possible.

In ultra-low anterior resection, the assistant keeps his fist on the perineum, to push the anal sphincter and levator ani into the pelvis to facilitate transection (Figure 23.7) at the level of anorectal ring/just at the level of levator ani. After transection of the rectum, the view of the pelvis is shown in Figure 23.8.

Specimen removal

The suprapubic port site is extended transversely (5 cm or more), depending on the size of the growth. The distal end of the bowel is brought outside the abdomen through a protective sheath, until the proposed level of transection of the bowel. The mesentery is divided and the bowel transected, keeping 5–6 cm of the bowel extending beyond the pubic symphysis, in order to avoid tension in the bowel after anastomosis, particularly in low rectal anastomosis. The size of the circular stapler is decided after division of the proximal colon and measuring its diameter. Usually we use a 31 or 29 Fr circular stapler according to the diameter of the colon. Proximal colon is repositioned into the peritoneal cavity. The Pfannenstiel incision is closed and pneumoperitoneum recreated.

Anastomosis (Figure 23.9)

Reconstruction following mesorectal excision of cancers of the rectum is usually of three types, namely low anterior resection, ultra-low anterior resection, and coloanal anastomosis depending on the distal limit of the tumor. Tumors located more than

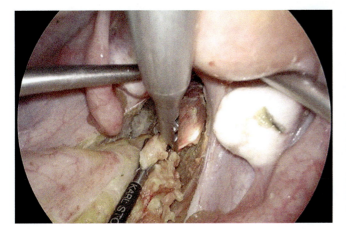

FIGURE 23.6 Sigmoidoscopic assessment of distal margin.

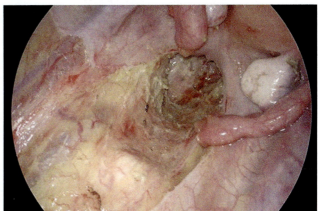

FIGURE 23.8 After total rectal transection in TME plane.

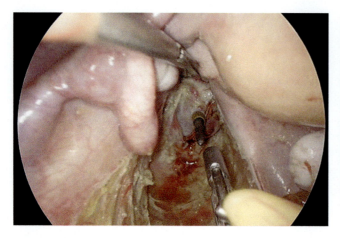

FIGURE 23.9   Colorectal anastomosis using a stapler.

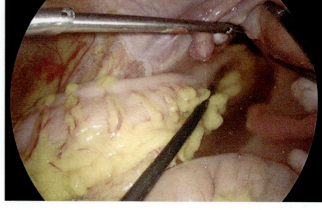

FIGURE 23.10   Assessing integrity using an air leak test.

8 cm proximal to the dentate line are suitable for low anterior resection, those within 6 cm of the dentate line are suitable for ultra-low anterior resection, and colo-anal anastomosis is suitable for growths located 2 cm from the dentate line.

Assessment of anastomosis

During this manoeuver the proximal colon is occluded with a clamp to prevent escape of air into the proximal part of colon. The pelvis is filled with saline to submerge the anastomotic line, and air insufflation of the rectum is performed with a syringe bulb to test for leakage. (Figure 23.10) The tissue donuts are checked for completeness and sent for histopathological analysis. A 24-size drainage tube is placed through the right lateral port for drainage. At the completion of the procedure, irrigation and a final examination of the peritoneal cavity is carried out to ensure hemostasis.

Intersphincteric resection

The mucosa of the anoderm is circumferentially opened, usually on or above the dentate line, and at least 1 cm from the distal margin of the tumor. A circular incision of the anal canal is started at the DL in partial-ISR, between the dentate line and inter sphincteric groove in subtotal-ISR, and at the inter sphincteric groove in total-ISR. Then a 1:200,000 adrenaline solution is infiltrated and the internal sphincter is circumferentially incised to enter the inter sphincteric plane, which is further dissected with electrocautery under direct vision (Figure 23.11). This dissection is continued to meet the already dissected intraperitoneal portion of the rectum. Specimens are extracted transanally (Figure 23.12). The pelvic cavity and the anal canal are irrigated with diluted 10% povidone iodine solution, followed by saline solution. After pull through of the descending colon, the coloanal anastomosis is performed between the colon, the external sphincter, and the anoderm with interrupted 2.0 PDS sutures keeping more than two thirds of the internal sphincter intact so that the postoperative quality of life will be good (Figure 23.13). At last a pelvic drain is placed laparoscopically.

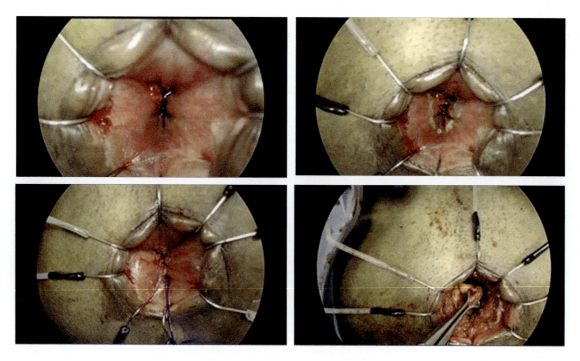

FIGURE 23.11   Mucosal incision and creation of space.

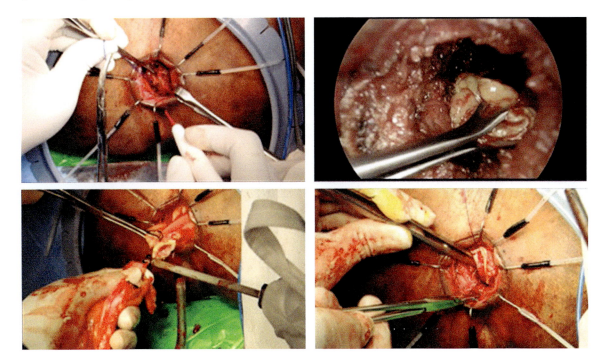

FIGURE 23.12   Per anal specimen extraction.

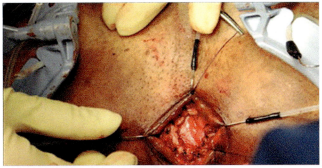

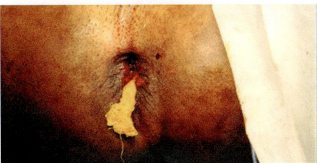

FIGURE 23.13   Completion of anastomosis final view.

Diversion ileostomy

We consider diversion only in coloanal anastomosis, ISR cases, and difficult ultra-low AR with doubtful donuts.

Postoperative care

Postoperatively, the patient is managed in HDU on the day of surgery and then shifted to the ward/room. The patient is started on liquids on the first postop day if he/she has an ileostomy, and on the second postop day for the others without ileostomy. The patient is started on a soft diet once he/she passes flatus and stool. The patient is discharged on the 4th or 5th postop day if he/she is not having any wound infections.

Postoperative follow-up

As with any colorectal malignancy, these patients are at a high risk of developing anastomotic site stricture postoperatively. So, frequent per rectal examinations are to be done in the follow-up visits.

Anal manometry should be done before ileostomy closure. Patients are made to hold increasing volumes of saline infused rectally in the weeks preceding the anticipated ileostomy closure. Ability of the patient to comfortably hold 200 mL of saline and ambulate without any leak indicates adequate sphincter function. It is also essential to rule out any distal obstruction prior to ileostomy reversal.

Discussion

The introduction of laparoscopy and other minimally invasive techniques to colorectal surgery has been a more gradual process. In particular, laparoscopy for the treatment of malignant colorectal disease was initially met with skepticism and controversy. Although much of this skepticism has been relieved since 2002 by the results of several large multicenter randomized controlled trials (RCTs), comparing laparoscopic and open colorectal cancer resections [2–6]. However, most of these studies have excluded rectal cancers from their studies due to the higher level of technical skill required to perform these surgeries.

In the COLOR II study [7], rates of positive CRMs after surgery for cancer located in the upper portion of the rectum were similar between groups. In this study, the rate of positive CRMs after laparoscopic resection of rectal cancer located within 5 cm from the anal verge was lower than that with open surgery. In the CLASICC trial, the occurrence of positive margins was 20%

after laparoscopic surgery and 27% after open APR. In patients who had APRs in the COREAN trial [8], positive margins were reported in 5.3% in the laparoscopic surgery group and 8.3% in the open surgery group.

In the ALaCaRT RCT, even though they were not able to establish the noninferiority of laparoscopy compared to open surgery, the pathological completion of TME in both groups was similar [9]. In the ACOSOG Z6051 RCT, short-term outcomes like length of stay, readmission rates, and complications were similar in both groups. But, the primary outcome of pathological completeness was inferior in the laparoscopic group [10].

The conversion rates vary from 3%–33% among the reported series. The morbidity of the procedure is around 25%–30% and has a minimal mortality of around 2% in many of the series. The conversion rates, morbidity, and leak rates have fallen due to the combination of experience, optimization of the technique, and technological advancements.

A systematic review of 17 studies found no negative impact of DRM <1 cm, or even <5 mm, in terms of local recurrence or overall survival in patients with good risk tumors, supporting sphincter preservation in even very low tumors [11]. Such advances enabled the use of ISR for tumors between 1 and 3 cm from the dentate line, and the combination of chemotherapy and neoadjuvant radiotherapy has been used with the objective to increase the opportunity to preserve the sphincter in patients with very low rectal tumors [12]. Tsukamoto et al. [13] compared the clinical results of intersphincteric resection and abdominoperineal resection for lower rectal cancer. They concluded that ISR is a feasible surgical procedure for T1–2 tumors (Tables 23.1 and 23.2).

Klose et al. [14] analyzed long-term results of oncological and functional outcomes after intersphincteric resection for low rectal cancer. They concluded that a majority of patients reported, after an ISR, improved fecal function, general satisfaction, and better quality of life after surgery. ISR remains an alternative surgical technique for low rectal cancer. Gokhan Cipe et al. [15] analyzed different studies on intersphincteric resection and found that the anastomotic leak rate ranged from 0.9% to 48% following intersphincteric resection.

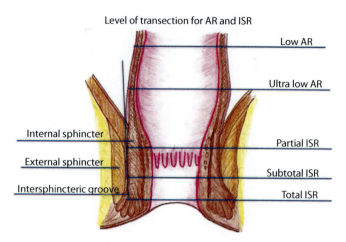

Level of transection for AR and ISR

FIGURE 23.14   Relevant anatomy.

The 5-year overall survival rate of intersphincteric resection is reported to range between 62% and 97%, and the disease free survival was 66%–87% in different studies [16].

Most of the studies comparing ISR and APR showed better survival following an ISR. Braun et al. compared the 5-year survival following an ISR and an APR for various stages of low rectal cancers and found similar 5-year survival rates in either group.

Laparoscopy comes with other advantages as well, which are as follows:

1. Greater patient comfort and early return to work.
2. *Improved visualization*: Magnification and clarity offered by the recent imaging equipments enable surgical precision and dissection in an otherwise difficult location in the narrow pelvis, where the surgeon has to struggle, and most often proceeds with the feel of tissues only. It is like a third eye for a surgeon:
   i. Identification and preservation of nerve plexus and branches.
   ii. Identification and entry into the holy plane of Heald.
   iii. Increased hemostasis due to minimally invasive sharp dissection.
3. *Enhanced teaching ability*: During conventional surgeries only the surgeon will be able to see the structures. Here, he has the ability to demonstrate the complete pelvic dissection to the entire team. The videos can be recorded and reviewed by the surgeon, or in the case of a resident, it can allow the consultant to offer practical advice and help in standardization of the surgery and to improve the outcomes.

Summary

Laparoscopic total mesorectal excision for tumors of the middle and distal one third of the rectum have proven to be feasible and safe in the hands of experienced laparoscopic colorectal surgeons, and the long-term results are comparable with conventional TME. With advancements on the technological front – such as better mechanical staplers (roticulating type), robots, and increased experience – both the short-term (conversion and anastomotic leak) and long-term results (survival and local recurrence) are likely to improve further.

TABLE 23.1: Type of Surgery in Low Rectal Tumors [17]

Type I	Supra-anal tumors (>1 cm from the anal sphincter)	Conventional coloanal anastomosis,
Type II	Juxta-anal tumors (<1 cm from anal sphincter) and	Partial intersphincteric resection
Type III	Intra-anal tumors (internal sphincter invasion)	Total intersphincteric resection
Type IV	Transanal tumors (external sphincter or levator ani muscles invasion)	APR

TABLE 23.2: Anterior Resection may be Further Subdivided into (Figure 23.14) [17]

High	Partial proctectomy with intraperitoneal anastomosis
Low	Extra peritoneal anastomosis
Ultra-low	Anastomosis at or just above the top of the levator ani muscle
Coloanal anastomosis	Anastomosis at or just above the dentate line

The ISR procedure appears to be oncologically and functionally acceptable as an alternative to APR in selected patients.

1. Preoperative chemoradiotherapy has to be considered for every patient planned for ISR.
2. Laparoscopic ISR for low rectal cancer is feasible and safe. The short-term surgical results and oncological outcomes are similar to those of the conventional open approach.
3. Indications have to be strict and patient selection is crucial to obtain optimal oncological and functional results.

Key points

- Laparoscopic total mesorectal excision for tumors of the middle and distal one third of the rectum have proven to be feasible and safe in the hands of experienced laparoscopic colorectal surgeons.
- Multiple RCTs and meta analyses have proven that laparoscopic resection of rectal cancer is safe and is associated with cancer-free survival similar to that obtained with traditional open rectal cancer surgery.
- Use of preoperative sigmoidoscopy preferably by the operating surgeon – to precisely identify the lower margin
- Patients scheduled for ISR should have anal manometry to assess anal function, for assessing resting pressures and squeeze pressures apart from DRE.
- The distal resection line: 2–5 cm distal to the tumor, and the mesorectum is dissected to at least 2–3 cm below the distal level of the tumor.
- The bowel is transected keeping 5–6 cm of the bowel extending beyond the pubic symphysis, in order to avoid tension in the bowel after anastomosis, particularly in low rectal anastomosis.
- The studies comparing ISR and APR showed better survival following ISR.

Videos

VIDEO 21 https://youtu.be/oh71URWukFs

Ultralow Resections and Coloanal Anastomosis for Low Rectal Cancers – Part 1.

VIDEO 22 https://youtu.be/7TIwRygOCMo

Ultralow Resections and Coloanal Anastomosis for Low Rectal Cancers – Part 2.

References

1. Ferlay J, Shin HR, Bray F, Forman D, Mathers C, Parkin DM. Estimates of worldwide burden of cancer in 2008: GLOBOCAN 2008. *Int J Canc* 2010;127(12):2893–917.
2. Lujan J, Valero G, Biondo S et al. Laparoscopic versus open surgery for rectal cancer: Results of a prospective multicentre analysis of 4,970 patients. *Surg Endosc* 2013;27:295–302.
3. Jayne DG, Guillou PJ, Thorpe H et al. Randomized trial of laparoscopic-assisted resection of colorectal carcinoma: 3-year results of the UK MRC CLASICC Trial Group. *J Clin Oncol* 2007;25:3061–8.
4. Van der Pas MH, Haglind E, Cuesta MA et al. Laparoscopic versus open surgery for rectal cancer (COLOR II): Short-term outcomes of a randomised, phase 3 trial. *Lancet Oncol* 2013;14:210–8.
5. Kang SB, Park JW, Jeong SY et al. Open versus laparoscopic surgery for mid or low rectal cancer after neoadjuvant chemoradiotherapy (COREAN trial): Short-term outcomes of an open-label randomised controlled trial. *Lancet Oncol* 2010;11:637–45.er. 2010;127:2893–917.
6. Lacy AM, Garcia-Valdecasas JC, Delgado S et al. Laparoscopy-assisted colectomy versus open colectomy for treatment of non-metastatic colon cancer: A randomised trial. *Lancet* 2002;359(9325):2224–9.
7. Jaap Bonjer H, Deijen CL, Abis GA et al. for the COLOR II Study Group*. A randomized trial of laparoscopic versus open surgery for rectal cancer. *N Engl J Med* 2015;372:1324–32.
8. SY, Park JW, Nam BH et al. Open versus laparoscopic surgery for mid-rectal or low-rectal cancer after neoadjuvant chemoradiotherapy (COREAN trial): Survival outcomes of an open-label, non-inferiority, randomised controlled trial. *Lancet Oncol* 2014;15:767–74.
9. Stevenson AR, Solomon MJ, Lumley JW et al. Effect of laparoscopic-assisted resection vs open resection on pathological outcomes in rectal cancer: The ALaCaRT randomized clinical trial. *JAMA* 2015;314:1356–63.
10. Fleshman J, Branda M, Sargent DJ et al. Effect of laparoscopic-assisted resection vs open resection of stage II or III rectal cancer on pathologic outcomes: The ACOSOG Z6051 randomized clinical trial. *JAMA* 2015;314:1346–55.
11. Bujko K, Rutkowski A, Chang GJ, Michalski W, Chmielik E, Kusnierz J. Is the 1-cm rule of distal bowel resection margin in rectal cancer based on clinical evidence? A systematic review. *Ann Surg Oncol* 2012;19:801–8.
12. Schiessel R, Novi G, Holzer B et al. Technique and long-term results of intersphincteric resection for low rectal cancer. *Dis Colon Rectum* 2005;48:1858–65.
13. Tsukamoto S, Kanemitsu Y, Shida D, Ochiai H, Mazaki J. Comparison of the clinical results of abdominoperanal intersphincteric resection and abdominoperineal resection for lower rectal cancer. *Int J Colorectal Dis* 2017;32:683–89.
14. Klose, J., Tarantino, I., Kulu, Y. et al. Sphincter-Preserving Surgery for Low Rectal Cancer: Do We Overshoot the Mark?. *J Gastrointest Surg* 2017;21:885–91. https://doi.org/10.1007/s11605-016-3339-0
15. Cipe G, Muslumanoglu M, Yardimci E, Memmi N, Aysan E. Intersphincteric resection and coloanal anastomosis in treatment of distal rectal cancer. *Int J Surg Oncol* 2012;2012:581258.
16. Saito N, Sugito M, Ito M et al. Oncologic outcome of intersphincteric resection for very low rectal cancer. *World J Surg* 2009 Aug;33(8):1750–6.
17. Rullier E, Denost Q, Vendrely V, Rullier A, Laurent C. Low rectal cancer: Classification and standardization of surgery. *Dis Colon Rectum* 2013;56(5):560–67.

Chapter 24

LAPAROSCOPIC CONVENTIONAL ABDOMINOPERINEAL (CAPE) AND EXTRA-LEVATOR ABDOMINOPERINEAL RESECTION (ELAPE)

Sanjiv Haribhakti and Deepak Govil

Contents

Learning objectives 154
Indications 154
Risk factors. 154
Staging workup (with emphasis on how MRI helps in loco-regional staging and preoperative planning) 154
Function after low anterior resection, and low anterior resection syndrome (LARS). 155
Surgical considerations 155
    LAR versus APR, sphincter preservation 155
    Conventional APR versus ELAPE 155
    ELAPE in supine versus prone position 156
        Perineal closure in ELAPE. 156
        Pelvic floor reconstruction after ELAPE. 156
        Laparoscopic ELAPE 156
    Preoperative preparation. 157
        Steps of the procedure: Tips and tricks. 157
        Options for perineal reconstruction 157
        Sacrectomy. 157
    Maintaining intestinal continuity after APE 157
Quality of life (QOL) issues 158
    Laparoscopic versus robotic rectal cancer surgery. 158
Summary 158
Key points 158
Videos. 158
References 158

Learning objectives

- Know which procedure is to be offered to which patient
- Know the staging work up and preoperative planning
- Know the risk factors involved in the procedures
- Know the difference between conventional APR vs. ELAPE and the different methods and steps of performing these procedure

The primary goal of surgical treatment of rectal cancer remains oncologic cure, while preserving sphincter function and maintaining intestinal continuity remain secondary goals.

Indications

An abdominoperineal resection is necessitated by lack of an adequate distal margin, loss of sphincter control as per clinical (digital) examination, and/or involvement of the sphincters on MRI. On the contrary, in a continent patient with an adequate distal margin and spared sphincters, sphincter preserving procedures should be attempted.

The indications for APR include

1. Anorectal adenocarcinoma
2. Squamous cell carcinoma anal canal
3. Other rectal malignancies, e.g., gastrointestinal stromal tumors, neuroendocrine tumors, and malignant melanoma
4. Rare etiologies including vascular malformations of the anorectum, and solitary rectal ulcer syndrome

Risk factors

A recent study [1] identified that age, BMI, interspinous distance, tumor distance from anal verge, prior abdominal surgery, preoperative chemoradiotherapy, and concurrent diseases influence the difficulty of performing laparoscopic abdominoperineal resection for ultra-low rectal cancer.

Staging workup (with emphasis on how MRI helps in loco-regional staging and preoperative planning)

Colonoscopy is advised for a patient suspected to have a low rectal growth. Besides obtaining a biopsy, a colonoscopy also helps in ruling out synchronous growth(s) or polyp(s). A biopsy from the growth can also be obtained with the help of a sigmoidoscope or proctoscope, which also helps in a more accurate assessment of the distal extent of the tumor. The staging workup for a rectal adenocarcinoma includes a contrast-enhanced computed tomography (CECT) scan of the abdomen and magnetic resonance imaging (MRI) of the pelvis. FDG PET scan is not used routinely for staging evaluation, rather it is employed in equivocal situations. Serum carcino-embryonic antigen (CEA) is a well-established tumor marker. Pretreatment CEA elevation is a marker of poor prognosis, as is also a failure of normalization of CEA after surgery. A serial rise in CEA in the follow-up period should prompt an evaluation for the same.

MRI is the investigation of choice to assess the loco-regional extent of the tumor. It is helpful in assessing the extent of mesorectal involvement, mesorectal fascia involvement as well as the mesorectal and lateral pelvic nodes,and sphincter involvement. MRI also helps in planning the treatment. Patients T3 and/or node positive disease are suitable candidates for neoadjuvant chemoradiation, especially patients with high risk features like positive circumferential margin and extramural venous invasion. MRI also provides a roadmap to select the appropriate surgical procedure – intersphincteric resection, conventional or extralevator APR, or exenteration procedures. MRI should be mandatory in planning radical surgery for rectal cancer. This improves R0 resection rates, and decreases local recurrences with improved oncological outcomes [2].

Function after low anterior resection, and low anterior resection syndrome (LARS)

While TME (commonly in conjunction with chemoradiation) has had a significant impact on local recurrence rates of rectal cancer, patients frequently experience varying degrees of altered bowel function. Low anterior resection syndrome (LARS) includes multiple bowel symptoms, may be associated with urinary or sexual dysfunction, varies in severity, and may impact quality of life. Patients report symptoms of urgency, incontinence, and difficult evacuation at rates of 12%–45%, 10%–71%, and 16%–74%, respectively [3]. Some degree of improvement with time is the norm, but symptoms can persist as late as 15 years postoperatively [4]. Postoperative factors contributing to the development of LARS include shortened intestinal length and a diminished rectal reservoir, as higher volumes of more liquid stool are delivered to a smaller neorectum. Anorectal manometry reveals reductions in urgent volume, maximal tolerable volume, and rectal compliance [5]. Other factors contributing to the development of LARS include damage to the sphincter complex or its innervation. Sympathetic nerves are at risk during high ligation of the inferior mesenteric artery (IMA), and parasympathetic nerves may be injured when the surgeon attempts to obtain wide negative CRMs. The levator ani nerve, arising from S3 and S4, runs on the superior surface of the pelvic floor, making it vulnerable to injury during dissection and potentially causing a dysfunctional pelvic floor postoperatively [6]. Despite the increased focus

on visualization and preservation of the pelvic autonomic nerve structures, symptoms consistent with pelvic floor dysfunction are common following TME. Of 178 participating patients with normal continence in the Dutch TME trial, 69 (39%) had new fecal incontinence after rectal cancer treatment, and 14% had new onset of combined fecal and urinary incontinence.

Surgical considerations

LAR versus APR, sphincter preservation

Sphincter preservation in rectal cancer – a goal worth achieving at all costs [7]? The answer must be no. While we should strive toward sphincter preserving options, we must recognize the limitations of currently available approaches and accept that sphincter preservation may not be the best overall option for each individual patient. Anorectal dysfunction and poor functional outcome are common following AR. The alternative of APE or low Hartmann's procedure imposes a permanent stoma. Quality of life following APE appears to be similar to that following AR. Given the choice, most patients would choose AR over APE. It is doubtful, however, that patients appreciate fully the functional outcome following AR, and also likely that patients harbor excessively negative misconceptions about life with a permanent stoma. Patients must be informed that function may not be as good as they expect after AR, and also that patients who have undergone APE positively appraise this option at follow-up. The morbidity associated with stoma reversal (following AR), and the significant risk of perineal wound problems following APE must also be considered.

Conventional APR versus ELAPE

In extralevator abdominoperineal excision (ELAPE) or cylindrical APE, the principles involve avoiding dissecting the mesorectum off the levator ani muscle and dividing the levators laterally at their point of insertion to the pelvic bony-ligamentous ring (Figure 24.1), thus reducing the chance of breaking into the tumor and waisting of the specimen (Figure 24.2). ELAPE involves the en bloc excision of the levator muscles and the rectum, in order to reduce the risk of tumor involvement in the circumferential resection margins (CRMs), and reduce the risk of tumor

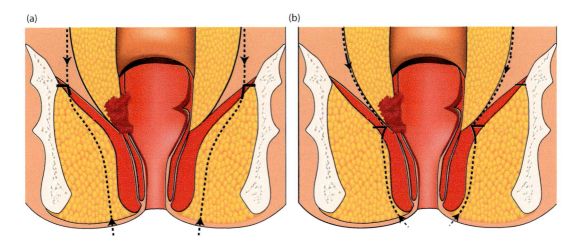

FIGURE 24.1 (a) Extralevator APE: Dividing the levators laterally at their point of insertion to the pelvic bony-ligamentous ring; (b) Conventional APE (dotted lines indicate line of dissection. Horizontal lines mark where the abdominal dissection and the perineal dissection meet).

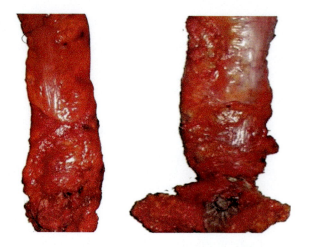

FIGURE 24.2 Specimen difference between extralevator APE with cylindrical specimen, and conventional APE with waisting of specimen.

perforation intraoperatively. This method has been demonstrated as leading to a wider surgical margin and, therefore, fewer positive CRMs [8,9]. A recent meta-analysis of five European randomized clinical trials on rectal cancer revealed that the APE procedure is a significant predictor for nonradical resections and increased risk of local recurrence with decreased cancer specific survival. Whenever possible, a more radical operation should be considered for low rectal cancer. There has been increasing awareness of the need to improve the outcome of APE for low rectal cancer. A recent multicenter analysis has reported on the use of ELAPE. It has reported a significant reduction in the rate of margin involvement and a reduced perforation rate when compared to the 'standard' technique [10].

A more recent review compared APE and ELAPE [11]. According to the findings and even though there are some publications recording a possible benefit in terms of reduction in CRM infiltration, iatrogenic perforations, or local recurrence, there is not enough evidence to affirm that the ELAPE leads to better oncological results when compared to conventional APE [12,13].

ELAPE in supine versus prone position

It is also possible to perform the ELAPE in a lithotomy position, but a prone jack-knife position is always preferred. The lithotomy position may result in poor visualization of the anatomy of the region, which may contribute to the increased risk of perforation of the specimen and a positive resection margin. With the patient in the prone position, these hazards may be easier to avoid. Any bleeding from the prostatic bed or vaginal wall is easy to control in prone position. Perhaps the prone dissection may reduce the incidence of sexual dysfunction, which is known to be higher after APE in the lithotomy position compared with low anterior resection (LAR). This may be partly related to the difficulty in visualizing the nerves in the lithotomy position. The prone position improves visualization of the operative field, and allows clear demonstration of the surgical anatomy for teaching [14].

The majority of shortcomings of the Lloyd-Davies position is related to the limited vision of the surgical site, which leads the dissection to be mostly blind and blunt, and does not follow the principle of the tumor-free technique. The prone jackknife position enables a sharp, standardized, and direct vision resection of the rectal stump, which ensures en bloc excision of the primary tumor, lesser CRM positivity, and lower perforation rates

[15,16]. Since the levator ani muscles have been resectioned by laparoscopic, the perineal phase in the prone jackknife position becomes easy; also, this modified technique reduces blood loss and operative time, and the benefits are oncologically equivalent to the ELAPE.

Perineal closure in ELAPE

The final part of the operation is to close the perineal wound. There is controversy regarding the best method for doing so. Some units prefer to use a muscle flap, particularly when the perineum has been irradiated. Other alternatives include primary closure, or closure with a biological collagen mesh. But the cost of biological mesh is quite high. Another indigenous method, which may be applicable in our country, is to pack the perineal gap with Gelfoam sponge (absorbable gelatine), and then place a prolene mesh over it, so that the small bowel cannot come into the direct contact with the prolene mesh.

Pelvic floor reconstruction after ELAPE

Various alternative techniques have been described to reconstruct the pelvic floor following ELAPE, with the aim to reduce perineal wound complications and hernias. The optimal method of perineal reconstruction remains a matter of debate. Myocutaneous flaps, such as those derived from the gluteus maximus [17], rectus abdominis, and latissimus dorsi muscles [18] have been used but are associated with donor-site morbidity, flap necrosis, prolonged operative time, additional resources, and increased cost. Biologic mesh has recently been introduced as an alternative form of reconstruction in order to improve perineal wound healing and reduce perineal hernia rates [19]. The mesh is usually placed as an inlay or bridge across the defect in the pelvic floor in close relation to the bony structures and sutured in 1-cm intervals to the origin of the levator muscles laterally [20]. The mechanism by which the use of a bridging prosthesis reduces perineal wound problems is not clear. It has been suggested that biological mesh allows native cellular ingrowth and promotes tissue remodeling, which in turn reduces perineal wound problems [21]. One recent review [22] suggested that overall, the use of a biologic mesh to close perineal defects has comparable complications rates to myocutaenous flaps, but may offer advantages – shorter operating time and early mobilization, which results in a more cost-effective repair.

In one recent review [23] biological mesh appears to be a valid option, at least in terms of hernia prevention, which can be reduced by up to 50%. While perineal infection is frequent in irradiated patients, the use of biological mesh seems logical, even if the evidence is scarce to draw definitive recommendations. On the other hand, perineal wound infection remains frequent and a perineal drain should be routinely used.

Laparoscopic ELAPE

An Indian study [24] described laparoscopic extralevator APE in the lithotomy position and concluded it reduces operative time significantly, as patient position change is not needed during the procedure. Another study [25] performed laparoscopic transabdominal transection of the levator muscles and the perineal part resection in a prone jackknife (PJK) position. The levator muscles in the tumor side arc are vertically cut under direct laparoscopic visualization, and the other side is mostly preserved. The dissection lines along the rectum meet at the apex of the coccyx bone. The R0 resections and no CRM involvement are required in the operation, it is defined as extralevator resection. A laparoscopic linear stapler was used to cut off the sigmoid colon, and the proximal colon is pulled out to make a colostomy . The patient's position was altered to a PJK position for the perineal resection, and dissection began first on the posterior side, performed behind the coccyx bone, as the levator muscles have been transected by the laparoscopic transabdominal approach. The dissection plane is relatively easy to find, and lateral dissection follows the levator ani muscle stump. The distal rectum is anteriorly pulled out from the pelvic cavity through the perineal wound. This approach allows to identify the boundary of the anterior rectal wall, vagina, or seminal vesicles/prostate with excellent visualization. Then a limited dissection is performed on the anterior; it must preserve the urethra in males and the posterior vaginal wall in females (perineal body). Since the dissection extent of the levator ani muscles has been modified, the pelvic and perineal incisions can easily be closed by suturing the subcutaneous tissue and the skin, and suturing the residue of the levator muscles if necessary.

Preoperative preparation (see Videos 23 and 26)
Steps of the procedure: Tips and tricks
Position the patient supine on the operating table with both arms tucked, padded, and protected at the sides. Place the patient in a modified lithotomy position using Allen stirrups (Lloyd-Davies or other designs may be used). It is imperative that the thighs be at or lower than the level of the abdominal wall to obviate difficulty in maneuvering the lower abdominal instruments. This position enables intraoperative colonoscopy, if needed, as well as the introduction of a circular stapler through the anus for construction of a low anastomosis. In general, the surgeon stands on the side of the patient opposite of the pathology and the site of dissection, with the first assistant standing across the table.

The procedure usually starts with the establishment of pneumoperitoneum through a supraumbilical incision. This can be achieved through an open approach, or by using Verre's needle. A 10 mm port is inserted and a thorough laparoscopy is performed to rule out distant metastases, especially peritoneal and on the liver. The surgical procedure consists of an abdominal phase and perineal phase.

Abdominal phase:
The port position used for the abdominal phase consists of *two working ports* on the right side of abdomen:

1. 12 mm port 2 finger breadth medial and superior to right anterior superior iliac spine (ASIS)
2. 5 mm port at the level of umbilicus of the right side, a hand breath away from the camera port, in line with the 12 mm port

Two assistant ports (5 mm in size) positioned on the left side of the abdomen are the mirror image of the right sided ports.

The assistant uses two atraumatic graspers, and the surgeon uses an atraumatic grasper, a spatula, and a harmonic scalpel.

1. *Medial to lateral dissection:* Division of the lateral peritoneal reflection.
2. *Splenic flexure mobilization:* Depending on the length and mobility of the sigmoid colon, it may not be necessary to mobilize the splenic flexure.
3. The level of vascular ligation may vary based on the same considerations.
4. Choose a point at which to divide the bowel. Serially divide the mesentery at this level using ultrasonically activated scissors, ligatures, clips, or a vascular stapler. At this site, the mesentery is serially divided to this level using either

the ultrasonically activated scissors, vessel loops, ligaclips, or vascular stapler.
5. Transect the bowel at the proposed site of division.
6. Grasp the distal colonic staple line and retract it anteriorly or inferiorly to expose the presacral space. The presacral space is entered posteriorly using either cautery scissors or an ultrasonic scalpel.
7. Dissect the presacral space posteriorly to the level of Waldeyer's fascia. Open this fascia to expose the levator muscles. Continue this dissection laterally on both sides.
8. Perform the anterior dissection last: retract the rectum superiorly and posteriorly. In females, retract the uterus (if present) anteriorly and inferiorly. Dissect the rectum from vagina (in females) or seminal vesicles and prostate (in males).
9. *Perineal part:* At this point, with the rectum fully mobilized intracorporeally, the perineal dissection is made. Make an elliptical incision around the external sphincter. Deepen this incision into the ischiorectal fat to expose the levator muscles. Posteriorly, place the levator plate at the level of the tip of the coccyx. Introduce a finger into the pelvis posteriorly and visualize it with the laparoscope. Divide the levators laterally and posteriorly. Insert a ring forceps into the pelvis from below. Under laparoscopic control, the tip of the rectum/sigmoid colon is handed to the perineal operator via the ring forceps. The rectosigmoid colon is then extracted from below. Complete the remaining dissection from the perineal aspect in the usual fashion.

Options for perineal reconstruction
Pass an endoscopic Babcock clamp via the trocar at the stoma site, and grasp the remaining end of the sigmoid colon. Excise a 2 cm disk of skin around the trocar site and enlarge the trocar site. Bring out the end of the colon as a colostomy. Mature this in the usual fashion. From the perineal wound, pass an endoscopic Babcock clamp into the abdomen and guide it up retrograde through the right lower quadrant trocar site. Grasp and pull an irrigation sump catheter through the trocar site and position it just above the levators. Close the levators and perineum, and complete the operation in the usual fashion.

Sacrectomy
The level of local involvement of the sacrum is a determinant of radicality and surgical morbidity. In cases of coccyx and S5 invasion, sacral resection is performed without major problems. However, if there is a more proximal involvement, it is more complex and can evolve with uncontrollable hemorrhage, neurological injury, and urinary complications [26].

Maintaining intestinal continuity after APE
Selected patients undergoing APRs may be able to maintain intestinal continuity. Several authors have described restoration of intestinal continuity following APR. Perineal colostomy, graciloplasty, and artificial sphincters provide pseudocontinence: intestinal continuity is maintained, but antegrade or retrograde colonic enemas may be required for defecation. Even though an immediate reconstruction at the time of APR could technically be performed, it is generally discouraged in favor of a secondary approach after the oncological long-term goals have been met. Restoration of intestinal continuity after APR is a challenge and the available procedures to achieve pseudocontinence are limited by relatively little experience and, in some cases, high rates of morbidity. However, these procedures may be appropriate for

well-informed, highly motivated patients who are not candidates for anterior or intersphincteric resection, and want to avoid a stoma at all costs.

Quality of life (QOL) issues

Quality of life (QOL) considerations are important when helping patients select the appropriate treatment for low rectal cancers. Many studies have addressed this issue over the past 20 years, comparing patients undergoing APR to those undergoing SSR. Initial reports demonstrated a QOL advantage for SSR. Williams and Johnston [27] showed that APR patients had considerably more sexual impairment, and only 40% returned to work, compared with 83% following SSR. Several other studies corroborated these findings [28,29].

However, as anastomoses became technically feasible more distally in the rectum, or upper anal canal, the differences in QOL diminished. Difficulties with evacuation and incontinence in very low SSR offset changes in sexuality found with APR [30]. Pachler and Wille-Jorgensen [31] examined 30 QOL studies and found 11 of sufficient merit to analyze, finding that in 6, QOL was not appreciably different when SSR and APR patients are compared. Vironen et al. [32] found that bowel and urogenital dysfunction in both SSR and APR patients, and not simply the presence of a stoma, was the biggest determinant of QOL deficits following rectal cancer surgery. An interesting study by Zolciak and colleagues [33] looked at patient preferences before and after rectal cancer resection. Approximately half the patients who underwent APR preferred that operation during a 4-year follow-up, suggesting a positive reappraisal of APR, once experienced.

Laparoscopic versus robotic rectal cancer surgery

A recent meta-analysis of RCT [34] evaluated eight RCTs involving 999 patients, where 495 of them underwent RP and 504 underwent LP. The results showed that the RP group had a longer operative time (P < 0.01), a lower conversion rate (P < 0.03), a longer distance to the distal margin (DDM) (P < 0.001), and a lower incidence of erectile dysfunction (P < 0.02). No significant differences were found between the two groups in perioperative mortality, complication rates, PRM, number of harvested lymph nodes, length of hospital stay, and time to first bowel movement. Current evidence suggests that RP is superior to LP in short-term clinical outcomes, and is similar to LP regarding pathological outcomes, and has better DDM outcomes.

The recently published ROLARR RCT [35] concluded that robotic rectal cancer surgery results in comparable outcomes to laparoscopic surgery. There is no statistical benefit in terms of conversion to open surgery, bladder or sexual function, pathological outcomes, or DFS and OS. The observed trend suggesting a reduced conversion in male patients requires further confirmation. Robotic rectal cancer surgery is not cost-effective compared to laparoscopic rectal cancer surgery, because the increased costs far outweigh any marginal benefit in QOL.

Summary

An abdominoperineal resection is necessitated by the lack of an adequate distal margin, loss of sphincter control as per digital examination, and/or involvement of the sphincters on MRI. The staging workup for a rectal adenocarcinoma includes a contrast-enhanced computed tomography (CECT) scan of the abdomen and magnetic resonance imaging (MRI) of the pelvis. Serum pretreatment CEA elevation is a marker of poor prognosis, as is also a failure of normalization of CEA after surgery. Postsurgery

perineal reconstruction to maintain intestinal continuity is important. QOL is important when helping patients select the appropriate treatment for low rectal cancers; patients who underwent APR preferred that operation during a 4-year follow-up, suggesting a positive reappraisal of APR, once experienced. The recently published ROLARR RCT concluded that robotic rectal cancer surgery results in comparable outcomes to those of laparoscopic surgery.

Key points

- Sphincter preservation in rectal cancer is a goal worth achieving at all costs? The answer must be NO.
- MRI should be mandatory in planning radical surgery for rectal cancer, this improves R0 resection rates, and decreases local recurrences with improved oncological outcomes.
- Avoid dissecting the mesorectum off the levator ani muscle and dividing the levators laterally, thus reducing the chance of breaking into a tumor.
- ELAPE has demonstrated a significant reduction in the rate of margin involvement and a reduced perforation rate.
- The optimal method of perineal reconstruction remains a matter of debate, with the options to use of myocutaneous flaps or biological collagen mesh or close by suturing the residue of the levator muscles.

Videos

VIDEO 23   https://youtu.be/DvmSJhWCCr0

Laparoscopic APE.

VIDEO 26   https://youtu.be/dKrkLAU4uqw

Extralevator APE.

References

1. Li Q, Li D, Jiang L et al. Factors Influencing Difficulty of Laparoscopic Abdominoperineal Resection for Ultra-Low Rectal Cancer. *Surg Laparosc Endosc Percutan Tech* 2017;27:104–9.
2. Saklani A, Bae S, Clayton A, Kim N. Magnetic resonance imaging in rectal cancer: A surgeon's perspective. *World J Gastroenterol* 2014;20(8):2030–41.
3. Bryant CL, Lunniss PJ, Knowles CH, Thaha MA, Chan CL. Anterior resection syndrome. *Lancet Oncol* 2012 Sep;13(9):e403–8.
4. Lundby L, Krogh K, Jensen VJ, Gandrup P, Qvist N, Overgaard J, Laurberg S. Long-term anorectal dysfunction after postoperative radiotherapy for rectal cancer. *Dis Colon Rectum* 2005 Jul;48(7):1343–9.
5. Lee SJ, Park YS. Serial evaluation of anorectal function following low anterior resection of the rectum. *Int J Colorectal Dis* 1998;13(5–6):241–6.
6. Wallner C, Lange MM, Bonsing BA, Maas CP, Wallace CN, Dabhoiwala NF, Rutten HJ, Lamers WH, Deruiter MC, van de Velde CJ; Cooperative Clinical Investigators of the Dutch Total Mesorectal Excision Trial. Causes of fecal and urinary

incontinence after total mesorectal excision for rectal cancer based on cadaveric surgery: A study from the Cooperative Clinical Investigators of the Dutch total mesorectal excision trial. *J Clin Oncol* 2008 Sep 20;26(27):4466–72.

7. Mulsow J, Winter A. Sphincter preservation for distal rectal cancer - a goal worth achieving at all costs? *World J Gastroenterol* 2011;17(7):855–61.

8. West NP, Anderin C, Smith KJ, Holm T, Quirke P, European Extralevator Abdominoperineal Excision Study Group. Multicentre experience with extralevator abdominoperineal excision for low rectal cancer. *Br J Surg* 2010;97(4):588–99.

9. Shihab OC, Heald RJ, Holm T et al. A pictorial description of extralevator abdominoperineal excision for low rectal cancer. *Colorectal Dis* 2012;14(10):e655–60.

10. Bebenek M. Abdominosacral amputation of the rectum for low rectal cancers: Ten years of experience. *Annals Surg Oncol* 2009;16(8):2211–7.

11. Serrano M, Sebastiano B. Abdominoperineal excision or extralevator abdominoperineal excision: Which is the best oncological treatment? *Ann Laparosc Endosc Surg* 2018;3:33.

12. Wang Q, Xu C, Wang J et al. Advantage of extralevator abdominoperineal excision comparing to the conventional abdominoperineal excision for low rectal cancer: A Meta-analysis. *Zhong Nan Da Xue Xue Bao Yi Xue Ban* 2017;42:320–7.

13. Prytz M, Angenete E, Bock D et al. Extralevator Abdominoperineal Excision for Low Rectal Cancer--Extensive Surgery to Be Used With Discretion Based on 3-Year Local Recurrence Results: A Registry-based, Observational National Cohort Study. *Ann Surg* 2016;263:516–21.

14. Mahadavan L, Veeramootoo D, Daniels I. Early results of porcine collagen membrane (Permacol) in pelvic floor reconstruction following prone cylindrical PAE. *Eur J Surg Oncol* 2008;34:1165.

15. Hu X, Cao L, Zhang J et al. Therapeutic results of abdominoperineal resection in the prone jackknife position for T3-4 low rectal cancers. *J Gastrointest Surg* 2015;19:551–7.

16. Mauvais F, Sabbagh C, Brehant O et al. The current abdominoperineal resection: Oncological problems and surgical modifications for low rectal cancer. *J Visc Surg* 2011;148:e85–93.

17. Habib K. Prevention of recurrent small bowel obstruction resulting from pelvic adhesions in patients who have previously undergone abdominoperineal excision of the rectum. *Tech Coloproctol* 2014;18(12):1179–80.

18. McMenamin DM, Clements D, Edwards TJ, Fitton AR, Douie WJ. Rectus abdominis myocutaneous flaps for perineal reconstruction: Modifications to the technique based on a large single-centre experience. *Ann R Coll Surg Engl* 2011;93(5):375–81.

19. Foster JD, Pathak S, Smart NJ et al. Reconstruction of the perineum following extralevator abdominoperineal excision for carcinoma of the lower rectum: A systematic review. *Colorectal Dis* 2012;14(9):1052–9.

20. Svane M, Bulut O. Perineal hernia after laparoscopic abdominoperineal resection – reconstruction of the pelvic floor with a biological mesh (Permacol™). *Int J Colorectal Dis* 2012;27(4):543–4.

21. Peacock O, Pandya H, Sharp T et al. Biological mesh reconstruction of perineal wounds following enhanced abdominoperineal excision of rectum (APER). *Int J Colorectal Dis* 2012;27(4):475–82.

22. Alam NN, Narang SK, Köckerling F, Daniels IR, Smart NJ. Biologic mesh reconstruction of the pelvic floor after extralevator abdominoperineal excision: A systematic review. *Front Surg.* 2016;3:9. doi:10.3389/fsurg.2016.00009

23. Schiltz B, Buchs NC, Penna M, Scarpa CR, Liot E, Morel P, Ris F. Biological mesh reconstruction of the pelvic floor following abdominoperineal excision for cancer: A review. *World J Clin Oncol* 2017 June 10;8(3):249–54.

24. Veerankutty F, Chacko S, Sreekumar VI, Krishnan P, Varma D, Kurumboor P. Exploring minimally invasive options: Laparoscopic transabdominal levator transection for low rectal cancers. *J Min Acc Surg* 2019:15;174–6.

25. Kai Ye, Jianan Lin, Yafeng Sun, Yiyang Wu, Jianhua Xu. Laparoscopic modify extralevator abdominoperineal resection for rectal carcinoma in the prone position. *Ann Laparosc Endosc Surg* 2016;1:6.

26. Pereira P, Ghouti L, Blanche J. Surgical treatment of extraluminal pelvic recurrence from rectal cancer: Oncological management and resection techniques. *J Visc Surg* 2013;150(2):97–107.

27. Williams NS, Johnston D. The quality of life after rectal excision for low rectal cancer. *Br J Surg* 1983;70(8):460–2.

28. Engel J, Kerr J, Schlesinger-Raab A, Eckel R, Sauer H, Holzel D. Quality of life in rectal cancer patients: A four year prospective study. *Ann Surg* 2003;238(2):203–13.

29. Guren MG, Eriksen MT, Wiig JN et al. Quality of life and functional outcome following anterior or abdominoperineal resection for rectal cancer. *Eur J Surg Oncol* 2005;31(7):735–42.

30. Schmidt CE, Bestmann B, Kucher T, Longo WE, Kremer B. Prospective evaluation of quality of life of patients receiving either abdominoperineal resection or sphincter-preserving procedure for rectal cancer. *Ann Surg Oncol* 2005;12(2):117–23.

31. Pachler J, Wille-Jorgensen P. Quality of life after rectal resection for cancer, with or without permanent colostomy. *Cochrane Database Syst Rev* 2005;(2):CD004323.

32. Vironen JH, Kairaluoma M, Aalto AM, Kellokumpu IH. Impact of functional results on quality of life after rectal cancer surgery. *Dis Colon Rectum* 2006;49(5):568–78.

33. Zolciak A, Bujko K, Kepka L, Oledzki J, Rutkowski A, Nowacki MP. Abdominoperineal resection or anterior resection for rectal cancer: Patient preferences before and after treatment. *Colorectal Dis* 2006;8(7):575–80.

34. Han C, Yan P, Jing W et al. Clinical, pathological, and oncologic outcomes of robotic-assisted versus laparoscopic proctectomy for rectal cancer: A meta-analysis of randomized controlled studies. *Asian J Surg* 2019, https://doi.org/10.1016/j.asjsur.2019.11.003

35. Jayne D, Pigazzi A, Marshall H et al. Robotic-assisted surgery compared with laparoscopic resection surgery for rectal cancer: The ROLARR RCT. *Efficacy Mech Eval* 2019;6(10).

Chapter 25

LAPAROSCOPIC SUBTOTAL/TOTAL/PROCTOCOLECTOMY

Sanjiv Haribhakti

Contents

Learning objectives 160
Introduction 160
Definition.. 160
Indications 160
    Synchronous colon cancer 160
    Lynch syndrome 160
    Obstructed left sided colon cancers 161
    Familial adenomatous polyposis (FAP)... 161
    Ulcerative colitis 162
    Crohn's disease 162
    Chronic severe constipation... 163
Contraindications.. 163
Summary 164
Key points 164
References 164

Learning objectives

- Select the right patient for the right procedure, with acceptable postop morbidity
- Know the indications of the procedure
- Know the contraindications of the procedure
- Understand the operative principles and techniques of the various procedures

Introduction

Laparoscopic or open subtotal, total, or proctocolectomy may be needed for a variety of indications such as synchronous colon cancers, selected patients with obstructed left colon cancers, selected cases of ulcerative colitis and Crohn's disease, selected patients with familial adenomatous polyposis, Lynch syndrome (hereditary nonpolyposis colon cancers), and a few selected patients with chronic severe slow transit constipation. The selection of patients to undergo either a segmental colectomy or restorative proctocolectomy, and total proctocolectomy and end ileostomy needs to be carefully done based on the patient's age, medical comorbidities and the extent of disease, general condition, and the expected functional outcomes based on sphincter tone.

Definition

Though there are no watertight definitions, the following are the generally acceptable definitions of the terminologies:

1. *Total colectomy*: Removal of the entire colon and performing an ileorectal anastomosis.
2. *Subtotal colectomy*: Total colectomy preserving a part or whole of the sigmoid colon and performing a colocolic anastomosis.
3. *Restorative proctocolectomy*: Total proctocolectomy preserving a small cuff of the rectum with a double-stapled pouch anal anastomosis, or a handsewn coloanal anastomosis after mucosectomy.

4. *Total proctocolectomy*: Complete removal of the colon and rectum with an end ileostomy.

Indications

Synchronous colon cancer

Synchronic cancers refer to a second primary colon cancer diagnosed at the same time, or within one year from when the index cancer is diagnosed [1]. It occurs in 4% of sporadic colon cancer cases [2]. Synchronic colon cancers can be treated with two separate resections or one extended resection; a subtotal or a total abdominal colectomy may be performed if there are synchronous neoplasms on the right and left sides of the colon (Figure 25.1).

The extent of resection is also influenced by any underlying colonic diseases. For example, carcinoma in a patient with chronic ulcerative colitis is usually treated with a proctocolectomy with or without an ileal pouch anal anastomosis (IPAA) [3]. For patients with hereditary nonpolyposis colorectal cancer (HNPCC, Lynch syndrome) who present with colon cancer, the procedure of choice is total abdominal colectomy with consideration for hysterectomy and bilateral salpingo-oophorectomy in females [4]. Total abdominal colectomy or proctocolectomy with IPAA are procedures that can be offered to patients with familial adenomatous polyposis (FAP) and MUTYH-associated polyposis.

Lynch syndrome

Lynch syndrome has important implications for management of colorectal neoplastic lesions due to the increased risk of metachronous colorectal cancer (CRC). In individuals with Lynch syndrome with colon cancer or an endoscopically unresectable adenoma, total abdominal colectomy with ileorectal anastomosis is the procedure of choice with continued annual endoscopic surveillance of the retained rectum. We advocate segmental colectomy with annual postoperative colonoscopic surveillance for individuals who are not candidates for total colectomy [5]. Individuals with Lynch syndrome, who undergo segmental colectomy for the first colon cancer diagnosis, have an increased risk of subsequent adenoma or CRC as compared with individuals who undergo subtotal colectomy

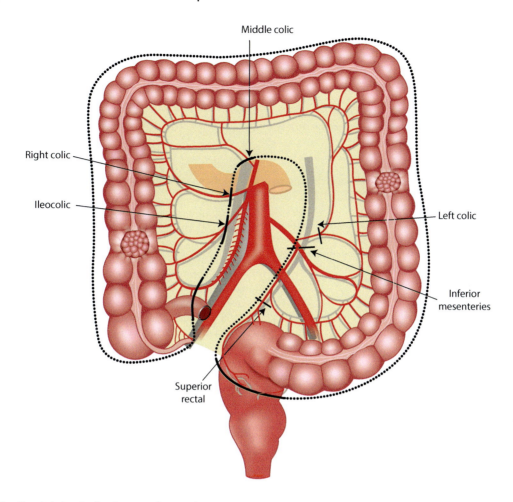

FIGURE 25.1   Total abdominal colectomy for synchronous cancers.

with ileorectal anastomosis [6–8]. Women undergoing colectomy should be offered concurrent prophylactic hysterectomy and bilateral salpingo-oophorectomy to prevent endometrial and ovarian cancer. The cumulative risk of metachronous CRC for carriers with segmental colectomy at 10, 20, and 30 years, was estimated to be 16%, 41%, and 62%, respectively. The risk of metachronous CRC is reduced by 31% for every 10 cm of bowel removed [7].

Obstructed left sided colon cancers

Some studies suggest that obstructing left-sided lesions can also be safely managed with a one-stage procedure while incurring acceptable morbidity [10,11]. As an example, in a retrospective study of 243 consecutive patients who underwent emergent surgery for obstructing colon cancer at Queen Mary's Hospital in Hong Kong, there were no statistically significant differences in hospital mortality or anastomotic leak rates among patients who underwent resection and primary anastomosis, regardless of tumor location (right- vs. left-sided) [10]. Nevertheless, many surgeons routinely perform a temporary proximal diverting colostomy following resection of an obstructing left-sided colon cancer. For patients who are not good candidates for surgery, a temporizing approach for an obstructing cancer is the endoscopic placement of an expandable metal stent.

Familial adenomatous polyposis (FAP)

Colectomy is recommended for patients with classic FAP, since the risk for developing CRC is considered to be 100%, and the high polyp number makes endoscopic control unrealistic. In patients with AFAP in whom endoscopic control is feasible, surveillance can obviate or delay the need for colectomy.

Indications for colectomy – Indications for colectomy in patients with FAP include:

- Documented or suspected colorectal cancer
- Severe symptoms related to colonic neoplasia (e.g., severe gastrointestinal bleeding)
- Adenomas with high-grade dysplasia, or multiple adenomas larger than 6 mm
- Marked increases in polyp number on consecutive exams
- Inability to adequately survey the colon because of multiple diminutive polyps

Surgical options for FAP patients include total proctocolectomy with end-ileostomy, total proctocolectomy with ileal pouch anal anastomosis (IPAA), or subtotal colectomy with ileo-rectal anastomosis (IRA). When choosing the extent of colon resection, the preventive effect is weighed against the impact on postoperative quality of life. A discussion regarding treatment options, risks, and the need for ongoing surveillance should take place with the patient.

In general, the preferred operation depends on the severity and distribution of colorectal adenomas. Other important factors to consider include the risk of desmoid tumors and the patient's age and comorbidities. The specific *APC* genotype may be useful in predicting which patients would be better suited for ileorectal anastomosis (IRA) versus total proctocolectomy with IPAA, by predicting the severity of colorectal polyposis and the risk of desmoid development [13]. IPAA is more extensive surgery compared to IRA and is associated with an increased risk of bleeding and reduction in fertility in women. Patients with an IRA who subsequently develop severe rectal polyposis will require a secondary proctectomy.

Guidelines suggest that a polyp number over 1000 is an indicator for a more extensive resection (proctocolectomy with IPAA vs. subtotal total colectomy with IRA). Another critical variable is the extent of rectal involvement.

- In cases with <10 rectal adenomas, we suggest subtotal colectomy with IRA, provided the rectal polyps can be managed endoscopically.
- In cases with profuse polyposis and >10 rectal adenomas, we suggest a proctocolectomy with IPAA.
- In patients at risk for desmoids, we suggest primary proctocolectomy with IPAA, as future conversion of IRA to IPAA might be difficult due to mesenteric desmoid tumors and shortening of the mesentery [14].

Elective colectomy can be deferred to the late teens or early twenties in patients with classic FAP who are in the second decade of life with only sparse (<10) or small (<5 mm) adenomas.

Ulcerative colitis

1. *Acute severe complications of ulcerative colitis*
   Fulminant ulcerative colitis: Patients with acute severe UC may progress to fulminant UC (or patients may present initially with fulminant colitis). The management of patients with fulminant UC is similar to treatment of patients with acute severe UC with the following additions. Patients who do not respond to initial treatment with glucocorticoids within three days are treated with either infliximab or cyclosporine. If the patient does not respond to second-line medical therapy within three days, colectomy is typically performed.
   Toxic megacolon: Toxic megacolon is a potentially lethal complication of IBD, especially UC, and is characterized by nonobstructive colonic dilatation plus systemic toxicity.
   Colonic perforation: Patients with UC who develop colonic perforation require colectomy, although this complication is rare.
2. *Chronic intractable ulcerative colitis*
   The current standard method for surgical treatment and cure in ulcerative colitis is restorative proctocolectomy and ileal pouch anal anastomosis (RPC IPAA). Total colectomy may be infrequently applied in ulcerative colitis.

Total abdominal colectomy with ileorectal anastomosis: A total abdominal colectomy with ileorectal anastomosis (TAC-IRA) removes the entire colon and connects the distal small bowel to the rectum. The rectum serves as the native pelvic reservoir for intestinal contents. As a result, TAC-IRA can produce normal bowel function and fecal continence.

A TAC-IRA is performed infrequently in patients with ulcerative colitis because it does not excise the diseased rectum and therefore leaves patients at risk for persistence of inflammatory symptoms and future malignancy. A retrospective analysis of 86 patients who underwent the TAC-IRA procedure found that the rectum was eventually resected in 46 patients (53%) for rectal dysplasia (17%), rectal cancer (8%), and refractory proctitis (28%) [15]. The risk of cancer development in the residual rectum has been reported to be 6% at 20 years and 15% at 30 years. This risk is significant considering that most patients with ulcerative colitis are young.

Potential candidates for the TAC-IRA procedure include:

- Patients who are not suitable for an IPAA but who refuse an ileostomy, or who have medical conditions for which an ileostomy is contraindicated (e.g., portal hypertension or ascites). It is important to note that such patients should have minimal rectal disease to be considered for a TAC-IRA.
- Young women who desire preservation of their fecundity.
- Patients with indeterminate colitis, in whom Crohn's disease cannot be excluded.
- Patients with ulcerative colitis and advanced colonic malignancy – who have a limited life expectancy.

Patients who choose to have a TAC-IRA need to have intensive endoscopic surveillance of the rectum and are often maintained on medical therapy. At 10 years, approximately 20% of patients will have required a completion proctectomy for either proctitis or rectal dysplasia/cancer.

Total abdominal colectomy with end ileostomy: A total abdominal colectomy with end ileostomy removes the entire colon but leaves behind a defunctionalized rectum as a Hartmann's pouch. It is a simple procedure that can be performed quickly and is favored in emergency or urgent situations.

Total proctocolectomy with end ileostomy: A total proctocolectomy with end ileostomy removes the entire colon and rectum without reestablishing gastrointestinal continuity. The end ileostomy is permanent and can be constructed in a continent (Kock) or incontinent (Brooke) fashion. A total proctocolectomy with permanent ileostomy is curative for ulcerative colitis, and can be performed laparoscopically as a 'scarless' or 'incisionless' procedure [16–18].

A total proctocolectomy with end ileostomy is primarily performed in patients who readily accept a permanent stoma – or those who cannot tolerate an IPAA because of comorbidities – and patients with poor anal sphincter function.

Crohn's disease

Surgical procedures commonly used to treat Crohn colitis or proctitis include segmental colectomy, total colectomy with ileorectal anastomosis, total proctocolectomy with end ileostomy, and proctectomy. The choice of procedures depends upon the location of the disease and the indication for surgery. Patients with Crohn's disease may undergo a segmental or a total colectomy, depending upon the extent of the disease. A segmental colectomy is adequate for treating isolated Crohn's disease of the colon, such as a colonic stricture that precludes endoscopic surveillance [19]. Patients with two or more involved colonic segments should undergo a total colectomy. In a meta-analysis that compared segmental colectomy with total colectomy for colonic Crohn's disease, the two procedures were equally effective, although patients developed earlier recurrences after a segmental colectomy than after a total colectomy [20].

Following a total colectomy, an ileorectal anastomosis (IRA) should be performed if the rectum is not involved with Crohn's disease [21]. Although the probability of clinical recurrence after IRA was 58% and 83% at 5 and 10 years, respectively, the probability of rectal preservation at 10 years was as high as 86% [22]. About one half of patients who had an end ileostomy and a defunctionalized rectum after a total colectomy because of rectal diseases required a secondary proctectomy in 6–10 years.

Proctectomy: A proctectomy can be performed for patients with refractory proctitis without colonic involvement. The entire rectum should be removed because cancer can develop in a rectal remnant [23].

In Crohn patients, an intersphincteric dissection with primary closure of the perineal wound, rather than a standard abdominal perineal resection, should be performed to minimize the risk of a nonhealing perineal wound or sexual dysfunction [24]. Crohn's disease of the rectum should not be confused with perianal Crohn's disease, which includes anal fistula, fissure, or abscess. Perianal Crohn's disease is treated medically or by nonresectional procedures [25].

Proctocolectomy: A total proctocolectomy with end ileostomy is performed in patients with longstanding Crohn's disease, who either have disease involvement of both the colon and rectum, or have malignant/premalignant lesions in either the colon or the rectum. Total proctocolectomy in properly selected patients has been associated with low morbidity, low risk of recurrence, and a long interval to recurrence [26]. It is important to note that a restorative procedure, such as IPAA, should generally not be performed in patients with Crohn's disease because of a high risk of disease recurrence, or pouch failure.

Chronic severe constipation

Subtotal colectomy with ileorectal anastomosis can dramatically ameliorate incapacitating constipation in carefully selected patients [27]. At least five criteria should be met prior to consideration for surgery:

- The patient has chronic, severe, and disabling symptoms from constipation that are unresponsive to medical therapy
- The patient has slow colonic transit of the inertia pattern
- The patient does not have intestinal pseudoobstruction, as demonstrated by radiologic or manometric studies
- The patient does not have pelvic floor dysfunction based on anorectal manometry, balloon expulsion testing, or defecography
- The patient does not have abdominal pain as a prominent symptom

A review of 13 studies of 362 patients who underwent colectomy, and who were followed for a mean of 106 months, reported a high degree of patient satisfaction (88%) [12].

1. There are no randomized trials focusing on the selection of constipated patients for surgery. A recent review and guidelines [9] suggest the most commonly described selection criteria for segmental, subtotal, or total colectomy as follows (Level V evidence, Grade C recommendation): ≤2 weekly defecations.
2. Duration of symptoms (mean 5–17 years).
3. The presence of symptoms such as abdominal bloating or pain, nausea, and vomiting that have a significant impact on the patient's quality of life.
4. Failure of behavioral, dietetic, pharmacological, and RTs to improve the symptoms.
5. Radiological evidence of slow transit constipation.
6. Exclusion of organic or functional pelvic floor disorders (obstructed defecation, Hirschsprung's disease) based on defecography and anorectal manometry.
7. Exclusion of upper gastrointestinal tract dysmotility based on functional (manometric, scintigraphic) examinations, if dyspeptic symptoms are present.
8. Normal results of psychological evaluation (patients with psychological disorders tend to show poor results after surgery for constipation).

Contraindications

1. Patients with *unresectable metastatic disease* are generally not candidates for resection of the primary colon tumor in the absence of symptoms or complications (e.g., perforation, obstruction) attributable to the primary tumor.
2. *Asymptomatic patients with incurable metastatic colon cancer*: Although several analyses suggested that resection of the primary tumor in the presence of incurable metastasis may slow disease progression and favorably impact survival, the studies are retrospective and potentially biased. Furthermore, these findings are not universal. Thus, until randomized trial results become available (two such studies are ongoing), the standard of care remains nonoperative management.
3. *Increasing age* may be accompanied by higher rates of medical comorbidity. Some patients may not be appropriate candidates for resection due to medical comorbidities.

Operative principles: These have been well described in the chapter on lap RPC IPAA for ulcerative colitis, including preoperative preparation and operative steps.

For subtotal/total colectomy the patient is placed in the low lithotomy position. The OR setup, port placements and the standardized operative technique of total colectomy have been well described in the Chapter 16. The procedure starts with left colon mobilization beginning with the medial to lateral dissection identifying the ureter, gonadal vessels, and duodenum on the right side. Subsequently IMA and IMV ligations are performed, followed by complete splenic flexure mobilization. Later, the lateral colonic attachments are divided and the splenic flexure mobilization is completed. For subtotal colectomy, the sigmoid colon is divided at the desired location based on the tumor. For total colectomy, the upper rectum is divided with a 60 mm straight stapler. The right colon is mobilized, and the hepatic flexure is completely mobilized. A minilaparotomy is performed, and the specimen is removed. Ileorectal anastomosis is performed with a circular stapled technique with a side-to-end anastomosis (Figure 25.2). Generally, no proximal diversion stoma is needed.

For proctocolectomy, rectal mobilization is started in the TME plane, and after complete circumferential rectal dissection is performed until the pelvic floor, the perineal dissection is commenced and the anorectal dissection is performed in the intersphincteric (in IBD) or extrasphincteric plane (in cancer), depending on the indication of the resection. After the specimen is removed, an end ileostomy is created in the right iliac fossa with an eversion.

Postoperative care and recovery, ERAS: Similar to all other laparoscopic colorectal resections.

Postoperative Complications: Have been dealt with in Chapter 10 on complications in details.

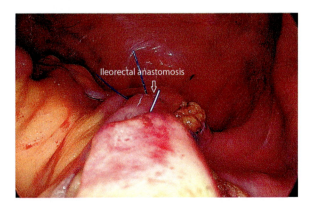

FIGURE 25.2 Ileorectal anastomosis with circular-stapled technique with a side-to-end anastomosis .

Functional results: Functional results after subtotal or total colectomy with ileorectal anastomosis are quite acceptable in the majority of patients. A majority of patients will have a normal bowel function with good continence. Elderly patients, those with poor sphincter tone or with irritable bowel syndrome, will have a higher frequency of stool and may develop minor incontinence.

After a proctocolectomy and end ileostomy, functional results are quite acceptable in the majority of patients provided they have been counselled adequately regarding their acceptance of the stoma before the surgery, and have been seen by a stoma therapist. Postoperatively, most patients will do well with the stoma if they do not have any stoma-related complications. Stoma-related issues and complications have been dealt in details in another Chapter 6.

Summary

Laparoscopic or open subtotal, total, or proctocolectomy may be needed for a variety of indications. As well, selection of the right patient for the right procedure – with acceptable postop morbidity – is important. With the early implementation of ERAS, patient care is not compromised and recovery to normalcy is fast. Patients need to be counselled adequately preoperatively regarding their acceptance of the stoma, and should be seen as well by a stoma therapist. Functional results after subtotal or total colectomy with ileorectal anastomosis are quite acceptable in a majority of patients and are based on preoperative sphincter tone. Postoperatively, most patients will do well with the stoma if they do not have any stoma-related complications.

Key points

- In ileo-rectal anastomosis, the functional outcomes are based on preoperative sphincter tone.
- The patient needs adequate preoperative counselling regarding his/her acceptance of the stoma, and should be seen by a stoma therapist.
- The anorectal dissection in APR is done in the intersphincteric (in IBD) or extrasphincteric plane (in cancer), depending on the indication of the resection.
- In Lynch syndrome, the risk of metachronous CRC is reduced by 31% for every 10 cm of bowel removed.
- In FAP, a polyp number over 1000 is an indicator for a more extensive resection (proctocolectomy with IPAA vs. subtotal total colectomy with IRA).
- Indications for colectomy in slow transit constipation is based on selection criteria for segmental, subtotal or total colectomy with a Level V evidence and Grade C recommendation.

References

1. Mekenkamp LJ, Koopman M, Teerenstra S, van Krieken JH, Mol L, Nagtegaal ID, Punt CJ. Clinicopathological features and outcome in advanced colorectal cancer patients with synchronous vs metachronous metastases. *Br J Cancer* 2010;103(2):159.
2. Thiels CA, Naik ND, Bergquist JR, Spindler BA, Habermann EB, Kelley SR, Wolff BG, Mathis KL. Survival following synchronous colon cancer resection. *J Surg Oncol* 2016;114(1):80.
3. Ross H, Steele SR, Varma M, Dykes S, Cima R, Buie WD, Rafferty J. Practice parameters for the surgical treatment of ulcerative colitis. *Dis Colon Rectum* 2014;57(1):5.
4. Herzig DO, Buie WD, Weiser MR, You YN, Rafferty JF, Feingold D, Steele SR. Clinical practice guidelines for the surgical treatment of patients with lynch syndrome. *Dis Colon Rectum* 2017;60(2):137.
5. Syngal S, Brand RE, Church JM, Giardiello FM, Hampel HL, Burt RW. ACG clinical guideline: Genetic testing and management of hereditary gastrointestinal cancer syndromes. *Am J Gastroenterol* 2015;110(2):223.
6. Kalady MF, McGannon E, Vogel JD, Manilich E, Fazio VW, Church JM. Risk of colorectal adenoma and carcinoma after colectomy for colorectal cancer in patients meeting Amsterdam criteria. *Ann Surg* 2010;252(3):507.
7. Parry S, Win AK, Parry B, Macrae FA, Gurrin LC, Jenkins MA. Metachronous colorectal cancer risk for mismatch repair gene mutation carriers: The advantage of more extensive colon surgery. *Gut* 2011;60(7):950–7.
8. Renkonen-Sinisalo L, Seppälä TT, Järvinen HJ, Mecklin JP. Subtotal solectomy for colon cancer reduces the need for subsequent surgery in lynch syndrome. *Dis Colon Rectum* 2017;60(8):792.
9. Bove A, Bellini M, Battaglia E et al. Consensus statement AIGO/SICCR diagnosis and treatment of chronic constipation and obstructed defecation (Part II: Treatment). *World J Gastroenterol* 2012 September 28;18(36):4994–5013.
10. Lee YM, Law WL, Chu KW, Poon RT. Emergency surgery for obstructing colorectal cancers: A comparison between right-sided and left-sided lesions. *J Am Coll Surg* 2001;192(6):719–25.
11. Chiappa A, Zbar A, Biella F, Staudacher C. One-stage resection and primary anastomosis following acute obstruction of the left colon for cancer. *Am Surg* 2000;66(7):619.
12. Pikarsky AJ, Singh JJ, Weiss EG, Nogueras JJ, Wexner SD. Long-term follow-up of patients undergoing colectomy for colonic inertia. *Dis Colon Rectum* 2001;44(2):179.
13. Nieuwenhuis MH, Mathus-Vliegen LM, Slors FJ, Griffioen G, Nagengast FM, Schouten WR, Kleibeuker JH, Vasen HF. Genotype-phenotype correlations as a guide in the management of familial adenomatous polyposis. *Clin Gastroenterol Hepatol* 2007;5(3):374.
14. Vasen HF, Möslein G, Alonso A et al. Guidelines for the clinical management of familial adenomatous polyposis (FAP). *Gut* 2008;57(5):704.
15. Da Luz Moreira A, Kiran RP, Lavery I. Clinical outcomes of ileorectal anastomosis for ulcerative colitis. *Br J Surg* 2010;97(1):65.
16. Nagpal AP, Soni H, Haribhakti S. Hybrid single-incision laparoscopic restorative proctocolectomy with Ileal pouch anal Anastomosis for ulcerative colitis. *Indian J Surg* 2010 Oct;72(5):400–3.
17. Fichera A, Zoccali M, Gullo R. Single incision ('scarless') laparoscopic total abdominal colectomy with end ileostomy for ulcerative colitis. *J Gastrointest Surg* 2011 Jul;15(7):1247–51.
18. Holubar SD, Privitera A, Cima RR, Dozois EJ, Pemberton JH, Larson DW. Minimally invasive total proctocolectomy with Brooke ileostomy for ulcerative colitis. *Inflamm Bowel Dis* 2009 Sep;15(9):1337–42.
19. Morimoto K, Watanabe K, Noguchi A et al. Clinical impact of ultrathin colonoscopy for Crohn's disease patients with strictures. *J Gastroenterol Hepatol* 2015 Mar;30(Suppl 1):66–70.
20. Tekkis PP, Purkayastha S, Lanitis S, Athanasiou T, Heriot AG, Orchard TR, Nicholls RJ, Darzi AW. A comparison of segmental vs subtotal/total colectomy for colonic Crohn's disease: A meta-analysis. *Colorectal Dis* 2006;8(2):82.
21. Lewis JD, Schoenfeld P, Lichtenstein GR. An evidence-based approach to studies of the natural history of gastrointestinal diseases: Recurrence of symptomatic Crohn's disease after surgery. *Clin Gastroenterol Hepatol* 2003;1(3):229.
22. Yamamoto T, Watanabe T. Surgery for luminal Crohn's disease. *World J Gastroenterol* 2014 Jan;20(1):78–90.
23. Cirincione E, Gorfine SR, Bauer JJ. Is Hartmann's procedure safe in Crohn's disease? Report of three cases. *Dis Colon Rectum.* 2000 Apr;43(4):544–7.
24. Zeitels JR, Fiddian-Green RG, Dent TL. Intersphincteric proctectomy. *Surgery* 1984 Oct;96(4):617–23.
25. Lewis RT, Bleier JI. Surgical treatment of anorectal crohn disease. *Clin Colon Rectal Surg* 2013 Jun;26(2):90–9.
26. Fichera A, McCormack R, Rubin MA, Hurst RD, Michelassi F. Long-term outcome of surgically treated Crohn's colitis: A prospective study. *Dis Colon Rectum* 2005;48(5):963.
27. Wofford SA, Verne GN. Approach to patients with refractory constipation. *Curr Gastroenterol Rep* 2000;2(5):389.

Chapter 26

LAPAROSCOPIC MANAGEMENT OF T4 TUMOR AND PELVIC EXENTERATION FOR LOCALLY ADVANCED TUMORS

Ajay Punpale

Contents

Learning objectives 165
Introduction 165
What is T4 colorectal cancers or LACRC? 165
Clinical presentation 165
Preoperative evaluation... 166
Colonoscopy 166
Radiological imaging 166
Selection of patients for neoadjuvant chemoradiation 166
Role of laparoscopy and surgical technique for T4 colorectal cancers/LACRC........ 166
Key operative steps in routine laparoscopic colorectal surgery...................... 166
Key differences in operative steps in T4 or LACRC................................. 167
In male patients.. 168
Specimen retrieval and formation of ileal conduit and stapler anvil head insertion in male patients 168
In female patients 169
Special situations 169
Summary 169
Key points 169
Videos.. 170
References 170

Learning objectives

- Is laparoscopic management of T4 colorectal cancer is safe and feasible?
- What kind of experience and operation theatre set-up is needed?
- What is the preoperative assessment of T4 colorectal cancers in terms of staging by radiological and endoscopic studies to decide operability, and also surgical approach?
- Is there any role of neoadjuvant chemoradiation in cases with threatened circumferential margins on radiological imaging?
- What is the most important predictive factor to improve overall survival and long-term disease-free interval in cases with T4 colorectal cancers?

Introduction

Colorectal cancer is the fourth most prevalent cancer worldwide, and metastatic disease is the predominant cause of death in this cancer. In spite of all advanced imaging modalities, 5%–10% of colorectal cancers are found to be locally advanced at the time of surgery, and curative resection with adequate margins is a challenge in such cases [1–4]. The negative resection margin remains the single-most predictive factor for local recurrences and disease-free survival [5–8]. Historically, pelvic exenterations or multivisceral resections for T4, or locally advanced cancers, remains the best chance of cure [9–10].

Over the last two decades, great progression has occurred in the management of colorectal cancers. Local, as well as distant, recurrence rates have dramatically declined due to the standardization of surgically replicable techniques and the use of neoadjuvant chemoradiation [11,12].

Early stage colorectal cancers are now managed by minimally invasive approaches with comparable oncological outcomes as open approaches, with all the advantages of minimal access surgery. Because of encouraging outcomes in early colorectal cancers, utility of the minimally invasive approach for locally advanced colorectal cancers (LACRC), as well as locally recurrent colorectal cancers, has been explored and laparoscopy is being increasingly used in such cases [13–25].

The surgical management of LACRC and locally recurrent rectal cancers has developed since Brunschwig first described pelvic exenteration for cervical cancer in 1948 [26].

Currently, the 5-year survival rate for LACRC is between 52%–65% [27,28]. Survival rate for LACRC is still worse if the tumor is not centrally located in the pelvis, especially if it extends to pelvic sidewalls, or high sacrum, making it anatomically unfavorable for resection [29].

What is T4 colorectal cancers or LACRC?

By definition (AJCC 7th edition), a T4 tumor is:

T4 a: The tumor invades through the visceral peritoneum (including gross perforation of the bowel through tumor and continuous invasion of tumor through areas of inflammation to the surface of visceral peritoneum); or

T4 b: The tumor directly invades or adheres to other adjacent organs or structures.

Clinical presentation

Most T4 or LACRC clinically present either with features of obstruction or perforation. T4 tumors of the rectosigmoid colon may present with a palpable mass in the left lower abdomen. Sometimes such tumors may invade the anterior abdominal wall and may present with local pain and sometimes signs of inflammation due to local perforation. Tumors invading the bladder may present with urinary symptoms, cystitis, but rarely hematuria. Low anterior rectal tumors invading the prostate may present with dysuria and symptoms of prostatitis.

Preoperative evaluation

Apart from a proper clinical examination and routine blood tests, all LACRC cases need evaluation by colonoscopy, CT scan of chest and abdomen or MRI, endo-ultrasound (if available), and preoperative CEA levels. Accurate preoperative multimodal staging is crucial in assessing potential resectibility of LACRC.

Colonoscopy

Upon colonoscopy, apart from taking tissue for histology, one needs to look for distance of the tumor from the anal verge, circumferential location (if tumor is on lateral, anterior, or posterior wall), degree of stenosis due to lesion, and if the lesion is negotiable. Complete colonoscopy should be done when the lesion is negotiable to rule out any synchronous lesions in the colon.

Radiological imaging

Preoperative imaging of the abdomen and pelvis using CT scan or MRI is needed to evaluate the extent of the disease. A CT scan of the chest should be performed to rule out pulmonary metastasis [30–32]. Endo-ultrasound, if available, may help for evaluation of involvement of adjacent organs in select cases. MRI is a reliable imaging technique to determine circumferential resection margin status with an accuracy of 91% and a negative predictive value of 93% [33,34]. Involvement of mesorectal fascia on MRI is an indication for neoadjuvant treatment in the form of chemoradiotherpy [35].

Detection of locally recurrent rectal cancers by radiology alone may be challenging in a postsurgical and postradiotherapy pelvis. In such cases, judicious use of PET scan may be advantageous, although further evidence is required for its routine recommendation [36].

Selection of patients for neoadjuvant chemoradiation

T4 colorectal cancers with acute clinical presentation of obstruction and perforation are not the candidates for neoadjuvant chemoradiation, as they need urgent surgical intervention. In select cases, a diversion stoma followed by neoadjuvant chemoradiation may be considered. As R0 resection is the single-most predictor of outcome after surgery for colorectal cancers, any surgery must be undertaken with the intention of achieving histologically clear surgical margins.

To achieve this goal, all T4 nonmetastatic colorectal cancers where margins are threatened – due to involvement of a tumor beyond the mesorectal fascia – or have involvement of adjacent organs – such as the prostate, bladder or seminal vesicles in males, or the uterus, vagina, and bladder in females – should be reviewed in multidisciplinary team meetings for evaluation and to plan neoadjuvant chemoradiation. Usually, these patients receive 50 Gys in 25 fractions of radiotherapy with concurrent Capecitabine to downstage the tumor. Post-neoadjuvant chemoradiation, circumferential resection margin (CRM) involvement is a predictor

of increased chances of local recurrence, development of distant metastasis, and decreased survival [37]. Neoadjuvant chemoradiotherapy is more effective in decreasing positive CRM than short course radiation [4,38,39,40].

Owing to poor outcome when CRM is positive, it is necessary to extend the resection beyond conventional total mesorectal excision (TME) to achieve a negative margin in such cases. In male patients with involvement of anterior mesorectal fascia, structures present anterior to the rectum such as the urinary bladder, seminal vesicles, prostate, and urethra should be excised partially or totally to achieve a negative margin, whereas in female patients, the uterus and the vagina are involved before invasion of the urinary bladder.

Role of laparoscopy and surgical technique for T4 colorectal cancers/LACRC

Over the last two decades, significant progress has been made in the treatment of colorectal cancers due to the advent of minimall access surgery. Many studies have shown comparable outcomes using laparoscopy for early colorectal cancers. Similarly, the role of laparoscopy is growing day-by-day, even for LACRC, with comparable oncological outcomes and with the added advantages of minimal access surgery such as early recovery, less postoperative pain, shorter hospital stay, and fewer adverse events in the postoperative period.

All patients planned for advanced laparoscopy procedures should undergo detailed cardio-respiratory evaluations. Whenever needed, adequate chest physiotherapy will help the patient to tolerate the procedure better. High definition laparoscopic camera systems with advanced energy sources and laparoscopic staplers are needed for all advanced colorectal cancer surgeries. Figure 26.1 elaborates on the OT set-up and the position of operating team members.

As shown in Figure 26.2, the patient is kept in a supine position with both legs split. A bolster below the hip will help break the abdomino-pelvic region, which aids the small bowel to fall back in the upper abdominal cavity. Port placement is as below (Figure 26.3a,b):

1. *Camera port (11 mm)*: The camera port can be put transumbilically, or one inch above umbilicus.
2. *Right-hand operating port*: 11 mm Versaport in the right lower quadrant one inch above and medial to the anterior superior iliac spine.
3. *Left-hand operating port*: 5 mm port in right midclavicular line below the level of the umbilicus and at least 4 finger breadth above the right-hand port.
4. *Retraction ports*: Two 5 mm ports for retraction are put in the left flank, mirroring the right flank ports.

Key operative steps in routine laparoscopic colorectal surgery

1. Exploratory laparoscopy and assessment of local disease for involvement of adjacent structures, and to rule out any distant metastasis
2. Medial to lateral mobilization of the rectosigmoid mesentery
3. Identification of the left ureter and left gonadal vessels
4. High ligation of the inferior mesenteric artery (IMA) pedicle at its origin
5. Medial to lateral mobilization of the left colonic mesenteric leaf off the Gerota's fascia until the tail of the pancreas and the inferior pole of the spleen is seen
6. Laterally, mobilization of the left colon until the splenic flexure

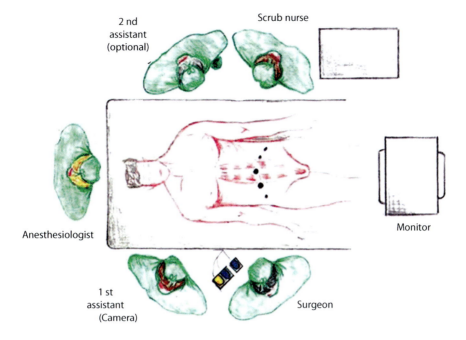

FIGURE 26.1   OT set-up.

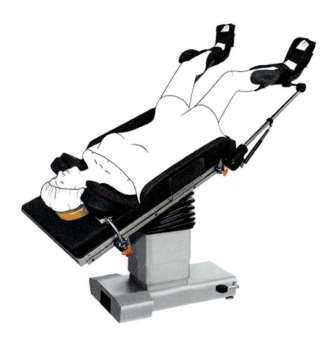

FIGURE 26.2   Patient position.

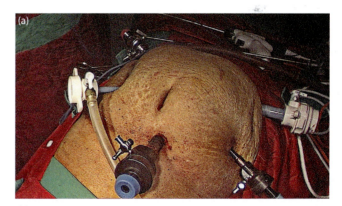

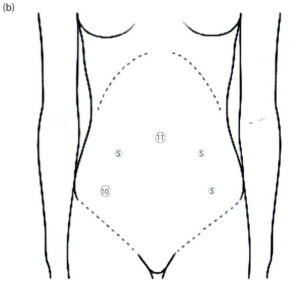

7. Late division of the inferior mesenteric vein to prevent the small bowel coming in an operative field during medial to lateral mobilization

8. Mobilization of the rectum in the pelvis on the lateral and posterior aspect, well beyond the level of growth

Key differences in operative steps in T4 or LACRC

Port placement and all steps of laparoscopic mobilization for LACRC remain nearly the same as for early colorectal cancers, with a few differences which depend on intraoperative findings and involvement of adjacent visceras (see Videos 27 and 28).

FIGURE 26.3   (a and b) Port placement.

After exploratory laparoscopy to rule off distant metastasis, the lesion is assessed – and its involvement with the prostate or bladder in males and with the uterus, adnexal structures, or bladder in females. Rectosigmoid growths may sometimes involve the small bowel loops, anterior abdominal wall, or bladder due to its mobility.

In male patients

Whenever bladder involvement is suspected by LACRC, on table cystoscopy should be done to assess the involvement of the bladder, which will help to decide if partial excision of the bladder along with the rectal growth is feasible. Such cases are suitable for en mass excision of a part of the bladder and rectal growth in the form of anterior resection (Figures 26.4, 26.5), primary closure of the bladder defect and stapled rectal anastomosis with or without a diversion stoma should be done.

Whenever the trigone of the bladder is involved along with the uretero-vesical junction and prostate, total pelvic exenteration with urinary diversion (Ileal conduit in right iliac fossa) and permanent colostomy in the left iliac fossa may have to be considered.

In select cases, where the rectal growth is involving the bladder and the prostate but the rectal growth is at least 5 cm from the anal verge, a cytsoprostatectomy with anterior resection of the rectal growth can be performed. The dissection is done in a clean plane anterior to the bladder going to the retropubic area, tackling the dorsal venous plexus, dividing the urethra and then dividing the rectum with laparoscopic articulating staplers to separate the complete specimen. An ileal conduit is made for urinary diversion, and stapled anastomosis for the rectum is then performed using circular staplers. If a protective diversion stoma is needed in such cases, then a transverse colon is used to form a stoma which may be closed later.

In select cases, where the anterior rectal tumors invade the anterior mesorectal fascia with loss of fat planes with prostate or seminal vesicles, then partial excision of prostatic tissue and capsule to get negative resection margin or excision of seminal vesicles along with rectal growth is followed by resection and stapled anastomosis of rectum.

Specimen retrieval and formation of ileal conduit and stapler anvil head insertion in male patients

When total pelvic exenteration is done in male patients with abdominoperineal resection and cystoprostatectomy, then the perineal wound itself provides passage for the removal of specimen. In cases where cystoprostatectomy is planned with anterior resection of the rectum, the specimen can be retrieved through a lower midline or Pfannelsteil incision. The ileal conduit, with ureteric implantation and insertion of the anvil of a circular stapler in the proximal end of the colon can be done through the same incision.

We have designed an innovative method to avoid an incision in such a situation. The site of ileostomy is marked for the proposed ileal conduit. After excision of the circle of skin for the stoma, a lateral cut is given to this circle at a 9'0 clock position for 5 cm (Figures 26.6, 26.7). Similarly, the cut on the rectus sheath and muscles is extended laterally. A wound protector is placed in the wound and the specimen is delivered from this wound, and the anvil is placed in the proximal colon. The distal ileum is exteriorized to form the ileal conduit and to perform ureteric

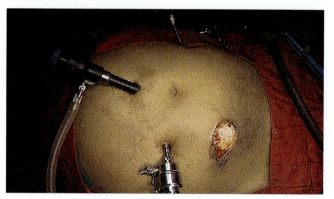

FIGURE 26.6 The site of ileostomy is marked for the proposed ileal conduit after excising the circle of skin for stoma.

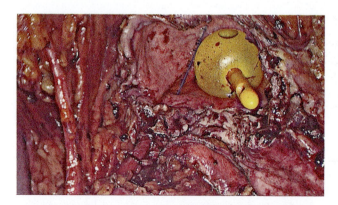

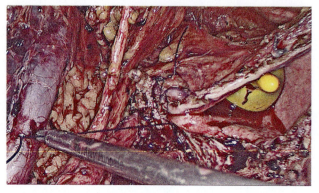

FIGURES 26.4 AND 26.5 Involvement of bladder from rectal growth needing partial bladder excision.

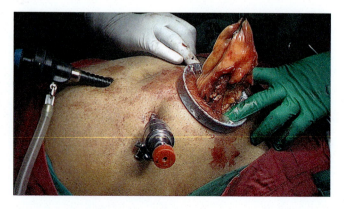

FIGURE 26.7 Distal ileum is out to form the ileal conduit.

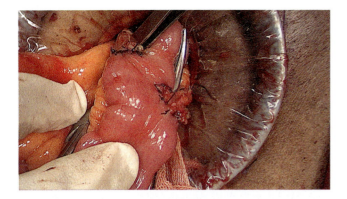

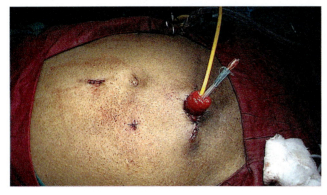

FIGURES 26.8 AND 26.9 Ureteric implantation in the ileal conduit, extracorporealy.

implantation in the ileal conduit extracorporealy (Figures 26.8, 26.9). After doing this, a glove can be put over the wound protector to create pneumoperitoneum, as then the stapled anastomosis can be carried out under vision using a circular stapler introduced through the distal rectal stump.

In female patients

In females, anterior rectal growths may involve the uterus and vagina while most of the time the bladder is spared. In such cases, posterior exenteration may be performed where uterus with bilateral adnexae, vagina and lower rectum are resected en mass and a permanent stoma can be performed in left iliac fossa. However, in a previously hysterectomised patient, anterior rectal growths may involve the bladder. In such cases, partial bladder excision or total pelvic exenteration where bladder, vagina and rectum may have to be resected enmass. Urinary diversion is done by an ileal conduit and a permanent colostomy is done.

In LACRC, whenever the rectal growth is at least 5 cm from the anal verge, anterior resection along with the involved organ like the uterus, vagina, bladder may be resected rather than doing total pelvic exenteration. In such cases, an ileal conduit will be needed when the complete bladder is removed.

Specimen retrieval in females is rather easy and the vagina provides a natural passage to remove specimens. When an ileal conduit is to be performed then the same technique, as described above for male patients, can be used.

Special situations

- Sometimes lateral rectal wall tumors may involve only the ureter without involvement of the bladder. In such cases,

excision of the ureter along with the lesion is sought. The ureter may be reimplanted or a Boari's bladder flap may be performed laparoscopically.
- Rectosigmoid growths may sometimes involve only loops of the small intestine without involvement of the bladder or uterus. In such cases, no attempt should be made to separate small bowel loops from rectal growth. In this situation, the trick is to do posterior and lateral dissection first, and to reach the distal level of the rectal division with TME and divide the rectum with laparoscopic staplers. Then, through a small lower midline incision, obtain the specimen with the involved small bowel loops out through a wound protector. Then complete the resection of the rectum and small bowel extracorporealy, and put the anvil head of the circular stapler in the proximal end of the colon to perform a stapled anastomosis with the distal rectal stump.
- Whenever lateral rectal wall tumors, or recurrent rectal tumors, involve the lateral pelvic wall, sciatic notch resection may be needed. Such cases may be anticipated beforehand and are best managed by an open approach in specialized centers.
- Similarly, posterior rectal tumors involving the sacral vertebrae may not be suitable for a laparoscopic approach; combined sacral resections may be planned by an open approach in specialized centers.

Summary

A minimally invasive approach is feasible and safe for the management of LACRC and for pelvic exenteration. Multimodal preoperative staging, multidisciplinary teamwork, the use of neoadjuvant chemoradiation, and experienced laparoscopic teams are needed to achieve good results. There are distinct advantages such as a fast recovery with less blood loss and fewer postoperative adverse events. Oncological outcomes are comparable to those of the open method, although long-term outcomes will need further studies and follow-up.

Key points

- Laparoscopic management of T4 colorectal cancer is safe and feasible, and has all the advantages of laparoscopy such as less blood loss or pain, shorter hospital stays, smaller scars, and fewer postoperative adverse events.
- Abundant experience with laparoscopic pelvic surgeries, good laparoscopic equipment units, and good teamwork are mandatory.
- Preoperative assessment of all cases with multimodal staging by radiological and endoscopic studies will help to decide on the operability and surgical approach.
- The negative circumferential resection margin is the most important predictive factor for overall survival and long-term disease-free interval.
- Neoadjuvant chemoradiation will help to improve negative circumferential margins in cases with threatened margins, as revealed by radiological imaging.
- Lateral rectal tumors invading the sciatic notch, or posterior rectal tumors invading the upper sacral vertebrae are not suitable for the laparoscopic approach and need to be managed by an open approach at specialized centers.

Videos

VIDEO 27 https://youtu.be/eS7_DIofpe0

Laparoscopic Pelvic Exenteration for Locally Advanced Rectal Tumours.

VIDEO 28 https://youtu.be/Ozpo5JDsr-E

Management of Locally Advanced Colon Cancer.

References

1. Patel UB, Taylor F, Blomqvist L et al. Magnetic resonance imaging-detected tumor response for locally advanced rectal cancer predicts survival outcomes: MERCURY experience. *J Clin Oncol* 2011;29:3753–60.
2. Harji DP, Sagar PM. Advancing the surgical treatment of locally recurrent rectal cancer, *Br J Surg* 2012;99:1169–71.
3. Sagar PM, Pemberton JH. Surgical management of locally recurrent rectal cancer. *Br J Surg* 1996;83:293–304.
4. Roh MS, Colangelo LH, O'Connell MJ et al. Preoperative multimodality therapy improves disease-free survival in patients with carcinoma of the rectum: NSABP R-03. *J Clin Oncol* 2009;27(31):5124–30.
5. The Expert Advisory Group on Cancer to the Chief Medical Officers of England and Wales. *A Policy Framework for Commissioning Cancer Services: A Report by the Expert Advisoy Group on Cancer to the Chief Medical Officers of England and Wales.* London, UK: Department of Health, 1995.
6. Nguyen DQ, McGregor AD, Freites O et al. Exenterative pelvic surgery – eleven year experience of the Swansea Pelvic Oncology Group. *Eur J Surg Oncol* 2005;31(10):1180–4.
7. Hunter JA, Ryan JA Jr, Schultz P. En bloc resection of colon cancer adherent to other organs. *Am J Surg* 1987;154(1):67–71.
8. Bhangu A, Ali SM, Darzi A, Brown G, Tekkis P. Meta-analysis of survival based on resection margin status following surgery for recur- rent rectal cancer. *Colorectal Dis* 2012;14(12):1457–66.
9. Ferenschild FT, Vermaas M, Verhoef C et al. Total pelvic exenteration for primary and recurrent malignancies, *World J Surg* 2009;33:1502–8.
10. Sagar PM, Gonsalves S, Heath RM, Phillips N, Chalmers AG. Composite abdominosacral resection for recurrent retal cancer. *Br J Surg* 2009;96:191–6.
11. MacFarlane JK, Ryall RD, Heald RJ. Mesorectal excision for rectal cancer. *Lancet* 1993;341:457–60.
12. van Gijn W, Marijnen CA, Nagtegaal ID et al. Dutch Colorectal Cancer Group. Preoperative radiotherapy combined with total mesorectal excision for resectable rectal cancer: 12–year follow-up of the multicentre, randomized controlled TME trial. *Lancet Oncol* 2011;12:575–82.
13. Lacy AM, Garcia-Valdecasas JC, Delgado S et al. Laparoscopy-assisted colectomy versus open colectomy for treatment of non-metastatic colon cancer: A randomised trial. *Lancet* 2002; 359(9325):2224–29.
14. Guillou PJ, Quirke P, Thorpe H et al. Short-term endpoints of conventional versus laparoscopic-assisted surgery in patients with colorectal cancer (MRC CLASICC trial): Multicentre, randomised controlled trial. *Lancet* 2005;365(9472):1718–26.
15. Veldkamp R, Kuhry E, Hop WC et al. Laparoscopic surgery versus open surgery for colon cancer: Short-term outcomes of a randomised trial. *Lancet Oncol* 2005;6(7):477–84.

16. Clinical Outcomes of Surgical Therapy Study Group. A comparison of laparoscopically assisted and open colectomy for colon cancer. *N Engl J Med* 2004;350(20):2050–59.
17. Chang GJ, Kaiser AM, Mills S, Rafferty JF, Buie WD, Standards Practice Task Force of the American Society of Colon Rectal Surgeons Practice parameters for the management of colon cancer. *Dis Colon Rectum* 2012;55(8):831–43.
18. Monson JR, Weiser MR, Buie WD et al. Practice parameters for the management of rectal cancer. *Dis Colon Rectum* 2013;56(5): 535–50.
19. Zerey M, Hawver LM, Awad Z et al. SAGES evidence-based guidelines for the laparoscopic resection of curable colon and rectal cancer. *Surg Endosc* 2013;27(1):1–10.
20. Bretagnol F, Dedieu A, Zappa M, Guedj N, Ferron M, Panis Y. T4 colorectal cancer: Is laparoscopic resection contraindicated? *Colorectal Dis* 2011;13(2):138–43.
21. Hemandas AK, Abdelrahman T, Flashman KG et al. Laparoscopic colorectal surgery produces better outcomes for high risk cancer patients compared to open surgery. *Ann Surg* 2010;252(1):84–9.
22. Kim KY, Hwang DW, Park YK, Lee HS. A single surgeon's experience with 54 consecutive cases of multivisceral resection for locally advanced primary colorectal cancer: Can the laparoscopic approach be performed safely? *Surg Endosc* 2012;26(2):493–500.
23. Huh JW, Kim HR. The feasibility of laparoscopic resection compared to open surgery in clinically suspected T4 colorectal cancer. *Adv Surg Tech A* 2012;22(5):463–67.
24. Vignali A, Ghirardelli L, Di Palo S, Orsenigo E, Staudacher C. Laparoscopic treatment of advanced colonic cancer: A case-matched control with open surgery. *Colorectal Dis* 2013;15(8): 944–48.
25. Nagasue Y, Akiyoshi T, Ueno M et al. Laparoscopic versus open multivisceral resection for primary colorectal cancer: Comparison of perioperative outcomes. *J Gastrointest Surg* 2013;17(7):1299–05.
26. Brunschwig A. Complete excision of pelvic viscera for advanced carcinoma. A one-stage abdominoperineal operation with end colostomy and bilateral ureteral implantation into the colon above the colostomy. *Cancer* 1948;1(2):177–83.
27. Yamada K, Ishizara T, Niwa K, Chuman Y, Aikou T. Pelvic exenteration and sacral resection for locally advanced primary and recurrent rectal cancer. *Dis Colon Rectum* 2002;45(8):1078–84.
28. Kecmanovic DM, Pavlov MJ, Kovacevic PA, Sepetkovski AV, Ceranic MS, Stamenkovic AB. Management of advanced pelvic cancer by exenteration. *Eur J Surg Oncol* 2003;29(9):743–6.
29. Yamada K, Ishizawa T, Niwa K, Chuman Y, Akiba S, Aikou T. Patterns of pelvic invasion are prognostic in the treatment of locally recurrent rectal cancer. *Br J Surg* 2001;88(7):988–93.
30. MERCURY Study Group. Diagnostic accuracy of preoperative magnetic resonance imaging in predicting curative resection of rectal cancer: Prospective observational study. *BMJ* 2006; 333(7572):779.
31. Augestad KM, Lindsetmo RO, Stulberg J et al. International Rectal Cancer Study Group (IRCSG) International preoperative rectal cancer management: Staging, neoadjuvant treatment, and impact of multidisciplinary teams. *World J Surg* 2010;34(11):2689–700.
32. Puli SR, Reddy JB, Bechtold ML, Choudhary A, Antillon MR, Brugge WR. Accuracy of endoscopic ultrasound to diagnose nodal invasion by rectal cancers: A meta-analysis and systematic review. *Ann Surg Oncol* 2009;16(5):1255–65.
33. Arya S, Das D, Engineer R, Saklani A. Imaging in rectal cancer with emphasis on local staging with MRI. *Indian J Radiol Imaging* 2015;25(2):148–61.
34. Al-Sukhni E, Milot L, Fruitman M et al. Diagnostic accuracy of MRI for assessment of T category, lymph node metastases, and circumferential resection margin involvement in patients with rectal cancer: A systematic review and meta-analysis. *Ann Surg Oncol* 2012;19:2212–23.
35. Shin DW, Shin JY, Oh SJ et al. The prognostic value of circumferential resection margin involvement in patients with extraperitoneal rectal cancer. *Am Surg* 2016;82(4):348–55.
36. Kamel IR, Cohade C, Neyman E, Fishman EK, Wahl RL. Incremental value of CT in PET/CT of patients with colorectal carcinoma. *Abdom Imaging* 2004;29(6):663–8.

37. Nagtegaal ID, Quirke P. What is the role for the circumferential margin in the modern treatment of rectal cancer. *J Clin Oncol* 2008;26:303–12.

38. Bujko K, Nowacki MP, Nasierowska-Guttmejer A, Michalski W, Bebenek M, Kryj M. Long-term results of a randomized trial comparing preoperative short-course radiotherapy with preoperative conventionally fractionated chemoradiation for rectal cancer. *Br J Surg* 2006;93:1215–23.

39. Rodel C, Grabenbauer GG, Matzel KE et al. Extensive surgery after high-dose preoperative chemoradiotherapy for locally advanced recurrent rectal cancer. *Dis Colon Rectum* 2000;43(3): 312–9.

40. Bosset JF, Calais G, Mineur L et al. Enhanced tumorocidal effect of chemotherapy with preoperative radiotherapy for rectal cancer: Preliminary results – EORTC 22921. *J Clin Oncol* 2005;23(24):5620–7.

Chapter 27

LAPAROSCOPIC SURGERY IN OBSTRUCTED AND RECURRENT TUMORS

Ramraj Vemala Nagendra Gupta and Govind Nandakumar

Contents

Learning objectives 172
Introduction 172
Clinical presentation 172
Management 172
Treatment.. 173
    Laparoscopic surgery in obstructed colorectal cancers... 173
    Laparoscopic surgery in recurrent colorectal cancers... 174
        Risk factors for recurrence 174
Classification of recurrences 175
Key steps for a safe surgery.. 176
Palliative resection 176
Postoperative care and follow-up 176
Summary 177
Key points 177
Video.. 177
References 177

Learning objectives

- Overview of clinical presentation and diagnosis
- Indications for laparoscopic resections
- Peri-operative preparation
- Types of resections
- Steps of surgery for a safe and effective outcome

Introduction

Colorectal cancer is the third most common cancer [1] and the second leading cause of cancer-related deaths. Despite recent advances, surgical resection remains the most reliable curative treatment modality. Laparoscopic and open colonic resections are now well accepted the world over for primary tumors. Short-term benefits of low perioperative morbidity and the long-term benefits of reduced incidence of intra-abdominal adhesions and consequent bowel obstructions are well acknowledged following laparoscopic resections [2,3].

Standard laparoscopic colorectal resections have stood the test of time and are part of the repertoire of most colorectal surgeons. However, the role of laparoscopic surgery in obstructed and recurrent colorectal cancers is not only ambiguous but is also challenging. This is because many landmark trials have excluded patients with obstructed and recurrent cancers [2].

Clinical presentation

Clinical manifestations indicate the site and morphology of a tumor to an extent and aid in planning treatment. Colorectal cancers typically present with altered bowel habits (74%), rectal bleeding (71%), unexplained iron deficiency anaemia (9.6%), or abdominal pain (3.8%) [4]. Altered bowel habits and hematochezia is more common with left-sided tumors and unexplained iron deficiency anaemia is more common with right-sided tumors [5]. Abdominal pain may arise from tumors at any site and usually indicate intestinal obstruction, perforation, or peritoneal dissemination.

Obstructive symptoms like abdominal distension, nausea, vomiting, and constipation are less common and are seen in approximately 30% of patients [6]. Constipation, as a primary symptom by itself, has been shown to have no direct link with prevalence of colorectal cancer. Intestinal obstructions are commonly seen in circumferential growths and are frequently identified as 'apple cores' on imaging. The median age of patients presenting with obstruction due to colorectal cancer is 73 years. Colorectal obstructions may be acute or chronic, and up to 70% of patients presenting with large bowel obstruction requiring emergency surgery have been found to have tumors in the rectosigmoid, rectum, or anus [7].

A majority (70%) of colonic obstructions occur due to tumors at, or distal, to the transverse colon and the splenic flexure is the most common site. As the right colon is wider in caliber and contents more liquid, lesions here are less likely to present with intestinal obstruction compared to left-sided colonic lesions [5]. Perforation may also coexist and is more commonly seen at the point of obstruction, likely due to tumor invasion or inflammatory reaction, rather than in the dilated proximal colon.

Recurrence of colon and rectal tumors are seen in 12%–20% of patients following curative resections [8]. Recurrence may be either local or distant. These tumors may either be picked up on routine surveillance, or patients with past resections can have a recurrence of symptoms. Pyrexia of unknown origin, pneumaturia, persistent back aches, sepsis, jaundice, dyspnea, altered sensorium, or seizures are other atypical presentations.

Management

A complete history, including previous medical and surgical history, along with a thorough examination is mandatory and of utmost importance (Table 27.1), especially in these special circumstances.

An unstable or septic patient with a high risk for general anesthesia is an absolute contraindication for any laparoscopic procedure. A grossly distended and tense abdomen with or without

TABLE 27.1: History and Physical Examination

Age, sex
Complete history of present ailment – onset, duration, associated symptoms
Medical comorbidities
Past surgical history
Family history
Physical examination
Vitals
General
Abdomen – Shape, surgical scars, palpable mass, peritoneal signs and bowel sounds
Digital rectal examination, vaginal examination

abdominal compartment syndrome, severe respiratory distress, and coagulation disorders are other absolute contraindications (Table 27.2). Abdominal scars, previous abdominal tuberculosis, disseminated disease, and large bulky growths are relative contraindications. A strong family history of malignancy, known syndromes, or genetic defects may require more extensive resections.

For diagnosis, standard protocols for evaluation should be followed. Although complete elaboration of each of them is beyond the scope of this chapter, a few salient points will be stressed upon.

Colonoscopy, a screening, diagnostic tests, and therapeutic modality helps in tumor localization, as well as tissue diagnosis and surveillance. In cases of obstruction, colonoscopy and tissue diagnosis is not mandatory. An impassable scope across the lesion is an indication for early surgery. However, in recurrent tumors colonoscopy is mandatory for localizing tumors, tattooing and also for identifying metachronous lesions. Histopathologic examination of the recurrent lesion is useful to rule out other unusual conditions. MSI, BRAF, MMR, and ctDNA tests on tissues obtained from colonoscopic biopsies are useful in planning adjuvant treatment and possible prognostication.

Imaging is an essential component in management. Although x-ray of the abdomen can indicate the presence of intestinal obstruction and the possible site of a tumor, CT scans can assess the depth of a tumor, invasion into adjacent structures (like nerves, ureters, vessels, bones, kidneys, mesentery and bowel), lymphatic spread, distant metastases, and complications like fistula, perforation, or obstruction. CT scans can also identify early recurrences, their extent, local spread, distant metastases, operability, and resectability. A CT scan is indicated in all patients presenting with possible colon-obstructing cancers. A transition point with a proximal dilated colon (>8 cm) and collapsed distal colon is diagnostic of a colonic obstruction [9].

TABLE 27.2: Contraindications for Laparoscopy in Obstructed or Recurrent Colorectal Cancers

Hemodynamically unstable patient
Coagulopathy and blood dyscrasias
Disseminated intraperitoneal disease or abdominal cocoon
Previous HIPEC
Associated cirrhosis of liver and portal hypertension
Multiple laparotomies
Pregnancy
Large abdominal aneurysm
Tumor perforation

MRI is important in staging rectal cancers. Though it has a limited role in the setting of an obstruction, it is indeed very essential for identifying recurrences in the rectum, delineating their relation to the sphincter complexes and lateral pelvic walls.

PET-CT is indicated in the presence of a high suspicion for distant metastases, progressively increasing CEA levels, and recurrent disease. PET may be useful in distinguishing postoperative fibrosis and scars from recurrences. Patients with grossly elevated CEA (>5 ng/mL) levels have worse prognosis, stage-by-stage, than those with lower levels [10].

Treatment

Laparoscopic surgery in obstructed colorectal cancers

Adhering to oncological principles and basics of laparoscopy are essential in these difficult and unpredictable clinical situations. After a complete clinical assessment and imaging, patients and family need to be consulted for their consent. Risks of bowel injury, possible conversion to open surgery, and the creation of a stoma should be discussed and stressed upon.

Surgeons should check laparoscopic equipment and ensure the availability of all instruments and accessories such as energy devices, sutures, staplers, and wound protectors before surgery. The technique of mobilization, the type of resection, the method of anastomosis, and possible site of stoma and incision to retrieve a specimen should be planned before embarking on the procedure.

Laparoscopic surgeries include either a single-stage procedure (resection and anastomosis) [11], a two-stage procedure (resection-anastomosis with proximal diversion stoma, or resection with end stoma followed by restoration of bowel continuity), or a three-stage procedure (proximal diversion, followed by resection with stoma and then restoration of continuity).

1. Right-sided obstructed colonic growths may require either:
   a. A standard right hemi-colectomy with ileo-colic anastomosis
   b. An extended right hemi-colectomy with ileo-colic anastomosis

Several retrospective trials have shown the benefits of laparoscopic resections, but randomized trials are lacking [12,13]. Primary anastomoses can be safely performed [14] since the right and transverse colon have low bacterial counts. Creation of a proximal diversion stoma depends on several factors such as the patient's general condition, nutritional status, extent of bowel dilatation, and the presence of extraluminal disease.

2. Left-sided obstructed colonic tumors may benefit from preoperative colonoscopic stenting to decompress the bowel. Stents can be used as a bridge to prepare the patient to proceed with laparoscopy. A randomized controlled trial by Cheung HY et al. [15], comparing endoluminal stenting followed by laparoscopic resection vs. immediate open surgical resection of obstructing left-sided colon cancers showed more patients in the stenting and laparoscopic resection group undergoing one-stage operations (66% vs. 37.5%; p = 0.04) and that no patients required colostomy, compared with 25% of patients in the open surgery group requiring an end colostomy. Patient selection is critical. Although the possibility of stoma creation can be reduced, colonoscopic self-expandable stents come with certain cost and a set of complications, including perforation, migration, and erosion.

Available surgical options for left-sided lesions include [16,17]:

a. End-colostomy and Hartmann pouch / procedure
b. Resection with on-table lavage and primary anastomosis with or without diversion stoma
c. Subtotal colectomy with ileorectal anastomosis

A retrospective study of 243 obstructed patients at Queens Mary hospital in Hong Kong, who underwent primary anastomosis, showed no statistically significant difference in mortality or anastomotic leaks [18]. It is important to note that an unprepared bowel is no more a contraindication for bowel anastomosis, as shown in multiple non-randomized trials, and a decision for anastomosis versus stoma must be individualized.

Intraoperative colonic lavage is another alternative option available to avoid multistage procedures in obstructed colorectal tumors. It is an antegrade bowel cleansing process, where a Foley's catheter is inserted into the appendix through an appendicostomy, which is used as an inlet, and a sterile anesthesia tubing connected to the proximal resected end of the colon, which is used as an outlet to clean the entire colon prior to anastomosis. Large volume saline, diluted povidone-iodine, or warm polyethylene glycol solutions have been used for lavage. Multiple studies have shown primary anastomosis performed after colonic resection and irrigation to be safe, with no increased risk in mortality or anastomotic leakage [19].

Tips for a safe surgery: [20]

- Preoperative bowel preparation should be avoided in obstructed lesions.
- Patient should be adequately strapped and positioned (supine, leg split, or semi-lithotomy/Lloyd-Davis position) as a complete Trendelenburg, reverse Trendelenburg, or even a sideward tilt may be required. Boots or stirrups with pads are useful to avoid nerve compression.
- Appropriate broad-spectrum antibiotic must be timed and administered.
- A Ryle's tube is inserted to avoid aspiration.
- Use two monitors, stationed on either side. Monitors must be movable as and when required.
- Open technique of port placement – Dilated bowel loops in an obstruction increases the possibility of injury; hence, an open technique with blunt trocars should be preferred.
- Low insufflation – Increased CO_2 pressure in presence of a distended gut might increase airway pressures.
- Diagnostic scopy is mandatory to assess the peritoneal cavity for any disseminated disease and for the localization of lesions.
- Secondary ports are to be inserted under vision.
- Avoid port placements over palpable masses.
- Atraumatic graspers should be preferred as distended bowels are thinned out and susceptible to injury.
- Movement of instruments should be precise, fine, and under vision to avoid any untoward injury of thinned out dilated bowels, especially while running the small intestines end-to-end.
- The oncologic principle of minimal tumor handling should be followed.
- Vessels are divided at their origin using preferable vessel sealing devices or clips. Suture ligation of vessels may be difficult due to limited operating space.
- High ligation of vessels ensures adequate lymphatic clearance.

- A low threshold to place additional ports, or even a hand port, is wise.
- Mobilization of the colon – Medial to lateral is preferred. Lateral to medial, or even caudo-cranial in case of a right hemi-colectomy are other options.
- Identify and dissect in the correct areolar tissue planes.
- Protect vital structures – Ureters, duodenum, gonadal vessels, etc. should be identified. Urinary bladder, seminal vesicles, uterus, and vagina encountered in case of low anterior resections or Abdomino-perineal resections should be identified and preserved whenever possible.
- Operative space should be reassessed to decide on laparoscopic versus open resection.
- If laparoscopic resection and anastomosis are decided, appropriate ports need to be upsized to accommodate a stapler.
- A white or a blue cartridge is preferred for dilated small bowel and colon, respectively.
- An incision is made at a convenient site, either midline or Pfannensteil, or even at the site of a planned stoma for specimen retrieval.
- Wound protectors are useful to avoid contamination with luminal contents and spillage of tumor cells.
- The resected or mobilized colon is exteriorized.
- If extracorporeal resection is planned, an obstructed bowel may be decompressed before anastomosis – Intraoperative irrigation/lavage.
- Orientation of the bowel should be checked, and a tension-free anastomosis must be ensured.
- The stoma is brought out through the marked site, and fashioned only after closure of the main wound to avoid contamination.
- Ports should be removed under vision and closed appropriately.

Laparoscopic surgery in recurrent colorectal cancers

Though recurrent rectal cancers have seen a significant decline since the advocation of total mesorectal excision (TME) by Heald in the 1990s [21], they continue to have very poor 5-year survival rates. It's also been observed that up to 20% percent of patients undergoing primary colorectal cancer resections with curative intent may develop recurrence [8]. About half of these recurrences are isolated and can be considered for either curative re-resection or palliative resections [22].

Management of these complex diseases requires a multidisciplinary team approach. Proper evaluation, planning, and involvement of other subspecialities are critical for optimal results. Laparoscopy, in this setting of recurrent colorectal malignancy – where tissue planes are lost and where traditional resections are not amenable, requires a higher level of expertise and a complete understanding of the disease process. Inadequate literature and lack of randomized trials has failed to provide definitive guidelines in such complex scenarios.

As mentioned earlier, all efforts should be made to gather information on prior interventions and surgeries, as this would be useful for planning further treatments.

Risk factors for recurrence

Most recurrences are now known to occur within the first two years after primary resection [23]. Multiple factors, either individually or together, may coexist to enhance the risk of recurrence in any given patient.

These factors are categorized as [24,25]:

Patient factors: Family history of colorectal malignancy, incomplete adjuvant treatment after previous resections, poor compliance for follow-up.

Treatment factors: Incomplete evaluation at the time of first malignancy, not advocating neoadjuvant or combined modality treatment with chemo- and radiotherapy in appropriate scenarios. R1/R2 resections during primary surgery. Tumor spillage or contamination of operative field.

Tumor factors: Bulky tumors (T3/T4), decreased distance between the tumor and surgical margins, close distal and circumferential or radial margins, poor differentiation, node positivity, and lymphovascular and perineural invasions.

Classification of recurrences

There are a variety of classifications (Table 27.3) being used to categorize recurrent colorectal cancers. Some of these are based on anatomical location, some on degree of fixation, and others on TNM systems.

Broadly, recurrences may be:

- Localized to the colon or rectum at the site of previous surgery
- Localized to the mesentery or nodes
- Locoregional or retroperitoneal recurrence with no distant metastases
- Isolated metastases to the liver and/or lung or ovary, with or without local recurrence
- Local recurrence with multiple distant metastases or disseminated disease

As the location of the tumor and its relation to adjacent structures seem to direct subsequent therapy, a classification based on location appears to be more realistic and easier to use.

Preoperative evaluation and restaging, as already elaborated, is essential in identifying the site of recurrence and the type of tumor. A complete pelvic examination to assess the rectum, anal canal, vagina, and sphincter tone is mandatory. Colonoscopy and tattooing of lesions are useful adjuncts for surgery, especially for the small and early recurrent tumors.

Imaging is crucial to select suitable candidates for surgery. Involvement of the small bowel mesentery, encasement of external iliac vessels, extension to the sacral promontory, growth into the greater sciatic notch and lateral pelvic sidewalls are contraindications for any radical resections (Table 27.4) [26,31,32].

Selected patients with local recurrence may benefit form a combined modality treatment (CMT), which includes chemotherapy, chemoradiotherapy, or intraoperative radiation therapy in addition to surgery. This is irrespective of receiving previous radiotherapy.

Surgery for recurrence depends on the clinical presentation, age of the patient, site of recurrence, stage of disease, response to neoadjuvant therapy, interval duration for recurrence, compliance, and nutritional and performance status. The risks and associated complications of radical resections must be weighed against the possible benefits.

Once evaluation is complete and a multidisciplinary decision is made as to the plan of treatment, patients and their family should be counselled in detail. Modalities of the treatment available, its duration, associated morbidity, mortality, expected quality of life, and life expectancy after completion of therapy must be communicated in detail and consented.

It is also useful to note that patients with initial stage II colorectal cancer have a better median survival after local recurrence

TABLE 27.3: Classifications Used in Pelvic Recurrence of Rectal Cancer

Memorial Sloan Kettering Cancer Center [26]	Based on location and involvement of other structures	*Axial*: Following low anterior resection, local following transanal-trans-sphincteric excision, or perineum following abdominoperineal resection. *Anterior*: Genitourinary tract including bladder, vagina, uterus, seminal vescicles, or prostate. *Posterior*: Sacrum and presacral fascia. *Lateral*: Lateral bony pelvis or sidewall structures including iliac vessels, ureters, lateral lymphnodes, autonomic nerves, and musculature
Yamada et al. [27]	Based on location	Localized (adjacent pelvic organs or connective tissue). Sacral (S3-5, coccyx, or periosteum). Lateral (lateral pelvic wall, S1/S2, sciatic nerve, or greater sciatic foramen)
Mayo Clinic [28]	Based on pain and degree of freedom or fixation	Pain (S0 = asymptomatic; S1 = symptomatic without pain; S2 = symptomatic with pain). Site (anterior, sacral, right or left) and Number of points of fixation (F0 = not fixed to any site; F1 = fixed to one site; F2 = fixed at two sites; F3 = fixed at three sites)
Wanebo et al. [29]	Based on TNM system	T_R1-2: Local recurrence at the primary resection site. T_R3: Anastomotic recurrence with full thickness penetration beyond the bowel wall and into perirectal soft tissue. T_R4: Invasion into anterior adjacent organs or presacral tissues (with tethering but not fixation). T_R5: Invasion of bony ligamentous pelvis including the sacrum, low pelvic/side walls, or sacrotuberous/ischial ligaments
Boyle KM et al. [30] Leeds group	Based on pattern of invasion	*Central*: Tumor confined to pelvic organs or connective tissue without contact or invasion into bone. *Sacral*: Tumor present in the presacral space and abuts into or invades into the sacrum. *Sidewall*: Tumor involving the structures on the lateral pelvic sidewall, including the greater sciatic foramen, and the sciatic nerve through to the piriformis and the gluteal region. *Composite*: Sacral and sidewall recurrence combined

Nerve root involvement at or above the level of S1-2
Proximal (S1, S2) sacral invasion extending to the sacral promontory (relative contraindication)
Involvement of the paraaortic lymph nodes
Tumor encasement of the external iliac vessels
Extension of tumor through the greater sciatic notch
Bilateral ureteral obstruction (relative contraindication)
Unresectable extra-pelvic disease
Circumferential involvement of the pelvic wall

than those with stage III (median 18 vs. 13 months). Survival is also better in those with a longer disease-free interval, and in those who did not receive FU-based adjuvant chemotherapy following resection of the primary tumor [33].

Laparoscopic surgical options include:

1. Salvage colectomy with or without anastomosis
2. Total procto-colectomy with end ileostomy
3. Total proctocolectomy with ileal pouch anal anastomosis
4. Abdomino-perineal resection
5. Pelvic exenteration (posterior or total pelvic exenteration for an anteriorly located recurrence, abdomino-sacral resection or partial sacrectomy for a posteriorly located recurrence)

R0 resection should be the goal and may entail – depending on type of involvement, a pelvic exenteration, ureteral resection, bladder resections, and distal or high sacrectomies. Laparoscopic total pelvic exenterations for locally recurrent rectal cancers, though technically challenging and having longer operative times, have been shown to be feasible and safe. Better vision, less blood loss, and smaller wounds are the other advantages of laparoscopic procedures [34,35]. In selected patients, the above procedures may be combined with liver or lung metastatectomies and bilateral oophorectomy with or without local peritonectomy.

Around 30% of patients with recurrent locoregional colon cancer will qualify and benefit from aggressive surgical resections. Achieving an R0 resection is the single-most important prognostic factor. In a systematic review by Chesney TR et al. [36], patients with an R0 resection were found to have a three-year overall survival of 58% (95% CI, 39% to 76%) and a five-year overall survival of 52% (95% CI, 32% to 72%). Five-year survival for patients with an R1 resection (microscopic positive margins), in the same review, was 11% and for R2 resection (macroscopic positive margins) 0%.

Hyperthermic intraperitoneal chemotherapy, or HIPEC, performed through open or laparoscopy procedure has been shown to be useful in certain specific situations with isolated peritoneal carcinomatosis [37].

Key steps for a safe surgery

- A multidisciplinary team discussion for a complete plan of treatment prior to any intervention should be the norm.
- An open technique of port placement is preferred to avoid inadvertent injury due to adhesions.
- Meticulous adhesiolysis, using a combination of sharp dissection and/or energy sources, should be completed and anatomy defined.

- The site of recurrence should be identified, and dissection continued. Typical avascular tissue planes as in primary surgery are usually lacking and every effort should be made to identify important structures. Preoperative ureteric stenting and indocyanine green injections aid in avoiding ureteric injuries.
- Additional ports, or a hand port, are beneficial in difficult cases.
- Tumor handling should be minimized.
- Intraoperative colonoscopy guides the level of resection with adequate margins.
- R0 resection should be the goal and the operating team must be prepared for composite or multivisceral resections.
- Involvement of urogenital organs may require an enbloc radical resection.
- Waldeyer's and Denonvilliers' fascia must be mobilized and care must be taken to protect the iliac vessels, posterior lumbo-sacral plexus, and obturator nerves.
- Presence of associated perineal recurrence will require laparoscopy to be combined with a transperineal approach for possible distal sacrectomy.
- A frozen section is useful for ensuring an R0 resection.
- Decision for anastomosis, intra/extra corporeal vs. stoma should be individualized.
- Orientation of intestines must be confirmed for a tension-free anastomosis.
- A pouch, if planned, is preferable after adjuvant chemoradiation.

Laparoscopic surgeries in these complex clinical situations are associated with certain morbidities and even mortality. Morbidity of up to 80% have been documented following surgery for recurrent rectal cancers – even in high volume centers. Complications can be immediate, early, or delayed.

Common complications include wound infection/disruptions (39%–86%), gastrointestinal fistula (8%), genitourinary fistula (10%), and ileus/intestinal obstruction (11%–33%) [39,40]. Chronic pain, stoma-related complications, re-recurrence of malignancy, loss of interest in sexual function, incontinence, and renal dysfunctions are other complications encountered.

Intraoperative radiotherapy, though debatable, has been used in high-risk patients. Both external beam radiation and brachytherapy have shown similar results. IORT may not be needed in patients if a frozen section shows a >5 mm negative margin [38]. IORT is contraindicated if the cumulative previous irradiation exceeds 64 Gy [41]. If therapy is contemplated, a dry bloodless operative filed must be ensured along with an adequate protection to the structures that are disease-free.

Palliative resection

Patients presenting with late-stage recurrent disease and with symptoms disturbing daily routine activities will benefit from palliative resections – where the goal is to palliate symptoms and minimize morbidity. Palliative resections can be performed laparoscopically in selected patients. Yeung RS et al. [42], in their study, have demonstrated that palliative exenteration can improve pain control and quality of life.

Postoperative care and follow-up

Early postoperative care of these patients is crucial. Prolonged duration of surgery and blood loss may warrant observation in an intensive care unit. Antibiotics as well as correction of fluid and electrolyte imbalances are important. Enteral nutrition should be instituted as soon as possible. Both mechanical and pharmacological prophylaxis against deep vein thrombosis are continued in the patient until adequately ambulant. Early mobilization and chest physiotherapy must be encouraged. Urinary catheters and abdominal drains must be removed appropriately to avoid infections. Stoma care education to patient and family is continued postoperatively and must be centered on possible complications. Surgical wounds should be inspected regularly. Enhanced recovery, ambulation, and early discharge should be aimed for.

As mentioned, R status is the single-most important factor to determine cure, as shown by multiple studies including Bhangu et al. [43], where in their meta-analysis of recurrent rectal cancers they have clearly demonstrated the survival advantage of R0 over R1 resection, and the same for R1 over R2. Regular postoperative follow-ups (monthly visit in the first year, quarterly CEA estimation, yearly imaging) with a multi-disciplinary team must be ensured in all patients and adjuvant therapy initiated appropriately.

Summary

Surgical management of obstructed and recurrent colorectal tumors requires adequate training, expertise, and a team-based approach. Though patient selection holds the key, laparoscopic surgery in these complex clinical situations is feasible and safe – provided all necessary safety precautions are followed. A low threshold for conversion should be the norm and must not be considered a failure.

Key points

- A majority (70%) of colonic obstructions occur due to tumors at or distal to the transverse colon, and the splenic flexure is the most common site.
- Recurrence of colon and rectal tumors are seen in 12%–20% of patients following curative resections.
- A laparoscopic approach can be used in obstructed and recurrent cancers, provided oncologic principles are followed, and the procedures carried out safely.

See Video 30.

VIDEO 30 https://youtu.be/bCDn5xTGWTE

Peritonectomy + HIPEC for Colorectal Cancer.

References

1. Siegel RL, Miller KD, Jemal A et al. *CA Cancer J Clin* 2019;69(1):7.
2. Bonjer HJ, Hop WC, Nelson H et al. Laparoscopically assisted vs open colectomy for colon cancer: A meta-analysis. *Arch Surg* 2007;142(3):298.
3. Jayne DG, Thorpe HC, Copeland J et al. Five-year follow-up of the Medical Research Council CLASICC trial of laparoscopically assisted versus open surgery for colorectal cancer. *Br J Surg* 2010;97(11):1638.
4. Majumdar SR, Fletcher RH, Evans AT. How does colorectal cancer present? Symptoms, duration, and clues to location. *Am J Gastroenterol* 1999;94(10):3039.
5. Goodman D, Irvin TT. Delay in the diagnosis and prognosis of carcinoma of the right colon. *Br J Surg* 1993;80(10):1327
6. Buechter KJ, Boustany C, Caillouette R et al. Surgical management of the acutely obstructed colon. A review of 127 cases. *Am J Surg* 1988 Sep;156(3 Pt 1):163–8.
7. Deans GT, Krukowski ZH, Irwin ST. Malignant obstruction of the left colon. *Br J Surg* 1994;81(9):1270.
8. Kruschewski M, Ciurea M, Lipika S et al. Locally recurrent colorectal cancer: Results of surgical therapy. *Langenbecks Arch Surg* 2012; 397:1059–67.
9. Taourel P, Kessler N, Lesnik A et al. Helical CT of large bowel obstruction. *Abdom Imaging* 2003 Mar;28(2):267–75.
10. Konishi T, Shimada Y, Hsu M et al. Association of Preoperative and Postoperative Serum Carcinoembryonic Antigen and Colon Cancer Outcome. *JAMA Oncol* 2018;4(3):309.
11. Breitenstein S, Rickenbacher A, Berdajs D et al. Systematic evaluation of surgical strategies for acute malignant left-sided colonic obstruction. *Br J Surg* 2007 Dec;94(12):1451–60.
12. Gash K, Chambers W, Ghosh A et al. The role of laparoscopic surgery for the management of acute large bowel obstruction. *Colorectal Dis* 2011 Mar;13(3):263–6.
13. Ng SS, Lee FY, Yiu YC et al. Emergency laparoscopic-assisted versus open right hemicolectomy for obstructing right-sided colonic carcinoma: A comparative study of short-term clinical outcomes. *World J Surg* 2008;32(3):454–8.
14. Veldkamp R, M Gholghesaei, HJ Bonjer et al. Laparoscopic resection of colon Cancer: Consensus of the European Association of Endoscopic Surgery (EAES). *Surg Endosc* 2004;18(8):1163–85.
15. Cheung, HY, Chung CC, Tsang WW et al. Endolaparoscopic approach vs conventional open surgery in the treatment of obstructing left-sided colon cancer: A randomized controlled trial. *Arch Surg* 2009;144(12):1127–32.
16. Lopez-Kostner F, Hool GR, Lavery IC. Management and causes of acute large-bowel obstruction. *Surg Clin North Am* 1997;77(6):1265–90.
17. The SCOTIA Study Group. Single-stage treatment for malignant left-sided colonic obstruction: A prospective randomized clinical trial comparing subtotal colectomy with segmental resection following intraoperative irrigation. Subtotal Colectomy versus On-table Irrigation and Anastomosis. *Br J Surg* 1995;82(12):1622–7.
18. Chiappa A, Zbar A, Biella F et al. One-stage resection and primary anastomosis following acute obstruction of the left colon for cancer. *Am Surg* 2000;66(7):619.
19. Awotar GK, Guan G, Sun W. Reviewing the management of obstructive left colon cancer: Assessing the feasibility of the one-stage resection and anastomosis after intraoperative colonic irrigation. *Clin Colorectal Cancer* 2017 Jun;16(2):e89–e103.
20. https://www.sages.org/publications/guidelines/guidelines-for-laparoscopic-resection-of-curable-colon-and-rectal-cancer/. 14th September 2019.
21. MacFarlane JK, Rayall RD, Heald RJ. Mesorectal excision for rectal cancer. *Lancet* 1993;341:457–60.
22. Heriot AG, Byrne CM, Lee P et al. Extended radical resection: The choice for locally recurrent rectal cancer. *Dis Colon Rectum* 2008;51:284–91.
23. Pilipshen SJ, Heilweil M, Quan SH et al. Patterns of pelvic recurrence following definitive resections of rectal cancer. *Cancer* 1984;53:1354–62.
24. Michelassi F, Block GE, Vannucci L et al. A 5- to 21-year follow-up and analysis of 250 patients with rectal adenocarcinoma. *Ann Surg* 1988;208:379–89.
25. Phillips RK, Hittinger R, Blesovsky L et al. Local recurrence following 'curative' surgery for large bowel cancer: II. The Rectum and rectosigmoid. *Br J Surg* 1984;71:17–20.
26. Moore HG, Shoup M, Reidel E et al. Colorectal cancer pelvic recurrences: Determinants of resectability. *Dis Colon Rectum* 2004;47:1599–606.
27. Yamada K, Ishizawa T, Niwa K et al. Patterns of pelvic invasion are prognostic in the treatment of locally recurrent rectal cancer. *Br J Surg* 2001;88:988–93.

28. Suzuki K, Dozois RR, Devine RM et al. Curative reoperations for locally recurrent rectal cancer. *Dis Colon Rectum* 1996;39:730–6.

29. Wanebo HJ, Antoniuk P, Koness RJ et al. Pelvic resection of recurrent rectal cancer: Technical considerations and outcomes. *Dis Colon Rectum* 1999;42:1438–48.

30. Boyle KM, Sagar PM, Chalmers AG et al. Surgery for locally recurrent rectal cancer. *Dis Colon Rectum* 2005 May;48(5):929–37.

31. Moriya Y, Akasu T, Fujita S et al. Total pelvic exenteration with distal sacrectomy for fixed recurrent rectal cancer in the pelvis. *Dis Colon Rectum* 2004;47:2047–53; discussion 43–4.

32. Dozois EJ, Privitera A, Holubar SD et al. High sacrectomy for locally recurrent rectal cancer: Can long-term survival be achieved? *J Surg Oncol* 2011;103:105–9.

33. O'Connell MJ, Campbell ME, Goldberg RM et al. Survival following recurrence in stage II and III colon cancer: Findings from the ACCENT data set. *J Clin Oncol* 2008;26(14):2336.

34. Akiyoshi T, Nagasaki T, Ueno M. Laparoscopic total pelvic exenteration for locally recurrent rectal cancer. *Ann Surg Oncol* 2015 Nov;22(12):3896.

35. Akiyoshi T. Technical feasibility of laparoscopic extended surgery beyond total mesorectal excision for primary or recurrent rectal cancer. *World J Gastroenterol* 2016 Jan 14;22(2):718–26.

36. Chesney TR, Nadler A, Acuna SA et al. Outcomes of resection for locoregionally recurrent colon cancer: A systematic review. *Surgery* 2016;160(1):54.

37. Verwaal VJ, Bruin S, Boot H et al. 8-year follow-up of randomized trial: Cytoreduction with Hyperthermic intra-peritoneal chemotherapy versus systemic chemotherapy and palliative surgery in patients with peritoneal carcinomatosis of colorectal cancer. *Ann Surg Oncol* 2008;15:2426–32.

38. Bouchard P, Efron J. Management of recurrent rectal cancer. *Ann Surg Oncol* 2010;17:1343–56.

39. Salom EM, Penalver MA. Pelvic exenteration and reconstruction. *Cancer J* 2003;9(5):415.

40. Berek JS, Howe C, Lagasse LD et al. Pelvic exenteration for recurrent gynecologic malignancy: Survival and morbidity analysis of the 45-year experience at UCLA. *Gynecol Oncol* 2005; 99(1):153.

41. Mohiuddin M, Marks G, Marks J. Long-term results of reirradiation for patients with recurrent rectal carcinoma. *Cancer* 2002;95:1144–50.

42. Yeung RS, Moffat FL, Falk RE. Pelvic exenteration for recurrent and extensive primary colorectal adenocarcinoma. *Cancer* 1993;72:1853–8.

43. Bhangu A, Ali SM, Darzi A et al. Meta-analysis of survival based on resection margin status following surgery for recurrent rectal cancer. *Colorectal Dis* 2012;14:1457–66.

Chapter 28

RESECTION FOR COLORECTAL LIVER METASTASIS

Palanisamy Senthilnathan, Srivatsan Gurumurthy Sivakumar, Srinivasan Muthukrishnan, and C Palanivelu

Contents

Learning objectives 179
Introduction 179
Evaluation of resectability.. 179
Management of resectable liver metastasis 180
    Timing of resection for synchronous liver metastases.. 180
    Laparoscopic major (right/left) hepatic resection 180
    Laparoscopic left lateral sectionectomy 182
    Laparoscopic segmentectomies/Nonanatomical resections.. 182
Radiofrequency ablation 182
Management of unresectable liver metastasis.. 182
Outcomes of laparoscopic resection for CRLM 182
Management flowchart for colorectal liver metastases.. 183
Summary 183
Key points 183
References 183

Learning objectives

- Evaluation of resectability
- Indications and timing for resection of colorectal liver metastasis (CRLM)
- Techniques for laparoscopic resection of resectable CRLM
- Outcomes of laparoscopic resection for CRLM
- Role of RF Ablation for CRLM
- Management of unresectable disease

Introduction

Colorectal cancer is a major health burden, ranking third in cancer incidence and fourth in cancer-related mortality worldwide [1]. Liver metastasis is one of the major causes of death in patients with CRC. Synchronous liver metastasis is observed in as many as 25% of patients and metachronous lesions in nearly 60% of patients on follow-up [2,3]. Multimodality treatment with surgery as a cornerstone considerably improves the overall survival in these patients [4]. But unfortunately, only about 20% of CRLM patients have resectable cancer [5]. The advent of highly effective chemotherapy and advances in the surgical techniques of liver resection (LR) has expanded the pool of resectable patients with CRLM, and metastatic lesions that were previously deemed terminal or nonsurgical are now being considered for surgical resection. According to recent reports, the 5-year survival rate of CRLM patients receiving surgery and neoadjuvant therapy has increased up to 50% [6].

The advantages of laparoscopic liver resection have been established for peripherally located tumors and minor hepatic resections. Robotic surgery has now made the minimally invasive approach possible even for major hepatic resections and lesions in difficult locations like the postero-superior segments.

Evaluation of resectability

Preoperative evaluation includes evaluation of the liver lesions and FLR, and a survey for extrahepatic metastatic disease (EHMD).

The imaging methods useful for evaluating LM include transabdominal ultrasound (US), contrast-enhanced computed tomography (CT), contrast-enhanced MRI, and positron emission tomography (PET). A meta-analysis has shown that the sensitivities of CT, MRI, and PET/CT for the diagnosis of CRLM are 82.1%, 93.1%, and 74.1%, respectively; while the specificities are 73.5%, 87.3%, and 93.9%, respectively [7]. A review of the literature indicates that MRI, especially gadoxetate disodium (Gd)-enhanced MRI, is more sensitive than CT for detecting a liver lesion of less than 1 cm, particularly 5 mm [8]. In clinical practice, despite having limited sensitivity, CT appears to be adequate for determining the resectability of CRLM for the majority of patients. The sensitivity and specificity of PET/CT for the detection of LM are similar to those of CT [9]. The currently established standard for planning liver surgery is contrast-enhanced CT, which as a rule enables appropriate resection planning, for example, a precise identification and localization of primary and secondary liver tumors, as well as the anatomical relationship to extrahepatic and/or intrahepatic vascular and biliary structures.

Preoperative evaluation of the FLR by virtual segmental volumetry, using 3D CT, has been found to be superior to that estimated using standard equations [10–12]. The FLR size should be at least 20% for patients with normal livers and 30%–40% in those who have received preoperative chemotherapy for more than a 12 weeks duration or more than eight cycles, in order to avoid postoperative liver failure [13,14].

Laparoscopic US can enhance the sensitivity of detection of additional LM not seen on routine preoperative imaging [15]. This may be particularly important during laparoscopic resections.

PET/CT is recommended for the detection of occult distant metastases as it can detect 25% of extrahepatic lesions and avoid worthless surgery in approximately 20% of patients [16]. Traditionally, EHMD was considered as one of the contraindications of CRLM resection because of its low 5-year survival rate [17]. A population-based study of 15,133 CRC patients showed that patients with isolated lung metastases had better cancer-specific survival and OS compared to patients with metastases to the liver, bone, and brain [18]; additionally, complete resection of concomitant hepatic and EHMD significantly prolongs survival. Therefore, limited EHMD such as pulmonary EHMD is now no longer a contraindication of LR and patients can receive an R0 resection, as long as the FLR is sufficient so that the patient can tolerate the major surgery of both the liver and EHMD [19–21]. However, unresectability of EHMD is a contraindication for curative LR, as it is extremely likely to result in a poor prognosis.

Management of resectable liver metastasis

The current criteria for resectability of CRLM are as follows: any tumor number, any tumor distribution in the liver, stable or resectable EHMD (excluding portal lymphadenopathy), functional liver remnant >20% of the total liver volume, venous involvement amenable to venous resection or reconstruction, and a tumor-free margin [22].

There is currently no consensus in the literature as to which patients with CRLM are suitable for LLR, although LLR has been performed for all liver segments in this context. Small tumors in the left lateral segments of the liver and patients with limited tumor burden (2 metastases or fewer) have been reported as advantageous in LLR. Similarly, patients with tumors involving the inferior vena cava, left or right portal veins, roots of any of the hepatic veins, or patients with multifocal or bilobar tumors are not good candidates for a minimally invasive liver resection [23].

Timing of resection for synchronous liver metastases

Optimal surgical management of patients with synchronous CRLM is still controversial. There are three main types of surgical strategies for synchronous CRLM patients [24]. The first type involves removal of the primary colorectal tumor, followed by chemotherapy and – about 3–6 months later – with resection of LM as the final step (classic or bowel-first). The second type is synchronous resection of the primary tumor and LM in the same surgical procedure (combined). The third approach, commonly termed as the reverse or liver first approach, involves liver metastasis (LM) resection as the first step, followed by chemo(radio) therapy, and removal of the primary tumor as the last step. The classical approach and the liver-first approach are both two-stage surgical procedures. In 2018, data from 1830 patients who lived in the United Kingdom showed that the percentages of patients who underwent the classical approach, the simultaneous approach, and the liver-first approach were 71.1%, 14.8%, and 14.2%, respectively [25].

There are no significant differences in the outcomes between these three approaches in patients with synchronous CRLM [25]. The current evidence is insufficient to decide upon the optimal strategy for a given patient with synchronous CRLM. The timing of the resection and the type of surgical approach should be based on patient characteristics and the protocols followed by individual centers. Individualized treatment should be offered by a multidisciplinary team after discussing the risks and benefits of each approach with the patient. We prefer concurrent surgery for eligible patients. Otherwise, we choose the classical approach or the liver-first approach based on the severity of the primary tumor and LM. In patients treated with neoCTx, there are chances of chemotherapy-related liver injury after receiving chemotherapeutic drugs. Hence, LR should be scheduled at 4–6 wk after the last day of conventional chemotherapy, or 7–8 wk after the last day of bevacizumab-based chemotherapy [26,27].

A wide RM (>1 cm) should be attempted whenever possible. LR should not be precluded if narrower margins are anticipated in patients with multiple lesions, or when resection borders are limited due to major vascular-biliary structures, since a submillimeter tumor-free margin may also improve survival [28].

Laparoscopic major (right/left) hepatic resection [29]

The patient is placed in a supine position with split legs. The table is usually kept in a reverse Trendelenberg's position with tilt maneuverability. The operating surgeon stands between the legs of the patient, while the camera surgeon stands on the right and the staff nurse on the left of the patient. The assistant surgeon changes his/her position according to need. The monitor is kept at the head end of the patient. The closed technique of creating pneumoperitoneum is achieved using a Veress needle. The camera port is placed above the umbilicus and toward the right of the midline. The right-hand working port (12 mm) is placed in the epigastric region and the left-hand working port (5 mm) is placed in the right mid-clavicular line, about 2 cm below the costal margin. Additionally, two more retraction ports (5 mm) are placed, one in the right anterior axillary line and the other in the left para-rectal line midway between the epigastric and supra-umbilical ports. Port placement is shown in Figure 28.1. The insufflation pressure is kept at 14 mmHg.

After thorough survey of the peritoneal cavity for signs of unresectable disease, we proceed with hepatic resection. We use a modified anterior approach. First, the falciform and round ligaments are divided using a harmonic scalpel (Ethicon endo-surgery, Cincinnati, USA) or ligasure (Valleylab, Boulder, CO). Separation of the falciform ligament from the anterior abdominal wall is extended cranially to expose the suprahepatic, infra-dia-phragmatic inferior vena cava (IVC). The divided end of the round ligament is then used to give cranial traction on the liver so that the porta hepatis and inferior surface of liver become clearly visible. The triangular and the coronary ligaments of the concerned side are divided last, after parenchymal transection and division of the hepatic veins. This maneuver of dividing these ligaments

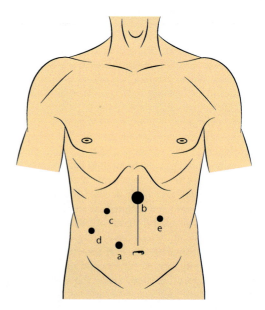

FIGURE 28.1 Port placement: a. Camera port (10 mm) supra-umbilical slightly on right side, b. Right-hand working port (12 mm) in epigastric region, c. Left-hand working port (5 mm) in right mid-clavicular line about 2 cm below the costal margin, d. Retraction port (5 mm) in right anterior axillary line, and e. Retraction port in left para-rectal line midway between epigastric and supra-umbilical ports.

helps in providing the necessary countertraction and support to the liver during the parenchymal division.

The next step is inflow control, which is achieved by the porta hepatis dissection. The liver is cranially retracted, and the porta can be clearly made out. Sometimes, downward retraction of the duodenum is necessary to have proper exposure of the porta. The peritoneal reflection along the free border of the lesser omentum is incised and dissected so as to expose the common bile duct, portal vein, and hepatic artery. The cystic duct and artery are dissected in the Calot's triangle, clipped, and divided. The divided gall bladder is then used to retract the liver cranially. As the dissection proceeds toward the hilum, the right and left branches of the portal vein and hepatic artery are identified. We generally follow extrahepatic dissection to achieve inflow control. The concerned hepatic artery is divided first after ligating it doubly with silk suture or applying plastic locking clips (Hem-o-lok; Teleflex Medical, Research Triangle Park, NC) (Figure 28.2). Next, the portal vein branch is dissected and divided using a vascular stapler (white cartridge, Endo GIA, Covidien, Mansfield, MA; Echelon Endopath Stapler, Ethicon Endo-Surgery). Alternately, if there is no space to apply the stapler, we ligate the portal vein branch doubly, using silk suture, and then divide it (Figure 28.3). Concerned hepatic duct branches are divided during the parenchymal transaction. Branches to caudate lobe are carefully

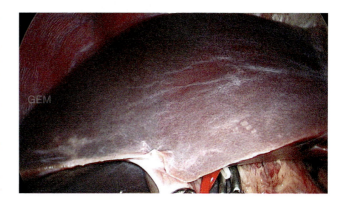

FIGURE 28.4 Demarcation becomes visible on the liver surface once portal supply is divided.

identified and preserved. Once the portal supply is divided, color changes become visible on the liver surface (Figure 28.4). At this stage, we reduce the insufflation pressure to 8–10 mmHg to minimize the risk of gas embolism.

The transection line is marked along the liver capsule with monopolar diathermy or a harmonic scalpel. After placing stay sutures on either side of the transection line along the inferior border of the liver for retraction, the liver parenchyma is divided for depth at 5–10 mm using a harmonic scalpel. For further parenchymal transection, we use laparoscopic CUSA with bipolar diathermy and ultrasonic shears. Vascular and biliary structures more than 3 mm are ligated applying titanium clips. In this way, the parenchyma is divided along the entire plane from the caudal to cranial and from anterior to posterior direction. The posterior Glisson's capsule is now divided along the anterior surface of the vena cava while systematically clipping and dividing the small bridging veins.

As the parenchymal division reaches the posterior surface of the liver, the major hepatic veins are encountered. Once the hepatic vein that is to be divided is visualized, it is dissected out clearly and its junction with IVC is identified. A vascular stapler is used to divide the hepatic vein concerned (Figure 28.5).

Finally, the triangular and coronary ligaments and diaphragmatic attachments are divided to complete the resection. The specimen is placed in a protective plastic retrieval bag and removed via a Pfannenstiel incision. The fascial layers are reapproximated, the pneumoperitoneum is reintroduced, and the operative site is lavaged and examined for hemostasis and biliary tract integrity. A closed drainage tube is placed in the Morrison's space, and the ports are closed.

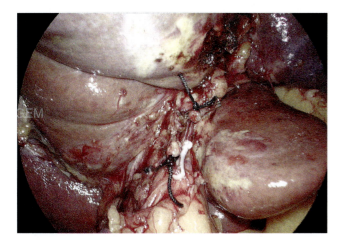

FIGURE 28.2 Left hepatic artery divided after ligating with silk suture and applying Hem-o-lok clip during left hepatectomy.

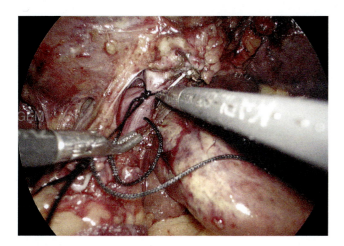

FIGURE 28.3 Left branch of the portal vein double ligated and divided during a left hepatectomy.

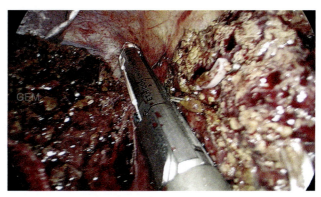

FIGURE 28.5 Left hepatic vein divided at the end of parenchymal transection using a vascular stapler.

We selectively use the Pringle maneuver to control blood flow to the liver, and we have used selective extra-glissonian pedicle clamping with a laparoscopic bulldog clamp for bleeding control. Postoperatively, all patients were monitored in the ICU. Oral fluids were started after return of bowel activity, usually on first postoperative day and solids on next day. Liver enzymes, bilirubin, and coagulation parameters were accessed on a daily basis. The drain was removed once output became minimal and nature becoming serous.

Laparoscopic left lateral sectionectomy

Removal of the anatomical left lobe segments (segments II and III) is far easier when compared to major resections such as right or left hepatectomies. The port positions are the same except that they are placed more on the left side. The round and falciform ligaments are divided. Pedicles to the segments II and III can be ligated either at the umbilical fissure or during parenchymal transection. The plane of division is along the line of attachment of the falciform ligament to the liver surface. Towards the end of parenchymal splitting, the left hepatic vein is encountered, which is divided using a vascular stapler. The division of parenchyma should end anterior to the caudate lobe. Finally, the left triangular ligament is divided and the specimen is retrieved.

Laparoscopic segmentectomies/ Nonanatomical resections

Tumors which are small and limited to a particular segment can be dealt with segmentectomy alone or nonanatomical resections, provided the margin is adequate. The segments II, III, IV, V, and VI can be easily accessed by laparoscopy while segments I, VII, and VIII are difficult to access. The principles governing these resections are the same as those of major hepatic resections. A laparoscopic ultrasound probe is used to identify the pedicles and plane of division. For left lobe segmentectomies (II, III, and IV) the falciform and round ligaments are divided and the undersurface of the liver is exposed. The pedicles can be ligated at the umbilical fissure or during the parenchymal division. As the parenchymal transection is proceeding, the corresponding hepatic vein branches of that particular segment are divided while preserving the major hepatic vein and other branches. For segment V resection, the parenchymal division is started at the anterior surface of the liver exactly at the Cantlie's line, and the right extent of the resection is at the right portal scissura. During resection, both middle and right hepatic veins should be preserved. Segment VI resection is performed with a left lateral tilt.

Radiofrequency ablation

RF ablation may be suitable for selected patients with an LM of less than 3 cm, tumors located deep in the liver parenchyma, patients with a high ASA score, or cardiopulmonary comorbidities. Furthermore, the heat-sink effect should be taken into consideration while treating LM located near vessels, as the size of the ablation zone is affected by the flow rate and the distance from the vessels [30].

Management of unresectable liver metastasis

The definition of unresectable CRLM is not widely recognized at this moment. In 2013, Takahashi and colleagues proposed a definition of unresectability as follows: multiple bilobar LM that require resection of more than 70% of the nontumorous liver for removal of all tumors leading to an inadequate FLR, tumors invading all three hepatic veins, tumors invading both the left and right branches of the hepatic artery or portal vein, and extrahepatic metastasis other than resectable pulmonary metastasis [31].

Tumor shrinkage and FLR hypertrophy are the two most-widely used approaches for converting unresectable CRLM to resectable disease. This can be achieved by a variety of modalities like chemotherapeutic and targeted biological agents (conversion chemotherapy), portal vein embolization (PVE), portal vein ligation (PVL), and ALPPS (associating liver partition and portal vein ligation for staged hepatectomy can help achieve FLR hypertrophy).

Liver transplantation (LT) for unresectable CRLM is gaining popularity with a 5-year OS rates reportedly reaching more than 50% in appropriately selected patients. With shortage of grafts and lots of ethical issues involved, defining the patient population that would benefit the most from liver transplantation is crucial. Selection strategies should be based on prognostic factors found to be favorable for survival: diameter of the largest CLM <55 mm, time interval of >2 years between colorectal and transplant operations, preliver transplantation carcinoembryonic antigen level <80 ng/mL, and responsive or stable disease under chemotherapy [32]. Further studies are needed to refine the risk stratification and optimize patient selection.

Outcomes of laparoscopic resection for CRLM

Compared to an open approach, benefits of LLR include decreased major and pulmonary complication rates, reduced intraoperative blood loss, and shorter hospital stay. So far, the laparoscopic approach has been described for most liver resections with respect to oncological principles, and has also been associated with a decreased morbidity and mortality in the elderly [33].

Laparoscopic LR (LLR), characterized by 'less invasiveness', is becoming increasingly popular for the treatment of primary and metastatic liver malignancies. The Oslo-Comet RCT compared laparoscopic and open LR for CRLM, and revealed that LLR was associated with a significantly lower postoperative complication rate (19% vs. 31%, $P = 0.021$), a shorter hospital stay (56 h vs. 96 h, $P < 0.001$), and a higher cost-efficiency; whereas there were no differences in the blood loss, operative time, resection margins, or 90-d mortality [34]. A recent meta-analysis demonstrated that a limited number (two or fewer) of metastases located in the left lateral segments are more suitable for LLR [23]. Moreover, the initial LLR for CRLM was associated with less inflammation, surgical stress, and postoperative adhesion, allowing a higher chance of repeated hepatectomies if recurrence occurred [35]. Concerning the technical difficulties and narrow operative field exposure, LLR was adopted less frequently for a major hepatectomy, but it was only attempted by a few specialized centers with a high volume of patients [36].

The da Vinci surgical system, also known as robot-assisted LR, is believed to overcome the disadvantages of a laparoscopy [37]. Robot-assisted LR is performed through a series of flexible mechanical arms, allowing more degrees of freedom, which can effectively avoid the 'fulcrum effect' caused by rigid laparoscopic instruments. What's more, the robotic approach makes the surgical procedure more precise by providing 3D vision and avoiding hand tremors. Therefore, robot-assisted LR can be used in narrow spaces or curved transections, and it is particularly suitable for the handling of metastases located in the posterior-superior segments [38]. Standard laparoscopy or robot-assisted LR for minor LRs can be performed with favorable perioperative

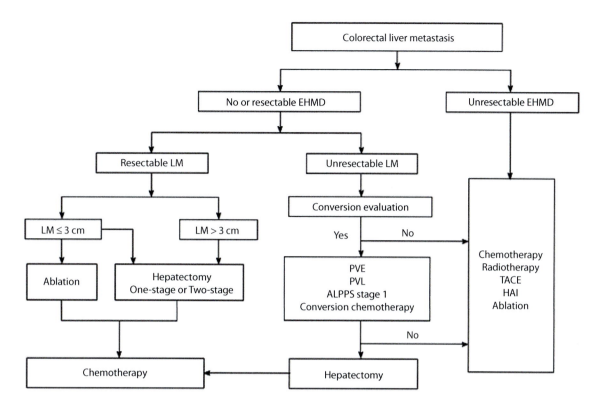

and long-term outcomes. Nevertheless, the robotic approach offers more benefits for a major hepatectomy and challenging cases [39].

Management flowchart for colorectal liver metastases [28]

EHMD: Extra-hepatic metastatic disease; LM: Liver metastases; PVE: Portal vein embolization; PVL: Portal venous ligation; ALPPS: Associated liver partition and PVL for staged hepatectomy; TACE: Transarterial chemoembolization; HAI: Hepatic artery infusion.

Summary

Management of CRLM is still a major challenge and requires multimodality treatment. Surgical resection with clear margins offers the best outcomes and has survival benefits even in the presence of resectable pulmonary metastasis. Laparoscopic and robotic surgery are feasible and safe for most lesions, and have comparable oncological outcomes to open surgery while they can be combined with primary tumor resection in synchronous lesions, offering benefits to patients in terms of early recovery and decreased morbidity.

Key points

- Resection for CRLM even in the presence of resectable extrahepatic metastatic disease offers survival benefits.
- Evaluation of resectability is done by a 3D Contrast Enhanced CT with volumetry and PET/CT.
- Laparoscopic resection is feasible and safe for most liver resections with respect to oncological principles, and

has also been associated with a decreased morbidity and mortality.
- Robotic surgery has expanded the use for major resections for postero-superiorly placed lesions.
- Conversion therapy can be attempted for unresectable disease using conversion chemotherapy, PVE, PVL, or ALPPS.

References

1. Ferlay J, Soerjomataram I, Dikshit R, Eser S, Mathers C, Rebelo M, Parkin DM, Forman D, Bray F. Cancer incidence and mortality worldwide: Sources, methods and major patterns in GLOBOCAN 2012. *Int J Cancer* 2015;136: E359–86.
2. Kemeny N. The management of resectable and unresectable liver metastases from colorectal cancer. *Curr Opin Oncol* 2010;22: 364–73.
3. Lupinacci RM, Andraus W, De Paiva Haddad LB, Carneiro D' Albuquerque LA, Herman P. Simultaneous laparoscopic resection of primary colorectal cancer and associated liver metastases: A systematic review. *Tech Coloproctol* 2014;18:129–35.
4. Chakedis J, Squires MH, Beal EW, Hughes T, Lewis H, Paredes A, Al-Mansour M, Sun S, Cloyd JM, Pawlik TM. Update on current problems in colorectal liver metastasis. *Curr Probl Surg* 2017;54:554–602.
5. Line PD, Hagness M, Dueland S. The Potential Role of Liver Transplantation as a Treatment Option in Colorectal Liver Metastases. *Can J Gastroenterol Hepatol* 2018;2018:8547940.
6. Hof J, Wertenbroek MW, Peeters PM, Widder J, Sieders E, de Jong KP. Outcomes after resection and/or radiofrequency ablation for recurrence after treatment of colorectal liver metastases. *Br J Surg* 2016;103:1055–62.
7. Choi SH, Kim SY, Park SH, Kim KW, Lee JY, Lee SS, Lee MG. Diagnostic performance of CT, gadoxetate disodium-enhanced MRI, and PET/CT for the diagnosis of colorectal liver metastasis: Systematic review and meta-analysis. *J Magn Reson Imaging* 2018;47:1237–50.

8. Ko Y, Kim J, Park JK, Kim H, Cho JY, Kang SB, Ahn S, Lee KJ, Lee KH. Limited detection of small (≤10 mm) colorectal liver metastasis at preoperative CT in patients undergoing liver resection. *PLOS ONE* 2017;12:e0189797.

9. Expert Panel on Gastrointestinal Imaging, Fowler KJ, Kaur H, Cash BD et al. ACR Appropriateness Criteria® Pretreatment Staging of Colorectal Cancer. *J Am Coll Radiol* 2017;14:S234–44.

10. Martel G, Cieslak KP, Huang R, van Lienden KP, Wiggers JK, Belblidia A, Dagenais M, Lapointe R, van Gulik TM, Vandenbroucke- Menu F. Comparison of techniques for volumetric analysis of the future liver remnant: Implications for major hepatic resections. *HPB (Oxford)* 2015;17:1051–7.

11. Pulitano C, Crawford M, Joseph D, Aldrighetti L, Sandroussi C. Preoperative assessment of postoperative liver function: The importance of residual liver volume. *J Surg Oncol* 2014;110:445–50.

12. Simpson AL, Geller DA, Hemming AW et al. Liver planning software accurately predicts postoperative liver volume and measures early regeneration. *J Am Coll Surg* 2014;219:199–207.

13. Shindoh J, Tzeng CW, Aloia TA et al. Optimal future liver remnant in patients treated with extensive preoperative chemotherapy for colorectal liver metastases. *Ann Surg Oncol* 2013;20:2493–500.

14. Takamoto T, Hashimoto T, Ichida A, Shimada K, Maruyama Y, Makuuchi M. Surgical Strategy Based on Indocyanine Green Test for Chemotherapy-Associated Liver Injury and Long-Term Outcome in Colorectal Liver Metastases. *J Gastrointest Surg* 2018;22:1077–88.

15. Boogerd LS, Handgraaf HJ, Lam HD, Huurman VA, Farina-Sarraqueta A, Frangioni JV, van de Velde CJ, Braat AE, Vahrmeijer AL. Laparoscopic detection and resection of occult liver tumors of multiple cancer types using real-time near-infrared fluorescence guidance. *Surg Endosc* 2017;31:952–61.

16. Viganò L, Lopci E, Costa G, Rodari M, Poretti D, Pedicini V, Solbiati L, Chiti A, Torzilli G. Positron Emission Tomography-Computed Tomography for Patients with Recurrent Colorectal Liver Metastases: Impact on Restaging and Treatment Planning. *Ann Surg Oncol* 2017;24:1029–36.

17. Scheele J, Altendorf-Hofmann A. Resection of colorectal liver metastases. *Langenbecks Arch Surg* 1999;384:313–27.

18. Luo D, Liu Q, Yu W, Ma Y, Zhu J, Lian P, Cai S, Li Q, Li X. Prognostic value of distant metastasis sites and surgery in stage IV colorectal cancer: A population-based study. *Int J Colorectal Dis* 2018;33:1241–9.

19. Creasy JM, Sadot E, Koerkamp BG et al. Actual 10-year survival after hepatic resection of colorectal liver metastases: What factors preclude cure? *Surgery* 2018;163:1238–44

20. Leung U, Gönen M, Allen PJ, Kingham TP, DeMatteo RP, Jarnagin WR, D'Angelica MI. Colorectal Cancer Liver Metastases and Concurrent Extrahepatic Disease Treated With Resection. *Ann Surg* 2017;265:158–65.

21. Imai K, Castro Benitez C, Allard MA, Vibert E, Sa Cunha A, Cherqui D, Castaing D, Bismuth H, Baba H, Adam R. Potential of a cure in patients with colorectal liver metastases and concomitant extrahepatic disease. *J Surg Oncol* 2017;115:488–96.

22. Abdalla EK, Vauthey JN, Ellis LM et al. Recurrence and outcomes following hepatic resection, radiofrequency ablation, and combined resection/ablation for colorectal liver metastases. *Ann Surg*;239:818–25.

23. Xie SM, Xiong JJ, Liu XT et al. Laparoscopic Versus open liver resection for colorectal liver metastases: A comprehensive systematic review and Metaanalysis. *Sci Rep* 2017;7:1012.

24. Ihnát P, Vávra P, Zonča P. Treatment strategies for colorectal carcinoma with synchronous liver metastases: Which way to go? *World J Gastroenterol* 2015;21:7014–21.

25. Vallance AE, van der Meulen J, Kuryba A, Charman SC, Botterill ID, Prasad KR, Hill J, Jayne DG, Walker K. The timing of liver resection in patients with colorectal cancer and synchronous liver metastases: A population-based study of current practice and survival. *Colorectal Dis* 2018;20:486–95.

26. Berardi G, De Man M, Laurent S et al. Radiologic and pathologic response to neoadjuvant chemotherapy predicts survival in patients undergoing the liver-first approach for synchronous colorectal liver metastases. *Eur J Surg Oncol* 2018;44:1069–77.

27. Lim C, Doussot A, Osseis M, Esposito F, Salloum C, Calderaro J, Tournigand C, Azoulay D. Bevacizumab improves survival in Surgery for colorectal liver metastases patients with synchronous colorectal liver metastases provided the primary tumor is resected first. *Clin Transl Oncol* 2018;20:1274–9.

28. Xu F, Tang B, Jin TQ, Dai CL. Current status of surgical treatment of colorectal liver metastases. *World J Clin Cases*. 2018 Nov 26;6(14):716–34.

29. Palanisamy S, Sabnis SC, Patel ND, Nalankilli VP, Vijai A, Palanivelu P, Ramkrishnan P, Chinnusamy P. Laparoscopic Major Hepatectomy-Technique and Outcomes. *J Gastrointest Surg*. 2015 Dec;19(12):2215–22.

30. Ringe KI, Lutat C, Rieder C, Schenk A, Wacker F, Raatschen HJ. Experimental Evaluation of the Heat Sink Effect in Hepatic Microwave Ablation. *PLOS ONE* 2015;10:e0134301.

31. Takahashi S, Konishi M, Kinoshita T, Gotohda N, Kato Y, Saito N, Sugito M, Yoshino T. Predictors for early recurrence after hepatectomy for initially unresectable colorectal liver metastasis. *J Gastrointest Surg* 2013;17:939–48.

32. Hagness M, Foss A, Line PD et al. Liver transplantation for nonresectable liver metastases from colorectal cancer. *Ann Surg* 2013;257:800–6.

33. Zarzavadjian Le Bian A, Tabchouri N, Bennamoun M et al. Fuks D After laparoscopic liver resection for colorectal liver metastases, age does not influence morbi-mortality. *Surg Endosc*. 2019 Nov;33(11):3704–10.

34. Fretland ÅA, Dagenborg VJ, Bjørnelv GMW et al. Laparoscopic Versus Open Resection for Colorectal Liver Metastases: The OSLO-COMET Randomized Controlled Trial. *Ann Surg* 2018;267:199–207.

35. Montalti R, Berardi G, Laurent S et al. Laparoscopic liver resection compared to open approach in patients with colorectal liver metastases improves further resectability: Oncological outcomes of a case-control matched-pairs analysis. *Eur J Surg Oncol* 2014;40:536–44.

36. Di Fabio F, Barkhatov L, Bonadio I, Dimovska E, Fretland ÅA, Pearce NW, Troisi RI, Edwin B, Abu Hilal M. The impact of laparoscopic versus open colorectal cancer surgery on subsequent laparoscopic resection of liver metastases: A multicenter study. *Surgery* 2015;157:1046–54.

37. Efanov M, Alikhanov R, Tsvirkun V, Kazakov I, Melekhina O, Kim P, Vankovich A, Grendal K, Berelavichus S, Khatkov I. Comparative analysis of learning curve in complex robot-assisted and laparoscopic liver resection. *HPB (Oxford)* 2017;19:818–24.

38. Nota CLMA, Molenaar IQ, van Hillegersberg R, Borel Rinkes IHM, Hagendoorn J. Robotic liver resection including the posterosuperior segments: Initial experience. *J Surg Res* 2016;206:133–8.

39. Wang WH, Kuo KK, Wang SN, Lee KT. Oncological and surgical result of hepatoma after robot surgery. *Surg Endosc* 2018;32:3918–24.

Chapter 29

SPECIMEN RETRIEVAL AFTER LAPAROSCOPIC COLECTOMY AND NOSE

Deep Goel, Ravindra Vats, Luv Gupta, Vipin Pal Singh, and Virandera Pal Bhalla

Contents

Learning objectives 185
Introduction 185
Mini-laparotomy or convenient incision 185
Criteria for site selection 185
Transabdominal 186
    BMI 186
    Type of incisions for retrieval 186
Issues with mini-laparotomies 186
NOSE 186
Background 186
Selection factors for NOSE 186
    Patient factors 186
        BMI 186
        Sex 187
    Anatomic location 187
    Specimen factors 187
Other potential factors 187
Summary 187
Key points 187
Video 187
References 187

Learning objectives

- Importance of specimen extraction after laparoscopic colonic resection
- Transabdominal mini-laparotomy for specimen extraction
- NOSE
    - Patient selection
    - Choosing transvaginal or transrectal route

Introduction

The first laparoscopic assisted colonic resection was described by Jacobs in 1991 [1]. Since then laparoscopic colonic resection is a preferred technique for both benign and malignant colorectal conditions [2]. Early in the development of laparoscopic colectomy for carcinoma, port-site metastasis was a major concern [3]. Presently, however, we know that the port-site metastasis incidence is 1%, which is the same as the incidence of incision site deposits following a laparotomy. The incision made on the abdomen for specimen retrieval, following laparoscopic colectomy, presents a challenge for the operating surgeon, who desires to keep the incision as small as possible in order to minimize postop morbidities such as pain, prolonged hospital stay, incisional hernia, surgical site infection, dissemination of tumor cells, and implantation of tumor cells in the wound [5]. Natural orifice specimen extraction (NOSE) is another [4] technique to extract specimens via a natural orifice that already communicates with the outside world such as the vagina or the rectum. This technique avoids mini-laparotomies, and there is an expectation that this may improve outcomes.

Currently, there is no standardized retrieval technique. Different types of incision are being used for specimen retrieval. All have their advantages and disadvantages.

Mini-laparotomy or convenient incision

Site of mini-laparotomy will depend upon the type of laparoscopic surgery:

a. *Total laparoscopic colo rectal surgery (TLCR):* Here mobilization, vascular ligation, and resection anastomosis are done completely intracorporeally.
b. *Laparoscopic assisted surgeries (LAS):* Mobilization is laparoscopic but vascular ligation and resection anastomosis are done through a most convenient incision.
c. *Hand-assisted laparoscopic surgery (HALS):* Mini-laparotomy is made for 'hand port' at some point to facilitate dissection and the rest of the procedure, and same incision is used to complete the procedure and specimen extraction.

Criteria for site selection (Table 29.1)

TABLE 29.1: Classification of Specimen Retrieval Sites

Transabdominal (Figure 29.1)	NOSE	Perineal
Pfannensteil incision	Transanal only in TLCR	Only in APR
Midline incision (peri umbilical)	Transvaginal only in TLCR	
Transverse incision (right/left iliac fossa)		
Stoma sites (ileostomy/ colectomy)		

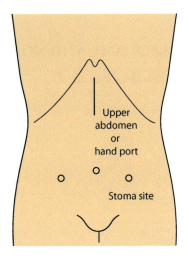 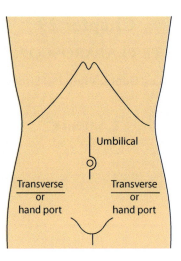 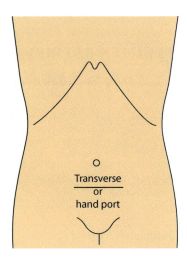

FIGURE 29.1 Different incisions for transabdominal specimen retrieval.

Transabdominal

BMI
- BMI is considered a significant factor; patients with higher BMI (male >30 kg/m² and females >35 kg/m²) are considered for transabdominal specimen extraction [6].

Type of incisions for retrieval
- If one is doing a total laparoscopic procedure and incision is required for only specimen extraction, then one can enlarge one of the port sites, or can use a separate suprapubic Pfannenstiel incision.
- In LAS, incision site is influenced by the type of colectomy. For right hemicolectomy the incision is made in upper abdomen as ileo-transverse anastomosis may be easy to perform through this route, and similarly for an anterior resection a suprapubic incision may be a better option.
- In hand-assisted laparoscopic surgery the hand port must be situated in a place where it will not obscure endo-vision and is generally placed away from midline. This site can be utilized for specimen extraction.
- One has to consider whether a stoma is required or not, because extraction can be done via the stoma site; however, this is associated with a higher incidence of parastomal hernias [7].

Issues with mini-laparotomies

1. *Incisional Hernia*: Incidence of incisional hernia is highest in midline (periumbilical) and least in supra-pubic (Pfannenstiel incision) [8,9]. The order is midline > stomal > transverse > suprapubic.
2. *Surgical site infection (SSI)*: Incidence of SSI is equal in all types of incisions [10].
3. Pain [11].
4. Prolonged hospital stay [10].
5. Extraction site metastasis [2,3].

NOSE

NOSE is an innovative technique which complements the cosmetic outcome of laparoscopic colonic resection.

Background

- Extraction of a colectomy specimen through the vagina was first reported in 1991 by Stewart et al. [4] for colonic leiomyosarcoma. The vaginotomy, also called posterior colpotomy, is a safe technique commonly employed by gynecologists [12]. A more recent series of right colectomies with NOSE via the vagina was described by Franklin et al. in 2013 [13]. This technique has been successfully used for specimen extraction operations for inflammatory bowel disease, diverticulitis, and malignancy.
- The first report of a colectomy specimen extracted through the anus was described in 1993 by Franklin et al. [14]. There have been many documented cases in which either the colon [15], rectum [13], anus [16], or vagina [4] has been used to remove both malignant and benign pathology.
- Technical difficulty is a barrier to the wider adoption of NOSE. Intracorporeal suturing and anastomosis skills are a prerequisite for those adopting NOSE. Removal of more proximal specimens, as in a right colectomy, requires the presence of a skilled endoscopist who can snare and pull the specimen endoluminaly. Furthermore, nonfamiliarity of surgeons with posterior colpotomy is another challenge preventing the more widespread acceptance of this route of specimen extraction.
- Randomized controlled trials and other large series now demonstrate some benefits of NOSE compared to conventional specimen extraction, particularly regarding postoperative analgesic use, time to first bowel function, cosmesis, and length of hospital stay [17,18]. Technical feasibility of this technique relies upon careful patient selection.

Selection factors for NOSE

Patient factors
Anatomical location
Specimen factors

Patient factors
BMI
Increased BMI is associated with increased visceral fat [19], which may be associated with considerable specimen bulk. Many series identified higher BMI as a main factor for NOSE failure and lower BMI (<30 kg/m²) as favorable factor [20,21].

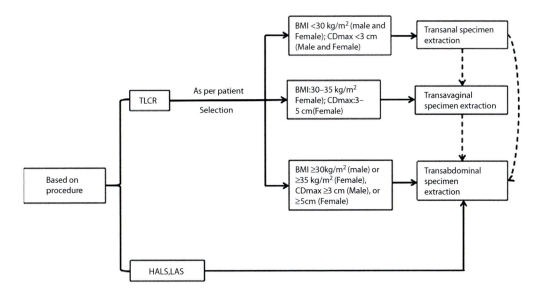

FIGURE 29.2   Algorithm for specimen extraction.

Sex

It is technically easier to extract the specimen transvaginally, through a posterior colpotomy, than via the anus. Karagul et al. [22] published a report in which 12 of 15 women who failed NOSE via the anus were able to have successful NOSE via the vagina.

The shape and anatomy of the pelvis differ between male and female. Pelvic geometry has however not been mentioned as a reason for NOSE failure (18). When transanal NOSE is compared between male and female, the success rate is similar in both. Most of the literature comparing these are in patients with a BMI <30 kg/m². It is possible that pelvic geometry becomes a more significant factor for patients with higher BMI.

Anatomic location

Distal lesions are most amendable to successful NOSE. As distance of the specimen from the anal verge increases, NOSE – via the transanal route – becomes more technically difficult. In right-sided colon pathology, many series have addressed this issue by removing the specimen transvaginally [22], this option is obviously available only in females.

Specimen factors

Specimen factors such as size and shape are also important in determining feasibility of successful NOSE [22,23], these factors can be determined preoperatively based on imaging investigations and on actual findings at surgery.

Other potential factors

a. History of prior operations.
b. Radiation exposure.
c. Coagulopathy has been set as an exclusion criterion in some NOSE colorectal studies. This should be considered as there is a reported rate of postoperative intraluminal hemorrhage of 4.5% [20] and intraperitoneal hemorrhage of 1.5%–3.7% [12].

Summary

Specimen retrieval can be done via the transabdominal or NOSE route, depending upon the type of procedure performed, and patient selection and specimen criteria. An algorithm for the same is shown in Figure 29.2 [24]. No single route can be considered ideal for specimen retrieval.

Key points

- Among transabdominal approaches, Pfannenstiel seems to be better in view of reduced chances of hernia and better cosmesis.
- Incidence of SSI among different transabdominal routes is equal.
- Preoperative maximum circumferential diameter of specimen (CD max) [24] and BMI should be calculated before planning for NOSE.
- Intracorporeal suturing and anastomosis skills are a must for performing NOSE.

See Video 29.

VIDEO 29   https://youtu.be/Gc5QetZBSA4

Specimen Extraction – Trans-abdominal and Natural Orifice.

References

1. Jacobs M, Verdeja JC, Goldstein HS. Minimally invasive colon resection (laparoscopic colectomy). *Surg Laparosc Endosc* 1991;1:144–150.
2. Jayne DG, Thorpe HC, Copeland J et al. Five-year follow-up of the Medical Research Council CLASICC trial of laparoscopically assisted versus open surgery for colorectal cancer. *Br J Surg* 2010;97(11):1638–45.
3. Berends FJ, Kazemier G, Bonjier HJ, Lange JF. Subcutaneous metastases after laparoscopic colectomy. *Lancet* 1994;344:58.
4. Stewert EA, Liau AS, Friedman AJ. Operative laparoscopy followed by colpotomy for resecting a colonic leiomyosarcoma: A case report. *J Reprod Med* 1991;36(12):883–884.

5. Buunen M, Veldkamp R, Hop WC et al. Survival after laparoscopic surgery versus open surgery for colon cancer: Long-term outcome of a randomised clinical trial. *Lancet Oncol* 2009;10(1):44–52.

6. Izquierdo KM, Unal E, Marks JH. Natural orifice specimen extraction in colorectal surgery: Patient selection and perspectivesm. *Clin Exp Gastroenterol* 2018 Jul 24;11:265–279.

7. Li, Wanglin, Benlice, Cigdem, Luca Stocchi et al. Does stoma site specimen extraction increase postoperative ileostomy complication rates?. *Surg Endosc* 2017;31:3552–3558.

8. Singh R, Omiccioli A, Hegge S et al. Does the extraction-site location in laparoscopic colorectal surgery have an impact on incisional hernia rates? *Surg Endsoc* 2008; 22:1596–2600.

9. Ihedioha U, Mackay G, Leung E et al. Laparoscopic colorectal resection does not reduce incisional hernia rates when compared with open colorectal resection. *Surg Endosc* 2008;22(3):689–692.

10. Winslow ER, Fleshman JW, Birnbaum EH et al. Wound complications of laparoscopic vs open colectomy. *Surg Endosc* 2002;16(10):1420–1425.

11. Kaminski JP, Pai A, Ailabouni L et al. Role of epidural and patient controlled analgesia in site-specific laparoscopic colorectal surgery. *JSLS* 2014;18(4):e2014.00207

12. Wolthuis AM, de Buck van Overstraeten A, D'Hoore A. Laparoscopic natural orifice specimen extraction-colectomy: A systematic review. *World J Gastroenterol* 2014;20(36):12981–12992.

13. Franklin ME Jr, Liang S, Russek K. Natural orifice specimen extraction in laparoscopic colorectal surgery: Transanal and transvaginal approaches. *Tech Coloprocto* 2013;17(Suppl 1):563–567.

14. Franklin ME Jr, Ramos R, Rosenthal D et al. Laparoscopic colonic procedures. *World J Surg* 1993;17(1):51–56.

15. Eshuis EJ, Voermans RP, Stokkers PC et al. Laparoscopic resection with transcolonic specimen extraction for ileocaecal Crohn's disease. *Br J Surg* 2010;97:569–574.

16. Marks J, Mizrahi B, Dalane S, Nweze I, Marks G. Laparoscopic transanal abdominal transanal resection with sphincter preservation for rectal cancer in the distal 3 cm of the rectum after neoadjuvant therapy. *Surg Endosc* 2010;24:2700–2707.

17. Wolthuis AM, Fieuws S, Van Den Bosch A et al. Randomized clinical trial of laparoscopic colectomy with or without natural-orifice specimen extraction. *Br J Surg* 2015;102(6):630–637.

18. Ma B, Huang XZ, Gao P et al. Laparoscopic resection with natural orifice specimen extraction versus conventional laparoscopy for colorectal disease: A meta-analysis. *Int J Colorectal Dis* 2015;30(11):1479–1488.

19. Camhi SM, Bray GA, Bouchard C et al. The relationship of waist circumference and BMI to visceral, subcutaneous, and total body fat: Sex and race differences. *Obesity (Silver Spring)* 2011;19(2):402–408.

20. Zhang X, Zhou H, Hou H et al. Totally laparoscopic resection with natural orifice specimen extraction for carcinoma of sigmoid colon and rectum: A feasible and innovative technique. *J Clin Gastroenterol* 2014;48(7):e57–e61.

21. Wolthuis AM, de Buck van Overstraeten A, Fieuws S, Boon K, D'Hoore A. Standardized laparoscopic NOSE-colectomy is feasible with low morbidity. *Surg Endosc* 2015;29(5):1167–1173.

22. Karagul S, Kayaalp C, Sumer F et al. Success rate of natural orifice specimen extraction after laparoscopic colorectal resections. *Tech Coloproctol* 2017;21(4):295–300.

23. Yagci MA, Kayaalp C, Novruzov NH. Intracorporeal mesenteric division of the colon can make the specimen more suitable for natural orifice specimen extraction. *J Laparoendosc Adv Surg Tech A.* 2014;24(7):484–486.

24. Guan CX, Zheng L, Antonio L et al. International consensus on natural orifice specimen extraction surgery (NOSES) for colorectal cancer. *Gastroenterology Report* 2019;7(1):24–31.

Section V
Robotic Colorectal Surgery

30 Robotic Colonic Cancer Surgery 190
31 Robotic Rectal Cancer Surgery... 196

Chapter 30

ROBOTIC COLONIC CANCER SURGERY

Varun Madaan, Rigved Gupta, Supreet Kumar, and Deepak Govil

Contents

Learning objectives 190
Introduction 190
Equipment 190
General principles 191
Right hemicolectomy.. 191
Left and sigmoid colectomy 192
Transverse colectomy 194
Robotic colectomy in the era of complete mesocolic excision (CME) 194
Summary 195
Key points 195
References 195

Learning objectives

- Learn the basic principles of robotic colonic surgery
- Know advantages and limitations of robotic colorectal surgery
- Compare the results of conventional laparoscopic and robotic colonic surgery
- Analyze its impact on the treatment of colorectal cancer

Introduction

A laparoscopic approach for colorectal resections has been used for many years with favorable outcomes compared to an open approach. Technical advancements have enabled colorectal surgeons to use laparoscopy for complex colorectal resections safely with shorter hospital stay and lower peri-operative morbidity. However, despite the favorable results, the number of laparoscopic colorectal resections performed overall remains low compared to laparotomy. The prime reason for this is the longer learning curve and extensive training often required before one can proceed with advanced laparoscopic procedures such as colorectal resections. Robotic surgery has been proposed as a feasible and safe alternative to laparoscopic colorectal surgery with the advantages of a favorable learning curve with improved vision and superior dissection at the difficult anatomic sites, while providing the similar benefits of minimal access surgery as laparoscopy.

Minimal access surgery with a laparoscopic approach has already been compared with the open technique for colonic surgery in various studies and randomized trials. The COST trial had shown faster postoperative recovery in terms of less postoperative hospital stay (5 vs. 6 d, $p < 0.001$), and less use of postoperative analgesia with laparoscopic surgery for colonic adenocarcinoma as compared to the open procedure. There were no differences in the oncological outcomes in terms of five-year overall survival (open: 74.6%, laparoscopic: 76.4%, $p = 0.93$), disease-free survival (open: 68.4%, laparoscopic: 69.2%, $p = 0.94$), and recurrence rates (open: 21.8%, laparoscopic: 19.4%, $p = 0.25$) [1,2]. Similarly, the COLOR trial has shown that laparoscopic colectomy was associated with earlier recovery of bowel function ($p = 0.0001$), the need for fewer analgesics, and a shorter hospital stay ($p = 0.0001$) compared to open colectomy at the cost of longer operating times for laparoscopic surgery. The oncological outcomes were comparable between the two groups [3,4].

As a modality for minimal access surgery, robotics were popularized during the last decade of twentieth century. Apart from urological, gynecological, and rectal surgery, robotic surgery has of late found a lot of applications in surgery for colonic diseases. The use of robotic surgery to perform colectomies has been described since 2002 [5]. Weber et al. had described the use and technique of robotic colonic surgery by publishing case reports of robotic-assisted sigmoid colectomy and robotic-assisted right hemicolectomy for benign diseases [5]. The robotic technique has been viewed as an approach to overcome the limitations of laparoscopic surgery. Robotic surgery offers an advantage with respect to operative dexterity, vision, and tissue handling as compared to a laparoscopic procedure. Robotic surgical systems with magnified high-definition 3D view and articulating instruments – with seven degrees of freedom of movement – help perform complex surgical procedures. The deterrents of robotic surgery have been the long operative time and loss of tactile feedback compared to open or laparoscopic procedures, and the need for multiple dockings in certain procedures like total colectomy. The operative time for most robotic colorectal surgeries has been in the range of 200–300 min [6]. It includes the docking time of up to 30 min in some cases, which can be substantially reduced with increasing case loads and experience. A large number of publications are showing the feasibility of robotics in colonic surgery. Robotic surgery has been compared to laparoscopic surgery in terms of operative time, blood loss, and complications with variable results.

Equipment

The Da Vinci™ surgical system is the only available robotic surgical system at present. It comes in the Si and the new Xi variants. The system consists of three parts:

1. Surgeon console
2. The patient cart
3. The vision cart

The surgeon sits on the surgeon console with 3D binoculars and a master controller for the operating instruments. The patient cart has four arms with especially designed articulating instruments and camera that are inserted inside abdominal cavity using adequate port placement. This patient cart is connected to the surgeon's console with multiple cables. The movements made by surgeon on the master controller are mitigated on the instruments at the patient cart to perform the various steps of the surgical procedure. The vision cart is a trolley that has an endovision camera controller, light source, insufflators, and a touch screen for the assistant and scrub nurse. The robotic arms are draped by sterile drapes and the patient cart is brought close to the operating table in alignment such that the camera, the target anatomy, and the central column of the patient cart lies in a straight line with the target anatomy in the center. The arms are then moved manually by using the buttons over the arms and are mounted on the adequately placed ports on the patient. This process is known as 'docking'. After docking, further movement of the patient cart is prohibited. The camera is inserted into the camera port through the camera arm and the instruments are then inserted into the ports under direct vision. The surgeon then starts the procedure by sitting on the console. Assistant surgeon and scrub nurse have two functions – one is help for retraction and suctioning and second is the help for changing instruments during the surgery. After completion of the surgery, or while changing the site of surgery, the patient cart is 'undocked'. In procedures like total colectomy, docking–undocking may be required multiple times.

General principles

1. General anesthesia in all cases
2. ERAS protocols are followed for preoperative preparation
3. Perioperative antibiotic coverage
4. Bowel preparation is given for most of the colorectal cases, as recommended by recent American Society of Colorectal Surgery guidelines [7]
5. Pneumoperitoneum is created either by an open technique or using a Veress needle
6. Careful tissue handling, avoiding excessive traction, sharp dissection, and meticulous hemostasis
7. Specimen is extracted by making a small Pfannensteil incision, or from the stoma site (if performed) after applying a wound protector, whenever required
8. Tension-free anastomosis at well-vascularized healthy bowel margins
9. Covering ileostomy is not done as a routine, and can be utilized on a case-by-case basis
10. Enteral feeding is started as early as the first postoperative day, depending upon the patient's recovery
11. Catheters, drains, and lines are kept to the minimum possible and are removed as early as possible postoperatively
12. DVT thrombo-prophylaxis is routinely added with low molecular weight heparin unless contraindicated
13. Early mobilization and early discharge

Right hemicolectomy

Position: Supine with arms by the side of the patient (Figure 30.1).
Port Placement: A 12-mm camera port in the periumbilical region and three 8-mm operating arms, as shown (Figure 30.2). An assistant port can be placed depending on the need of the surgeon (Figure 30.2).

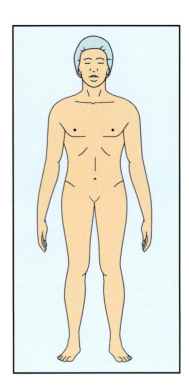

FIGURE 30.1 Patient position.

Docking: The robot can be brought in from either the right side of the patient, or from the upper-right abdomen depending on the surgeon's preference and the need for extensive transverse colon mobilization.

Procedure: Three robotic arms are used for traction and dissection. Depending upon the requirement, an assistant port can be placed for suctioning and application of clips and staplers. The right hemicolectomy proceeds as in a laparoscopic procedure. The ileocecal region is lifted and the ileocolic pedicle is skeletonized. The ileocolic artery and vein are clipped separately using

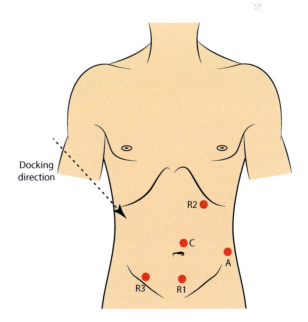

FIGURE 30.2 Port position for robotic right hemicolectomy.

hemolock clips and are divided. Clipping is done at the origin to follow the principle of central vessel ligation for oncological clearance in case of malignant disease. Then a medial to lateral mobilization of the ascending colon is performed. The right colic vessels, if encountered, are also clipped and divided in the same way. The hepatic flexure is mobilized after opening the lesser sac and careful dissection of the transverse mesocolon is achieved. Utmost care is required for proper identification of the duodenum and to avoid any injury to it. The right branch of the middle colic pedicle is clipped and divided. The right colon is lifted from the retroperitoneum using principles of complete mesocolic excision. The margins of resection of the bowel are then marked and divided. The proximal margin is at 10 cm proximal to ileocaecal junction and the distal margin at proximal one-third of the transverse colon. Vascular perfusion of the divided ends can be checked using intraoperative intravenous injection of the indocyanine green dye and visualization of fluorescence under near-infrared light. The ileocolic anastomosis can be performed either intracorporeally or extracorporeally using staplers. With the help of 3D vision, important structures like the right ureter, the duodenum, and the pancreatic head can be visualized and protected, despite the lack of tactile feedback [8].

Results: Robotic right hemicolectomy (RRH) is considered by most surgeons as the initial learning platform before proceeding to complex colorectal surgery. There are a lot of studies highlighting the use of robotic surgery for right hemicolectomy. Park et al., in a randomized trial, compared robot-assisted right hemicolectomy (RAC) versus standard laparoscopic right colectomy in 71 patients (35 in each group). Hospital stay, surgical complications, postoperative pain score, resection margin clearance, and number of lymph nodes harvested were similar in both groups. The duration of surgery was longer in the RAC group (195 vs. 130 min; p < 0·001). No conversion to open surgery was needed in either group. Overall hospital costs were significantly higher for RAC (US $12,235 vs. $10,320; p = 0·013); the higher costs were attributed primarily to the costs of surgery, including consumables. They concluded that robotic-assisted laparoscopic right colectomy was feasible but provided no benefit to justify the greater cost [9]. The results of robotic versus laparoscopic right colectomies have been compared in a meta-analysis. Huirong Xu et al., in their meta-analysis of seven studies, compared 234 robotic with 415 laparoscopic right hemicolectomies. They concluded that RRC had longer operative times (p < 0.00001), lower estimated blood loss (p = 0.0002), lower postoperative overall complications (p = 0.02), and significantly faster bowel function recovery (p < 0.00001). There were no differences in the length of hospital stay (p = 0.12), conversion rates to open surgery (p = 0.48), postoperative ileus (p = 0.08), anastomosis leakage (p = 0.28), and bleeding (p = 0.95) [10]. A similar meta-analysis by Niccolò Petrucciani et al., which included six studies, compared 168 patients undergoing RRC with 348 patients undergoing LRC. They concluded that the only significant difference between the two groups was a longer operative time in case of RRC [11]. The mode of bowel anastomosis can either be intracorporeal or extracorporeal. The intracorporeal anastomotic technique has also been compared to the extracorporeal anastomotic technique. Intracorporeal anastomosis is associated with a faster postoperative recovery and less overall morbidity at the cost of longer operating times [12]. In a recent report from MSKCC, robotic right colectomy with CME was associated with a better lymph node yield than laparoscopic or open approaches, concluding that robotic right colectomy may facilitate a better CME [13]. Robotic right hemicolectomy can, thus, be considered a safe and feasible procedure. It is an ideal initial learning step before proceeding to complex pelvic bowel procedures.

Left and sigmoid colectomy

Position: Supine or semi-lithotomy position with arms by the side of the patient (Figure 30.3).

Port Placement: A 12-mm camera port in the periumbilical region and three 8-mm operating arms, as shown in the figure. An assistant port can be placed depending on the need of the surgeon (Figure 30.4).

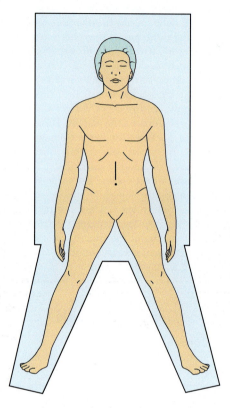

FIGURE 30.3   Patient position for left and sigmoid colectomy.

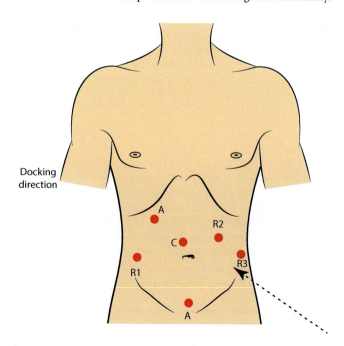

FIGURE 30.4   Port position for robotic left hemicolectomy/sigmoidectomy.

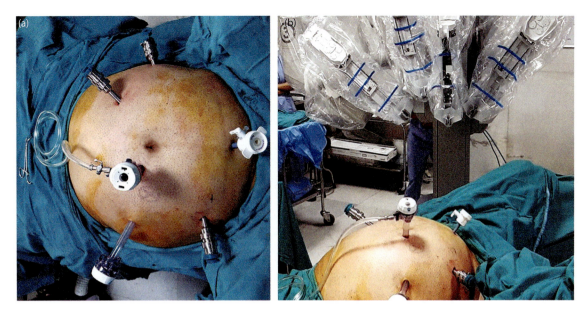

FIGURE 30.5 Port position (a) For robotic sigmoidectomy/left hemicolectomy, and (b) direction of docking.

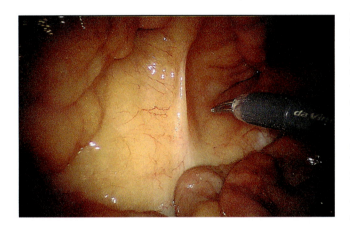

FIGURE 30.6 Identification and ligation of the inferior mesenteric vessels in sigmoidectomy.

Docking: The robot is brought in from either the left of the abdomen, or diagonally from the left thigh region (Figure 30.5).

Procedure: Sigmoid colectomy is relatively simpler and is performed in a fashion similar to laparoscopy. The sigmoid mesentery is lifted up and the inferior mesenteric artery is identified, clipped, and cut. Next, the inferior mesenteric vein is encountered more laterally and is dealt with similarly (Figure 30.6). Then the dissection is begun in the mesentery, which should have opened up with the pneumoperitoneum. Medial to lateral dissection is done, taking care not to injure the left ureter. The superior and inferior dissections performed similarly, and the desired level of dissection is obtained. After division of the bowel ends using staplers, the specimen is extracted through a small Pfannensteil incision or through the stoma site (if planned) after applying a wound protector. Depending on the level of inferior dissection, the anastomosis can either be performed with a linear or circular stapler.

Robotic left hemicolectomy is considered more cumbersome than the sigmoid colectomy or right hemicolectomy, as there is a need to operate in more than one quadrant of the abdomen. Splenic flexure dissection and mobilization is the trickiest part of the procedure (Figure 30.7). Different docking methods have been described for the left hemicolectomy [14].

1. *Hybrid technique*: This technique involves initial laparoscopic mobilization of the splenic flexure followed by docking of the robot in the left lower quadrant to proceed with the left colonic mobilization.

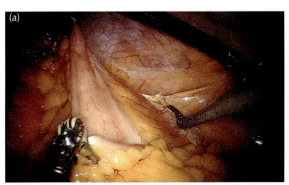
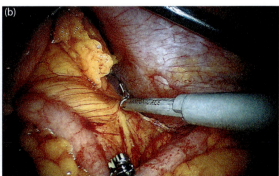

FIGURE 30.7 (a) Lateral dissection of the descending colon, (b) splenic flexure mobilization.

2. *Single-docking technique (described by Kim SH)*: This technique involves single docking of the robot in the left lower quadrant with mobilization of the second and third robotic arm for the different parts of the procedure (splenic flexure mobilization and for the pelvic dissection).

3. *Double-docking technique (described by KY Lee and BS Min)*: This technique involves dual docking, once for the left hemi-abdomen for dissection of the splenic flexure, and then changing the docking to the left lower quadrant for pelvic dissection.

Results: There are a lot of reports of left colectomies and sigmoid colectomies performed robotically. There are reports of sigmoidectomy being done with a single-port technique as well. Rami Makhoul et al. have reported four cases of single-incision robotic colectomy (SIRC) for sigmoid colon. All the procedures were performed for diverticulitis diseases. They used only two operating arms with a SILS port at the umbilicus. The mean operating time was 250 min with a mean blood loss of 75 cc. They concluded that SIRC is safe and feasible in such cases [15]. A systematic review and meta-analysis, conducted by Laura Lorenzon et al., evaluated a total of 400 left hemicolectomies, of which 143 were robotic and 257 were laparoscopic. The only significant difference noted was a lesser blood loss in robotic surgery compared to the laparoscopic group [16]. Robotic left hemicolectomy can be considered a safe and feasible option for both benign and malignant diseases.

Transverse colectomy

Position: Supine with arms by the side of the patient (Figure 30.1).

Port Placement: A 12-mm camera port in the periumbilical region, and three 8-mm operating arms, as shown in the figure. An assistant port can be placed depending on the need of the surgeon (Figure 30.8).

Docking: The robot is brought in from the head end of the table.

Procedure: The transverse colon is lifted up with its omentum. The lesser sac is entered by creating a window in the omentum.

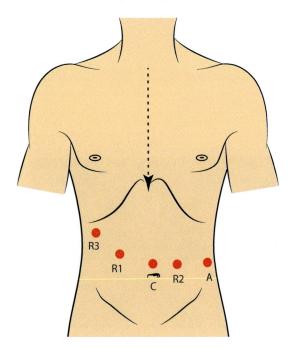

FIGURE 30.8 Port position for robotic transverse colectomy.

The middle colic pedicle is visualized, clipped, and cut. The rest of the root of the transverse mesocolon is then dissected off the duodenum and pancreas. Enhanced vision helps the surgeon prevent injuring these structures. The splenic and hepatic flexure are then dissected and mobilized as per requirement for a tension-free anastomosis. The proximal and distal ends are divided after proper margins from the tumor. Colo-colic anastomosis can then either be performed by intracorporeal suturing, stapling, or extracorporeal means. The ease of intracorporeal anastomosis does not warrant extensive mobilization of the hepatic and splenic flexure.

Results: There are relatively few studies on pure robotic transverse colectomy. Kyung Uk Jung et al., in their series of 162 colectomies, had only three cases of pure transverse colectomies. The mean operative time for those cases was in the range of 300 min. They had no major complications and were able to use intracorporeal suture anastomosis [17]. There will only be a few occasions where pure transverse colectomy is required, but as the procedure requires single docking and operating in a single quadrant, the robotic procedure may be useful.

Robotic colectomy in the era of complete mesocolic excision (CME)

The benefits of robotic colectomy, discussed previously, are likely to be enhanced with the advent of complete mesocolic excision for colonic malignancies, akin to total mesorectal excision for rectal cancers. Complete mesocolic excision with central vascular ligation, especially for right-sided cancers, has been shown to provide better oncological outcomes compared to standard lymphadenectomy and this may translate into better survival rates. The performance of CME with traditional rigid laparoscopic instruments is difficult. Robotic surgery offers technical advantages over laparoscopy in terms of improved dexterity, freedom of movement, and 3D vision, which may result in a better dissection around the central vessels during CME. However, literature regarding the benefits of robotic CME over conventional laparoscopic colectomy with CME is still lacking, with no randomized trials comparing them. Single center studies have shown that robotic CME can be safely performed, and results in better lymph node yield compared to laparoscopic CME. Yozgatli et al. [18] compared robotic complete mesocolic excision (CME) for right-sided colon cancer with conventional laparoscopic right hemicolectomy and found that robotic CME was safe and effective in terms of short-term outcomes. The overall complication rates were similar in both groups while robotic CME resulted in a significantly higher number of harvested lymph nodes and longer length between the vascular tie and colonic wall. Spinoglio et al. [19] reported on the short-term outcomes and 5-year survival rate for robotic versus laparoscopic right colectomy with CME. They showed a statistically significant reduction in the conversion rate while performing CME with a robotic approach, with a longer operative time. However, there was no difference in the perioperative clinical or pathological outcomes. Five-year survival was 77 and 73 months for robotic versus laparoscopic CME (p = 0.64), respectively. However, for UICC stage III patients, there was a trend toward a better 5-year disease-free survival (but not statistically significant) for the robotic group (81 vs. 68 months; p = 0.122). Ozben et al. [20] have also shown the feasibility of robotic CME for transverse colon cancers. With upcoming evidence in favor of robotic CME, it is likely that robotic colectomy may soon become the standard approach for resection of colon cancers. However, this needs to be established through high-quality studies with a larger number of patients. Presently, it is evident that robotic CME is feasible and safe, providing technical superiority over laparoscopic CME. Whether it results in improved oncological outcomes compared to the laparoscopic approach remains to be proven.

Summary

Robotic colonic surgery is a feasible option as an alternative to laparoscopic surgery with the benefits of improved ergonomics, 3D vision, and instrument handling at the expense of greater healthcare cost and prolonged operating time. Proper port positioning and docking are essential to successfully completing this procedure, which requires learning and experience. Most of the literature has shown equivalent outcomes for robotic surgery when compared to laparoscopic colectomies. Cost factor is the issue that precludes its widespread use. With the growing technology and innovations in the field of robotic surgery, the cost of the equipment and procedure may decrease in the near future.

Key points

- Robotic colorectal surgery is a safe and feasible option.
- Robotic surgery has shown comparable or even better post-surgery outcomes than coventional laparoscopy.
- The longer operating time and higher cost are hindrances to full adoption of robotic surgery.

References

1. Nelson H, Sargent DJ, Wieand HS et al. A comparison of laparoscopically assisted and open colectomy for colon cancer. *N Engl J Med.* 2004;350(20):2050–9.
2. Fleshman J, Sargent DJ, Green E et al. Laparoscopic colectomy for cancer is not inferior to open surgery based on 5-year data from the COST Study Group trial. *Ann Surg.* 2007;246(4):655–62.
3. Veldkamp R, Kuhry E, Hop WC et al. Laparoscopic surgery versus open surgery for colon cancer: Short-term outcomes of a randomised trial. *Lancet Oncol.* 2005;6(7):477–84.
4. Buunen M, Veldkamp R, Hop WC et al. Survival after laparoscopic surgery versus open surgery for colon cancer: Long-term outcome of a randomised clinical trial. *Lancet Oncol.* 2009;10(1):44–52.
5. Weber PA, Merola S, Wasielewski A, Ballantyne GH, Delaney CP. 'Telerobotic-assisted laparoscopic right and sigmoid colectomies for benign disease.' *Dis Colon Rectum.* 2002;45(12), 1689–96.
6. Tsoraides SS, Huettner F, Rawlings AL, Crawford DL, *Robotic Surgery of the Colon: The Peoria Experience.* Robot Surgery, Book edited by: SeungHyukBaik.
7. Migaly J, Andrea CB, Todd DF et al. The American Society of colon and rectal surgeons clinical practice guidelines for the use of bowel preparation in elective colon and rectal surgery. *Dis Colon Rectum.* 2019 January;62(1).
8. Witkiewicz W, Zawadzki M, Rząca M, Obuszko Z, Czarnecki R, Turek J, Marecik S. Robot-assisted right colectomy: Surgical technique and review of the literature. *Videosurgery Miniinv.* 2013;8(3):253–7.
9. Park JS, Choi GS, Park SY, Kim HJ, Ryuk JP. Randomized clinical trial of robot-assisted versus standard laparoscopic right colectomy. *Br J Surg.* 2012;99:1219–26.
10. Xu H, Li J, Sun Y, Li Z, Zhen Y, Wang B, Xu Z. Robotic versus laparoscopic right colectomy: A meta-analysis. *World J Surg Oncol.* 2014;12:274.
11. Petrucciani N, Sirimarco D, Nigri GR et al. Robotic right colectomy: A worthwhile procedure? Results of a meta-analysis of trials comparing robotic versus laparoscopic right colectomy. *J Minim Access Surg.* January-March 2015;11(1).
12. Cleary RK, Kassir A, Johnson CS et al. Intracorporeal versus extracorporeal anastomosis for minimally invasive right colectomy: A multi-center propensity score-matched comparison of outcomes. *PLOS ONE.* 2018 October 24;13(10):e0206277.
13. Widmar M, Keskin M, Strombom P, Beltran P, Chow OS, Smith JJ, Nash GM, Shia J, Russell D, Garcia-Aguilar J. Lymph node yield in right colectomy for cancer: A comparison of open, laparoscopic and robotic approaches. *Colorectal Dis.* 2017;19(10):888–94.
14. Parra-Davila E, Diaz-Hernandez JJ. Totally robotic left colectomy. *J Robotic Surg.* 2011;5:57–64.
15. Makhoul R, Obias V. Robotic single-incision sigmoid colectomy: Initial case series. *J Robotic Surg.* 2014;8:375–8.
16. Lorenzon L, Bini F, Balducci G, Ferri M, Salvi PF, Marinozzi F. Laparoscopic versus robotic-assisted colectomy and rectal resection: A systematic review and meta-analysis. *Int J Colorectal Dis.* 2016;31(2):161–73.
17. Jung KU, Park Y, Lee KY, Sohn SK. Robotic transverse colectomy for mid-transverse colon cancer: Surgical techniques and oncologic outcome. *J Robot Surg.* June 2015;9(2):131–6.
18. Yozgatli TK, Aytac E, Ozben V et al. Robotic complete mesocolic excision versus conventional laparoscopic hemicolectomy for right-sided colon cancer. *J LaparoendoscAdvSurg Tech A.* 2019;29(5):671–76.
19. Spinoglio G, Bianchi PP, Marano A et al. Robotic versus laparoscopic right colectomy with complete mesocolic excision for the treatment of colon cancer: Perioperative outcomes and 5-year survival in a consecutive series of 202 patients. *Ann SurgOncol.* 2018 November;25(12):3580–6.
20. Ozben V, de Muijnck C, Esen E et al. Is robotic complete mesocolic excision feasible for transverse colon cancer? *J LaparoendoscAdvSurg Tech A.* 2018 December;28(12):1443–50.

Chapter 31

ROBOTIC RECTAL CANCER SURGERY

Somashekhar SP and Ashwin K Rajagopal

Contents

Learning objectives 196
Introduction 196
Preoperative preparation and precautions... 196
Position, port placement, and instrumentation 197
Steps of surgery.. 197
    Nerves... 198
    Margins... 198
    Vascularity 198
Robotics in rectal cancer 198
    Conversion rate 199
    Learning curve.. 199
    Short-term clinical outcomes.. 199
    Sexual and urinary functions 199
Oncological outcomes.. 199
Cost.. 199
Advantages of robot-assisted TME for rectal cancer... 199
Summary 200
Key points 200
Videos... 200
References 200

Learning objectives

- Step-by-step explanation of the technique for performing optimal TME.
- Detailed technical specifications, operative tips, current status, and future perspectives of robotics for rectal cancer surgery.
- Clarify the delimitation of the mesorectum and anatomic landmarks of the correct surgical plane in rectal cancer surgery. Demonstrate the anatomy of the ureters and pelvic autonomic nerves in relation to the vessels and mesorectal fascial planes.
- Accurate determination of the resection line of the bowel using an indocyanine green (ICG) fluorescence technique and an optimal site of anastomosis.
- Differences between laparoscopic and robotic rectal surgery.

Introduction

Minimally invasive surgery (MIS) has revolutionized surgical practice, especially surgery of the gastrointestinal tract. The well-known benefits of such an approach include reduced postoperative pain, shorter hospital stays, and an improved cosmetic outcome [1].

Total mesorectal excision (TME) with autonomic nerve preservation – the gold standard procedure for rectal cancer – was popularized by Heald [2]. The oncologic outcome has improved greatly in terms of local recurrence and cancer-specific survival with the introduction of TME [3]. Rectal cancer surgery is challenging since the rectum has a dual arterial blood supply and venous drainage, has extensive lymphatic drainage, and is located in the bony pelvis in close proximity to urogenital and neurovascular structures that are invested with intricate fascial covering. The pelvic size is regarded as a direct relating factor to the quality of the resected rectum [4].

The biologic behavior and management of rectal cancer differ significantly from those of colon cancer. In order to eradicate the primary rectal tumor and control regional disease, the rectum, the area of lymph node drainage, and the surrounding tissue must be completely excised while maintaining an intact fascial envelope around the rectum [5].

Laparoscopy was a significant technological advance in gastrointestinal surgery when introduced in the last quarter century. The success of laparoscopic surgery for benign surgeries, notably cholecystectomy and appendectomy, laid the foundations of the modern use of this technique in a variety of diseases, especially cancer. Though slower to gain acceptance, laparoscopic cancer surgery – in experienced hands – is now regarded as a safe and feasible alternative to open surgery. The safety, feasibility, and clinical benefits of laparoscopy have been demonstrated over open approaches by many studies. Despite these proven benefits, laparoscopic surgery has not achieved high acceptance by the surgeons, especially for rectal cancer surgery. The long learning curve, together with inherent difficulties such as 2D imaging, limited dexterity, and diminished tactile sense, have meant that the application of laparoscopic surgery to technically demanding pelvic procedures continues to present a challenge, in particular for restorative resection of mid and low rectal cancers [6,7].

Preoperative preparation and precautions

All patients who present with newly diagnosed rectal cancer undergo rigid sigmoidoscopy to identify the tumor location. Abdominal pelvic computerized tomography is performed to assess distant metastases. According to our institution protocol, all patients undergo pelvic MRI to assess local infiltration and nodal metastasis. Patients with local invasion (T3-T4) or node involvement are reviewed by multidisciplinary teams and receive neoadjuvant chemo-radiotherapy. They receive a 50.4 Gy dose of EBRT in 28 fractions over five and a half weeks, along with systemic 5-flurouracil-based chemotherapy followed by surgery 6–8 weeks later [8].

Preoperatively, the patient is admitted 12 hours before surgery and is advised to take clear liquids with an oral antibiotic (Ciprofloxacin + Tinidazole) from two days prior to surgery. The night before the surgery after admission, a proctoclysis enema and two bisacodyl tablets are given orally. We do not administer a bowel prep at our institution because we found it causes bowel dilatation.

The da Vinci® Surgical System (Intuitive Surgical, Mountain View, CA) consists of a console, which is placed where the surgeon sits while operating, and the robotic cart with its three or four robotic arms, which is in close proximity to the patient. Various instruments, attached to the robotic arms, are inserted into the patient through small incisions. The console provides a magnified high-definition 3D view of the operating field through a stereoendoscope fitted to one of the robotic arms, whose visual field and angle of vision are adjustable. The surgeon manipulates two-finger joysticks (finger and wrist movements) at the console while watching the surgical field through the visual system. Movements of the surgeon's hands are transmitted through the robot to the robotic arms, so that equivalent but scaled movements of the surgical instruments are made within the surgical field. The instruments have seven degrees of movement freedom and hand tremor is filtered out [9,10]. The da Vinci® system overcomes many of the problems that characterize laparoscopic rectal resection. Initially, the 3D high-definition camera is under the direct control of the surgeon, and the double optical system makes consistently clear vision more likely. Furthermore, the tremor-filtered, multiple-degree-of-movement instruments, which can be scaled relative to the surgeon's hand movements, permit more precise dissection in narrow spaces and render the more difficult steps of the operation easier. Tissue retraction with the robot is also easier, since the third arm can be used as a fixed retractor, and is always manipulated by surgeon [11]. These potential advantages within the narrow space of the pelvis have been shown to be translated into concrete advantages for robotic radical prostatectomy [12], and in our opinion the excellent ergonomics and precise dissection offered by the robotic system can also be helpful in colorectal surgery for vessel ligation and flexure mobilization. This is why we have standardized a 'fully robotic' technique for resection [13].

Position, port placement, and instrumentation (see Video 32)

The robotic surgery was performed using the four-arm Da Vinci® X surgical system (Intuitive Surgical Inc., Sunnyvale, CA). Total robotic colorectal mobilization and resection anastomosis is performed in all patients at our center. We used two types of port placements in our patients. Initially, we used the port placement as provided with intuitive procedure card, but it needed dual docking. For the subsequent cases, we modified the port placement as follows (Figure 31.1). In the modified port placement, dual docking is not needed and only port hopping is sufficient (Figure 31.1).

The patient is placed supine on the operating table. After induction of general anesthesia and insertion of an oral gastric tube and Foley catheter, the patient is rotated with the left side up and right side down, to approximately a 25°–30° tilt. The patient is then placed in the Trendelenburg position; this helps gravitational migration of the small bowel away from the operative field.

A 12-mm camera port is placed 3–4 cm above the umbilicus and 2–3 cm to the right side from the midline with an optical trocar. The rest of the ports are placed after insufflating the abdomen

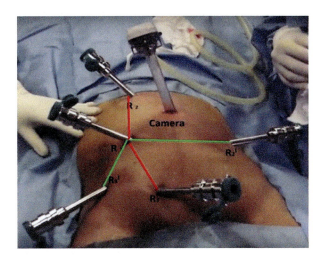

FIGURE 31.1 Modified port positions for robotic rectal cancer surgery to avoid dual docking.

with gas and marking the port measurements. Arm one (8 mm) port is placed on patient's right side, at the crossing of the midclavicular line (MCL) and spino-umbilical line. Arm two (8 mm) port is placed on the patient's left side, similarly to arm 1. The third arm (8 mm) is placed 3 cm below the right costal margin and 2 cm medial to the right MCL. An additional port (8 mm) is placed on the patient's right side, 2 cm superior to the ASIS used for pelvic surgery, and which is used by the bedside assistant during the abdominal surgery. Another port (8 mm) is placed on the right mid-inguinal point for abdominal surgery, and later converted to an assistant port (12 mm) for stapler firing.

Manipal port modification: Here the camera is placed in the midline about 3 cm from the umbilicus. The R1 port is placed along the spino-umbilical line at the level of the midclavicular line. The R2 port is placed 2 cm to the right of the midline at the subcostal region. The R2I port is placed similarly to R1 at the left side along the spino-umbilical line at the level of the midclavicular line. The R3 is then placed 3 cm right of the midline just above the inguinal ligament. The R3I port is place laterally. The advantage of using the second approach is less arm clashing, easier mobilization of the left colon up to the splenic flexure, and easier application of the linear stapler through the R3 port, which is then converted to an assistant port during pelvic dissection [14].

Steps of surgery

The low anterior resection is a technically demanding procedure in robotic-assisted colorectal surgery because it is a multi-quadrant surgery. It features both abdominal and pelvic dissections. The abdominal part entails central quadrant surgery for high vascular ligation, and a left upper quadrant approach for splenic flexure mobilization. The pelvic part entails mesorectal excision and anastomosis. A 30-degree down-facing camera is used and hot shears are used in R1, Cadiere forceps in R2, and a double fenestrated grasper in R3.

Robotic dissection is performed in the following steps [15]:

1. Initial metastatic survey of the abdomen
2. Identification and isolation of the inferior mesenteric artery and vein
3. Safeguarding autonomic nerves followed by high ligation/clipping and transection of the inferior mesenteric artery and vein

4. Medial to lateral dissection (identification of the ureter and gonadal vessels)
5. Left colon mobilization up to the splenic flexure
6. *Pelvic dissection and mesorectal excision*: Pelvic dissection is performed sequentially as follows: Posterior dissection, deep posterior dissection, posterolateral dissection, anterior dissection, and finally circumferential pelvic dissection toward the pelvic floor
7. ICG fluorescence for identifying the line of transection
8. Distal transection, exteriorization of specimen
9. Anastomosis

The underlying principle for a TME is the meticulous and precise dissection of an avascular plane between the presacral fascia and the fascia propria of the rectum.

Nerves

Urinary and sexual dysfunctions are common problems after rectal cancer surgery due to damage to the pelvic autonomic nerves during surgery. Attention has been focused on preserving the autonomic nerves without compromising on the radicality of total mesorectal excision. The nerve-sparing techniques involve the dissection and exposure of the pelvic splanchnic nerves and the inferior hypogastric plexus. Knowledge of the topographic anatomy and awareness of the landmarks for avoiding intraoperative nerve injuries are the most important factors in avoiding postoperative bladder and sexual dysfunction.

The autonomic nerves consist of the paired sympathetic hypogastric nerve, sacral splanchnic nerves, and the pelvic autonomic nerve plexus. The superior hypogastric plexus is located ventrally to the abdominal aorta a t the origin of IMA and later bifurcates to form right and left hypogastric nerves just proximal to at the sacral hollow. The hypogastric nerves, which derive from the superior hypogastric plexus, carry the sympathetic signals to the internal urethral and anal sphincters, as well as to the pelvic visceral proprioception. The pelvic splanchnic nerves from S2 to S4 carry nociceptive and parasympathetic signals to the bladder, rectum, and colon. The hypogastric and pelvic splanchnic nerves merge into the pararectal fossae to form the inferior hypogastric plexus [16].

Margins

TME completeness is a representative of the quality of rectal cancer surgery. The two crucial parameters of TME completeness are CRM involvement and DRM distance. Involvement of CRM is defined as when the tumor is located ≤ 1 mm from the CRM [17].

Park et al. proposed that the rate of CRM involvement is mainly influenced by two factors: The location of the tumor in the rectum and the quality of the surgery. Because the location of the tumor is random and a key factor is the quality of dissection, robotic surgery is more dominant in the macroscopic grading than in conventional laparoscopic surgery [18]. However, the results of two studies were not statistically different between the groups [19,20].

Vascularity

Poor vascular perfusion is one of the most common causes for postoperative anastomotic leakage, with preoperative concurrent chemo-radiotherapy being the most important risk factor. Intraoperative assessment of the bowel transection line and selection of an optimal site for anastomosis has been dependent on the surgeons' gross visual inspection. Intestinal perfusion and viability estimation is based on clinical parameters, such as the color of the bowel wall, presence of bowel peristalsis, bleeding from the edges of the bowel, and pulsations of the mesenteric arteries. However, this assessment is subjective and based on the surgeons' experience. The surgeons' ability to predict anastomotic leakage is low in gastrointestinal surgery, with a sensitivity of 61.3% and a specificity of 88.5% [21].

Fluorescence imaging has been increasingly used as an intraoperative tool in routine practice to ensure adequate perfusion at the time of anastomosis. Recent literature shows the potential benefit of fluorescence imaging in lowering leak rates by changing the bowel transection line [22–24].

Intraoperative ICG-enhanced fluorescent angiography provides information about in situ vascular perfusion during colorectal surgery. This accurate determination of the resection margin of the viable bowel may help to reduce anastomotic leakage. It is a feasible and readily achievable technique, with minimal added intraoperative time. Larger further randomized prospective trials, like PILLAR-III, are awaited to validate this new technique.

Laparoscopic surgery in rectal cancer [8,26]:

- Two trials, the CLASICC trial, which recruited colon and rectal cancer patients, and the COREAN trial, which recruited rectal cancer patients only, showed feasibility and oncological safety.
- In the CLASICC tria,l higher rate of CRM involvement among rectal cancer patients in the laparoscopic arm (12.4%) compared with the open arm (6.3%) especially in distal rectal cancer was seen.
- In the CLASICC trial, with a 34% conversion rate, the morbidity and mortality rates were high among laparoscopic cases (colon and rectal cancer) converted to open surgery (Table 31.1).

Laparoscopic rectal surgery could not achieve a high impact mainly because of the following: Unstable video camera platforms, 2D imaging, limited dexterity of instruments, fixed tips of instruments, amplification of tremor leading to steep learning curves, high rates of conversion, and the technical challenge of working in a narrow pelvis with limited instrument maneuverability, especially in the obese and in patients treated by preoperative chemo-radiation [27] (Table 31.2).

Robotics in rectal cancer

The benefits of robotic surgery, as a minimally invasive surgical technique, parallel those of traditional laparoscopy, with the added advantages of overcoming several barriers to the use of laparoscopy, such as limitations of the human hand (seven degrees of movement and elimination of hand tremors), elimination of the fulcrum effect

TABLE 31.1: Results of Comparision between CLASICC and COREAN Trial for Laparoscopic Colorectal Cancer Surgery

	CLASICC [8]	COREAN [26]
Conversion rate	82/242 (34%)	2/170
30-day morbidity in converted patients	48/82 (59%)	N/A
CRM involvement	30/193 (16%)	5/170 (2.9%)
Mean procedures per surgeon	20	75
Participating centers	27	3
Mean BMI	25	24.1

TABLE 31.2: Comparision of Robotic and
Laparoscopic Surgeries

	Robotic Surgery	Laparoscopic Surgery
Binocular stereoscopic vision with camera, which is stable	Yes	No
High definition 3D camera	Yes	No
12x magnification	Yes	No
Stability of camera	Yes	No
Endowrist technology	Yes	No
Degree of precision	Very high	Operator dependent
Ease of intracorporeal knotting	Very easy	Long learning curve
Multitasking instruments	Yes	No
Surgeon comfort	Very high	Fatigue
Elimination of tremors	Yes	No
Learning curve	Short	Long

of laparoscopy (the robotic arms imitate the movements of the surgeon's hand), improved visualization (3D stereoscopic imaging), and increased independence of the operating surgeon, thus enabling the surgeon to achieve a more complete mesorectal excision with better autonomic nerve preservation, leading to superior bladder and sexual functions. Due to these advantages, robotic-assisted management of rectal cancer has been more widely utilized.

Initial published studies are small, not randomized, single center series. Most of the published studies are mainly retrospective or prospective single center series, comparing mainly robotic rectal resection to laparoscopy. Five meta-analyses have already been published on this technique, indicating the marked interest in robotic surgery for rectal cancer. The operative approaches were evaluated in terms of various parameters.

Conversion rate
In comparison with standard laparoscopy, the most important finding for robotic rectal surgery is the lower rate of conversion to open surgery. Conversion to open surgery is an important indicator of proficiency, generally being ~10%–15% in laparoscopic rectal surgery, except for the COREAN trial, where the conversion rate was 1.1%. A preliminary publication of the COLOR II trial reported a 17% conversion rate to open surgery [28]. An RCT (robotic vs. laparoscopic resection for rectal cancer [ROLARR]) – comparing laparoscopic with robotic rectal resection for cancer – is ongoing, and its first end-point is the conversion rate to open surgery [29].

In a meta-analysis, robotic rectal resection was associated with a significant reduction of conversion rate in comparison with laparoscopy [30]. In another meta-analysis, conversion rates and estimated blood loss were significantly lower in robotic rectal cancer patients than in rectal cancer patients undergoing conventional laparoscopic resection [31].

Learning curve
The learning curve for minimally invasive surgery is a crucial issue, because laparoscopic colorectal surgery has a steep learning curve, particularly for rectal cancer, and robotic surgery seems to reduce the learning curve to 15/20 cases. This is an important benefit as the conversion is directly related to a higher rate of postoperative complications and mortality, as shown by the CLASICC trial [8,32,33].

Short-term clinical outcomes
In comparison with open surgery, robot-assisted surgery maintains all the advantages of minimally invasive procedures. Considering short-term clinical outcomes, robotic surgery did not show significant differences compared to the laparoscopic technique. Overall complications rate and length of hospital stay are similar for both techniques [34,35].

Sexual and urinary functions
Laparoscopy did not add an advantage in terms of sexual/urinary dysfunctions preservation. In fact, the MRC CLASICC trial raised a concern that laparoscopic TME may be associated with increased rates of male sexual dysfunction. Anatomic variability and inability to visualize the small caliber fibers in laparoscopy underlines the reasons that some postoperative visceral and sexual dysfunction occur in spite of careful dissection and adequate surgical technique. Only three studies evaluating genitourinary function, after robotic rectal surgery, have been published. A similar trend for sexual function has been observed, with a decrease at one month after surgery and subsequent progressive recovery [36]. Surgeons agree that the robotic system provides an easier identification of the nerves and of the planes of dissection.

Oncological outcomes

A multivariate analysis that included potent parameters, that is SSO types, preoperative CRT, T-category, and growth pattern, showed that patients with a distal resection margin ≥2 cm were significantly more likely to be in the robotic than in the open group (OR, 2.415; 95% CI, 1.233–4.73; P=0.01) [35]. The mean number of harvested lymph nodes and lymphovascular or perineural invasion was similar in the two groups. Concern about the CRM involvement was reported in CLASICC trial. Studies available so far demonstrate oncologic results comparable to laparoscopy.

Cost

Robotic surgery is expensive, due to the cost of robot purchase, maintenance, and instruments. Therefore, a careful analysis of costs and of cost-effectiveness is mandatory, even if it is difficult to perform because of the lack of available data about the potential benefits of robotic surgery. A recent cost analysis demonstrates that robotic surgery is more expensive than laparoscopic surgery, but said the cost-effectiveness of robotic rectal cancer surgery should be assessed based on oncologic outcomes and functional results especially in lower rectal cancer surgery [37]. The average reduction in total direct cost is difficult to define due to the increasing cost over time, making the comparisons between studies conducted over a time range of more than 10 years challenging.

Advantages of robot-assisted TME for rectal cancer

- Precise pelvic dissection especially for the narrow male pelvis
- Preservation of bladder and sexual function
- Low conversion rate
- Rectal transection under robotic setting
- Transanal specimen extraction and single-stapling anastomosis [25]

Summary

Oncosurgical practice has evolved tremendously in the past decade due to technological advancements. An important example is the introduction of robotic surgery to overcome the technical limitations of laparoscopic surgery and further optimize patient outcomes for complex surgeries. The robot is an extension of the surgeon, helping to provide maximum range of motion with unprecedented control and precision. With increasing emphasis on optimizing and measuring surgical quality, it is imperative that robotic surgery become a mainstay to perform complex surgeries in confined places like the pelvis or thorax.

Key points

- The surgeon's knowledge of the anatomy of these nerves is the main factor for complete mesorectal excision with better autonomic nerve preservation.
- The use of the da Vinci® robotic system has been postulated to compensate for the technical limitations of laparoscopy.
- The robotic technique is safe and more easily reproducible, and is associated with a higher rate of preservation of functions while not compromising the oncological outcomes.

See Video 33.

Videos

VIDEO 32   https://youtu.be/hX8ot4KOWz8

Robotic LAR.

VIDEO 33   https://youtu.be/ufnPGgbn07o

Robotic LAR.

References

1. Martel G, Boushey RP. Laparoscopic colon surgery: Past, present and future. *Surg Clin N Am* 2006;86:867–97.
2. Heald RJ. A new approach to rectal cancer. *Br J Hosp Med* 1979;22:277–81.
3. Heald RJ, Ryall RD. Recurrence and survival after total mesorectal excision for rectal cancer. *Lancet* 1986;1:1479–82.
4. Baik SH, Kim NK, Lee KY et al. Factors influencing pathologic results after total mesorectal excision for rectal cancer: Analysis of consecutive 100 cases. *Ann Surg Oncol* 2008;15:721–8.
5. Kulaylat MN. Mesorectal excision: Surgical anatomy of the rectum, mesorectum, and pelvic fascia and nerves and clinical relevance. *World J Surg Proced* 2015;5(1):27–40.
6. Cadiere GB, Himpens J, Germay O, Izizaw R, Degueldre M, Vandromme J, Capelluto E, Bruyns J. Feasibility of robotic laparoscopic surgery: 146 cases. *World J Surg* 2001;25:1467–77.
7. Berguer R, Rab GT, Abu-Ghaida H, Alarcon A, Chung J. A comparison of surgeon's posture during laparoscopic and open surgical procedures. *Surg Endosc* 1997;11:2139.
8. Guillou PJ, Quirke P, Thorpe H et al. Short-term endpoints of conventional versus laparoscopic assisted surgery in patients with colorectal cancer (MRC CLASICC trial): Multicentre, randomised controlled trial. *Lancet* 2005;365:1718–26.

9. Spinoglio G, Summa M, Priora F et al. Robotic laparoscopic surgery with the da Vinci® system: An early experience. *Surg Technol Int* 2009;18:70–4 PMID: 19579191.
10. Taylor GW, Jayne DG. Robotic applications in abdominal surgery: Their limitations and future developments. *Int J Med Robot* 2007;3:3–9. Review DOI: 10.1002/rcs.115 PMID: 17441019
11. Bianchi PP, Ceriani C, Locatelli A et al. Robotic versus laparoscopic total mesorectal excision for rectal cancer: A comparative analysis of oncological safety and short-term outcomes. *Surg Endosc* 2010;24(11):2888–94. DOI: 10.1007/s00464-010-1134-7
12. Ficarra V, Novara G, Ahlering TE et al. Systematic review and meta-analysis of studies reporting potency rates after robot-assisted radical prostatectomy. *Eur Urol* 2012;62(3):418–30. DOI: 10.1016/j.eururo.2012.05.046
13. Luca F, Cenciarelli S, Valvo M et al. Full robotic left colon and rectal cancer resection: Technique and early outcome. *Ann Surg Oncol* 2009;16:1274–78. DOI: 10.1245/s10434-009-0366-z
14. Somashekhar SP, Deshpande AY, Ashwin KR, Gangasani R, Kumar R. A prospective randomized controlled trial comparing conventional Intuitive® procedure card recommended port placement with the modified Indian (Manipal) technique. *J Minim Access Surg* 2020;16(3):246–50. DOI: 10.4103/jmas.JMAS_18_19
15. Somashekhar SP, Ashwin KR, Rajashekhar J, Zaveri S. Prospective randomized study comparing robotic-assisted surgery with traditional laparotomy for rectal cancer – Indian study. *Indian J Surg* 2015;77(Suppl 3):788–94. DOI: 10.1007/s12262-013-1003-4
16. Kim NK, Kim YW, Cho MS. Total mesorectal excision for rectal cancer with emphasis on pelvic autonomic nerve preservation: Expert technical tips for robotic surgery. *Surg Oncol* 2015;24(3):172–80.
17. Adam IJ, Mohamdee MO, Martin IG et al. Role of circumferential margin involvement in the local recurrence of rectal cancer. *Lancet* 1994;344(8924):707–11.
18. Park EJ, Cho MS, Baek SJ et al. Long-term oncologic outcomes of robotic low anterior resection for rectal cancer: A comparative study with laparoscopic surgery. *Ann Surg* 2015;261(1):129–37.
19. Leonard D, Penninckx F, Fieuws S et al. PROCARE, a multidisciplinary belgian project on cancer of the rectum. Factors predicting the quality of total mesorectal excision for rectal cancer. *Ann Surg* 2010;252(6):982–8.
20. Jayne DG, Thorpe HC, Copeland J, Quirke P, Brown JM, Guillou PJ. Five-year follow-up of the medical research council CLASICC trial of laparoscopically assisted versus open surgery for colorectal cancer. *Br J Surg* 2010;97(11):1638–45.
21. Karliczek A, Harlaar NJ, Zeebregts CJ et al. Surgeons lack predictive accuracy for anastomotic leakage in gastrointestinal surgery. *Int J Colorectal Dis* 2009;24:569–76.
22. Bae SU, Min BS, Kim NK. Robotic low ligation of the inferior mesenteric artery for rectal cancer using the firefly technique. *Yonsei Med J* 2015;56(4):1028–35.
23. Boni L, David G, Dionigi G, Rausei S, Cassinotti E, Fingerhut A. Indocyaninegreenenhanced fluorescence to assess bowel perfusion during laparoscopic colorectal resection. *Surg Endosc* 2016;30(7):2736–42.
24. Foppa C, Denoya PI, Tarta C, Bergamaschi R. Indocyanine green fluorescent dye during bowel surgery: Are the blood supply 'guessing days' over? *Tech Coloproctol* 2014;18(8):753–8.
25. Trastulli S, Farinella E, Cirocchi R, Cavaliere D, Avenia N, Sciannameo F, Gullà N, Noya G, Boselli C. Robotic resection compared with laparoscopic rectal resection for cancer: Systematic review and meta-analysis of short-term outcome. *Colorectal Dis* 2012;14:e134–56.
26. Kang SB, Park JW, Jeong SY et al. Open versus laparoscopic surgery for mid or low rectal cancer after neoadjuvant chemoradiotherapy (COREAN trial): Short-term outcomes of an open-label randomised controlled trial. *Lancet Oncol* 2010;11(7):637–45. DOI: 10.1016/S1470-2045(10)70131-5
27. Ramos JR. Current status of robotic rectal cancer surgery. *J Coloproctol (Rio J.)* 2014;34(3):129–30. https://doi.org/10.1016/j.jcol.2014.06.001
28. Color II Study Group, Buunen M, Bonjer HJ et al. COLOR II. A randomized clinical trial comparing laparoscopic and open surgery for rectal cancer. *Dan Med Bull* 2009;56(2):89–91.

29. Collinson FJ, Jayne DG, Pigazzi A et al. An international, multi-centre, prospective, randomised, controlled, unblinded, parallel-group trial of robotic-assisted versus standard laparoscopic surgery for the curative treatment of rectal cancer. *Int J Colorectal Dis* 2012;27;(2):233–41. DOI:10.1007/s00384-011-1313-6

30. Memon S, Heriot AG, Murphy DG, Bressel M, Lynch AC. Robotic versus laparoscopic proctectomy for rectal cancer: A meta-analysis. *Ann Surg Oncol* 2012;19(7):2095–101. DOI:10.1245/s10434-012-2270-1

31. Yang Y, Wang F, Zhang P et al. Robot-assisted versus conventional laparoscopic surgery for colorectal disease, focusing on rectal cancer: A meta-analysis. 2012. In: Database of Abstracts of Reviews of Effects (DARE): Quality-assessed Reviews [Internet]. York (UK): Centre for Reviews and Dissemination (UK); 1995. Available from: https://www.ncbi.nlm.nih.gov/books/NBK114606/.

32. Bokhari MB, Patel CB, Ramos-Valadez DI, Ragupathi M, Haas EM. Learning curve for robotic-assisted laparoscopic colorectal surgery. *Surg Endosc* 2011;25:855–60.

33. Jiménez-Rodríguez RM, Díaz-Pavón JM, de la Portilla de Juan F, Prendes-Sillero E, Dussort HC, Padillo J. Learning curve for robotic-assisted laparoscopic rectal cancer surgery. *Int J Colorectal Dis* 2013;28:815–21.

34. Park JS, Choi GS, Lim KH, Jang YS, Jun SH. S052: A comparison of robot assisted, laparoscopic, and open surgery in the treatment of rectal cancer. *Surg Endosc* 2011;25:240–8.

35. Kim JC, Yang SS, Jang TY, Kwak JY, Yun MJ, Lim SB. Open versus robot-assisted sphincter-saving operations in rectal cancer patients: Techniques and comparison of outcomes between groups of 100 matched patients. *Int J Med Robot.* 2012;8(4):468–75.

36. Morino M, Parini U, Allaix ME, Monasterolo G, Brachet Contul R, Garrone C. Male sexual and urinary function after laparoscopic total mesorectal excision. *Surg Endosc* 2009;23:1233–40.

37. Baek S, Kim S, Cho J et al. Robotic versus conventional laparoscopic surgery for rectal cancer: A cost analysis from a single institute in Korea. *World J Surg* 2012;36(11):2722–9.

Section VI
Transanal Surgery

32 Transanal Minimally Invasive Surgery (TAMIS)... 203
33 Transanal Total Mesorectal Excision for Rectal Cancer................................ 211
34 Combined Endoscopic-Laparoscopic Surgery (CELS) for Colorectal Polypectomy........ 224

Chapter 32

TRANSANAL MINIMALLY INVASIVE SURGERY (TAMIS)

Sanjeev Patil and Shrikant Makam

Contents

Learning objectives 203
Introduction 203
Indications 204
Reach of TAMIS 204
Risks of TAMIS 204
Contraindications 205
    Evaluation of the lesion 205
    Preparation of the lesion 205
    Bowel preparation 205
    Deep venous thrombosis prophylaxis 205
    Prevention of urinary retention 205
    Equipment and operative set-up 205
Equipment: Articulated stabilizing arm 205
    Operative proctoscopes 205
    Optics 206
    Long instruments 206
    Insufflator/suction/irrigation/light/electrocautery machines 206
Adaptable laparoscopic instruments 206
    Harmonic scalpel 206
    LigaSure 206
Resection options 206
    Mucosectomy 206
    Partial rectal wall excision 206
    Full-thickness excision 206
    Full-thickness excision with perirectal fat 206
Procedure 206
Complications 208
    Peritoneal entry 208
    Bleeding 208
    Dehiscence 209
    Conversion to laparotomy 209
    Urinary 209
    Anal incontinence 209
    Recto-vaginal fistula 209
Summary 209
Key points 209
Video 209
References 209

Learning objectives

- Understand the indications and contraindications of trasanal minimally invasive surgery
- Learn about the risks of TAMIS
- Learn about the evaluation, preparation of the lesion, and bowel preparation
- Equipment and operative set-up
- Know the options for resection
- Prevent and manage complications

Introduction

Globally, colon and rectal cancer rank third for the incidence of cancer. For developed countries, they are ranked second for incidence and mortality, and in developing countries, they are ranked fourth for incidence and mortality. In addition, colorectal adenomas are known to lead to colorectal cancer, especially when they possess a villous component and grow larger [1].

Following the popularization of colorectal cancer screening, the incidence of large rectal polyps and early stage cancer is increasing [1]. Surgical treatment of rectal tumors has traditionally required an abdominal approach, but is associated with considerable mortality rate (2%–3%) and morbidity (20%–30%) like anastomotic leakage, sepsis, temporary or permanent stoma, genitourinary disorders, sexual dysfunction, and abnormalities in defecation [2–4]. Several goals are important in the management of patients with rectal cancer: Local control and prevention of distant metastases, long-term survival, preservation of the anal sphincter and bladder, sexual functions, and maintenance of quality of life.

High complication rates and possible sacrifice of the anal sphincter after radical dissection have led clinicians to reconsider the role of local excision. Sessile rectal adenomas are usually treated by snare diathermy excision, as a total specimen, or by piecemeal excision. It is better to remove large rectal adenomas by per-anal submucosal or full-wall thickness excision with distinct margins of clearance, using anal retractors to ensure complete removal of the neoplasia [5]. Various surgical techniques are still under discussion for the treatment of early rectal carcinomas. The gold standard procedures, such as anterior and abdomino-perineal resection, show excellent results regarding local recurrence and survival rates [6], but are associated with high incidence of complications [7] and impaired quality of life (anorectal, sexual, and urinary dysfunction) [8]. Additionally, some of the patients require temporary diverting enterostomies.

On the other hand, there are conventional sphincter-preserving techniques that were carried out because downward spread of rectal carcinomas was confirmed to be limited to within 2 cm in 95% of all cases [9,10]. So transanal surgery came to the foreground, such as conventional transanal resection with Park's retractor [11], which preserves sphincter function and has low morbidity and mortality. But, its limitations are low level of the lesion (7–8 cm from the anal verge) and limited visualization [11], and they are associated with an almost unacceptably high recurrence rate of up to 29% [12]. The primary factor limiting the effectiveness of local treatment for early rectal cancer is lymph node invasion. Depths of invasion into the rectal wall, grade or degree of differentiation, as well as vascular, lymphatic, and neural invasion are independent predictors of the risk of nodal metastasis. Since initial studies by Morson [13] and Hermanek [14], large series of resected rectal cancers have shown that well-differentiated tumors confined to the submucosa (T1) without vascular, lymphatic, or neural invasion carry a 4% risk of nodal metastasis [15,16].

In 1980, Buess et al. [17] introduced the technique of transanal endoscopic microsurgery (TEM/TEMS), which allows resection of the lesion up to 18–20 cm from the anal verge. It is associated with low morbidity and safe technique from both oncologic and surgical points of view in select patients. This technique of local resection of rectal and anal polyps, and T1 tumors, is found to be as effective as radical surgery with no significant morbidity. Now with advanced set-ups, this procedure is being termed as transanal minimal invasive surgery (TAMIS). This technique is technically challenging and requires specialized instrumentation. This procedure is performed in a few centers in India, but there are still no convincing data published regarding indications for TAMIS surgery, how it is used, and what are the outcomes. TAMIS allows greater versatility and options for the operating surgeon.

Indications

By far, the most common uses of TAMIS are for resection of colonoscopically unresectable rectal adenomas and carefully selected rectal cancers. It should be stressed that even though TAMIS extends the reach of conventional transanal resections, it should not change the stringent indications for resection, especially with regard to rectal cancer.

Resection of rectal and distal sigmoid adenomas is the most appealing indication for TEM or TAMIS. These are benign lesions in which patients can be spared the morbidity of an unnecessary mesorectal dissection. Smaller adenomas without evidence of high-grade dysplasia may be removed by submucosal dissection. Larger adenomas or those with high-grade dysplasia are at high

TABLE 32.1: Indications for Transanal Endoscopic Microsurgery by Disease Process

Adenoma	Diverticulum
Carcinoma	Epithelioid cell granuloma
Carcinoid	Hyperplastic polyp
Rectal prolapse	Stricture
Rectal ulcer	Rectal stump excision
Non-Hodgkin's lymphoma	Endometrioma
Angiodysplasia	Enterovaginal fistula

risk of harboring invasive adenocarcinoma and should be excised in full thickness with a 10-mm resection margin. Still others recommend full-thickness resection with en bloc removal of the adjacent mesorectum when resecting cancer with curative intent [8]. When there is suspicion, but not confirmation, of a malignant rectal polyp in a patient unfit for or unwilling to undergo major abdominal surgery, TAMIS can be useful in resecting the entire lesion in one piece for complete histological assessment. Prompt radical surgery, if indicated, can be performed without significantly increasing morbidity (Table 32.1).

TAMIS may also be useful as a palliative tool in patients with extensive metastatic disease, or those medically unfit to withstand radical surgery. Neoadjuvant radiation therapy, when used in conjunction with resection either for cure or palliation, does not appear to increase complications following TAMIS [18].

Reach of TAMIS

The limited access and visibility afforded by traditional transanal retractors have restricted their use to resection of rectal polyps and cancers that are mobile, less than 8–10 cm from the anal verge, are smaller than 3–4 cm, and occupy less than 40% of the rectal circumference [9,10]. The TAMIS technique permits access to the entire rectum; including lesions with a proximal margin located 20 cm from the anal verge. Resections of larger or more proximal lesions are technically more demanding, but with experience, these, as well as circumferential sleeve resections, can be performed safely [19,20].

The inferior limit for effective use of the TAMIS instrument is the upper anal canal, approximately 3–4 cm proximal to the anal verge. When the surgeon is operating this low, the aperture of the operating proctoscope is prone to slipping downward and out of the anal canal. This results in escape of the CO_2 pneumorectum, collapse of the operative field, and loss of adequate exposure of the target lesion. Low rectal lesions, however, are good opportunities for surgeons to gain TAMIS operative experience, for if the TAMIS experience does not proceed as planned, excision can be performed with conventional transanal techniques [20].

Risks of TAMIS

The resection of anterior rectal lesions requires special attention. Full-thickness excision of the anterior and even lateral rectum carries the risk of inadvertent dissection into the vagina, urethra, or bladder. Though rare, failure of adequate closure may lead to a rectourethral or rectovaginal fistula.

In an interesting in vitro anatomical study, Najarian et al. [21] documented the mean distance from the anal verge to peritoneal reflection (Table 32.2). This information should be considered in preoperative planning for TAMIS as intraperitoneal access, while unusual, may occur during full-thickness resection of more proximal rectal lesions.

TABLE 32.2: Average Mean Anterior, Lateral, and Posterior Length Measurements from the Anal Verge to the Peritoneal Reflection [21]

	Women	Men
Anterior (cm)	9 (5.5–13.5)	9.7 (7–16)
Lateral (cm)	12.2 (8.5–17)	12.8 (9–19)
Posterior (cm)	14.8 (11–19)	15.5 (12–20)

Intraperitoneal entry carries a risk of injuring intra-abdominal structures, of bacterial and potential cytologic contamination, and of anastomotic leak. Initially regarded as a complication, with experience, intraperitoneal excision with secure closure of the rectal defect can be performed without increased short-term morbidity [22]. If there is concern about the adequacy of an intraperitoneal closure, the patient may be observed overnight for signs of a leak and undergo a water-soluble contrast enema the following morning.

Bulky lesions such as large pedunculated or circumferential polyps can be challenging to manage with any transanal technique, including TEM [23]. These larger specimens can be difficult to see around, and are prone to fragmentation and bleeding.

Contraindications

Contraindications for TAMIS are few and include patients unfit for general or regional anesthesia, uncorrected coagulopathy, rectal varices, and anal stenosis. A careful history of prior surgery with pelvic mesh placement should also be sought, as this may hinder access of the operating proctoscope. Caution should also be taken in patients with a remote history of high-dose pelvic radiation therapy for gynecologic or urologic malignancies. Chronic radiation-induced changes are known to predispose patients to decreased rectal compliance, stenosis, friability, and impaired wound healing.

Evaluation of the lesion
Full colonic evaluation is done preoperatively to identify any synchronous lesions, and the lesion is examined by endorectal ultrasound to determine the depth of penetration into the rectal wall, and the presence of suspicious lymph nodes. Endorectal ultrasound has an accuracy for depth of invasion ranging from 75% to 90% and can be used to identify patients with T2 lesions who may require adjuvant chemo-radiotherapy, and T3 lesions not appropriate for curative TEM.

Preparation of the lesion
In order to facilitate TAMIS excision of a lesion, it is sometimes necessary to manipulate the lesion itself preoperatively. This might include tattooing of the site or debulking of the lesion. The timing of these techniques will depend a lot on the nature of the lesion itself. The timing of TAMIS excision from the original polypectomy at colonoscopy can be crucial. If done too soon, dissection planes will be distorted from the inflammation secondary to the polypectomy itself. If TAMIS excision proceeds too late, the polypectomy site can be completely healed, making identification of the site difficult or impossible. Tattooing is important if a small lesion has been removed and further excision is warranted. Such a situation can arise if polypectomy during colonoscopy results in a pathologic diagnosis of adenocarcinoma with questionable margins. Since this finding will likely have been unsuspected at the time of the colonoscopy, the polypectomy site could heal and potentially become unidentifiable in the near future, particularly

if there is a delay between diagnosis and referral to the surgeon. This becomes especially pertinent if TAMIS cannot be scheduled expeditiously. A tattoo in the area is useful to direct further excision. Patients should be brought back for tattooing as soon as possible. Once they have been tattooed, further excision can be scheduled at a more leisurely pace. Ideally, the surgeon who will perform the TAMIS excision should do the tattooing so the India ink can be placed appropriately. An indiscriminate tattoo at the site can make TAMIS excision more difficult, turning all the tissue black and making the planes difficult to see. The preferred technique is to inject circumferentially a short distance away from the lesion, preferably at the margin of excision. This leaves an 'outline' around the lesion, but no ink left within the actual lesion site itself. Injections should be in the submucosal plane and not mucosa as the mucosa will rapidly turn over, causing the tattoo to disappear.

Bowel preparation
Mechanical bowel preparation is done to have clean rectum during surgery to avoid contamination and difficulty during procedure.

Deep venous thrombosis prophylaxis
As indicated.

Prevention of urinary retention
By urinary catherization.

Equipment and operative set-up
The insufflation/suction/irrigation machine provides the exposure necessary to carry out the cutting, dissect, and sew. The equipment is fitted with locking gaskets and caps to maintain a gas-tight system, thus keeping the rectum insufflated to facilitate operative exposure.

Equipment: Articulated stabilizing arm

The patient is placed in left lateral, right lateral, lithotomy, or prone position based on the location of the tumor (Figure 32.1). The articulated arm, also known as the Martin arm (Figure 32.2), attaches to the operating table and serves as a brace to hold the operating proctoscope firmly in place, allowing for secure fixation of the proctoscope without interfering with the surgeon's ability to manipulate the instruments.

Operative proctoscopes
The operating proctoscope is 4 cm in diameter and is available in two lengths, 12 and 20 cm, and allows for access throughout the

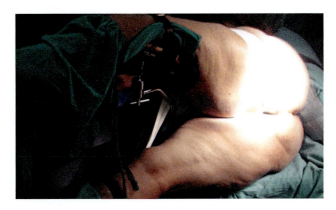

FIGURE 32.1   Patient position.

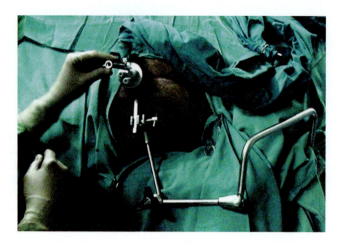

FIGURE 32.2 Martin arm in position.

rectum. The handle has a port to which a hand-bulb insufflator can be attached, or to which a tube is connected for monitoring the CO_2 pressure.

Optics

A 30°, 5-, or 10-mm scope is inserted within the stereoscope and is attached to a laparoscopic camera to allow viewing on a video monitor.

Long instruments

Long instruments are needed to reach up into the rectum via the operating proctoscopes. The instruments include an electric knife (electrocautery), straight and angled forceps, scissors, suction probe, clip applicator, needle holder, and retractable needle. The long, rigid, high-frequency electric knife has an angled, pointed tip that is insulated so that only the distal 2–3 mm conducts the electric current. The electrocautery machine is connected to a foot control, which has the alternative of a cutting or cautery pedal. The pistol grip, utilizing the ulnar grip portion of the hand, is ergonometrically designed for operations that require holding the knife for prolonged periods.

The suction probe is a long, double-curved, rigid tube that is designed to be inserted through the proctoscope and sit to the side of the scope away from the center of the operative field. The suction is generally placed through the lower, center operating port, and can be used by the surgeon or assistant to remove blood, liquid stool, and smoke. There is a connection for attaching the electrocautery. Clips are placed at the beginning and the end of running sutures, replacing the need for knot tying, using a clip applicator.

Insufflator/suction/irrigation/light/ electrocautery machines

The video monitor and machines for CO_2 insufflation, water injection, light, and suction are stacked on a portable cart. An electro-coagulation machine may be placed in the stack of machines on the cart, or a standard operating room machine may be employed. Water may be switched on using a pedal.

Adaptable laparoscopic instruments

Harmonic scalpel

It is a high-energy ultrasonic vibrator (55,500 cycles/s), which mechanically denatures tissue proteins, resulting in cavitation and sealing of blood vessels. The shears coagulate most vessels up to a 5-mm diameter with minimal vapor production [24].

LigaSure

LigaSure is a vessel-sealing device that delivers electrical energy through special graspers. A high coaptive pressure with a temperature greater than 100°C denatures collagen and elastin, permanently sealing blood vessel walls.

The operation is performed in designated minimally invasive surgery (MIS) suites equipped with movable flat screen monitors and recording facilities. This allows the circulating nurse to have a monitor of his or her own to efficiently follow progress of the operation. The surgeon typically operates seated with the assistant at the left to wash the laparoscope lens as needed, alter the degree of the angled laparoscope, and provide suction. The primary monitor is placed over the patient's torso directly in front of the surgeon.

Patients included have T1 rectal cancers or large tubulo-villous adenomas involving less than one-third of the circumference of the rectum. Ideal locations are in the middle or upper third of the rectum, although lower-third lesions are not a contraindication. All patients with suspected pT2 lesions are sent first for neoadjuvant therapy. Local resection for cure is contraindicated in pT3 lesions, unless comorbidities prohibit radical resection or the patient refuses an operation resulting in a permanent colostomy.

Resection options

Mucosectomy

Removing the mucosa, including the polyp from the inner circular layer of the muscularis; a suitable technique for sessile adenomas.

Partial rectal wall excision

Removal of a portion of the rectal wall separating the inner circular layer from the longitudinal muscle of the rectal wall.

Full-thickness excision

Removal of all layers of the rectal wall in the plane just superficial to the perirectal fat – for the majority of lesions localized in the extraperitoneal rectum.

Full-thickness excision with perirectal fat

A full-thickness excision is performed that includes the adjacent perirectal fat-containing lymph nodes. This excision is indicated in cases of malignant lesions or very large polyps with suspected malignancy. For posterior lesions, the perirectal fat is removed, dissecting in the holy plane outside the mesorectum. In the case of anterior tumors, the excision must reach the vaginal septum or the prostatic capsule. Once the excision is completed, the shape of the specimen is a 'truncated pyramid'.

Procedure (see Video 34)

We use a proctoscope of 12 cm length (for lesions less than 15 cm from the anal verge), and the 20 cm long proctoscope is reserved for higher rectal lesions as it is more difficult to suture through. Once positioning is satisfactory, the proctoscope is fixed to the operating table using the Martin arm. This arm can be manipulated easily during the operation if the operating field needs to be modified.

For full-thickness resection, the following current indications are mentioned in the literature:

1. Rectal adenomas (sessile polyps of the rectum)
2. Rectal carcinomas T1 well or moderately well differentiated (G1–G2)

3. Rectal carcinomas T1 poorly differentiated (G3) after neo-adjuvant treatment
4. Rectal carcinomas T2–N0–M0 (smaller than 3 cm) after neoadjuvant treatment
5. Rectal carcinomas independent of the stage as palliative treatment in high-risk patients for major surgery, or with a diffuse metastatic disease, or in patients who refused a Miles operation

Wide margins of resection (at least 1 cm) are carefully marked circumferentially using an angled needle cautery. Wider margins are used for known cancers. The marks are approximately 1 cm apart. The submucosal and perirectal planes are injected using diluted epinephrine solution to aid in hemostasis (Figure 32.3). A monopolar needle cautery at a standard electrocautery setting is used for the resection. The marks are used to outline the lesion and then are connected, dividing the rectal wall perpendicular to the mucosa (Figure 32.4). The mucosa is divided using the cutting function of the cautery, and the 'blend' setting is used for deeper tissues (Figure 32.5). The submucosal plane is the most vascular plane and the continuous suction probe is used to maintain adequate visualization. The layers of the rectal wall are divided perpendicular to the mucosa to maintain full-thickness margins, making the incision deep into the perirectal fat

(Figure 32.6). Whenever possible, one should create the proximal incision early to prevent undermining during the deep dissection. As opposed to a known benign lesion, where a simple flap is elevated, the dissection is continued perpendicular and deep, to include a wedge of perirectal fat with the specimen. Great care should be taken not to manipulate the lesion itself, grasping only the resection margin edges. Dissection continues until the extra rectal plane or the peritoneum is entered. The deep margins of the resection that are exposed are therefore the presacral plane posterior, pelvic sidewalls lateral, or the vaginal wall or prostate anteriorly. Particular care is taken with anterior lesions where the prostatic or vaginal wall is in close proximity. If there is uncertainty, an 'on table' vaginal examination may be performed. In male patients with anterior lesions, a urethral catheter should be placed to facilitate visualization of any urethral injuries. The perirectal tissue is removed in continuity with the lesion to allow accurate pathologic staging and risk stratification.

Intraperitoneal resections require particular attention. If the resection is into the mesentery, a generous wedge of the mesentery is removed along with the rectosigmoid wall – being careful with larger blood vessels, which may require control or division with ultrasonic or bipolar technologies. If the resection

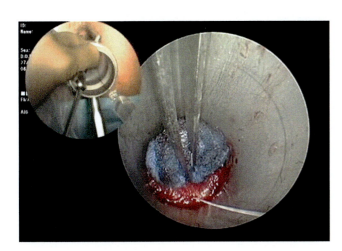

FIGURE 32.3 Submucosal adrenaline injection.

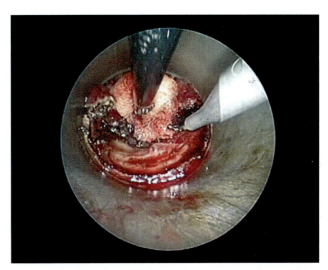

FIGURE 32.5 Rectal dissection.

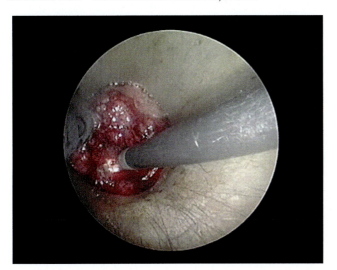

FIGURE 32.4 Marking with electrocautery.

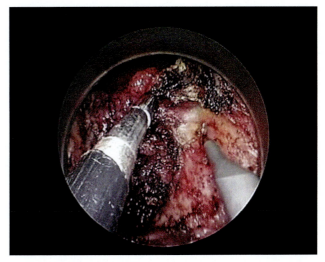

FIGURE 32.6 Rectal dissection completed.

is free into the peritoneal cavity, one must avoid injury to adjacent small bowel. Adequate relaxation must be maintained by anesthesia to prevent the bowel from herniating through the defect. Placing the patient in a Trendelenberg position may also be helpful. Again, if the adjacent mesentery is visible through the rectotomy, a sample may be resected by pulling it into the rectal lumen and dividing it hemostatically (Figure 32.7). After the resection is complete, a washout of the resection bed is performed with a tumoricidal agent, such as diluted betadine solution (Figure 32.8).

Obviously after such an extended resection, particularly if the peritoneal cavity was entered, a secure closure of the excision site must be performed (Figure 32.9). Repair of the excision site is performed transversely, along the lines of a Heinike–Miculitz stricturoplasty, to avoid narrowing of the rectum. A running absorbable suture is used with metallic clips for securing the suture in place (Figure 32.10).

Since its inception, there has been an extensive global experience with TAMIS that substantiates its effectiveness and associated low morbidity rate [15]. The morbidity and mortality associated with TAMIS have been evaluated widely.

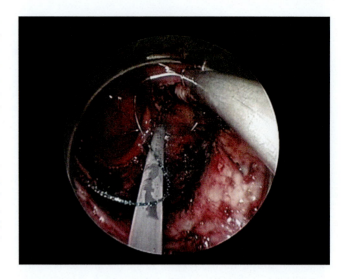

FIGURE 32.9   Suturing the defect.

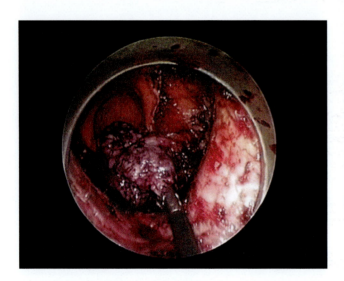

FIGURE 32.7   Removal of the specimen.

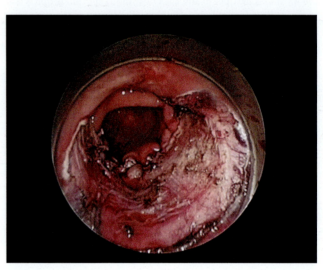

FIGURE 32.10   Completed defect closure.

Complications

Peritoneal entry

Peritoneal entry during TAMIS can be expected during inadvertent or intentional full-thickness excision of anterior rectal tumors located more than 8 cm from the anal verge. Entrance into the peritoneal cavity during resection of a rectal tumor by TAMIS will cause a loss of optimal distention, and has been cited as a cause for a laparotomy. At laparotomy, the defect may be sutured closed after appropriate excision of the tumor.

Conversion to laparotomy may be needed for the repair of peritoneal entry that cannot be repaired through the resectoscope. Other reasons for conversion to laparotomy cited by Salm et al. are hemorrhage, problems with suturing technique, defective instruments, patient positioning, lack of adequate visualization, and lesion size.

Bleeding

Intraoperative bleeding during TAMIS is exceedingly rare, owing to the use of the monopolar high-frequency needle electro-cautery knife.

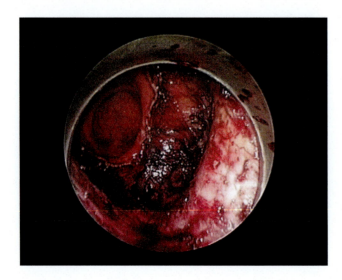

FIGURE 32.8   Defect seen after specimen removal.

Dehiscence

Dehiscence of the site of excision in the rectal wall after sutured repair ranges from 0% to 15% [25].

Conversion to laparotomy

Conversion to laparotomy, for reasons other than a complication, occurs infrequently in TAMIS and decreases as experience is gained [26].

Urinary

The most commonly reported urinary complications are retention requiring catheterization, with a frequency of up to 8% [27], and urinary tract infection, with a similar rate [28]. Almost all cases of urinary retention are transient and merely require temporary catheterization of the bladder [29].

Anal incontinence

This complication is usually transient [26,30]. Most of the dysfunction or incontinence after surgery is reported as fecal soilage or incontinence to gas, as opposed to frank fecal incontinence.

Recto-vaginal fistula

Recto-vaginal fistula is a complication that arises after excision of tumors from the anterior wall of the rectum in female patients.

Summary

In conclusion, with current findings it can be stated that local excision of T1 rectal cancer avoids major surgery or colostomy without compromising the oncologic results. If the tumor invades the muscularis propria (T2), neoadjuvant treatment using high-dose radiation combined with adequate full-thickness local excision shows the same oncologic results as TAMIS, and it also appears to be a promising option in the management of highly selected patients with small T2 rectal cancer.

This minimally invasive approach minimizes the risks of postoperative morbidity and mortality, as well as the need for stomas that may be associated with traditional surgery. It is good technique for full-thickness excision of the large rectal adenomas and getting accurate histopathological results – saving patient's and physician's time, thus avoiding multiple biopsies, and leading to proper management of the patients' disease. Hospital stay is also remarkably reduced, and the quality of life is improved in our opinion; these benefits may be achieved by close collaboration within a multidisciplinary team, correct image staging and careful patient selection, use of good instrumentation, and an adequate local excision by the TAMIS.

Key points

- It should be stressed that even though TAMIS extends the reach of conventional transanal resections, it should not change the stringent indications for resection, especially with regard to rectal cancer.
- When there is suspicion, but not confirmation, of a malignant rectal polyp in a patient unfit for or unwilling to undergo major abdominal surgery, TAMIS can be useful in resecting the entire lesion in one piece for complete histologic assessment.
- The TAMIS technique permits access to the entire rectum – including lesions with a proximal margin located 20 cm from the anal verge.
- The timing of TAMIS excision from the original polypectomy at colonoscopy can be crucial.

Video

VIDEO 34   https://youtu.be/nEEvUPrwmCc

Transanal Full Thickness Resections.

References

1. Logan RFA, Patnick J, Nickerson C et al. Outcomes of the Bowel Cancer Screening Programme (BCSP) in England after the first 1 million tests. *Gut* [Internet] 2012 October 1 [cited 2018 June 8];61(10):1439–46. Available from: http://www.ncbi.nlm.nih.gov/pubmed/22156981
2. Blair S EJ. Transanal excision for low rectal cancers is curative in early stage of disease with favorable histology. *Am Surg Atlanta* 2000;66(9):817–20.
3. Law WL, Chu KW. Anterior resection for rectal cancer with mesorectal excision: A prospective evaluation of 622 patients. *Ann Surg* 2004 August;240(2):260–8.
4. Chiappa A, Biffi R, Bertani E et al. Surgical outcomes after total mesorectal excision for rectal cancer. *J Surg Oncol* 2006 September 1;94(3):182–93.
5. Parks AG. A technique for excising extensive villous papillomatous changes in the lower rectum. *Proc R Soc Med* 1968;61:441–2.
6. Bulow S, Christensen IJ, Harling H, Kronborg O, Fenger CNH. Recurrence and survival after mesorectal excision for rectal cancer. *Br J Surg* 2003;90:974–80.
7. Enker WE, Merchant N, Cohen AM et al. Safety and efficacy of low anterior resection for rectal cancer: 681 consecutive cases from a specialty service. *Ann Surg* 1999 October;230(4):544–52; discussion 552-4.
8. Havenga K, Maas CP, DeRuiter MC, Welvaart K, Trimbos JB. Avoiding long-term disturbance to bladder and sexual function in pelvic surgery, particularly with rectal cancer. *Semin Surg Oncol* 2000 April;18(3):235–43.
9. Williams W. The rationale for preservation of the anal sphincter in patients with low rectal cancer. *Br J Surg* 1984;71.
10. McDermott FT, Hughes ES, Pihl E, Johnson WRP, Price AB. Local recurrence for rectal cancer in a series of 1008 patients. *Br J Surg* 1985;72:34–7.
11. Parks AG. A technique for the removal of large villous tumours in the rectum. *Proc R Soc Med* 1970;63(Suppl 1):89–91.
12. Madbouly KM. Recurrence after Transanal excision of T1 rectal cancer: Should we be concerned? *Dis Colon Rectum* 2006;48(4):711–21.
13. Morson BC. Histological criteria for local excision. *Br J Surg* 1985;53(4).
14. Hermanek P, Marzoli GP. *Lokale Therapie des Rektumkarzinoms: Verfahren in kurativer Intention.* Springer-Verlag; 2013.
15. Brodsky JT, Richard GK, Cohen AM, Minsky MB. Variables correlated with the risk of lymph node metastasis in early rectal cancer. *Cancer* 1992;69:322–6.
16. Blumberg D, Paty PB, Picon AI et al. Stage I rectal cancer: Identification of high-risk patients. *J Am Coll Surg* 1998 May 1;186(5):574–80.
17. Buess G, Theiss R, Günther M, Hutterer F, Pichlmaier H. [Transanal endoscopic microsurgery]. *Leber Magen Darm* 1985 November;15(6):271–9.
18. Lezoche E, Guerrieri M, Paganini AM et al. Transanal endoscopic versus total mesorectal laparoscopic resections of T2–N0 low rectal cancers after neoadjuvant treatment: A prospective randomized trial with a 3-years minimum follow-up period. *Surg Endosc Other Interv Tech* 2005 Jun 4;19(6):751–6.
19. Mentges B, Buess G, Schäfer D, Manncke K, Becker HD. Local therapy of rectal tumors. *Dis Colon Rectum* 1996 August;39(8):886–92.
20. Saclarides TJ. Transanal endoscopic microsurgery. *Dis Colon Rectum* 1992;35:1183–91.

21. Najarian MM, Belzer EG, Cogbill TH, Mathiason MA. Determination of the peritoneal reflection using intraoperative proctoscopy. *Dis Colon Rectum* 2004 December;47(12):2080–5.
22. Gavagan JA, Whiteford MH, Swanstrom LL. Full-thickness intraperitoneal excision by transanal endoscopic microsurgery does not increase short-term complications. *Am J Surg* [Internet] 2004 May 1 [cited 2018 May 27];187(5):630–4. Available from: http://www.ncbi.nlm.nih.gov/pubmed/15135680
23. Stipa F, Lucandri G, Ferri M, Casula G, Ziparo V. Local excision of rectal cancer with transanal endoscopic microsurgery (TEM). *Anticancer Res* 2004 March 1;24(2C):1167–72.
24. Langer C, Markus T, Liersch T, Füzesi L, Becker H. UltraCision or high-frequency knife in transanal endoscopic microsurgery (TEM)? *Surg Endosc* 2001 May 21;15(5):513–7.
25. Schäfer H, Baldus SE, Hölscher AH. Giant adenomas of the rectum: Complete resection by transanal endoscopic microsurgery (TEM). *Int J Colorectal Dis* 2006 September 20;21(6):533–7.
26. Salm R, Lampe H, Bustos A, Matern U. Experience with TAMIS in Germany. *Endosc Surg Allied Technol* 1994 October;2(5):251–4.
27. Katti G. An evaluation of transanal endoscopic microsurgery for rectal adenoma and carcinoma. *JSLS J Soc Laparoendosc Surg* 2004;8(2):123–6.
28. Demartines N, von Flüe MO, Harder FH. Transanal endoscopic microsurgical excision of rectal tumors: Indications and results. *World J Surg* 2001 July;25(7):870–5.
29. Smith LE, Ko ST, Saclarides T, Caushaj P, Orkin BA, Khanduja KS. Transanal endoscopic microsurgery. *Dis Colon Rectum* 1996 October;39(Sup 1):S79–84.
30. Steele RJC, Hershman MJ, Mortensen NJM, Armitage NCM, Scholefield JH. Transanal endoscopic microsurgery – Initial experience from three centres in the United Kingdom. *Br J Surg* 1996 February;83(2):207–10.

Chapter 33

TRANSANAL TOTAL MESORECTAL EXCISION FOR RECTAL CANCER

Daniel Peyser and Patricia Sylla

Contents

Learning objectives 211
Transanal TME history and results 211
Preoperative evaluation 213
   Indications and contraindications 213
Preoperative assessment 214
Operative approach 214
Positioning 214
Abdominal dissection 215
Transanal dissection 215
'Rendez-vous' 217
Anastomosis 217
Complications of taTME 217
   Urethral injury 218
   Carbon dioxide embolism 219
   Anastomotic leaks 220
Summary 221
Key points 221
Videos 221
References 221

Learning objectives

- Review optimal selection criteria for taTME, including inclusion and exclusion criteria
- Review taTME technique for low and mid-rectal cancer
- Review the current literature on outcomes of taTME
- Understand complications specific to transanal TME and how to prevent them

Transanal TME history and results

Colorectal cancer is the third-most common cancer worldwide with an estimated 1.8 million new cases and over 860,000 deaths in 2018 [1]. Rectal cancer accounts for approximately 40% of these cancers. Surgery for rectal cancer is a challenge due to the difficulty in obtaining access to and exposure of the distal rectum, particularly in obese male patients. Surgical treatment of rectal cancer has progressed significantly since Miles described the abdominoperineal resection (APR) in 1908 [2]. In the 1980s, Heald popularized the technique of total mesorectal excision (TME), which has now become the gold standard for oncologic resections [3]. TME dissection along the fascia propria ensures an intact mesorectum with negative distal (DRM) and circumferential resection margins (CRM), both of which are associated with decreased locoregional recurrence and improved disease-free survival [4,5].

Laparoscopic TME was introduced in the 1990s and has been shown to improve short-term postoperative outcomes. A number of randomized control trials comparing laparoscopic TME to open TME have demonstrated that a laparoscopic approach is associated with reduced postoperative pain, reduced wound infection rates, and decreased length of hospital stay [6]. The COREAN [7] and COLOR II [8] trials demonstrated equivalent oncologic outcomes relative to open TME. However, the ACOSOG Z6051 [9] and ALaCaRT [10] trials failed to show noninferiority of laparoscopic TME compared to open TME with respect to short-term oncologic outcomes. In these two trials, the positive CRM rate for laparoscopic TME was 6.7%–12.1%, versus 2.9%–7.7% for open TME. Additionally, relatively high conversion rates were reported with laparoscopic TME in the COLOR II and ACOSOG Z6051 trials; that is 17% and 11.3%, respectively [8,9]. The three most common factors contributing to conversion in the COLOR II trial were a narrow pelvis, obesity, and tumor fixation [8]. Investigations into patient and tumor-related factors predictive of intraoperative difficulty and positive CRM included male sex, obesity, narrow pelvis, bulky tumors, and advanced T-stage [11,12]. These factors can complicate both laparoscopic and open TME by limiting visualization of and access to the mesorectal plane and dissection within the confined space of the narrow pelvis, leading to dissection in the wrong tissue plane, incomplete TME, and worse oncologic outcomes.

Transanal TME (taTME), via a 'bottom up' approach to pelvic dissection, overcomes some of the limitations of abdominal TME by providing more direct access to the distal rectum and unobstructed exposure of the TME planes, which should allow for a more accurate oncologic resection and improved completeness of TME specimens. In 2010 Sylla et al. reported on the first clinical case of taTME with laparoscopic assistance, and over the past decade taTME has been increasingly adopted worldwide [13]. Studies on the procedural safety and initial long-term oncologic outcomes of taTME have been promising [14].

When evaluating data from taTME series with n ≥ 50 cases, the 30-day postoperative morbidity ranges from 13.4% to 52.5%, with major complications ranging between 10% and 24.5% and mortality from 0.3% to 5.6% (Table 33.1). Rates of complete and near-complete TME grading are 86%–100%, with 0.6%–7% rates

TABLE 33.1: Perioperative and Oncologic Outcomes of Published taTME Series with N > 50 Patients

Series	N	Perioperative	Oncologic	Local Recurrence
Veltcamp HM [32] 2016	80	Morbidity – 39% Major – 12%	Complete/near-complete – 97% + CRM – 2.5% + DRM – 0%	Follow-up period – 2 years Local recurrence – 2.5%
Tuech [33] 2014	56	Morbidity – 26%	Complete/near-complete – 100% + CRM – 5.3% + DRM – 0%	Mean follow-up – 29 months Local recurrence – 1.7%
Lacy [17] 2015	140	Morbidity – 34.2% Major – 10%	Complete/near-complete – 99.2% + CRM – 6.4% + DRM – n/a	Mean follow-up – 15 months Local recurrence – 2.3%
Chen [34] 2016	50	Morbidity – 20%	Complete/near-complete – n/a + CRM – 4% + DRM – n/a	Follow-up – n/a Local recurrence – n/a
Burke [35] 2016	50	Morbidity – 36%	Complete/near-complete – 98% + CRM – 4% + DRM – 2%	Mean follow-up – 15.1 months Local recurrence – 4%
Perdawood [15] 2017	100	Morbidity – 36% Mortality – 2%	Complete/near-complete – 86% + CRM – 7% + DRM – 0%	Follow-up – n/a Local recurrence – n/a
Marks [36] 2017	373	Morbidity – 13.4% Mortality – 0.3%	Complete/near-complete – 96% + CRM – 6% + DRM – 1.4%	Mean follow-up – 5.5 years Local recurrence – 7.4%
de Lacy [37] 2018	186	Morbidity – n/a	Complete/near-complete – 97.3% + CRM – 8.1% + DRM – 3.2%	Follow-up period – 5 years Local recurrence – n/a
International taTME Registry [40] 2019	2653	Morbidity – n/a	Complete/near-complete – 91.2% + CRM – 4% + DRM – 1%	Follow-up period – n/a Local recurrence – n/a
D'Andrea [38] 2019	54	Morbidity – 42.6% Mortality – 5.6%	Complete/near-complete – 94.4% + CRM – 3.7% + DRM – 0%	Mean follow-up – 28 months Local recurrence – 3.9%
Hol [39] 2019	159	Morbidity – 52.5% Major – 24.5%	Complete/near-complete – 97.5% + CRM – 0.6% + DRM – 0%	Mean follow-up – 54.8 months Local recurrence (3 yr) – 2% Local recurrence (5 yr) – 4%

Abbreviations: CRM: Circumferential resection margin; DRM: Distal resection margin; n/a: Data not available

of positive CRM, and 0%–3.2% rates of positive DRM. Thus far, few data report local recurrence rates (LR) ranging from 1.7% to 7.4% with a mean follow-up time between 15 and 54.8 months [15,17,32–40].

A case-matched study, comparing 100 patients undergoing taTME to patients undergoing laparoscopic TME and open TME, demonstrated that taTME was associated with decreased operative time, blood loss, and lower rates of incomplete TME relative to laparoscopic TME but not open TME [15]. The complication rates, mortality, and rate of successful resection were comparable between the three groups.

A 2019 meta-analysis of 14 studies comparing taTME (495 patients) to laparoscopic TME (547 patients), demonstrated lower morbidity (both overall and major), anastomotic leak rate, and lower CRM involvement with taTME. Additionally, taTME was associated with decreased length of stay and readmission rate. There was no difference in operative time, conversion rate, DRM involvement, TME grade, lymph node harvest, or local recurrence rates [41].

In 2019, the most recent update from the International taTME Registry reported on 2653 patients with rectal cancer and reported a positive CRM and DRM rate of 4.0% and 1.0%,

respectively, with 91.2% of TME specimens being graded as complete/near-complete [40]. Previous data from the international registry had reported a 96.6% TME specimen grading of complete/near-complete and this decrease in specimen quality is likely a reflection of the increased adoption of taTME and the significant learning curve. Additionally, postoperative morbidity and mortality of taTME according to the International taTME Registry were 35.4% and 0.6%, respectively, comparable to the historical 40%–57% morbidity and 0.4%–4% mortality rates reported for laparoscopic TME in previous studies [8–10,20,42].

Preliminary long-term oncological results of taTME have also been promising. Recently published results from the Netherlands on 159 patients, who underwent taTME for rectal cancer, reported local recurrence rates of 2% and 4%, disease-free survival of 92% and 81%, and overall survival of 84% and 77% at three and five years, respectively. These results compare favorably to historical long-term oncologic outcomes of laparoscopic TME [43–45].

Most recently, however, concern was raised regarding the high incidence of LR following taTME in Norway. A moratorium was issued and a national audit of all taTME procedures for rectal cancer performed over four years was conducted. The results of this audit determined an LR rate of 7.6% following taTME among

157 patients, with an estimated local recurrence rate at 2.4 years of 11.6%, compared to a 2.4% local recurrence rate among the national Norwegian Colorectal Cancer Registry [64]. The majority of patients (152/157), including the 12 patients who developed LR, had surgery performed at one of four hospitals (case range 32–57). The operating surgeons had attended international workshops and completed structured training programs on taTME before implementing taTME at their institutions, with one center having been proctored. Of 152 patients who survived more than 100 days after surgery, 12 developed LR. Multifocal recurrences occurred in 6 patients, extensive LR occurred in 2 patients, staple line recurrence in 1 patient, and presacral recurrence in 1 patient. Additionally, concurrent distant metastases occurred in 3 patients. Of the 12 patients, 10 patients had pT3 or pT4 disease, and 8 patients had node positive disease, yet only one patient had received preoperative neoadjuvant therapy. With regard to the resection, 4 patients had an R1 resection and the remaining 8 had an R0 resection at time of surgery. Median time to recurrence was 9.5 months (range 2–23) and 50% of the patients who developed LR were deceased at the time of the audit. The hazard ratio for LR after taTME compared to the national registry cohort was 5.7 (CI 2.70–12.06) with no change when adjusted for sex, age, and CRT. When adjusted for tumor distance, pT, and pN stage, the hazard ratio increased to 6.71 (CI 2.94–15.32). In addition to the local recurrence rate, the Norwegian national audit also revealed an anastomotic leak rate of 8.4% in the taTME group, compared to 4.5% in the national registry group, and a 30-day mortality rate of 2.3% after taTME compared to 0.3% for the comparison group [64].

The Norwegian results highlight safety concerns regarding adoption of a highly complex procedure with a significant learning curve. Questionable selection criteria for taTME and technical factors at the time of taTME may account for the rate of LR observed in Norway, including improperly secured distal purse-string suture, which may result in the spread of contaminants and tumor cells during transanal insufflation. The authors reported 7 rectal perforations, 2 urethral, and 1 bladder injury during procedures, and video review of these cases would likely highlight wrong-plane dissection as a potential contributor to negative oncologic outcomes. While 152/157 taTME cases in Norway were performed in one of four hospitals, the total number of cases was 32–57 over the 4-year period and the actual annual volume at each hospital is unknown. Assuming an equal number of cases per year, the annual case volume may have been only 8–14 taTME cases per year at these four hospitals, well below the volume to be considered a high-volume center, and a number of studies have shown a relationship between volume and clinical outcomes. A 2016 study comparing low volume (≤30 total cases) versus high volume taTME centers (>30 total cases) demonstrated higher conversion rates (4.3% vs. 2.7%), lower rates of complete TME (80.5% vs. 89.7%), and higher rates of local recurrence (8.9% vs. 2.8%) at low volume centers [46]. Evaluation of the learning curve for taTME, defined as a decrease in major postoperative complications and anastomotic leak rates, occurs once a surgeon's experience exceeds 40 patients [47]. Another study reported a minimum of 45–51 cases to reach proficiency in producing high-quality TME with the taTME approach [48]. This case volume is not sustainable for most surgeons who wish to adopt taTME, and many surgeons are unlikely to gain the technical competency required for taTME due to low case volume. In the United States, over 400 surgeons have received taTME training, but only 25 of those could be considered high-volume rectal cancer surgeons. Current training pathways for taTME adoption vary by country with no standardization in training. A national training pathway was established in the Netherlands in 2014, and required a

number of prerequisites including: (1) expertise in laparoscopic rectal cancer surgery (>50 laparoscopic TME cases), (2) experience in transanal endoscopic surgery, (3) case volume of ≥20 taTME cases per year, and (4) adequate equipment for taTME, with strong recommendation for a two-team approach. The training program consisted of a two-day course with didactic courses, live taTME surgery, hands-on training with box trainers, and a cadaveric course performing taTME with faculty guidance. Following the course, the trainees were proctored by experienced taTME surgeons until proficiency was determined by the proctor for the trainee to proceed alone [49]. Similar training pathways have been described by other institutions, and are agreed upon by experts in taTME [19,50,51].

Preoperative evaluation

Indications and contraindications

Appropriate case selection for taTME is determined by both patient and tumor characteristics, and should be based on multidisciplinary tumor-board assessment of the case both before and after neoadjuvant treatment. The first taTME consensus statement from 2014 included indications for taTME, including malignant disease requiring accurate dissection of the mid- to distal rectum, male gender, tumor located less than 12 cm from the anal verge, narrow or deep pelvis, tumor diameter >4 cm, obesity (visceral or BMI >30), prostatic hypertrophy, distorted or scarred tissue planes from neoadjuvant radiation, and impalpable and low tumors. Contraindications to taTME included T4 tumors, obstructing tumors, and emergency resection [16]. Tumors staged cT4 are considered a relative contraindication because many studies have excluded T4 tumors that could warrant pelvic exenteration. However, some studies have included cT4 tumors that demonstrated clinical and radiologic downstaging following neoadjuvant therapy [17,18]. Based on the expert's experience as well as recent reports of taTME-specific procedural complications such as urethral injury, it is recommended that taTME be avoided for cT4 tumors, recurrent tumors, and in patients with prior prostatectomy or a history of prostate seeds, and as well in cases where prior pelvic surgery or radiation may have resulted in major distortion of the perineal and pelvic anatomy. This is particularly recommended in surgeons who are along their learning curve, which has been estimated to be between 40–51 cases [47,48]. More experienced surgeons who are well beyond their learning curve may consider taTME on a case-by-case basis, and only when the benefits of a taTME approach outweigh procedural and oncologic risks, and as discussed with patients during the informed consent [38].

In 2017, a multidisciplinary consensus statement by experts in taTME confirmed that taTME is the preferred approach for patients with a narrow pelvis, obese patients, and patients with a bulky, mid-to-distal rectal tumor [19]. For patients with distal and ultra-low tumors, an intersphincteric resection can be performed with taTME to preserve sphincter function, as these tumors benefit from the enhanced visualization of the lower rectum associated with taTME, ensuring a negative DRM and avoiding permanent colostomy.

One of the most promising uses of taTME is in ultra-low rectal tumors and its role in sphincter preservation surgery. The distal limit of rectal cancer surgery was revolutionized when it was realized that the internal sphincter muscle could be partially or completely sacrificed with intersphincteric resection (ISR), decreasing the minimal distal margin requirement of 5 cm to 2 cm [65]. The 2-cm rule was ended in 2005, when Rullier reported that distal rectal cancer treated with ISR was feasible without oncologic compromise [52]. Sphincter preservation for patients with ultra-low rectal tumors is not dependent on distal extent, but involvement of the external anal sphincter. The Rullier Classification System is used for ultra-low tumors and includes four classifications: Type I, which are supra-anal tumors located >1 cm from the anorectal ring; Type II, which are juxta-anal tumors located <1 cm from the anorectal ring; Type III, which are intra-anal tumors involving the internal anal sphincter; and Type IV, where tumors invade into the levator ani muscle, or external anal sphincter [53]. When performing sphincter-preserving surgery for ultra-low tumors, it is recommended that an ultra-low anterior resection be performed for Type I. Type II and III tumors require ISR – partial for Type II and a total for Type III. Type IV tumors are not amenable to sphincter-preserving surgery and will require an APR. One of the advantages of taTME is that it can be combined with ISR. For ultra-low rectal tumors abutting the anorectal ring and/or involving only the internal anal sphincter, partial or total ISR is first performed using a standard perineal approach followed by purse-string closure of the anorectal stump, insertion of the transanal endoscopic platform, and completion of the taTME. The advantage of the taTME approach for ultra-low tumors has been the ability to extend the ISR dissection further cephalad toward the TME planes under significantly improved visualization relative to standard perineal dissection.

Overall, based on experts' experience to date, taTME is most impactful for low and mid-rectal tumors, when an abdominal approach is anticipated to be technically difficult due to tumor location and/or patient anatomy. Most agree that taTME is a less desirable approach for upper rectal tumors (>10 cm), where an abdominal approach should result in satisfactory outcomes, unless the patient is an obese male.

Preoperative assessment

The first step in assessing a patient for taTME is a thorough history and physical examination. Many patients with rectal cancer are asymptomatic, but symptoms may include rectal bleeding, rectal pain, tenesmus, change in bowel habits or stool caliber, weight loss, nausea, or fatigue. Prior pelvic surgery, such as prostate or gynecological surgery, and/or pelvic radiation can affect TME dissection planes and increase the complexity of transanal dissection and the risk of wrong-plane surgery. Information about baseline urinary and sexual function are important to document because of the risks of pelvic autonomic nerve injury associated with TME. Likewise, a history of fecal incontinence is critical in preoperative evaluation, as fecal incontinence would preclude a patient from sphincter preservation surgery. A comprehensive medical history should identify other medical conditions that may warrant additional assessment to optimize the patient prior to surgery. Diabetes, obesity, immunosuppression, and smoking have been associated with anastomotic leak in taTME and should be addressed before surgery [20]. Laboratory studies should include complete blood count, electrolyte panel, coagulation studies, and type and screen. Serum carcinoembryonic antigen (CEA) should be obtained to facilitate postoperative surveillance.

Digital rectal examinations are essential for assessment of tumor size, mobility, location, and relationship to the anal sphincter complex. Distance of the tumor from the anal verge and anorectal ring should be measured, and the tone of the sphincter muscles should be assessed. Endoscopic assessment, preferably with rigid proctoscopy, is essential to accurately measure the distance of the tumor from the anal verge. All patients diagnosed with rectal cancer should have a complete colonoscopy to exclude synchronous cancers.

Preoperative imaging, in accordance with the National Comprehensive Cancer Network (NCCN) guidelines, is necessary for rectal cancer staging. A CT of the chest, abdomen, and pelvis is obtained to assess for distant metastasis to the liver, lungs, and other organs, while a pelvic MRI is obtained to assess local T and N stage of the rectal tumor [54]. Patients should be presented at a multidisciplinary team tumor board (MDT), where the patient's presentation, imaging, and pathology can be reviewed to create an individualized treatment plan. For patients determined to benefit from neoadjuvant therapy, a posttreatment pelvic MRI should be obtained to assess tumor response. The patient is then re-presented at the MDT to optimize the surgical plan.

Before surgery, patients should meet with an enterostomal therapist to be marked for potential ostomy sites, as research has shown that patients with preoperative stoma markings have better quality of life and fewer postoperative stoma complications [21].

Although ERAS (enhanced recovery after surgery) pathways vary between hospitals, all incorporate preoperative, intraoperative, and postoperative components to allow for earlier discharge home without risk of readmission or complications. All patients undergoing taTME should undergo mechanical and antibiotic bowel preparation, which allows for better bowel manipulation. Additionally, parenteral preoperative antibiotics are given to decrease the risk of surgical site infection. Other preoperative components of most ERAS pathways include patient education, preoperative analgesia, and carbohydrate-loading fluids consumed the morning of surgery. Intraoperative ERAS components include utilization of a minimally invasive approach, intraoperative fluid restriction, venous thromboembolism (VTE) prophylaxis, and minimization of opioids through locoregional blocks. Postoperative components include early feeding and advancement of diet, early mobilization, postoperative fluid restriction, and multimodal analgesia to avoid opioids.

Operative approach

The feasibility of pure NOTES and hybrid (laparoscopic-assisted) taTME was established in animal [22,23] and human cadaver models [24,25] before the first clinical case in 2010 [13]. Although single-team taTME was originally described, the most common approach involves an abdominal team and a transanal team working simultaneously. The current consensus among taTME experts is that a two-team approach decreases operative time and improves visualization of TME planes and coordination between the two teams [19]. The abdominal approach can be performed open, laparoscopic, or robotically. As described by Penna et al., taTME can be broken down into five critical steps: (1) placement of the distal purse string to close the rectal lumen, (2) full-thickness rectotomy, (3) TME dissection, (4) specimen extraction, and (5) anastomosis [26].

Positioning (see Video 35)

After induction of general endotracheal anesthesia, the patient is positioned in lithotomy position with adjustable stirrups and padding to protect from peroneal nerve injury. During the case, the lithotomy positioning is adjusted to facilitate both teams working simultaneously. Abdominal and perineal teams, laparoscopic towers, and instrument tables are set up ergonomically to facilitate procedures (Figure 33.1). Intravenous antibiotic prophylaxis covering aerobic and anaerobic bacteria is given within 60 minutes prior to incision to minimize the risk of surgical site infection [27]. Subcutaneous heparin is administered and sequential compression devices are placed to decrease the rate of

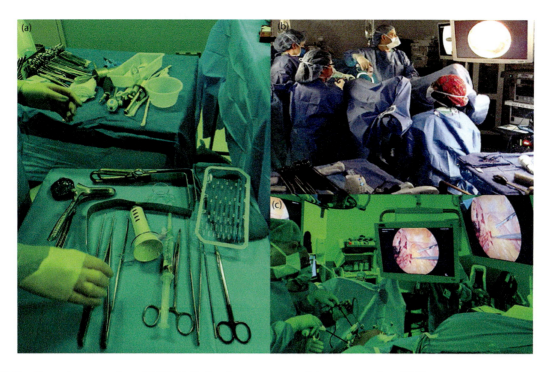

FIGURE 33.1 Operating setup for taTME. (a) Perineal team setup and instrumentation. (b) Two-team operative setup. Lithotomy position is adjusted to facilitate both teams working simultaneously. (c) One-team abdominal setup. Ergonomic position of monitors facilitates completion of procedures. When the transanal team initiates dissection, one of the monitors is dedicated to the transanal view.

venous thromboembolism [28], and a urinary catheter is inserted. Ureteral stents are not routinely recommended, and can be considered in reoperative pelvic surgery, or in cases where there is concern for ureteral injury.

Abdominal dissection

The abdominal team begins the operation by establishing pneumo-peritoneum and placing trocars as for a laparoscopic low-anterior resection. A 12-mm trocar can be placed at the site of the future ileostomy in the right lower quadrant, or along a planned lower midline or Pfannenstiel extraction site. The abdominal team assesses the abdomen for any evidence of liver or peritoneal metastases, and then cross-clamps the distal sigmoid colon while the transanal team places the distal purse-string suture. Once the rectum has been washed out with a betadine solution and the purse-string suture confirmed to be airtight, both teams can work simultaneously (Figure 33.1b). Many surgeons prefer not to initiate the transanal dissection until high ligation of the inferior mesenteric artery (IMA) and inferior mesenteric vein (IMV) have been performed (Figure 33.1c).

The abdominal team performs a medial to lateral dissection of the rectosigmoid mesentery. The IMA is ligated close to its origin off the aorta, taking care to identify and protect the left ureter. The IMV is then identified and ligated near the inferior border of the pancreas. The descending colon is medialized by releasing it from its retroperitoneal attachment, by dissecting along the white line of Toldt. The splenic flexure is typically mobilized to ensure adequate reach of the colonic conduit in preparation for coloanal anastomosis or end-colostomy. The abdominal team then turns toward the pelvis and begins upper TME dissection until convergence with the transanal team. In cases with an exceedingly narrow pelvis, in an effort to avoid an incomplete TME specimen, mesorectal dissection is interrupted until transanal dissection has been completed and carried out as far superiorly as possible

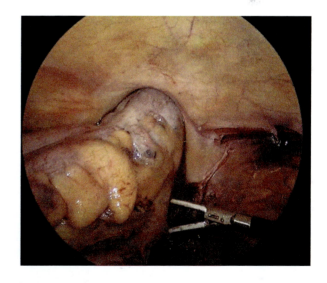

FIGURE 33.2 Abdominal view of a very narrow pelvis precluding safe abdominal TME.

(Figure 33.2). The abdominal team can also assist the transanal team by retracting the rectum to facilitate transanal dissection.

Transanal dissection

The transanal team begins by irrigating the rectum with povidone-iodine and performing digital rectal examination to confirm tumor location and distance from anal verge. An anal retractor system is then placed to expose the anal canal. For tumors of the mid-rectum, the tumor is best visualized endoscopically, and the distal purse string is placed through a transanal access platform after establishing pneumorectum. This requires the abdominal team to occlude the sigmoid until the purse-string is secured to prevent colonic distension. For tumors of the lower rectum, the purse string can be placed directly under vision through an anoscope, or through the transanal platform. If an intersphincteric resection is performed, it is done first, prior to purse-string closure of the anorectal stump (Figure 33.3). If a transanal APR (taAPR) is to be performed then standard perineal dissection is performed. Transanal endoscopic setup for taTME is carried out as shown in Figure 33.4, with a TEO (Karl Storz, Tuttlingen Germany) platform. Extralevator dissection is more amenable to taAPR, and once the appropriate landmarks are identified (i.e., the puborectalis posteriorly and the transverse perineal muscles anteriorly) the transanal platform is inserted and fixated before dissection continues.

The distal purse-string suture is placed at least 1 cm distal to the lower edge of the tumor in order to ensure a negative DRM. It is critical that the purse string be airtight and completely occlude the rectal lumen; failure to place an adequate purse string will lead to colonic insufflation and contamination with liquid stool and tumor cells, increasing the risk of locoregional recurrences,

and possibly increasing the risk of multifocal pelvic recurrences. The level of planned rectotomy is marked out circumferentially with cautery on the rectal mucosa, just distal to the purse-string suture. This is followed by full-thickness dissection through the rectal wall with monopolar cautery. Full-thickness dissection is continued until the avascular TME plane is reached. The CO_2 pneumorectum is usually maintained between 12 and 15 mmHg of pressure using high-flow insufflators, which help maintain a stable pneumorectum, evacuate smoke build-up, and help distend tissue planes. Dissection occurs along the mesorectal 'holy plane' between the parietal endopelvic fascia and mesorectal envelope, as described by Heald [3]. The TME dissection continues cephalad, alternating between posterior, anterior, and lateral dissection. Even and circumferential dissection helps avoid dissecting too far in one direction and distorting the anatomy. Care must be taken to identify anatomic landmarks early to avoid wrong plane surgery. Posteriorly, dissection must remain just above the endopelvic fascia to avoid injury to the presacral venous plexus and hypogastric nerves (Figure 33.5). Anteriorly, the rectoprostatic/rectovaginal plane must be dissected carefully, and the prostate/

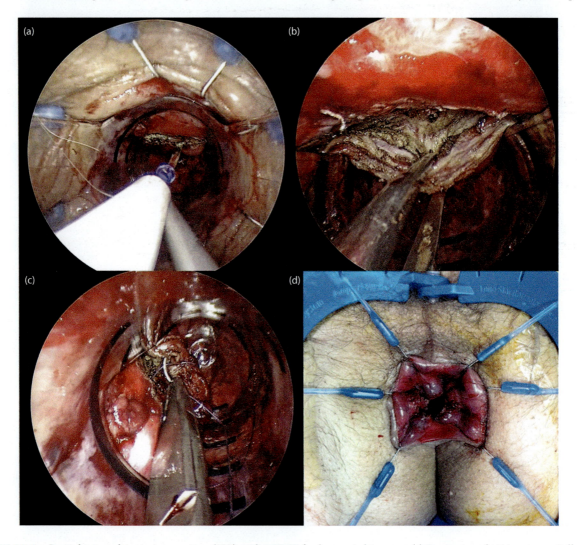

FIGURE 33.3 Partial intersphincteric resection (ISR) with taTME for low rectal tumors. (a) For tumor abutting or partially invading the internal anal sphincter (IAS), in which sphincter preservation is deemed oncologically and functionally acceptable, partial ISR is started first. (b) ISR proceeds cephalad under direct visualization until the puborectalis is identified posteriorly and laterally, and the rectourethral muscle and/or prostate is identified anteriorly. (c) The anorectal stump is then closed with an airtight purse-string suture, which may need to be reinforced. (d) Following completion of ISR, the transanal endoscopic platform is inserted and taTME is carried out under laparoscopic visualization.

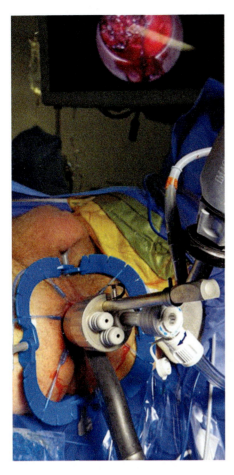

FIGURE 33.4 Transanal endoscopic setup for taTME. The short 7.5-cm TEO platform (Karl Storz, Tuttlingen Germany) is inserted and sealed with the multiport faceplate. The 8-mm airseal trocar (Conmed, Edison NJ) is inserted, and taTME is initiated.

vagina identified early, in order to avoid wrong-plane surgery, and the risk of perforation of the rectum – if the dissection is carried out too low anteriorly, or urethral injury – if the dissection is carried out too high anteriorly (Figure 33.6). Laterally, dissection too close to the pelvic sidewall will put the pelvic plexus at risk for injury. Anterolaterally, care must be taken to avoid injury to the neurovascular bundles, where injury will result in brisk bleeding and urinary and erectile dysfunction. As dissection is carried out superiorly, the peritoneal reflection is usually breached and the peritoneal cavity entered by the transanal team (Figure 33.6d).

'Rendez-vous'

The abdominal and the transanal teams continue to work simultaneously, and can assist each other with retraction until the anterior and posterior dissections are complete, at which point the two teams complete the 'rendez-vous' at the level where the peritoneal cavity has been entered. The fully mobilized specimen can be extracted either transanally or transabdominally. Advantages of transanal extraction include decreased risk of incisional hernias and surgical site infections, as well as improved postoperative pain and cosmesis. Transanal extraction should not be attempted for large bulky tumors, or in a narrow pelvis, as the specimen and sphincter complex may be at risk for damage, or undue tension on the mesentery of the colonic conduit during extraction, which may result in injury to the marginal artery

and lead to colonic conduit ischemia. In most cases, the specimen should be extracted via a Pfannenstiel incision, or planned ileostomy creation site, through a wound protector to reduce the risk of wound infection and tumor implantation. When transanal extraction is appropriate, the rectum and sigmoid are pulled through the anus and transected. Indocyanine green fluorescence can help confirm the viability of the colon at the level of planned proximal transection (Figure 33.7).

Anastomosis

When an anastomosis is completed, it should be performed transanally with either a hand-sewn coloanal, or a double purse-string stapled anastomosis (Figure 33.8). The configuration of the anastomosis is based on surgeon's preference and includes end-to-end, side-to-end, or colonic J pouch, but should always ensure a tension-free and well-vascularized anastomosis. A number of anastomotic techniques have been described following taTME [55]. Hand-sewn anastomosis is commonly performed for very low coloanal anastomoses, or if an intersphincteric resection was performed. If oncologically safe, a rectal cuff above the internal sphincter is preferential to ensure a better functional outcome. A common technique is the double purse-string circular stapled anastomosis. A full-thickness purse-string suture, using 2-0 monofilament polypropylene suture, is placed to close the open rectal stump, taking care to avoid incorporation of the vagina in female patients. This purse string can be placed either endoscopically, through the transanal platform, or in an open fashion using an anal retractor and circular dilator. A 28- or 31-mm circular stapler anvil is secured to the proximal colon. A 10 Fr drain is inserted through the purse string, with its distal end attached to the stapler, and advanced into the pelvis where it acts as a guide to ensure the stapler is placed through the center of the purse string. The drain is then removed laparoscopically, and the anvil is connected to the stapler to perform the anastomosis under laparoscopic visualization.

As the transanal team constructs the anastomosis, the abdominal team can perform a transversus abdominis plane (TAP) block. A drain may be placed in the pelvis, based on surgeon's preference, and a diverting loop ileostomy is usually created at the previously marked stoma site, unless APR is performed, in which case an end-colostomy is matured.

The specimen is subsequently processed by pathology according to standard TME protocol. Briefly, the fresh specimen is grossly examined to assess the quality of the mesorectum (complete, near-complete, or incomplete) and the specimen is photographed from the anterior, posterior, and lateral aspects (Figure 33.9). The specimen is inked and opened 2 cm above and below the tumor and fixed for 48 hours before cross-sectional slicing of the specimen transversely (3–5 mm thickness). The cross-sectional rings are laid out and the quality of the mesorectum is assessed again, as well as the relationship of the tumor to the lateral margin. Additionally, at least 12 lymph nodes should be identified in the TME specimen.

Complications of taTME

Early postoperative complications for taTME series, with ≥50 cases, have shown rates of early anastomotic leak ranging from 1.1% to 9.5%, urethral injury rates of 1%–11%, and rectal perforation or vaginal injury rates between 1.3% and 3.7% (Table 33.2) [15,17,20,32–36,38,39]. Although colorectal surgeons are well versed with traditional 'top down' pelvic anatomy, the 'bottom-up' approach can be disorienting, even for experienced

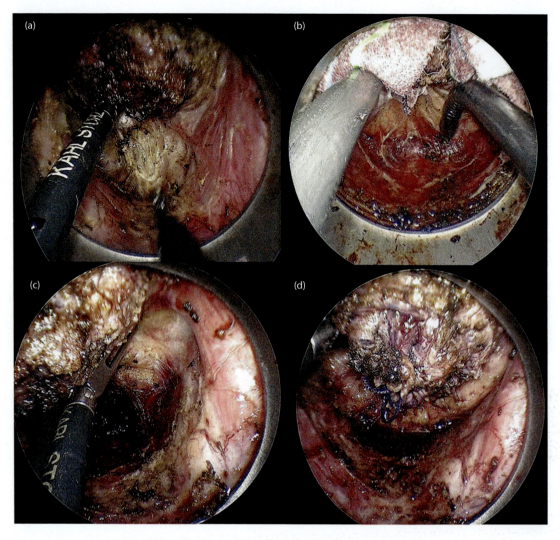

FIGURE 33.5 Posterior and lateral transanal dissection. (a) Posteriorly, intersphincteric dissection is completed, the sacrococcygeal ligament is divided, and the bottom of the mesorectum is identified. (b) Dissection is carried out along the plane between the mesorectal fascia and the endopelvicfacia, taking care to preserve the hypogastric nerves. (c) Lateral dissection proceeds superiorly, with attention to preservation of the pelvic plexus. (d) Circumferential mobilization of the rectum and mesorectum is completed until dissection from the abdominal and transanal are merged.

surgeons. Knowing the anatomic landmarks can avoid pitfalls, and ensure a complete TME while avoiding potential intraoperative complications.

In both abdominal TME and taTME, identification of the extrafascial plane of the mesorectum is crucial for an intact TME dissection. In taTME, the location of the tumor will determine the location of the distal purse string and rectotomy. If the rectotomy is created above the anorectal junction, the TME dissection will begin on the cranial side of the endopelvic fascia in the correct plane. When the rectotomy is created at the anorectal junction, there is little mesorectum, which makes identification of the correct plane difficult. The surgeon must correctly identify Waldeyer's fasica and remain anterior to the endopelvic fascia. The presacral venous plexus is deep to Waldeyer's and the endopelvic fascia. Deeper dissection along the wrong plane posteriorly can lead to profuse bleeding, which can be difficult to control.

Urethral injury

The anterior dissection differs in difficulty between male and female patients. In female patients, the rectovaginal septum is well defined, and although perforation of the vagina is a risk during wrong-plane surgery anteriorly, injury to the urethra is exceedingly rare. In male patients, the prostate, seminal vesicles, and urethra are at risk for injury. The most feared complication in male patients is urethral injury, an injury that does not occur during abdominal TME, and that is otherwise only reported during perineal dissection of an APR [56–59]. The urethra can be injured due to inadvertent mobilization of the prostate. In difficult cases, the surgeon may have difficulties identifying the correct plane anteriorly, and preferentially mobilizes the rectum and mesorectum posteriorly and laterally. This further distorts the anatomy and makes correct plane identification more complicated. Downward retraction of the rectum pulls the prostate inferiorly, and if dissection occurs too anteriorly, or too anterolaterally, the prostate is at risk of becoming mobilized en bloc with the rectum. The membranous urethra becomes at risk of being exposed, as the dissection continues anteriorly [29]. Injury to the urethra can have devastating sequelae, when the injury is not identified intraoperatively, or when initial repair fails. The International LOREC taTME Registry reported urethral injury in 12/1594 cases for an estimated incidence of 0.8% [20]. However, this number is likely

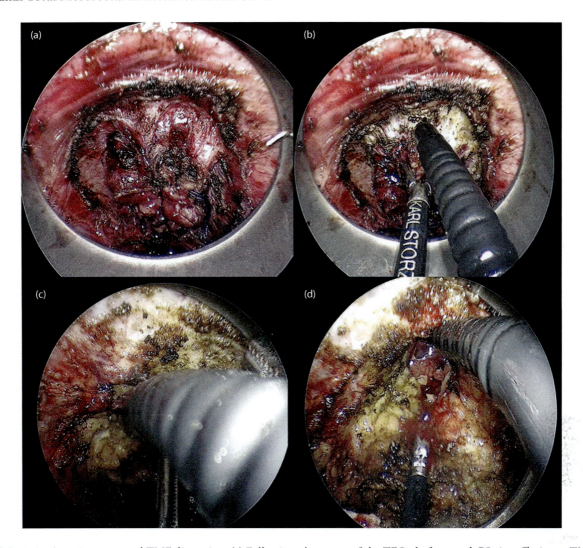

FIGURE 33.6 Anterior transanal TME dissection. (a) Following placement of the TEO platform and CO_2 insufflation, taTME dissection proceeds circumferentially. (b) Anteriorly, dissection proceeds cautiously, with division of the rectourethral muscle and identification of the posterior prostate or vagina. (c) Anterior dissection proceeds along the rectoprostatic or rectovaginal plane with care to preserve the mesorectum anteriorly, and avoid rectal perforation. (d) Superiorly, anterior dissection is extended to the peritoneal reflection, which is opened and the abdominal cavity is entered from below.

an underrepresentation of the true incidence, as a recent international report of self-reported urethral injuries during taTME reported 34 urethral injuries, with 15% requiring permanent urinary diversion. Urethral injuries were also associated with long-term erectile dysfunction in 59% of patients [29].

Three anatomic landmarks have been described to avoid urethral injury in males during taTME [30]. The first is the paired neurovascular bundles of Walsh (NVB), which can be identified between the rectum and the prostate, and are located at the 10 and 2 o'clock positions. Dissection must remain posterior to both the NVB and Denonvilliers' fascia during taTME. The second landmark is the inferior lobe of the prostate, which can be identified by its smooth, spherical, and symmetric shape. Prior pelvic radiation, prostatic hypertrophy, or large anterior tumors can severely distort the rectoprostatic plane. The third landmark the surgeon should recognize is the cylindrical shape of the preprostatic urethra. Failure to recognize these anatomic landmarks can lead to urethral injury. Another important landmark is the rectourethral muscle (RUM). This band of smooth muscle fibers extends from the muscular propria of the rectum anteriorly to the

external urethral sphincter. In taTME for low rectal tumors, the RUM must be divided close to the rectum in order to enter the plane between the anterior rectum and the posterior surface of the prostate. Dividing the muscle too anteriorly can lead to dissection along the inferior lobe of the prostate toward the membranous urethra, risking injury [31].

Carbon dioxide embolism

Carbon dioxide embolism is a rare but potentially deadly complication of laparoscopic surgery, and has been reported to occur during taTME [60,61]. Data from the LOREC and OSTRiCH registries reported 25 cases of carbon dioxide embolism out of 6375 total taTME cases, with an estimated incidence of 0.4% [62]. Notably, all cases occurred during the transanal dissection, and 84% reported visible bleeding at the time of the carbon dioxide embolism event. Hemodynamic compromise was reported in 52% of them, with two patients requiring CPR. Fortunately, no deaths were reported and the operation could be continued in 84% of cases, although 28% were converted to open procedures, and 52% were converted from a taTME to a laparoscopic TME.

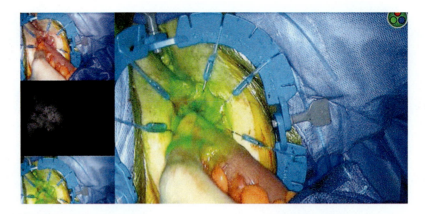

FIGURE 33.7 Perfusion assessment of the colonic conduit. Following specimen extraction, the colonic conduit is pulled transanally, with care to avoid injuring the marginal artery. Adequate perfusion of the colonic conduit is assessed with indocyanine green fluorescence prior to completion of the anastomosis.

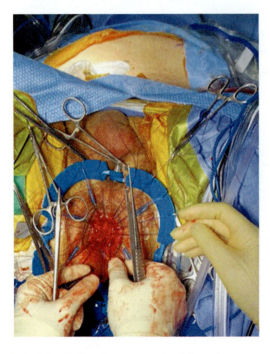

FIGURE 33.8 Coloanal anastomosis. Coloanal anastomosis is performed end-to-end using a hand-sewn technique.

Contributing factors to carbon dioxide embolism include high CO_2 insufflation pressure, venous bleeding, small operative field during the transanal phase, and Trendelenburg positioning.

Anastomotic leaks

According to the International taTME Registry, among 1540 cases of taTME, the rate of anastomotic failure was 15.7%. This figure includes early leaks (<30 days postoperatively; 7.8%), delayed leaks (>30 days postoperatively; 2%), pelvic abscess (4.7%), anastomotic fistula (0.8%), chronic sinus (0.9%), and anastomotic stricture (3.6%). When looking at only early anastomotic leaks, the rate is similar to the results from previous randomized trials comparing open and laparoscopic TME (10%–13%) [8,42]. Risk factors for early anastomotic leak were identified and included both patient and technical factors such as male sex, obesity, current smoker, diabetes, large tumor (>25 mm maximum diameter), tumor height >4 cm from anorectal junction, and intraoperative blood loss of >500 mL. Additionally, significantly

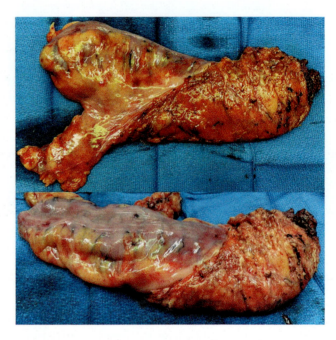

FIGURE 33.9 TME specimen. Assessment of TME grade is performed by pathology. This specimen was graded as complete.

TABLE 33.2: Early Postoperative Complications from Published taTME Series with N > 50 Patients [15,17,20,32–36,38,39]

Outcome	Complication Rate (%)
30-day morbidity major complications	13.4–52.5
	10–24.5
30-day mortality	0.3–5.6
Early anastomotic leak	1.1–9.5
Rectal perforation	1.3–3.7
Vaginal injury	1.9–2
Urethral injury	1–11

more patients without a diverting loop ileostomy developed an anastomotic leak compared to those who were diverted (12.4% vs 7.2%, p = 0.015). Previous studies have demonstrated that diverting stomas do not prevent anastomotic leaks, but rather reduce the sequela of anastomotic leak [63]. Initial results from the International taTME Registry reported an anastomotic leak rate of 5.4%; this increase in anastomotic leak rates is multifactorial and likely the result of the increase in surgeons performing taTME, many at the beginning of their learning curve. The registry reports that 35% of centers that have joined the registry have performed fewer than five cases. This highlights the importance of case volume and surgeon experience in taTME, and the importance of regulated training pathways.

Summary

Transanal TME, when performed by an experienced surgeon at a high-volume center, is a novel technique in the surgical treatment of rectal cancer that has the potential to benefit obese, male patients, and those with mid- to low rectal tumors. Complications from taTME are associated with its significant learning curve, as more regulated training pathways are needed. The short-term results show taTME to be safe, producing adequate TME specimen quality. The current debate regarding local recurrence will likely be resolved as long-term oncologic data become more available from the ongoing multicenter trials.

Key points

- Case selection for taTME is determined by both patient and tumor characteristics, and should be based on a multidisciplinary tumor board assessment of the case both before and after neoadjuvant treatment.
- One of the most promising uses of taTME is in ultra-low rectal tumors, and in sphincter preservation surgery.
- One of the advantages of taTME is that it can be combined with ISR.
- The first step in assessing a patient for taTME is a thorough history and physical examination.
- History of fecal incontinence is critical in preoperative evaluation.
- Although colorectal surgeons are well versed with traditional 'top down' pelvic anatomy, the 'bottom-up' approach can be disorienting, even for experienced surgeons.
- The surgeon must correctly identify Waldeyer's fasica, and remain anterior to the endopelvic fascia.

See Video 37.

Videos

VIDEO 35 https://youtu.be/9nbtHEtti0s

Transanal TME for Rectal Cancers.

VIDEO 37 https://youtu.be/xyhDQunn-PM

Single Access Laparoscopic and Transanal TME.

References

1. Bray F, Ferlay J, Soerjomataram I, Siegel RL, Torre LA, Jemal A. Global cancer statistics 2018: GLOBOCAN estimates of incidence and mortality worldwide for 36 cancers in 185 countries. *CA Cancer J Clin* 2018;68(6):394–424.
2. Miles WE. A method of performing abdomino-perineal excision for carcinoma of the rectum and of the terminal portion of the pelvic colon (1908). *CA Cancer J Clin* 1971;21(6):361–4.
3. Heald RJ, Husband EM, Ryall RD. The mesorectum in rectal cancer surgery-the clue to pelvic recurrence? *Br J Surg* 1982;69:613–6.
4. Birbeck KF, Macklin CP, Tiffin NJ et al. Rates of circumferential resection margin involvement vary between surgeons and predict outcomes in rectal cancer surgery. *Ann Surg* 2002;235:449–57.
5. Martling A, Singnomklao T, Holm T et al. Prognostic significance of both surgical and pathological assessment of curative resection for rectal cancer. *Br J Surg* 2004;91:1040–5.
6. Breukink S, Pierie J, Wiggers T. Laparoscopic versus open total mesorectal excision for rectal cancer. *Cochrane Database Syst Rev* 2006;(4):CD005200. doi:10.1002/14651858.CD005200.pub2.
7. Jeong SY, Park JW, Nam BH et al. Open versus laparoscopic surgery for midrectal or low-rectal cancer after neoadjuvant chemoradiotherapy (COREAN trial): Survival outcomes of an open-label, non-inferiority, randomized controlled trial. *Lancet Oncol* 2014;15:767–74.
8. van der Pas MH, Haglind E, Cuesta MA et al. Laparoscopic versus open surgery for rectal cancer (COLOR II): Short-term outcomes of a randomised, phase 3 trial. *Lancet Oncol* 2013;14:210–8.
9. Fleshman J, Branda M, Sargent DJ et al. Effect of laparoscopic-assisted resection vs open resection of stage II or III rectal cancer on pathologic outcomes: The ACOSOG Z6051 randomized clinical trial. *JAMA* 2015;314:1346–55.
10. Stevenson AR, Solomon MJ, Lumley JW et al. Effect of laparoscopic-assisted resection vs open resection on pathological outcomes in rectal cancer: The ALaCaRT randomized clinical trial. *JAMA* 2015;314:1356–63.
11. Targarona EM, Balague C, Pernas JC et al. Can we predict immediate outcome after laparoscopic rectal surgery? Multivariate analysis of clinical, anatomic, and pathologic features after 3-dimensional reconstruction of the pelvic anatomy. *Ann Surg* 2008;247:642–9.
12. Oh SJ, Shin JY. Risk factors of circumferential resection margin involvement in the patients with extraperitoneal rectal cancer. *J Korean Surg Soc* 2012;82:165–71.
13. Sylla P, Rattner DW, Delgado S et al. NOTES transanal rectal cancer resection using trans-anal endoscopic microsurgery and laparoscopic assistance. *SurgEndosc* 2010;24:1205–10.
14. Penna M, Hompes R, Arnold S, Wynn G, Austin R, Warusavitarne J, Moran B, Hanna GB, Mortensen NJ, Tekkis PP, TaTME Registry Collaborative. Transanal total mesorectal excision: International registry results of the first 720 cases. *Ann Surg* 2017 Jul;266(1):111–7.
15. Perdawood SK, Thinggaard BS, Bjoern MX. Effect of transanal total mesorectal excision for rectal cancer: Comparison of short-term outcomes with laparoscopic and open surgeries. *Surg Endosc* 2018 May;32(5):2312–21.
16. Motson RW, Whiteford MH, Hompes R, Albert M, Miles WF. Current status of trans-anal total mesorectal excision (TaTME) following the second international consensus conference. *Colorectal Dis* 2016 Jan;18(1):13–8.
17. Lacy AM, Tasende MM, Delgado S et al. Transanal total mesorectal excision for rectal cancer: Outcomes after 140 patients. *J Am Coll Surg* 2015;221:415–23.
18. Deijen CL, Velthuis S, Tsai A et al. COLOR III: A multicenter randomized clinical trial comparing transanal TME versus laparoscopic TME for mid and low rectal cancer. *SurgEndosc* 2016;30:3210.
19. Adamina M, Buchs N, Penna M, Hompes R, St. Gallen Colorectal Consensus Expert Group. St. Gallen consensus on safe implementation of transanal total mesorectal excision. *Surg Endosc* 2018;32:1091–103.

20. Penna M, Hompes R, Arnold S et al. Incidence and risk factors for anastomotic failure in 1594 patients treated by transanal total mesorectal excision results from the international TaTME registry. *Ann Surg* 2019 Apr;269(4):700–11.

21. Person B, Ifargan R, Lachter J, Duek S, Kluger Y, Assalia A. The impact of preoperative stoma site marking on the incidence of complications, quality of life, and patient's independence. *Dis Colon Rectum* 2012;55(7):783–7.

22. Sylla P, Willingham FF, Sohn DK, Gee D, Brugge WR, Rattner DW. NOTES rectosigmoid resection using transanal endoscopic microsurgery (TEM) with transgastric endoscopic assistance: A pilot study in swine. *J Gastrointest Surg* 2008;12:1717–23.

23. Trunzo JA, Delaney CP. Natural orifice proctectomy using a transanal endoscopic microsurgical technique in a porcine model. *SurgInnov* 2010;17:48–52.

24. Whiteford MH, Denk PM, Swanstrom LL. Feasibility of radical sigmoid colectomy performedas natural orifice transluminal endoscopy surgery (NOTES) using transanal endoscopic microsurgery. *SugEndosc* 2007;21:1870–4.

25. Sylla P, Kim M, Dursun A et al. NOTES rectosigmoid resection using transanal endoscopicmicrosurgery (TEM): Experience in human cadavers. *Dis Colon Rectum* 2010;53:640.

26. Penna M, Cunningham C, Hompes R. Transanal total mesorectal excision: Why, when, and how. *ClinColon Rectal Surg* 2017 Nov;30(5):339–45.

27. Rosenberger LH, Politano AD, Sawyer RG. The surgical care improvement project and prevention of postoperative infection, including surgical site infection. *Surg Infect* 2011;12(3):163–8.

28. McNally MP, Burns CJ. Venous thromboembolic disease in colorectal patients. *Clin Colon Rectal Surg Today* 2012;42:613–24.

29. Sylla P, Knol JJ, D'Andrea AP et al. On behalf of the International taTME urethral injury collaborative urethral injury and other urologic injuries during transanal total mesorectal excision. *Ann Surg* 2019. doi: 10.1097/SLA.0000000000003597

30. Atallah S, Albert M. The neurovascular bundle of Walsh and other anatomic considerations crucial in preventing urethral injury in males undergoing transanal total mesorectal excision. *Tech Coloproctol* 2016;20:411–2.

31. Uchimoto K, Murakami G, Kinugasa Y, Arakawa T, Matsubara A, Nakajima Y. Rectourethralis muscle and pitfalls of anterior perineal dissection in abdominoperineal resection and intersphincteric resection for rectal cancer. *AnatSci Int* 2007 Mar;82(1):8–15.

32. Veltcamp HM, Deijen CL, Velthuis S, Bonjer HJ, Tuynman JB, Sietses C. Transanal total mesorectal excision for rectal carcinoma: Short-term outcomes and experience after 80 cases. *SurgEndosc* 2016 Feb;30(2):464–70.

33. Tuech JJ, Karoui M, Lelong B, De Chaisemartin C, Bridoux V, Manceau G, Delpero JR, Hanoun L, Michot F. A step toward NOTES total mesorectal excision for rectal cancer: Endoscopic transanal proctectomy. *Ann Surg* 2015 Feb;261(2):228–33.

34. Chen CC, Lai YL, Jiang JK, Chu CH, Huang IP, Chen WS, Cheng AY, Yang SH. Transanal total mesorectal excision versus laparoscopic surgery for rectal cancer receiving neoadjuvant chemoradiation: A matched case-control study. *Ann Surg Oncol* 2016 Apr;23(4):1169–76.

35. Burke JP, Martin-Perez B, Khan A, Nassif G, de Beche-Adams T, Larach SW, Albert MR, Atallah S. Transanal total mesorectal excision for rectal cancer: Early outcomes in 50 consecutive patients. *Colorectal Dis* 2016 Jun;18(6):570–7.

36. Marks JH, Myers EA, Zeger EL, Denittis AS, Gummadi M, Marks GJ. Long-term outcomes by a transanal approach to total mesorectal excision for rectal cancer. *Surg Endosc* 2017 Dec;31(12):5248–57.

37. de Lacy FB, van Laarhoven JJEM, Pena R, Arroyave MC, Bravo R, Cuatrecasas M, Lacy AM. Transanal total mesorectal excision: Pathological results of 186 patients with mid and low rectal cancer. *Surg Endosc* 2018 May;32(5):2442–7.

38. D'Andrea AP, McLemore EC, Bonaccorso A, Cuevas JM, Basam M, Tsay AT, Bhasin D, Attaluri V, Sylla P. Transanal total mesorectal excision (taTME) for rectal cancer: Beyond the learning curve. *Surg Endosc* 2019 Oct 10. [Epub ahead of print]

39. Hol JC, van Oostendorp SE, Tuynman JB, Sietses C. Long-term oncological results after transanal total mesorectal excision for rectal carcinoma. *Tech Coloproctol* 2019 Sep;23(9):903–11.

40. Roodbeen SX, de Lacy FB, van Dieren S, Penna M, Ris F, Moran B, Tekkis P, Bemelman WA, Hompes R, International TaTME Registry Collaborative. Predictive factors and risk model for positive circumferential resection margin rate after transanal total mesorectal excision in 2653 patients with rectal cancer. *Ann Surg* 2019 Nov;270(5):884–91.

41. Aubert M, Mege D, Panis Y. Total mesorectal excision for low and middle rectal cancer: Laparoscopic versus transanal approach: A meta-analysis. *Surg Endosc* 2019 Oct 15. https://doi.org/10.1007/s00464-019-07160-8

42. Guillou PJ, Quirke P, Thorpe H, Walker J, Jayne DG, Smith AM, Heath RM, Brown JM, MRC CLASICC trial group. Short-term endpoints of conventional versus laparoscopic-assisted surgery in patients with colorectal cancer (MRC CLASICC trial): Multicentre, randomised controlled trial. *Lancet* 2005 May 14–20;365(9472):1718–26.

43. Bonjer HJ, Deijen CL, Abis GA et al., COLOR II Study Group. A randomized trial of laparoscopic versus open surgery for rectal cancer. *N Engl J Med* 2015 Apr 2;372(14):1324–32.

44. Stevenson ARL, Solomon MJ, Brown CSB, Lumley JW, Hewett P, Clouston AD, Gebski VJ, Wilson K, Hague W, Simes J, Australasian Gastro-Intestinal Trials Group (AGITG) ALaCaRT investigators. Disease-free survival and local recurrence after laparoscopic-assisted resection or open resection for rectal cancer: The Australasian laparoscopic cancer of the rectum randomized clinical trial. *Ann Surg* 2019 Apr;269(4):596–602.

45. Fleshman J, Branda ME, Sargent DJ et al. Disease-free survival and local recurrence for laparoscopic resection compared with open resection of stage II to III rectal cancer: Follow-up results of the ACOSOG Z6051 randomized controlled trial. *Ann Surg* 2019 Apr;269(4):589–95.

46. Deijen CL, Tsai A, Koedam TW, Veltcamp HM, Sietses C, Lacy AM, Bonjer HJ, Tuynman JB. Clinical outcomes and case volume effect of transanal total mesorectal excision for rectal cancer: A systematic review. *Tech Coloproctol* 2016 Dec;20(12):811–24.

47. Koedam TWA, Veltcamp HM, van de Ven PM, Kruyt PM, van Heek NT, Bonjer HJ, Tuynman JB, Sietses C. Transanal total mesorectal excision for rectal cancer: Evaluation of the learning curve. *Tech Coloproctol* 2018 Apr;22(4):279–87.

48. Lee L, Kelly J, Nassif GJ, deBeche-Adams TC, Albert MR, Monson JRT. Defining the learning curve for transanal total mesorectal excision for rectal adenocarcinoma. *Surg Endosc* 2020;34(4):1534–42.

49. Veltcamp HM, van Oostendorp SE, Koedam TWA et al. Structured training pathway and proctoring; multicenter results of the implementation of transanal total mesorectal excision (TaTME) in the Netherlands. *Surg Endosc* 2020;34(1):192–201.

50. McLemore EC, Harnsberger CR, Broderick RC et al. Transanal total mesorectal excision (taTME) for rectal cancer: A training pathway. *Surg Endosc* 2016 Sep;30(9):4130–5.

51. Abbott SC, Stevenson ARL, Bell SW, Clark D, Merrie A, Hayes J, Ganesh S, Heriot AG, Warrier SK. An assessment of an Australasian pathway for the introduction of transanal total mesorectal excision (taTME). *Colorectal Dis* 2018 Jan;20(1):O1–6.

52. Rullier E, Laurent C, Bretagnol F, Rullier A, Vendrely V, Zerbib F. Sphincter-saving resection for all rectal carcinomas: The end of the 2-cm distal rule. *Ann Surg* 2005 Mar;241(3):465–9.

53. Rullier E, Denost Q, Vendrely V, Rullier A, Laurent C. Low rectal cancer: Classification and standardization of surgery. *Dis Colon Rectum* 2013 May;56(5):560–7.

54. National Comprehensive Cancer Network. Rectal Cancer (Version 3, 2019). Available from: https://www.nccn.org/professionals/physician_gls/pdf/rectal.pdf. Accessed December 5, 2019.

55. Penna M, Knol JJ, Tuynman JB, Tekkis PP, Mortensen NJ, Hompes R. Four anastomotic techniques following transanal total mesorectal excision (TaTME). *Tech Coloproctol* 2016 Mar;20(3):185–91.

56. Stitt L, Flores FA, Dhalla SS. Urethral injury in laparoscopic-assisted abdominoperineal resection. *Can Urol Assoc J* 2015 Nov-Dec;9(11–12):E900-2.

57. Sawkar HP, Kim DY, Thum DJ, Zhao L, Cashy J, Bjurlin M, Bhalani V, Boller AM, Kundu S. Frequency of lower urinary tract injury after gastrointestinal surgery in the nationwide inpatient sample database. *Am Surg* 2014 Dec;80(12):1216–21.

58. Ng KH, Ng DC, Cheung HY, Wong JC, Yau KK, Chung CC, Li MK. Laparoscopic resection for rectal cancers: Lessons learned from 579 cases. *Ann Surg* 2009 Jan;249(1):82–6.

59. Andersson A, Bergdahl L. Urologic complications following abdominoperineal resection of the rectum. *Arch Surg* 1976 Sep;111(9):969–71.

60. Ratcliffe F, Hogan AM, Hompes R. CO_2 embolus: An important complication of TaTME surgery. *Tech Coloproctol* 2017 Jan;21(1):61–2.

61. Harnsberger CR, Alavi K, Davids JS, Sturrock PR, Zayaruzny M, Maykel JA. CO_2 embolism can complicate transanal total mesorectal excision. *Tech Coloproctol* 2018 Nov;22(11):881–5.

62. Dickson EA, Penna M, Cunningham C, Ratcliffe FM, Chantler J, Crabtree NA, Tuynman JB, Albert MR, Monson JRT, Hompes R, International TaTME Registry Collaborative. Carbon dioxide embolism associated with transanal total mesorectal excision surgery: A report from the international registries. *Dis Colon Rectum* 2019 Jul;62(7):794–801.

63. McDermott FD, Heeney A, Kelly ME, Steele RJ, Carlson GL, Winter DC. Systematic review of preoperative, intraoperative and postoperative risk factors for colorectal anastomotic leaks. *Br J Surg* 2015 Apr;102(5):462–79.

64. Wasmuth HH, Faerden AE, Myklebust TÅ et al. Transanal total mesorectal excision for rectal cancer has been suspended in Norway. *Br J Surg* 2020 Jan;107(1):121–30.

65. Williams NS, Dixon MF, Johnston D. Reappraisal of the 5 centimetre rule of distal excision for carcinoma of the rectum: A study of distal intramural spread and of patients' survival. *Br J Surg* 1983 Mar;70(3):150–4.

Chapter 34

COMBINED ENDOSCOPIC-LAPAROSCOPIC SURGERY (CELS) FOR COLORECTAL POLYPECTOMY

Miguel E Gomez and Parul J Shukla

Contents

Learning objectives 224
Introduction 224
CELS polypectomy surgical technique... 224
Benefits and limitations of CELS polypectomy... 226
Current research on CELS polypectomy 227
Summary 227
Key points 228
References 228

Learning objectives

- Understand why combined endoscopic-laparoscopic surgery is used for polypectomy in certain cases
- Determine the benefits and limitations of combined endoscopic-laparoscopic surgery for polypectomy
- Review and analyze current studies on combined endoscopic-laparoscopic surgery that assess its efficacy in removing polyps
- Describe the combined endoscopic-laparoscopic surgery technique and how it facilitates the removal of certain polyps
- To explore the short-term and long-term outcomes of combined endoscopic-laparoscopic surgery for polypectomy

Introduction

Combined endoscopic-laparoscopic surgery (CELS) is a type of procedure that uses laparoscopy and colonoscopy techniques in conjunction. In the context of polypectomy, it is used to remove complex polyps that cannot be removed through colonoscopic methods [1]. Complex polyps can be large, broad-based, lodged within intestinal folds, and/or situated in areas with increased risk of bowel perforation [2]. In these cases, endoscopic removal is difficult, as ensnaring the polyp becomes tricky. CELS facilitates the removal of these polyps through gentle prodding of the external wall of the colon using laparoscopic tools, allowing the polyp to stick out and providing more surface area for the endoscope to snare [3]. CELS has been lauded as a safe and effective way of approaching polypectomy for these complex polyps. In general, this procedure is considered minimally invasive, and is seen as a promising alternative to bowel resection surgeries.

CELS polypectomy surgical technique

Before beginning the surgery, all necessary equipment for colonoscopic polypectomy, laparoscopic polypectomy, and open colectomy are acquired in case the surgeon decides to switch procedures. After putting the patient under general anesthesia, Venodyne boots, a nasogastric tube, and a Foley catheter are placed accordingly for the surgery. For this type of surgery, the patient is placed in a modified lithotomy position, where the patient's legs are fitted into padded yellow fin stirrups, facilitating the insertion and maneuvering of the colonoscope [4]. Next, the

patient's arms are tucked at their sides and their hands and wrists are also padded. Heparin and antibiotics are administered to the patient before proceeding with the initial incision [4].

In addition, the placement of the laparoscopic monitors will depend on the particular location of the polyp. Monitors are placed at the patient's right side and toward the head of the bed, if the patient has a right colon polyp, while the monitors for patients with left colon polyps are placed at the patient's left side, and toward the foot of the bed. However, in the case of a transverse colon polyp or flexure lesion, the monitors are situated at the head of the bed, while the colonoscopist stands in between the patient's legs [4]. Carbon dioxide colonoscopy also needs to be available in the operating room. This is because doing combined endoscopic laparoscopic surgery with room air presents the surgeon with a couple of technical challenges, including a concealed laparoscopic view and compromising exposure of the polyp [5]. Therefore, it is recommended to have carbon dioxide insufflation during laparoscopy, as the bowel tends to absorb carbon dioxide much faster than room air, which will facilitate good visualization of the polyp during the procedure. The patient's abdomen is then prepared using a sterile technique and the lesion is located first using the carbon dioxide colonoscopy technique [11]. A colonoscopy is performed before the laparoscopy in order to truly assess whether the polyp in question can be removed through an endoscopic method alone (Figure 34.1). Once the colonoscope is established, dilute indigo carmine solution is used to mark the location of the polyp while protruding it for better visualization [6] (Figure 34.2).

At this point in time, it is important for the surgeon to definitively recognize whether the polyp in question shows possible malignancy. In addition, polyps that have been removed before will show signs of scarring and/or be difficult to lift. If any of these are present, the surgeon has the option to switch procedures to a formal colectomy [4]. Laparoscopy is added only if endoscopic methods alone are not working (Figure 34.3). Once laparoscopy is determined to be necessary for the procedure, a periumbilical incision is made. The fascia is entered into the abdomen at a sharp angle, and a 5 mm port is placed within the abdomen to establish pneumoperitoneum. The abdomen is then explored laparoscopically by the surgeon, and the location of the polyp found using the markings from the dilute indigo carmine solution. Once this is done, two extra 5 mm trocars are placed depending on the location of the procedure. For right colon polyps, trocars are placed within the left lower quadrant of the abdomen above the pubis,

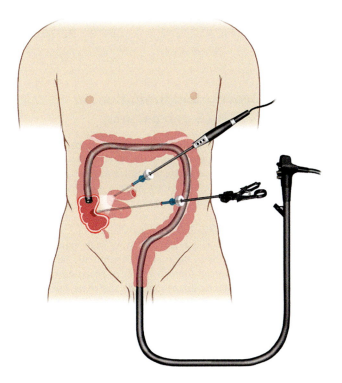

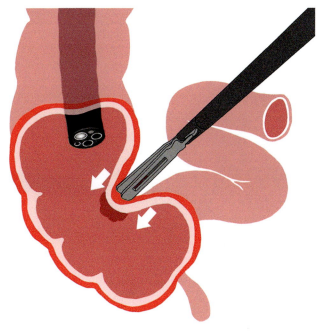

FIGURE 34.3 Laparoscopic manipulation for endoscopic polypectomy.

FIGURE 34.1 Schematic view of endoscopic and laparoscopic assessment of colonic polyp.

while trocars for left colon polyps are placed in the right lower quadrant of the abdomen, also above the pubis. However, if it is a transverse colon polyp, the trocars are placed on both sides of the abdomen in both the lower and upper quadrants [4,7]. The position is confirmed by the laparoscopist with transillumination and/or endoscopic visualization during laparoscopic manipulation of the colon (Figure 34.4). However, before the polyp can be truly maneuvered, the colon needs to be mobilized properly to

obtain the best angle to remove the polyp [6]. This could result in the entire colon being mobilized in order to facilitate exposure. Once this is done, the polyp is lifted via the dilute carmine solution. This will facilitate endoscopic resection and will prevent full-thickness injury. If the polyp does not lift properly, the surgery must transition to colectomy, no matter the circumstances. The process of polypectomy is done using an electrosurgical snare (Figure 34.5). For flat polyps in a difficult location, laparoscopic manipulation of the polyp during snare polypectomy eases the polyp into the endoscope's snare (Figure 34.3). During this

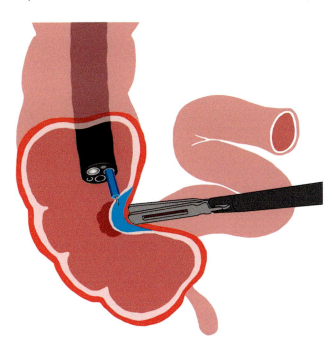

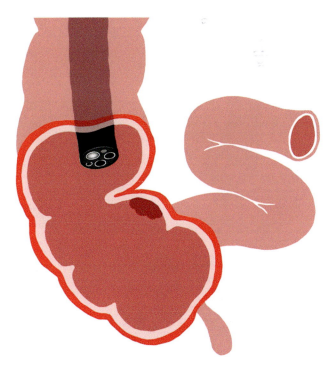

FIGURE 34.2 Endoscopic submucosal injection to elevate the polyp.

FIGURE 34.4 Endoscopic views of colonic polyp.

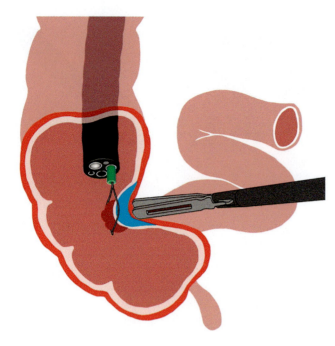

FIGURE 34.5 Endoscopic snare polypectomy.

process, deterioration of the muscle layers is monitored and the area is reinforced to avoid partial or full-thickness injuries during the postoperative period. Overall, this procedure allows for a more aggressive approach to polypectomy, due to potential intraoperative damage being repaired using laparoscopy [6].

After the polyp is retrieved (Figure 34.6), via an endoscopic roth net or through a suction device on the colonoscope, the patient is monitored diligently for months thereafter [9]. Follow-up colonoscopies are conducted three-months postprocedure. This is to check for possible recurrent polyps, even though CELS generally leads to a low polyp recurrence rate (5%–10%). If a recurrent polyp is found, then surgeon can decide whether to remove

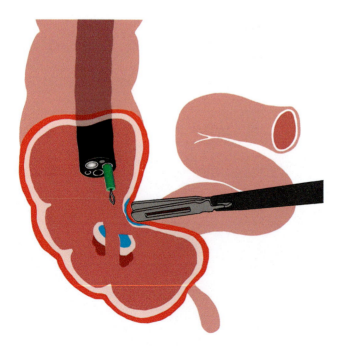

FIGURE 34.6 Completed endoscopic snare polypectomy.

it with colonoscopic polypectomy, CELS again, or laparoscopic segmental colectomy. Choice of procedure for the recurrent polyp will depend upon the polyp's location, size, and difficulty in removal [4].

Benefits and limitations of CELS polypectomy

CELS provides colorectal surgeons with an innovative way of performing polypectomies. Among the colorectal surgical community, CELS is viewed as a safe and efficient method of removing polyps, especially those that are difficult to remove through endoscopic methods alone. CELS polypectomy has many benefits to offer, ranging from the minute details of the procedure to long-term postoperative outcomes for patients [10].

To start off, the procedure allows for the underlying colon to be invaginated, assisting in the snaring of a difficult flat polyp. By manipulating the colon to allow the polyp to protrude, colorectal surgeons can facilitate its placement into the snare for removal, therefore preventing the need for resection [11]. In addition, laparoscopic mobilization and angulation of the colon provide better access to, and exposure of, the polyp in question. This again facilitates manipulation of the polyp, while also providing better visualization of the lesion [12]. The laparoscopic component of CELS also allows for easy detection and repair of full-thickness injury to the colon [4]. Therefore, surgeons can treat this possible injury, while also ensuring that patient postoperative complications are minimal. Having laparoscopic equipment readily available also facilitates conversion of the surgery to laparoscopic resection, in case the polyp cannot be removed endoscopically, or is deemed to be suspicious of malignancy during the intraoperative period [13]. The possibility of potentially switching procedures during surgery provides surgeons with flexibility and less stress, as they are better able to tailor their surgical approach to the unique conditions of the patient. Moreover, visualization of both the external and internal wall of the colon provides simple verification of the complete excision of the polyp and of any unexpected bleeding or perforation that can be immediately addressed [11].

Many studies have also shown that the benefits of CELS extend into the postoperative healing period, where long-term outcomes for patients – who underwent CELS polypectomy – are excellent [14]. Successful CELS polypectomies are associated with decreased levels of postsurgery morbidity in patients, decreased costs/financial burden, and shorter hospital stays allowing patients to return home anywhere from the same day as the procedure to 2–3 days after the procedure [15]. This is especially the case when comparing to the postoperative outcomes of patients who received a segmental colectomy for polyp removal. Complications are also minimal, as infectious complication rates and gastrointestinal motility issues are commonly low among patients who underwent CELS polypectomy. Most importantly, polyp recurrence rates are low after CELS (5%–10% average rate) [16].

Although benefits of CELS polypectomy greatly outweigh its detriments, there are still a few limitations that prevent CELS polypectomy from being widely used across the field of colorectal surgery. To start off, there are some risks associated with the details of the CELS procedure. Port placement during CELS causes a risk of abdominal wall or intraabdominal injury, and must be performed carefully. Although generally low, there is still a risk of perforation of the bowel during CELS; therefore all laparoscopies done within CELS must be completed carefully by a surgeon with expertise in the technique [17,18]. In addition, laparoscopic light transillumination can distort the endoscopic view, and must be turned away periodically.

Another major limitation of CELS involves the possible presence of malignancy after polypectomy. This is because of the potential risk of invasive cancer in the patient, which is why CELS should be strictly limited to benign polyps [19]. Evaluation of the polyp for malignancy, via frozen section, adds time to the procedure and may not even be consistent with the final pathologic evaluation. If this discrepancy exists, it can necessitate subsequent bowel resection, rendering the initial CELS procedure futile [17].

The CELS procedure also requires equipment for both laparoscopic and colonoscopic techniques, in case the surgeon determines that the procedure must be switched intraoperatively. CELS is therefore more resource-heavy and will require the hospital to have all the necessary materials for operation. There is also the potential for the wasting of equipment if the surgeons believe endoscopic methods alone should suffice. CELS also has a learning curve, and requires two skilled doctors in the operating room to perform the procedure safely and efficiently. Adept surgeons are required for visualization of lesions, and establishment of a coordinated manipulation of the bowel by the laparoscopist and the endoscopist [13]. Therefore, it is not used as frequently – most surgeons are not as comfortable with the technique – compared to resection, or other forms of bowel surgery. Last, since CELS is a relatively new procedure, there is a lack of standardized criteria, making it difficult to compare results of research done with CELS. Standardized criteria are still evolving, thus deterring less experienced surgeons from using this technique [13].

Current research on CELS polypectomy

Currently, there is a lot of research being conducted on CELS polypectomy, to demonstrate its effectiveness and persuade more surgeons to use the technique as an alternative to bowel resection. One study, conducted by Jayaram et al., looked at the financial benefits of the CELS procedure by performing a cost analysis of CELS compared to bowel resection. They found that the length of hospital stay and median OR times for the CELS procedure were much lower than those of a laparoscopic right colectomy (1 vs. 3.82 d for length of stay, and 166.73 vs. 204.73 min for operating times) [20]. Therefore, they calculated the total cost required to take care of the CELS patient, compared to the colectomy patient, and found the cost to be significantly less for CELS (~$5500 vs. $12,600), indicating that CELS provides a financial benefit for both the patient and the surgeon [20].

Subramaniam et al.'s 2017 study addresses difficult colorectal polyps, and how to deal with them without performing a colectomy. In their article, they describe CELS as a promising technique for this, stating its success rate to be between 69% and 87% for benign polyps, and the recurrence rates of removed polyps to be between 0% and 13% [2]. Although the procedure is still changing, Subramaniam et al. recommend that surgeons begin adopting this technique, as it is associated with lower morbidity for the patient, while providing a way to remove pesky polyps that could become malignant in the future. The results found by Subramaniam et al. are also supported by a study conducted in Denmark by Jensen and Rud. They found CELS to be successful in removing benign polyps 65%–97% of the time, while recurrence remained extremely low (0%–5%) [8]. However, Jensen and Rud also remark that CELS should be limited to medical centers with the necessary equipment and surgical expertise. This is because CELS poses the risk of invasive cancer if

done incorrectly, and if the polyp turns out to be cancerous. Therefore, endoscopic screening must be done meticulously to ensure the absence of malignant tissue [8]. A 2017 study by Placek and Nelson also agrees with the previous studies, indicating that CELS is an efficient and safe way of treating difficult benign colorectal polyps. CELS not only is relatively successful but also allows the surgeons to tailor their surgical approach to the patient, verify the complete removal of the polyp, and immediately address any intraoperative complications that can occur with polypectomy – including perforation of the bowel and unexpected bleeding. Thus, Placek and Nelson encourage gastroenterologists, and surgeons performing colonoscopies, to consider CELS when encountering complicated colorectal polyps [11].

At Weill Cornell Medicine, extensive research has been done in the colorectal department on the efficacy of CELS for the treatment of complex benign polyps. In a study by Nakajima et al., CELS was deemed as an excellent option for benign polypectomy, stating that its minimally invasive nature reduces morbidity in patients, improves patient outcomes, and reduces the economic burden involved with polyp removal [13]. The study does outline that improving the standardization of CELS polypectomy technique will bring CELS closer to being used in the mainstream, as it will be easier for surgeons-in-training to learn about the procedure [13]. In another study at Weill Cornell, Garrett and Lee explored many patient outcomes after CELS polypectomy. To start off, the study outlines postcomplication rates of CELS of around 4%, with most postoperative complications being urinary retention and hematoma. In addition, Garrett and Lee reported no full-thickness injury during the procedure, noting that if it did occur, it would be easy to fix with the already available laparoscopic equipment. In terms of long-term follow-up, the study reported excellent outcomes for patients, indicating a fast recovery and relatively low recurrence rate (less than 10%) [4].

Current research shows that CELS is a relatively new technique with a lot of potential. It can help reduce the number of colectomies performed for benign colon polyps, thus improving patient outcomes and reducing morbidity. It can also further improve cancer screening by removing all benign polyps with the possibility of becoming malignant. CELS has been shown to be a successful, safe, and effective method for polypectomy, and a great alternative to colectomy and bowel resection. In the future, the standardization of the CELS technique should be developed so that more surgeons, across different hospitals, can begin using it for polypectomies.

Summary

CELS polypectomy is used to remove complex polyps through the use of endoscopic and laparoscopic methods working in conjunction. In 1993, it was described by surgeons as an alternative to bowel resection that would greatly reduce the morbidity of patients with benign complex polyps. Since then, there have been many studies published describing CELS as a safe and effective method for preventing and screening for possible colorectal cancer by removing difficult colon polyps [21]. The benefits of CELS greatly outweigh its detriments, where patients who undergo this procedure instead of a colectomy have far better long-term outcomes. Although proven to be successful, CELS is still not widely used by many surgeons due to the lack of standardization of the technique, and the requirement for surgeons to be especially adept in both laparoscopic and endoscopic methods [21].

Key points

- CELS is an effective and safe way of performing a polypectomy, specifically for benign polyps.
- CELS is seen as a promising minimally invasive technique, and offers a viable alternative to colectomy and/or other bowel resection procedures that are more life-threatening.
- CELS polypectomy possesses both key benefits (i.e., easier to fix intraoperative complications, excellent long-term outcomes for patients, less morbidity in patients post-surgery) and limitations (i.e., possible malignancy of polyp during CELS, very resource-heavy, steep learning curve, and requires skilled surgeons). However, based on the opinions of the surgical community, the benefits of CELS greatly outweigh its detriments, and it should always be strongly considered when working with difficult benign polyps.
- Many studies indicate that CELS polypectomy is effective, with success rates hovering around an average of 87%, and recurrence rates as low as 5%–10%.
- One component missing from CELS polypectomy is the standardization of the technique, which has yet to be developed due to the procedure's relative novelty. Once CELS is standardized, it will become much easier for surgeons around the world to begin adopting it as a way to treat benign colon polyps, and prevent possible colon cancers in the future.

References

1. Tholoor S, Tsagkournis O, Basford P, Bhandari P. Managing difficult polyps: Techniques and pitfalls. *Ann Gastroenterol.* 2013;26(2):114–21.
2. Subramaniam S, Bhandari P, Pidala MJ, Cusick MV. The Difficult Colorectal Polyp. *Frontline Gastroenterol.* 2017;97(3):515–27.
3. Thirumurthi S, Raju GS. How to deal with large colorectal polyps: Snare, endoscopic mucosal resection, and endoscopic submucosal dissection; resect or refer? *Curr Opin Gastroenterol.* 2016;32(1):26–31.
4. Garrett KA, Lee SW. Combined Endoscopic and Laparoscopic Surgery. *Clin Colon Rectal Surg.* 2015;28(3):140–5.
5. Nakajima K, Lee SW, Sonoda T, Milsom JW. Intraoperative carbon dioxide colonoscopy: A safe insufflation alternative for locating colonic lesions during laparoscopic surgery. *Surg Endosc.* 2005;19(3):321–5.
6. Crawford AB, Yang I, Wu RC, Moloo H, Boushey RP. Dynamic article: Combined endoscopic-laparoscopic surgery for complex colonic polyps: Postoperative outcomes and video demonstration of 3 key operative techniques. *Dis Colon Rectum.* 2015;58(3):363–9.
7. Lee SW, Garrett KA, Shin JH, Trencheva K, Sonoda T, Milsom JW. Dynamic article: Long-term outcomes of patients undergoing combined endolaparoscopic surgery for benign colon polyps. *Dis Colon Rectum.* 2013;56(7):869–73.
8. Jensen S, Rud B. Combined endoscopic laparoscopic colon polypectomy. *Ugeskr Laeger.* 2017;179(15). doi: 10.1016/j.suc.2017.01.003
9. Yan J, Trencheva K, Lee SW, Sonoda T, Shukla P, Milsom JW. Treatment for right colon polyps not removable using standard colonoscopy: Combined laparoscopic-colonoscopic approach. *Dis Colon Rectum.* 2011;54(6):753–8.
10. Wilhelm D, von Delius S, Weber L, Meining A, Schneider A, Friess H, Feussner H. Combined laparoscopic-endoscopic resections of colorectal polyps: 10-year experience and follow-up. *Surg Endosc.* 2009;23(4):688–93.
11. Placek SB, Nelson J. Combined Endoscopic Laparoscopic Surgery Procedures for Colorectal Surgery. *Clin Colon Rectal Surg.* 2017;30(2):145–50.
12. Kandiah K. Polypectomy and advanced endoscopic resection. *Surg Endosc.* 2017;8(2):110–4.
13. Nakajima K, Sharma SK, Lee SW, Milsom JW. Avoiding colorectal resection for polyps: Is CELS the best method? *Surg Endosc.* 2016;30(3):807–18.
14. Franklin ME, Jr. Portillo G. Laparoscopic monitored colonoscopic polypectomy: Long-term follow-up. *World J Surg.* 2009;33(6):1306–9.
15. Goh C, Burke JP, McNamara DA, Cahill RA, Deasy J. Endolaparoscopic removal of colonic polyps. *Colorectal Dis.* 2014;16(4):271–5.
16. Lee MK, Chen F, Esrailian E, Russell MM, Sack J, Lin AY, Yoo J. Combined endoscopic and laparoscopic surgery may be an alternative to bowel resection for the management of colon polyps not removable by standard colonoscopy. *Surg Endosc.* 2013;27(6):2082–6.
17. Hamdani U, Naeem R, Haider F, Bansal P, Komar M, Diehl DL, Kirchner HL. Risk factors for colonoscopic perforation: A population-based study of 80118 cases. *World J Gastroenterol.* 2013;19(23):3596–601.
18. Zhou PH, Yao LQ, Qin XY. Endoscopic submucosal dissection for colorectal epithelial neoplasm. *Surg Endosc.* 2009;23(7):1546–51.
19. Anderloni A, Jovani M, Hassan C, Repici A. Advances, problems, and complications of polypectomy. *Clin Exp Gastroenterol* 2014;7:285–96.
20. Jayaram A, Barr N, Plummer R, Yao M, Chen L, Yoo J. Combined endo-laparoscopic surgery (CELS) for benign colon polyps: A single institution cost analysis. *Surg Endosc.* 2019;33(10):3238–42.
21. Lin AY, O'Mahoney PR, Milsom JW, Lee SW. Dynamic article: Full-thickness excision for benign colon polyps using combined endoscopic laparoscopic surgery. *Dis Colon Rectum,* 2016;59(1):16–21. doi: 10.1097/dcr.0000000000000472

Section VII
Hand-Assisted and Single-Incision
Laparoscopic Colorectal Surgery

35 Hand-Assisted Laparoscopic Colorectal Surgery. 230
36 Single-Incision Laparoscopic Colorectal Surgery 236

Chapter 35

HAND-ASSISTED LAPAROSCOPIC COLORECTAL SURGERY

Deeksha Kapoor, Amanjeet Singh, and Adarsh Chaudhary

Contents

Learning objectives 230
Introduction 230
HAL colorectal resections. 230
Indications 230
Preoperative preparation. 231
Surgical instruments 231
Surgical steps. 231
Position. 231
Incision and trocar placement 231
    Camera port. 231
    Working port 232
Surgical procedure 232
Modifications. 234
Summary 234
Key points 234
Video. 234
References 235

Learning objectives

- Philosophy of HALS
- Indications of HAL colorectal resection
- Hand port and its placement, other instruments required
- Port placements for various resections
- Colorectal mobilization
- Division of vascular pedicles
- Restoration of continuity
- Modifications in HAL colorectal surgery

Introduction

The first laparoscopic-assisted colectomy was reported in 1991 [1], and has subsequently gained momentum despite being technically challenging, while imposing a long learning curve. Laparoscopic-assisted surgery has been associated with decreased postoperative pain, shorter hospital stays, and a quicker recovery of bowel function [2,3]. Initial studies, such as CLASICC [4] and a long-term follow-up of the COLOR trial [5], had suggested similar oncological outcomes in comparison to open surgery, in terms of survival and disease recurrence. But recent studies, like the ALaCaRT trial [6] and ACOSOG Z6051 trial [7], have failed to prove the noninferiority of laparoscopic rectal resections for carcinoma rectum, when compared to open surgery.

Laparoscopic colorectal surgery is a challenging operation, involving work in more than one quadrant of abdomen, and is associated with a long learning curve. Hand-assisted laparoscopic surgery (HALS) has been advocated as a useful alternative to total laparoscopy. This hybrid technique allows introduction of the surgeon's nondominant hand in the abdominal cavity, restoring tactile feedback. The incision, which would have been performed for specimen delivery, is placed earlier on during the surgery for hand insertion. HALS has been found to have similar short-term advantages compared to laparoscopic surgery, along with suggested decreased conversion rates to open surgery. HALS not only facilitates traction, countertraction, and decreases operative time, but also shortens the learning curve of laparoscopic surgery [8]. It improves adaptability to difficult surgeries, like those for diverticular disease or inflammatory bowel disease – where phlegmon formation and dense adhesions are expected [9–11].

HAL colorectal resections

Depending on the segment of colon resected, the various surgical procedures can be described as:

- HAL right hemicolectomy
- HAL left hemicolectomy
- HAL sigmoidectomy
- HAL anterior resection
- HAL low anterior resection
- HAL abdominoperineal resection
- HAL subtotal colectomy
- HAL total proctocolectomy
- HAL transanal TME (hybrid procedure)

Depending on the primary disease and type of resection required, a stoma in the form of an ileostomy or colostomy may be added. When surgery is being performed for ulcerative colitis, an IPAA may also be performed via HALS [12,13].

Indications

Indications for HALS are similar to those for conventional open methods. Most common indications in our practice include elective procedures for colorectal malignancies, diverticular disease, inflammatory bowel disease, and polyposis syndromes. We prefer a conventional open approach for emergency cases, although data now suggest the feasibility of laparoscopic methods for these [10,11].

Preoperative preparation

Preoperative workup is determined by the suspected primary pathology. Diagnostic and staging workup includes computerized tomography (CT) scan of the abdomen and pelvis, with or without CT chest scan, and colonoscopy/ sigmoidoscopy with or without biopsy. In case of a small tumor or sessile polyp, preoperative colonoscopic clipping or tattooing may help in intraoperative identification of the lesion. Routine preoperative investigations are carried out, with certain specific tests dictated by patient's comorbidity status. Although the role of preoperative bowel preparation for colonic surgery is debated, we prefer giving mechanical bowel preparation in the afternoon, on the day prior to elective surgery. The patient is kept on a liquid diet and DVT prophylaxis, with a single dose of parenteral low molecular weight heparin, given the evening before surgery. Sites of permanent colostomy, or temporary ileostomy/colostomy, are marked preoperatively after confirming in at least three positions. Hair clipping and skin preparation are done in the operation theater, and a combination of second- or third-generation cephalosporin with metronidazole is given at the time of induction.

Surgical instruments

- *Hand port*: Multiple hand-port devices are available, like the Ethicon Endosurgery (Cincinnati, OH) hand port, which is available in three different sizes, according to the thickness of the abdominal wall of the patient. In our institute, we have improvised this technique we call the 'Medanta hand port method.' The wound protector system (SURGI SLEEVE, Covidien, Dublin, Ireland), along with a double-gloved technique, is used as a hand port (Figure 35.1). The bottom ring gets inserted inside the abdominal wall and fits snuggly, allowing an airtight

seal. The upper ring is rolled to fit snuggly on the skin of the anterior abdominal wall, sandwiching the abdominal wall between the two rings. The operating surgeon wears two gloves on the nondominant hand, inserting the hand through the wound protector, and inverting the outer glove over the outer ring of the device, forming an airtight, yet flexible seal over the hand – providing enough mobility at the wrist joint for the surgeon.
- *Energy devices*: Multiple energy devices, such as the harmonic scalpel (Ethicon Endosurgery), or LigaSure (Medtronic), monopolar electrocautery are available, and their use depends entirely on the surgeon's preference and comfort.
- *Trocars*: One to two disposable 12-mm or 10-mm trocars, one to two disposable 5-mm trocars.
- *Endostaplers*: Usually one to two linear cutter endostaplers are needed with or without vascular loads.
- Circular staplers for colorectal anastomosis deep in the pelvis.
- *Laparoscopic tower and monitor*: It is preferable to use two monitors to avoid changing position of the monitors while working in different quadrants of the abdomen.
- *Laparoscopic camera*: We prefer a 30-degree laparoscopic camera, although some surgeons may be comfortable with 0 degrees as well. Additional facilities like an indocyanine green camera may be used, if available, to assess bowel vascularity.

Surgical steps (see Video 36)

The steps for HAL low anterior resection for rectal malignancy are described here. Modifications for other resections are discussed subsequently. The procedure is carried out under general anesthesia with endotracheal intubation, with or without epidural analgesia. DVT pumps are applied for all patients before positioning. Nasogastric or orogastric tubes may be placed, and a per-urethral catheter is placed for all patients.

Position

With arms tucked by the sides, the patient is placed in a low lithotomy, or modified Lloyd Davies position. For rectal dissection, the patient is placed in a deep Trendelenberg position, with the left side tilted upward. The operating surgeon stands on the patient's right side, with the camera assistant to the left of the operating surgeon.

Incision and trocar placement (Figure 35.2)

A 5-cm periumbilical midline incision is used for placement of the wound manager as a hand port. In case of tall male patients with narrow pelvises, the incision may be placed more caudally to prevent hand fatigue due to excessive pull and strain. A slightly bigger incision may be required, depending on the size of surgeon's hand. Alternatively, a low transverse Pfannenstiel incision may be used for placement of the hand port. After placing the surgeon's nondominant hand in the abdominal cavity, other trocars are placed under guidance. We usually use two trocars in the right lower quadrant for performing a rectal resection or sigmoidectomy. A third 5-mm trocar may be placed in the left lower quadrant, as needed, for retraction or smoke evacuation (Figure 35.2).

Camera port

A 10-mm trocar is placed on the right side, 6–8 cm below the right subcostal margin, in the midclavicular line. Placement of

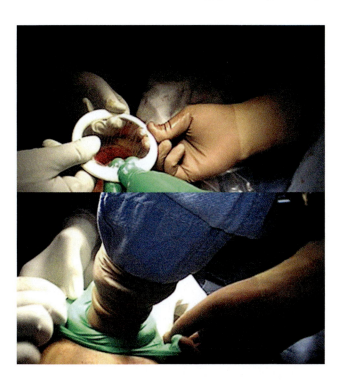

FIGURE 35.1 Medanta hand port method: A wound protector is used, with a double-gloved technique. The outer glove is everted over the external ring of the wound protector.

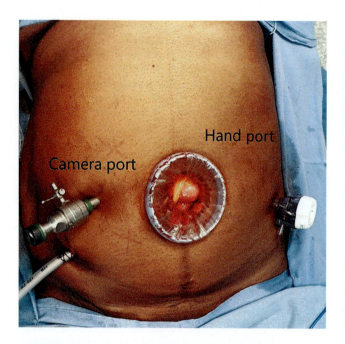

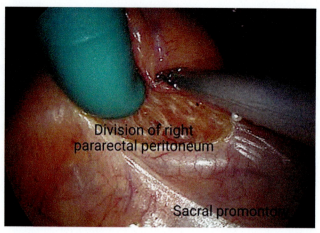

FIGURE 35.3 With the nondominant hand of the surgeon in the abdominal cavity, the rectosigmoid is held retracted cephalad, making the pararectal peritoneum prominent. The sacral promontory is palpated and the peritoneum incised, and retro-mesenteric dissection is commenced.

FIGURE 35.2 Hand port and trocar placement for hand-assisted laparoscopic low anterior resection. A 10-mm trocar is used on the right side in the midclavicular line as the camera port. This site can be subsequently used for making the stoma trephine. A working port (12 mm) is placed in the right anterior axillary line, lower than the camera port – a drain has been placed via the same at the end of the procedure, in this figure. An additional 5-mm port can be placed in the left lower quadrant, for retraction or smoke evacuation.

this trocar is often attempted at the site of diversion stoma, if needed subsequently. Subsequent trocars are placed after creation of pneumoperitoneum via this port. The abdomen is insufflated with CO_2, and pressure is maintained at 13–15 mm Hg.

Working port

Another 12-mm trocar is inserted about 4–5 cm below the first port in the right anterior axillary line. Placement of this port is determined by the height of the tumor in the rectum and the pelvic anatomy. For a low tumor in a narrow and deep male pelvis, this port may be placed more medially and cranially, to avoid clashing with the right pelvic brim. This port is used for dissection and passing stapling devices for bowel transection and anastomotic stapling.

Surgical procedure

- With the 30-degree camera and the surgeon's hand in the abdominal cavity, the abdomen is inspected for any evidence of distant disease, and local resectability of the tumour. The small bowel is displaced to the right upper quadrant, and dissection is commenced at the sacral promontory. The sacral promontory is palpated and the rectosigmoid lifted to make the right pararectal fascia taut. Using a harmonic scalpel, we incise the right pararectal fascia, which allows air to enter between the rectosigmoid mesentery anteriorly and the presacral fascia posteriorly, exposing the crisscrossing fibroareolar tissue (Figure 35.3). Dissection is continued in this avascular plane, medially to laterally, identifying the left ureter and gonadal vessels posteriorly. Once this tunnel is created, we prefer placing

a gauze piece, which not only helps with hemostasis, but also acts as an indicator while releasing the lateral peritoneal attachments. The colon is now flipped medially, the reflection of the gauze noted, and the lateral peritoneal attachments released. This dissection is continued cranially, along the descending colon, and inferiorly up to the upper rectum.

- Alternatively, a lateral to medial dissection can be undertaken, in which the lateral attachments of the sigmoid colon are released by dissecting along the white line of Toldt. As the dissection proceeds medially, the left ureter and gonadal vessels are identified posteriorly (Figure 35.4).

- As dissection in this plane proceeds cranially, on stretching the sigmoid mesentery the inferior mesenteric pedicle becomes prominent, and is easily identified just superior to the aortic bifurcation. At this juncture, the ureter and

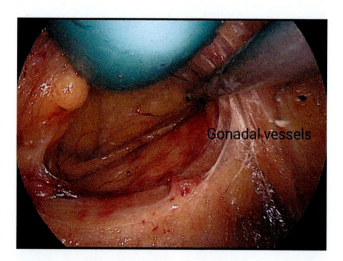

FIGURE 35.4 The tunnel is created medially to laterally, pushing the retroperitoneal fat, left ureter, and left gonadal vessels posteriorly. The left gonadal vessels can be seen in this figure, and the left ureter has already been pushed behind. The nondominant hand of the surgeon maintains adequate traction, and blunt finger dissection helps to remain in the correct plane.

pelvic plexus of nerves must have been displaced posteriorly into the retroperitoneum. The pedicle is dissected and divided using a vascular endostapler, or divided after application of hemoclips. At this point, the DJ flexure must be safeguarded, as thermal injuries during pedicle dissection are possible. With the colon in the nondominant hand, the mesentery is separated from the anterior surface of Gerota's fascia and the retroperitoneum, using a harmonic scalpel.

- *High versus low ligation*: Although oncological superiority of one technique over the other is not proven, we prefer a tumor-specific ligation of the inferior mesenteric pedicle. When the left colic artery is spared a low ligation is performed, and when sacrificed, a high ligation performed [14,15].
- *Rectal dissection*: Once vascular control is achieved, pelvic dissection is carried out by continuing in the same avascular plane, safeguarding the hypogastric plexus below. Once proceeding in the correct plane, the chances of nerve damage and bleeding are minimized. With the nondominant hand retracting the rectosigmoid anteriorly and laterally, toward the left anterior abdominal wall, the loose areolar fibers of the avascular plane become prominent, and can be easily divided using a harmonic scalpel, or electrocautery. During dissection, sweeping movements are made toward the mesorectum, so as to avoid tears and breech of the mesorectal fascia. The operating surgeon should remember that the 'fat belongs to the rectum,' and the mesorectal fascia should not be incised. As the dissection proceeds inferiorly, the surgeon alternates between anterior and lateral dissection before proceeding to a lower posterior dissection at a later stage. This is best facilitated by using the 'rule of triangles.'
- *Anterior dissection* (Figure 35.5): Anterior dissection is different in male and female patients. An additional retractor

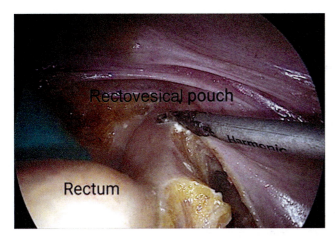

FIGURE 35.5 Anterior dissection: Anterior dissection is started after dissecting the upper rectum off from the sacral curve. At this point, the surgeon alternates between anterior and lateral dissection to completely free the rectum on all sides. The mesorectal fat is sparse anteriorly, and therefore, one should be cautious of remaining in the correct plane. The rectovesical pouch is incised and dissection continued inferiorly, exposing the posterior aspect of seminal vesicles. Hand-assisted laparoscopy has a particular advantage, while dissecting in a narrow male pelvis. The traction maintained by the hand is rather uniform as against the traction provided by laparoscopic instruments in pure laparoscopy. In our experience, this maintains the quality of the TME specimen, by avoiding tears in the mesorectal fascia due to improper traction.

from the left side may aid in opening the rectovesical pouch in male patients. In females, the uterus may have to be hitched to the anterior abdominal wall. Additionally, a vaginal swab over a Kelly clamp, placed vaginally, may facilitate traction and countertraction for anterior dissection.

- In males, the rectovesical pouch is incised, and dissection proceeds on the posterior surface of the seminal vesicles. In case of anteriorly placed tumors, the Denonvillier's fascia may be excised with the resection specimen.
- *Lateral dissection*: With adequate traction on the rectum, pulling the rectum out from its sacral curve, the lateral attachments get exposed. For dissection of the right lateral attachments, the rectum is retracted to the left and the apex of the attachments are divided in a posterior to anterior direction. For releasing the attachments on the left side, the same maneuver is done, with the rectum being pulled to the right. As the so-called lateral ligaments are approached, some bleeding may be encountered, which is controlled by Ligaclips. This is best understood using the 'rule of triangles." Dissection should be done at the apex of the triangle created by traction and countertraction.
- *Inferior dissection*: Once the rectum has been mobilized from the sacral curve, the inferior extent of dissection is assessed by performing a rectal examination to assess the distal tumor margin. The contribution of a trained assistant is paramount at this stage, as camera work with a 30-degree laparoscope can provide excellent vision for the operating surgeon. The surgeon may perform a bimanual palpation to decide the distal transection margin, at which point division of the mesorectum is undertaken – perpendicular to the rectal wall. Once the lateral and posterior mesorectum is divided, a linear cutter endostapler is passed through the 12-mm trocar and rectal division completed.
- The rectal stump and sacral curve are inspected for adequate hemostasis, and the specimen along with the colon is delivered through the wound.
- After dividing the mesentery and assessing vascularity, colonic resection is completed. The proximal cut-end of the colon is assessed for good vascularity, and the anvil of the circular stapler (29 or 31 mm) is applied using a purse-string polypropylene suture. The colon, with the anvil applied at its end, is repositioned in the abdominal cavity.
- *Splenic flexure mobilization*: At this point, the surgeon may want to mobilize the splenic flexure, to allow adequate and tension-free descent of the colon into the pelvis for a stapled colorectal anastomosis.
- *Anastomosis*: After the sphincter is dilated, the assistant places the shaft of the circular stapler transanally. The surgeon directs the stapler posteriorly, so that the stapler pin is released posterior to the staple line. Under laparoscopic vision, the anvil is attached to the pin. Before tightening the stapler, the lie of the colonic mesentery should be assessed for any traction, rotation, or twists. The stapler is then closed, especially safeguarding the posterior vaginal wall in women. Before firing the stapler, a pervaginum examination may be done to rule out pinching of the vaginal mucosa into the staple line.
- The stapler is fired, completing the double-stapled, end-to-end colorectal anastomosis. With gentle rotatory movements, the stapler is disengaged, withdrawn, and donuts inspected. Depending on institutional policy, a leak test may be performed. The pelvic cavity is filled with water and air, insufflated transrectally, and a note is made of any

air bubbles that escape from the staple line, indicating the site of leak.

- Hemostasis is ensured, and instrument and sponge counts confirmed before releasing pneumoperitoneum, and withdrawing ports.
- A diversion stoma may be constructed in the right iliac fossa depending on surgeon's preference, vascularity of the bowel, and integrity of the anastomosis.

Modifications

- *Splenic flexure mobilization*: All sigmoid or anterior resections may not warrant splenic flexure mobilization. To mobilize the splenic flexure, the surgeon stands between the legs of the patient and inserts an additional 5-mm port on the left side. The transverse colon is pulled caudally and the avascular plane between the colon and gastrocolic omentum incised. After entering the lesser sac, the surgeon palpates the avascular plane between the omentum and colonic mesentery, incising it with a harmonic scalpel. Once this is complete, the only attachment remaining is the lienocolic ligament. With the colon in the left hand and medial traction, the glistening lienocolic ligament is divided and the splenic flexure reflected down. At this point, the inferior aspect of the tail of the pancreas may be identified in the lesser sac.
- *HAL right hemicolectomy*: With arms tucked by the sides, patient is placed in reverse Trendelenberg position, with the right side tilted upward. The surgeon and the assistant stand on the left side of the patient, with the laparoscope console on the right side, head-end corner. We prefer to use a periumbilical midline hand port, with two additional ports. A 10-mm camera port and a 5-mm working port are used in the epigastrium and left upper abdomen. Dissection may be attempted medial to lateral, or lateral to medial. In medial to lateral dissection, with the small bowel swept to the left lower quadrant, the hepatic flexure and transverse colon are held and retracted cephalad. This maneuver exposes the right colon mesentery and the duodenum, which is an important landmark. With traction of the ileocecal region, the ileocolic pedicle becomes prominent, and can be identified just at the base of the duodenum. The pedicle is dissected and ligated at a level determined by the nature of the disease. The right colic pedicle, if present, is ligated in a similar manner. Once vascular control is achieved, a medial to lateral retromesenteric dissection is undertaken. The duodenum is bluntly swept down and plane dissected laterally up to the white line. The retroperitoneum and Gerota's fascia are swept posteriorly, and the colonic mesentery lifted toward the cecum inferiorly and the hepatic flexure superiorly. The mesocolon is lifted from the pancreatic head, taking care of the venous bleeding. The gastrocolic omentum is divided, safeguarding the right gastro epiploic pedicle. At this point, the entire right colon, along with the ileocolic region, should be free and can be delivered in the wound. The middle colic pedicle can be approached either extracorporeally after delivering the bowel, or intracorporeally. For an intracorporeal approach, the transverse colon mesentery is held taut by the nondominant hand, and the middle colic pedicle is palpated at its base. Depending on the site of the tumor, the middle colic pedicle or the right branch of the middle colic may be dissected and divided. HALS is especially useful in obese patients, where the pedicles may be hidden under the fat-laden mesentery. The intracorporeal nondominant hand helps in palpation and easy identification of the vascular structures, while maintaining the advantage of laparoscopy.
- The bowel is then delivered into the wound and an anastomosis performed. We routinely prefer a hand-sewn anastomosis; however a stapled anastomosis can be undertaken according to surgeon's preference.
- *HAL abdominoperineal resection*: TME is performed as in HAL low anterior resection, and distally continued up to the levator ani muscles. The perineal phase is performed in the standard fashion, and the descending end colostomy is performed in the left upper abdomen at the preoperatively marked site.
- *HAL total proctocolectomy/subtotal colectomy*: A total proctocolectomy requires the surgeon to operate in various quadrants of the abdomen, requiring frequent positional changes. The patient is placed in a low lithotomy position, and at least two monitors are used for comfortable dissection. This procedure involves maneuvers of both anterior resection and right hemicolectomy, as described previously.
- *HAL transanal TME*: Transanal TME can also be performed as a hybrid, hand-assisted procedure. This surgery involves an additional transanal phase, which involves identification of the distal resection margin, followed by a bottom-to-top approach for rectal dissection [16].

Summary

HALS is a useful technique, which combines the advantage of laparoscopic surgery, while restoring the tactile feedback of open surgery. It helps in conforming to the same oncological standards as the open approach for colorectal malignancy [17]. With HALS, operative time is significantly reduced, while maintaining the short-term benefits of laparoscopy. HALS is a useful substitute to pure laparoscopy, and is associated with lower conversion rates. Although the technique faces criticism as not being pure laparoscopy, the incision required for specimen delivery, when taken earlier, works to the advantage of both the surgeon and patient.

Key points

- HALS is the balance between pure laparoscopy and open surgery, which combines the best of both worlds.
- Site of hand port, port placement, and position of the surgeon depends on the location of the lesion and the quadrant of abdomen in which the surgery is envisaged.
- For HAL low anterior resection, the surgery can be divided into mobilization of left colon, rectal resection, colon division, and anastomosis.
- Splenic flexure mobilization is undertaken selectively.
- The hand-assisted technique can also be used for right hemicolectomy, total proctocolectomy, or subtotal colectomy.

Video

VIDEO 36   https://youtu.be/bHw-MSEInOg

Hand Assisted Laparoscopic TME.

References

1. Cooperman AM, Katz V, Zimmon D, Botero G. Laparoscopic colon resection: A case report. *J Laparoendosc. Surg* 1991;1:221–24.

2. Abraham NS, Young JM, Solomon MJ. Meta-analysis of short-term outcomes after laparoscopic resection for colorectal cancer. *Br J Surg* 2004 September;91(9):1111–24.

3. Tong G, Zhang G, Liu J, Zheng Z, Chen Y, Cui E. A meta-analysis of short-term outcome of laparoscopic surgery versus conventional open surgery on colorectal carcinoma. *Medicine* 2017 December;96(48):e8957.

4. Green BL, Marshall HC, Collinson F et al. Long-term follow-up of the Medical Research Council CLASICC trial of conventional *versus* laparoscopically assisted resection in colorectal cancer: Conventional *versus* laparoscopically assisted surgery for colonic and rectal cancer. *Br J Surg* 2013 January;100(1):75–82.

5. Deijen CL, Vasmel JE, de Lange-de Klerk ESM et al. Ten-year outcomes of a randomised trial of laparoscopic versus open surgery for colon cancer. *Surg Endosc* 2017 June;31(6):2607–15.

6. Stevenson ARL, Solomon MJ, Lumley JW et al. Effect of laparoscopic-assisted resection vs open resection on pathological outcomes in rectal cancer: The alacart randomized clinical trial. *JAMA* 2015 October 6;314(13):1356.

7. Fleshman J, Branda M, Sargent DJ et al. Effect of laparoscopic-assisted resection vs open resection of stage II or III rectal cancer on pathologic outcomes: The ACOSOG Z6051 randomized clinical trial. *JAMA* 2015 Oct 6;314(13):1346.

8. Romanelli JR, Kelly JJ, Litwin DE. Hand-assisted laparoscopic surgery in the United States: An overview. *SeminLaparosc Surg* 2001 June;8(2):96–103.

9. Aalbers AGJ, Biere SSAY, van Berge Henegouwen MI, Bemelman WA. Hand-assisted or laparoscopic-assisted approach in colorectal surgery: A systematic review and meta-analysis. *Surg Endosc* 2008 August;22(8):1769–80.

10. Letarte F, Hallet J, Drolet S et al. Laparoscopic emergency surgery for diverticular disease that failed medical treatment: A valuable option? Results of a retrospective comparative cohort study. *Dis Colon Rectum* 2013 December;56(12):1395–402.

11. Wu K-L, Lee K-C, Liu C-C, Chen H-H, Lu C-C. Laparoscopic versus open surgery for diverticulitis: A systematic review and meta-analysis. *Dig Surg* 2017;34(3):203–15.

12. Shimada N, Ohge H, Yano R et al. Hand-assisted laparoscopic restorative proctocolectomy for ulcerative colitis. *World J Gastrointest Surg* 2016;8(8):578.

13. Zhu P, Xing C. Hand-assisted laparoscopic restorative proctocolectomy with ileal pouch-anal anastomosis for ulcerative colitis. *J Minim Access Surg* 2017;13(4):256.

14. Yasuda K, Kawai K, Ishihara S et al. Level of arterial ligation in sigmoid colon and rectal cancer surgery. *World J Surg Oncol [Internet]* 2016 December [cited 2019 August 6];14(1). Available from: http://wjso.biomedcentral.com/articles/10.1186/s12957-016-0819-3

15. Zeng J, Su G. High ligation of the inferior mesenteric artery during sigmoid colon and rectal cancer surgery increases the risk of anastomotic leakage: A meta-analysis. *World J Surg Oncol* 2018 August 2;16(1):157.

16. Vignali A, Elmore U, Milone M, Rosati R. Transanal total mesorectal excision (TaTME): Current status and future perspectives. *Updates Surg* 2019 March;71(1):29–37.

17. Taggarshe D, Attuwaybi BO, Matier B, Visco JJ, Butler BN. Hand-assisted laparoscopic (HAL) multiple segmental colorectal resections: are they feasible and safe? *Int Surg* 2015 April;100(4):632–7.

Chapter 36
SINGLE-INCISION LAPAROSCOPIC COLORECTAL SURGERY
Muralidhar Kathlagiri

Contents

Learning objectives 236
Introduction 236
SILS ports and equipment 236
Robotic SILS 237
Single-incision laparoscopic appendectomy 237
    Surgical tips 237
Single-incision laparoscopic right hemicolectomy. 237
    Surgical tips 237
Single-incision laparoscopic left hemicolectomy 237
    Surgical tips 237
Single-incision laparoscopic anterior resection 238
Single-incision laparoscopic total colectomy 238
    Surgical tips 238
Summary 238
Key points 238
Videos 238
References 238

Learning objectives

- Learn the advantages of SILS
- Know surgical tips of various colorectal SILS

Introduction

Minimally invasive surgery has been one of the major advances in surgery over the last three decades. It has specific advantages in various gastrointestinal surgeries, including colorectal surgery. SILS seems to be a natural progression of laparoscopic surgery. This format of surgery is performed by multiple instruments inserted simultaneously via a large-caliber single-port device placed through a single skin incision, or via small adjacent ports placed into a single skin incision – but with multiple fascial incisions. There are multiple terminologies describing this kind of surgical access: SILS, single-access laparoscopic surgery (SALS), single-port access (SPA) surgery, single laparoscopic incision transabdominal (SLIT) surgery, one-port umbilical surgery (OPUS), natural orifice transumbilical surgery (NOTUS), and embryonic natural orifice transumbilical endoscopic surgery (E-NOTES). There appears to be a consensus on the term laparo endoscopic single site surgery (LESS) [1]. In this chapter, LESS will be referred to as SILS.

Laparoscopic surgery has definite advantages over open surgery with respect to reduced pain of retraction and incision, better cosmesis, fewer adhesions, and earlier recovery. Yet, certain complications of laparoscopic surgery are related to the port site, which include adhesions, bleeding, trauma to internal structures, and torque at the port site. As SILS has a reduced number of ports, and a decreased overall length of incision, it reduces the complications related to multiple ports. Having a single incision at the umbilicus, or at the site of stoma, makes it cosmetically more acceptable.

There are advantages of SILS specific to colorectal surgery. This surgery can be performed from the site of the planned stoma, with either ileostomy or colostomy, which can also be used to extract specimen and perform anastomosis, virtually making it a zero-scar surgery.

SILS surgery comes with a set of limitations, as well as technical and ergonomic challenges. It poses difficulties in the triangulation of instruments, manipulation, and retraction. Clashing of instruments is a major disadvantage in performing this surgery. The reduced range of movement makes it difficult to perform certain steps. Crossing of the surgeon's hands is a challenge while performing the surgery with conventional laparoscopic instruments. Also, it has a longer learning curve compared to conventional laparoscopic surgery.

The European Association's consensus statement on the ergonomics of single-incision endoscopic surgery is based on controlled trials, systematic reviews, and expert opinions. Their findings included:

a. Head trunk rotation and viewing direction are better with single-incision endoscopic surgery.
b. Workload, muscle activity, and the wrist's ulnar and radial range of movements are increased with single-incision surgery, compared to conventional laparoscopic surgery.
c. Workload, muscle activity, and the wrist's radial and ulnar range of movements are increased with articulating instruments, compared to straight instruments [2].

The level of evidence is weak, as there is a lack of randomized controlled trials.

SILS ports and equipment

SILS surgery needs special equipment and ports to perform the surgery. There is a wide range of equipment and ports available; any of the following may be selected:

- There are two types of SILS ports available
- Disposable single-use port – SILS port (Covidien), Olympus triport+

- Multiuse single-incision port – X cone (Storz), Endocone (Storz)

The equipment spectrum available to facilitate SILS includes:

- Long 5-mm scope for visualization
- 5-mm flexible-tip high-definition laparoscope (Olympus)
- L-connector for the light cable connections to the laparoscope
- SILS hand instruments (Covidien)
- Cuschieri deviating instruments
- Cambridge endo instruments

A varying combination of the aforementioned can be used based on the procedural demand and the surgeon's preference. The use of equipments of varying lengths can minimize clashes.

Robotic SILS

SILS colectomy has been performed using the da Vinci robotic assistance platform [3]. Intuitive Surgicals is developing new SILS platforms, for SILS surgeries. Robotics may well help overcome multiple shortcomings inherent to SILS surgery, thus making the procedure more ergonomically sound.

Single-incision laparoscopic appendectomy

Appendicitis is a common surgical emergency. Conventional laparoscopic appendectomy (CLA) is shown to have fewer wound infections, reduced pain, and shorter hospital stays compared to open appendectomy for acute appendicitis [4]. Single-incision appendectomy (SILA) has been found to be equivalent to CLA [5].

SILS appendectomy can be performed through either a transumbilical single incision or a suprapubic single incision. Suprapubic incision is better for a retrocaecal and gangrenous appendix.

Surgical tips
The patient's position is supine, with a left tilt. The surgeon stands on the left of the patient, while the camera assistant stands toward the head, and the scrub nurse toward the leg end.

The umbilicus is everted to reach the base, using Kelly's or Alli's forceps. The umbilical skin is opened vertically about 2.5 cm. The SILS port is inserted with the help of large Kelly's forceps. One 10 mm and two 5 mm ports are inserted. The insufflator is connected to the inlet port. A transabdominal sling can be used to hold the appendix to facilitate mesoappendix dissection. The mesoappendix can be dissected, and the appendicular artery can be clipped or coagulated with an ultrasonic vessel sealer device. The base of the appendix is ligated with suture or a stapler. Additional ports may need to be inserted if there are difficulties in dissection. An appendix specimen is retrieved through the SILS port site and put in an endobag.

There is no difference found between the morbidities of CLA and SILA, as well as for resting and overall pain score or complications. There is a slight increased need for intravenous analgesic in SILA. Also, standing pain and pain on activity is slightly increased in SILA [5].

Single-incision laparoscopic right hemicolectomy (see Videos 38 and 39)

Single-incision laparoscopic colectomy (SILC) is gaining in popularity despite the technical challenges it poses. Right colectomy is suited for the SILS approach; however, it may be technically challenging in obese patients and for bulky tumors.

Surgical tips
General anesthesia is the preferred modality. Position of patient is supine, with 30-degrees right side up. The surgical team stands to the left of the patient, and the camera assistant stands toward the head end of the patient. The surgeon is in the middle, and the scrub nurse toward the foot end. The laparoscopic rack or the monitor is placed in front of the surgeon, on the right side of the patient. The abdomen is accessed through a 2.5–3 cm transumbilical incision. A SILS (Covidien) port is used at the center. Two 5 mm ports and one 10 mm port are used. The instruments and camera can be shuffled between ports to suit the surgical steps being performed. Initial laparoscopic exploration is carried out, and the patient is then put into a 20-degree Trendelenburg position. Surgery begins by exposing the ileocolic pedicle, which can be accomplished by retracting the ileocecal junction. It can be further achieved by taking a transabdominal suture with a straight needle on the transverse colon, and pulling it upward toward the anterior abdominal wall. The peritoneum is opened below the ileocecal pedicle and dissected to identify the duodenum. Medial-to-lateral dissection is performed between Toldt's and Gerota's fascia, with blunt and vessel sealer devices. There is an avascular plane between the mesentery and retroperitoneum. Care should be taken not to go too deep, which is indicated by bleeding, and it puts the ureters and gonadal vessels at risk. The ileocecal pedicle can be cut by LigaSure, as well as by vascular stapler or between vascular clips. The caecum is mobilized from the lateral attachments, and the mesentery is freed up to the terminal ileum to the point of transection. The ileum is sectioned with endo GIA. Caecal mobilization is continued upward up to the hepatic flexure, and then mobilized by dividing the hepatocolic attachments with vessel sealer devices. The omentum attached to the transverse colon up to the site of transection is divided. The transverse colon is divided with an endoscopic stapler. Specimens can be extracted through the umbilical incision in an endobag. Anastomosis can be performed outside with sutures or a stapler. The bowel is then repositioned, and the SILS port is reinserted to check for hemostasis. The fascial closure is performed with monofilament and delayed absorbable suture, while the skin is closed with absorbable suture. Local anesthetic infiltration, carried out at the port site, helps in postoperative analgesia.

Available data suggest that the SILC is feasible and safe, and that oncologic outcomes in terms of margins and lymph node harvest are comparable to conventional laparoscopic surgery.

Single-incision laparoscopic left hemicolectomy

Single-incision left hemicolectomy must be performed by an experienced surgeon.

Surgical tips
The patient is in a supine position with legs apart and a urinary catheter and Ryle's tube are inserted. The surgeon is on the right of the patient. The assistant stands to the left of the surgeon, and the assistant comes to the right during splenic flexure mobilization. The monitor is placed in front of the surgeon on the patient's left, near the left thigh. The scrub nurse stands between the legs of the patient. Here, a foot controlled vessel-sealing device gives more freedom to perform the SILC.

The abdomen is accessed through the umbilicus through a SILS port with a 3-cm fascial incision. The patient is placed into a reverse Trendelenberg position. The sigmoid colon, descending colon, and splenic flexure are mobilized. Gerota's fascia is separated from Toldt's fascia. The ureters and gonadal vessels are identified. At this point, there may be clashing of equipment in this step. The dissection should be extended as close to the parieto-colic ligament as possible. The patient is then shifted to a Trendelenberg position. The inferior mesenteric vein is isolated and transacted below the inferior border of the pancreas. The inferior mesenteric artery (IMA) is isolated and transected 2 cm distal to the origin from the aorta, after the branching of the left colic artery. In benign conditions, IMA may be preserved. The rectum sigmoid junction is transected with an articulate linear stapler. The left colon is divided extracorporeally, after getting the colon out through the umbilicus incision with a wound protector. The head of a 33-mm circular stapler is inserted into the proximal colonic segment, and sutured with a 2-0 polypropylene suture. The proximal colon with the circular stapler head is replaced inside, and the SILS port is reinserted. Colorectal anastomosis is accomplished with an EEA stapler intracorporeally. A leak test is performed with hydropneumatic testing. The umbilical incision is closed with monofilament delayed absorbable suture, and the skin is closed with poliglecaprone suture.

Single-incision laparoscopic left colectomy is found to be safe and feasible when performed by experienced surgeons [6].

Single-incision laparoscopic anterior resection

Single-port total mesorectal excision was first published in 2011 by Hamzaoglu I et al. [7]. They published a series of four cases of total mesorectal excision. The position of the patients was similar to that in the left colectomy. The access was transumbilical with a multichannel single port. The sigmoid colon was hung to the left lateral abdominal wall to achieve the medial dissection, and ligate the IMA pedicle. The mesorectum was sharply dissected up to the pelvic floor, and the sutures were subsequently removed for the sigmoid, descending colon, and splenic flexure mobilization. The rectum and proximal colon were transacted with an endoscopic roticulating linear stapler, and the specimen was retrieved through the umbilicus. Anastomosis was performed by circular stapler or pull-through hand-sewn anastomosis. A diverting stoma was not performed in this series.

Alternatively, when an ileostomy is planned, the SILS port can be inserted at the planned site of stoma, and surgery can be accomplished. An additional port may be needed to complete the splenic flexure mobilization. This can be used to remove the drain.

The transabdominal transanal approach, with hand-sewn coloanal anastomosis, is planned for low rectal tumors, and large pelvic tumors where transanal TME, up to 5–6 cm above the dentate line, is performed. Subsequently, transabdominal single-port TME is performed. The specimen is retrieved from the anal canal. Hand-sewn anastomosis is then accomplished from below.

TME should be performed by experienced surgeons.

Single-incision laparoscopic total colectomy

SILS is suited to perform total colectomy, as all quadrants are accessible through a single incision.

Surgical tips

The access can be through the umbilicus, or through the ileostomy site. Monitors are needed on both sides of the patient, and there has to be adequate room around the patient for the surgeon to move to the left or right, as per the segment being operated. The surgery begins with mobilization of the right colon,

from the caecum up to the transverse colon. The left side colon is subsequently mobilized, starting from the sigmoid colon to the transverse colon. The site of transection at the sigmoid colon, or sigmoid rectum junction, is decided and transacted with endoscopic roticulating linear stapler. The mesenteric dissection is decided by the primary indication.

Summary

SILC and CLC were found to be similar in terms of operative time, length of hospital stays, lymph node harvest rates, postoperative morbidity, postoperative mortality, surgical site infection, anastomotic leak, conversion rate, and reoperation rate [8]. SILC has a smaller incision length, and better patient satisfaction index compared to CLC [9]. Case selection is important. Single-incision colectomy is safe and feasible for: <T4 tumors less than 5 cm, BMI less than 35, and no previous surgery. Single-incision TME for rectal tumors is safe and feasible for tumors <4 cm, and BMI <30 [8]. SILC is a technically demanding procedure, and should be performed by experienced surgeons. SILS surgery is a good addition to the minimal access surgeons' armamentarium.

Key points

- SILA has been found to be equivalent to CLA
- Oncological outcome of SILC – for right hemicolectomy – is comparable to conventional laparoscopic surgery in terms of margins and lymph node harvest
- Single-incision laparoscopic left colectomy is found to be safe and feasible with experienced surgeons
- SILS TME should be performed by experienced surgeons

Videos

VIDEO 38   https://youtu.be/KXmVZG1uZ-0

SILS Right Hemicolectomy – Part 1.

VIDEO 39   https://youtu.be/GG7g7b-Ow6U

SILS Right Hemicolectomy – Part 2.

References

1. Gill IS, Advincula AP, Aron M et al. Consensus statement of the consortium for laparoendoscopic single-site surgery. *Surg Endosc* 2010;24:762–8.
2. European association for endoscopic surgery (EAES) consensus statement on single-incision endoscopic surgery. *Surg Endosc* April 2019;33(4):996–1019.
3. Ostrowitz MB, Eschete D, Zemon H, DeNoto G. Robotic-assisted single-incision right colectomy: Early experience. *Int J Med Robot Comput Assist Surg* December 2009;5(4):465–70.
4. Sauerland S, Jaschinski T, Neugebauer EA. Laparoscopic versus open surgery for suspected appendicitis. *Cochrane Database Syst Rev* 2010;(10):CD001546.

5. Cho MS, Min BS, Hong YK et al. Single-site versus conventional laparoscopic appendectomy: Comparison of short-term operative outcomes. *Surg Endosc* 2011;25:36–40.

6. Maggiori L, Gaujoux S, Tribillon E, Bretagnol F, Panis Y. Single-incision laparoscopy for colorectal resection: A systematic review and meta-analysis of more than a thousand procedures. *Colorectal Dis* 2012;14(10):e643–54.

7. Hamzaoglu I, Karahasanoglu T, Baca B, Karatas A, Aytac E, Kahya AS. Single-port laparoscopic sphincter-saving mesorectal excision for rectal cancer: Report of the first 4 human cases. *Arch Surg* 2011;146:75–81.

8. Hebbar M, Riaz W, Sains P, Baig MK, Sajid MS. Meta-analysis of randomized controlled trials only exploring the role of single incision laparoscopic surgery versus conventional multiport laparoscopic surgery for colorectal resections. *Transl Gastroenterol Hepatol* 2018;3:30.

9. Liu X, Li J-B, Shi G, Guo R, Zhang R. Systematic review of single-incision versus conventional multiport laparoscopic surgery for sigmoid colon and rectal cancer. *World J Surg Oncol* 2018;16:220.

INDEX

A

Abdominal dissection, 215
Abdomino-perineal resection (APR), 4, 154, 211
    maintaining intestinal continuity after,
        157–158
Accessories, 22
Acetaminophen, 40
Acute complicated diverticulitis, management
    of, 69–70
Acute diverticulitis, 68–69
    choice of procedure, 69
    diagnosis, 69
    Hinchey classification for, 69
    laparoscopic lavage in acute diverticulitis,
        71–72
    laparoscopic sigmoid colectomy in, 72–73
Adaptable laparoscopic instruments, 206
Adjuvant chemotherapy, 24
Alvimopan, 39
American College of Surgery National Surgical
    Quality Improvement Program
    (ACS NSQIP), 35
American Society for Enhanced Recovery
    (ASER), 36
American Society of Anesthesiologists (ASA), 38
American Society of Colon and Rectal
    Surgeons (ASCRS), 10, 36
Anal incontinence, 209
Anal manometry, 78
Anal transition zone (ATZ), 105
    dysplasia, 105
    inflammation, 105
Anastomosis, 136, 149, 217
    assessment, 150
    of rectum, 143–144
Anastomotic dehiscence and leaks, 53–54
Anastomotic leak (AL), 30, 35, 220–221
Anesthetic agents, 39
Anesthetic management
    anesthetic techniques and intraoperative
        monitoring, 45–46
    morbidity and mortality, 46
    pain control, 46
    physiological changes occurring during
        laparoscopic surgery, 45
    preoperative assessment and
        optimization, 44
    preoperative preparation, 44–45
    recovery, 46
Animal and human cadaver training
    models, 9
Anterior mobilization, 148–149
Anterior rectopexy, 4
Anterior sling rectopexy, 80
Antibiotic prophylaxis, 39
Antitumor-necrosis-factor (anti-TNF), 105
Appendectomy, 62
Appendicular lump, 66
Appendicular perforation, 66
Arc of Riolan, 132
Arterial supply, 13–14
Artery of Moskowitz, *see* Arc of Riolan
Articulated stabilizing arm, 205–206
Associating liver partition and portal vein
    ligation for staged hepatectomy
    (ALPPS), 182

Atraumatic endoclinch grasper, 20–21
Autonomic nerve preservation (ANP), 51

B

Benign colorectal condition, evolution of
    laparoscopic surgery for, 4–5
Benign strictures, 54
Bipolar energy, 22
Bladder injury, 50–51
Bleeding, 208
Blood transfusion (BT), 18, 46
Body mass index (BMI), 110, 186
Bowel obstruction, 31
Bowel preparation, 38
    in colorectal surgery, 35
    contraindications for, 36
    evidence, 35
    guidelines, 36
    history, 35–36
    types, 36

C

C-reactive protein (CRP), 40
Caecal volvulus, 60
Carbohydrate-rich drink, 39
Carbon dioxide embolism, 219–220
Carcino-embryonic antigen (CEA), 123, 154, 214
Cardiac output (CO), 45
Cardiopulmonary exercise testing (CPET), 44
Cardiovascular system, effect on, 45
Cecum, 59
Central venous oxygen saturation ($ScvO_2$), 46
Chemoradiation therapy (CRT), 120
Chowbey, Dr Pradeep, 3
Chronic obstructive pulmonary disease
    (COPD), 110
Chronic presacral sinus, 54
Chronic severe constipation, 163
Circumferential resection margin (CRM), 119,
    155, 166, 211
CLASICC trial, 198
Clear liquids, 38
Cold light system, 3
Coloanal anastomosis, 4, 24
Colon
    embryological development, 12–13
    fascias of, 14–15
    lymphatic drainage, 14
    posterior relationships, 16
    vascular anatomy, 13–14
Colonic diverticulosis, 68
Colonic transit study, 78
Colonoscopy, 154, 166
Colorectal cancer (CRC), 123, 146, 160, 165,
    172, 211; *see also* Rectal cancer
    evolution of laparoscopy for, 4
Colorectal liver metastasis (CRLM), 179
    evaluation of respectability, 179–180
    management flowchart for, 183
    management of resectable liver metastasis,
        180–182
    outcomes of laparoscopic resection for,
        182–183
    radiofrequency ablation, 182
Colorectal surgery (CR surgery), 44, 46

COLOR II trials, 119
Colostomy, 30, 86
    operative approach, 87
    sigmoid, 86–87
    sigmoid stoma reversal, 87
    SILS stoma, 88
    transverse, 87
Combined endoscopic-laparoscopic surgery
    (CELS), 224
    benefits and limitations of, 226–227
    current research on CELS polypectomy, 227
    polypectomy surgical technique, 224–226
Combined modality treatment (CMT), 175
Competency Assessment Tool (CAT), 10
Complete mesocolic excision (CME), 14, 17,
    132–133, 194
    robotic colectomy in era of, 194–195
Complications in laparoscopic colorectal
    surgery
    anastomotic dehiscence and leaks, 53–54
    bladder injury, 50–51
    chronic presacral sinus, 54
    classification of, 48–49
    early postoperative small bowel obstruction
        and postoperative ileus, 50
    female infertility, 52
    fistulas, 54
    incidence, 48
    major bleeding, 53
    major vessel injury, 49
    minor bleeding, 52–53
    pancreatic and gastric injury, 49
    presacral bleeding, 50
    sexual dysfunction, 51–52
    small bowel and duodenal injury, 49
    splenic injury, 49
    SSI, 49–50
    strictures, 54
    ureteral injury, 50
    urethral injury, 51
    urinary dysfunction, 51
    wound disruptions, 50
Computed tomography (CT), 63, 123, 179, 231
Contrast-enhanced computed tomography
    (CECT), 154
Contrast-enhanced CT, 179
Conventional APR, 155–156
Conventional laparoscopic appendectomy
    (CLA), 237
COREAN trials, 119, 198
Crohn's disease, 162–163
Cybernetic surgery, 121
Cyclooxygenase-2 specific inhibitor (COX-2
    specific inhibitor), 40

D

Da Vinci™ surgical system, 182, 190–191
Deep vein thrombosis prophylaxis, 39
Defecography, 78
Dehiscence, 209
Dentate line (DL), 147
Descending colon
    medial to lateral mobilization of, 148
    mobilization of lateral attachments of, 148
Distal gut, 12
Distal occlusion, 149

Distal rectal transaction, 143–144
Distance to distal margin (DDM), 158
Diversion ileostomy, 151
Diverticular disease, 5
Diverticulitis, 27–28
Docking, 191
Double-docking technique, 194
Duodeno-jejunal flexure (DJ flexure), 134

E

Early postoperative small bowel obstruction
    and postoperative ileus, 50
Electromyography (EMG), 78
Embryological development of colon and
    rectum, 12–13
Embryonic natural orifice transumbilical
    endoscopic surgery (E-NOTES), 236
End-tidal carbon dioxide ($ETCO_2$), 45
Endoclinch type graspers, 21
Endoloop, 66
Endoscopic ultrasound (EUS), 147
Endotrainer box, 9
Enhanced recovery after surgery program
    (ERAS program), 38, 214
    components of ERAS protocols and current
    recommendations, 38–41
European Hernia Society (EHS), 110
European Society of Coloproctology (ESCP), 36
Extended lymphadenectomy (EL), 120
Extended right hemicolectomy (ERH), 133
External rectal prolapse (ERP), 76
Extracorporeal
    knot, 66
    procedure, 144
Extrahepatic metastatic disease (EHMD), 179
Extralevator abdominoperineal excision
    (ELAPE), 155–156
    laparoscopic, 156–157
    pelvic floor reconstruction after, 156
    perineal closure in, 156
    in supine versus prone position, 156
Extraperitoneal approach, 111

F

Familial adenomatous polyposis (FAP), 90,
    160–161
Familial polyposis (FAP), 106
Fascia, 140
    of colon and rectum, 14–15
Fast-track surgery, *see* Enhanced recovery after
    surgery program (ERAS program)
Fasting guidelines, 38
Fecal incontinence, 104–105
Fellowships in MAS or advanced laparoscopy, 10
Female infertility, 52, 105
Finger dissection, 4
Fistulas, 54
Fulcrum effect, 182
Full-thickness excision, 206
    with perirectal fat, 206
Full-thickness rectal prolapse (FTRP), 75

G

Gadoxetate disodium (Gd), 179
Gastrointestinal (GI)
    effect, 45
    tract, 117
Goal-directed fluid therapy, 46
Granulomas, 32

H

Hand-assisted laparoscopic surgery (HALS),
    185, 230
    colorectal resections, 230
    incision and trocar placement, 231–232
    indications, 230
    modifications, 234
    position, 231
    preoperative preparation, 231
    surgical instruments, 231
    surgical procedure, 232–234
    surgical steps, 231
Hand-assisted techniques, 118
Haray maneuver, 142–143
Harmonic scalpel, 206
Hartmann's procedure, 4
Hartmann's reversal, 87
High-flow insufflators, 216
High-output ileostomy, 32
High dependency unit (HDU), 46
High inspired oxygen concentrations, 39
Highly structured training courses, 10
Hybrid technique, 193
Hypothermia prevention, 39–40

I

Ibuprofen, 40
Ileal pouch anal anastomosis (IPAA), 23–24,
    90, 105, 160–161
Ileocecal area, applied anatomy and physiology
    of, 59–60
Ileocecal resection, 59
Ileocolic artery (ICA), 14
Ileorectal anastomosis (IRA), 24, 91, 161
Ileostomy, 24, 30
Incisional hernia, 186
Indocyanine green (ICG), 121, 196
Inferior mesenteric artery (IMA), 12, 131, 135,
    140, 155, 166, 215, 238
    ligation, 95, 142
    ligation after ureter visualization, 21
Inferior mesenteric pedicle, division of,
    147–148
Inferior mesenteric vein (IMV), 14, 132,
    134–135, 140, 215
    ligation, 140–141
Inferior vena cava (IVC), 180
Inflammatory bowel disease (IBD), 4–5, 106
Insufflator/suction/irrigation/light/
    electrocautery machines, 206
Internal anal sphincter (IAS), 147
Internal rectal prolapse (IRP), 76
Intersphincteric dissection, 24
Intersphincteric groove (ISG), 147
Intersphincteric resection, 4, 150
Intra-abdominal pressure (IAP), 45
Intracorporeal knots, 66
Intraoperative fluid management, 39
Intraoperative monitoring, 45–46
Intraperitoneal mesh repair, 112–113

J

J-pouch, 106

K

Ketorolac, 40
'Key-hole' technique, 112–113

L

Laparo endoscopic single site surgery (LESS),
    236
Laparoscopic-assisted techniques, 118
Laparoscopic access and exposure, 134
Laparoscopic anterior resection and low anterior
    resection for rectal cancers, 23
Laparoscopic appendectomy, 62
    absolute contraindications, 62
    indications, 62
    operative steps, 63–66
    OR setup, 63
    postoperative complications, 66
    postoperative course and recovery, 66
    preoperative preparation, 62–63
    relative contraindications, 62
    selection of patients, 62
    SILS appendicectomy, 66–67
Laparoscopic APR for ultra-low rectal cancers,
    22–23
Laparoscopic assisted surgeries (LAS), 185
Laparoscopic colectomy, 185
Laparoscopic colon replacement for corrosive
    strictures, 24
Laparoscopic colorectal cancer resection,
    evidence for quality of life after,
    118–119
Laparoscopic colorectal surgery (LCS), 8, 230
    basic principles, 18–19
    breakthrough trials, 118
    complications, 25
    conversion in, 24
    in emergency situations, 5
    energy sources, 22
    future of, 120–121
    future of, 5–6
    general surgery apprenticeship and
    traineeship programmes, 10
    historical perspectives, 117–118
    initial entry and initial assessment, 20–21
    instrumentation, 21–22
    knowledge of basic laparoscopic surgical
    skills, 9
    laparoscopic surgery in colorectal diseases,
    8–9
    learning tools, techniques and
    methodologies, 9
    OR setup, 20
    patient preparation, 20
    potential benefits, 18
    standard operative steps, 22–24
    standard port placements, 20
    standard training models for teaching
    advanced laparoscopic skills in
    colorectal surgery, 10–11
    staplers and accessories, 22
    techniques and adjuncts, 24
    training in, 18
Laparoscopic ELAPE, 156–157
Laparoscopic ileocecal resection
    applied anatomy and physiology of
    ileocecal area, 59–60
    contraindications, 60
    difference in resection between benign and
    malignant indications, 60
    indications, 60
    preoperative preparation, 60
    results and consequences of resection, 60
    right hemicolectomy for ileocaecal
    tuberculosis, 22
Laparoscopic ileostomy and colostomy, 85

Laparoscopic lavage in acute diverticulitis, 71
  complications, 72
  conversion to laparoscopic colectomy, 72
  operative steps, 72
  patient positioning, 71
  port placement, 71–72
Laparoscopic left hemicolectomy, 134
  for descending colon cancer, 23
Laparoscopic left lateral sectionectomy, 182
Laparoscopic LR (LLR), 182
Laparoscopic major hepatic resection, 180–182
Laparoscopic posterior sutured rectopexy (LPSR), 82
Laparoscopic rectal cancer surgery, 158
Laparoscopic rectopexy (LR), 75
  goals of surgery, 76
  historical perspective, 75–76
  indications for surgery, 76
  long-term functional results, 81–82
  operative principles for posterior suture/mesh/resection rectopexy, 78
  operative steps, 79
  operative techniques, 79–80
  ORPG, 76
  OR setup, 78
  port placements, 78
  postoperative care and early outcomes, 80
  postoperative complications, 80–81
  preoperative evaluation, 77–78
  preoperative preparation, 78
  rectal prolapse, 75–76
  robotic rectopexy, 82
  selection of approach and controversies, 77
  surgical options, 76–77
Laparoscopic resection rectopexy (LRR), 81
Laparoscopic restorative proctocolectomy, 23–24
Laparoscopic reversal of Hartmann's operation, 24
Laparoscopic right hemicolectomy for right colon cancer, 23
Laparoscopic segmentectomies/nonanatomical resections, 182
Laparoscopic sigmoid colectomy
  in acute diverticulitis, 72–73
  for sigmoid colon cancer, 22
Laparoscopic stoma formation, 86
Laparoscopic subtotal/total/proctocolectomy, 160
  contraindications, 163–164
  indications, 160–163
Laparoscopic surgery, 2; *see also* Single incision laparoscopic surgery (SILS)
  advantages of, 67
  disadvantages of, 67
  evolution, 2–4
  evolution of laparoscopic surgery for benign colorectal condition, 4–5
  evolution of laparoscopy for colorectal cancers, 4
  filling gap between open and, 118
  in obstructed colorectal cancers, 173–174
  physiological changes occurring during, 45
  in recurrent colorectal cancers, 174–175
  technical evolution of rectal cancer surgery, 4
  technological evolution, 2
Laparoscopic suture rectopexy (LSR), 81
Laparoscopic suture rectopexy for rectal prolapse, 22
Laparoscopic total colectomy, 24

Laparoscopic total mesorectal excision, 147–151, 211
Laparoscopic total proctocolectomy, 24
Laparoscopic transverse colectomy, 23
  steps of, 129
Laparoscopic ventral mesh rectopexy (LVMR), 79–82
Laparoscopic *vs.* open approach, 70, 105
  advantages, 70
  disadvantages, 71
  prerequisites for, 71
  technical challenges, 71
Laparoscopic *vs.* open repair, 113
Laparoscopy, 60, 85
Laparosopic surgery, 40
Laparotomy conversion, 209
LAPCO programme, 10
Lap posterior mesh rectopexy, 79
Lap resection rectopexy, 79
Lap suture rectopexy, 79
Lateral colonic attachment, 96–97
Lateral pelvic lymph nodes (LPLN), 120
Left-sided tumors, 28
Left and sigmoid colectomy, 192–194
Left colic artery, 131
Left colon, 131
  lymphatic drainage, 132
  mobilization, 94–97
  resection templates for left colon cancer, 133–134
  surgical steps, 134–137
  vascular anatomy, 131–132
Left hemicolectomy (LH), 134
Left segment colectomy (LSC), 134
Length of stay (LOS), 35, 41
Lesser sac, 142
LigaSure, 206
Liver metastasis resection (LM resection), 180
Liver resection (LR), 179
Liver transplantation (LT), 182
Locally advanced colorectal cancers (LACRC), 165
Locally advanced rectal disease, 120
Long instruments, 206
Loop ileostomy, 86
Loop stoma reversal, 86
Low anterior resection (LAR), 155
  function after, 155
Low anterior resection syndrome (LARS), 155
Low molecular weight heparin (LMWH), 39
Low rectal division, 99–100
Low rectal tumors, 28
Lung-protective ventilation, 39
Lymphatic drainage
  of colon and rectum, 14
  of left colon, 132
Lymph node (LN), 66
Lynch syndrome, 160–161

M

Magnetic resonance imaging (MRI), 63, 78, 154
Major bleeding, 53
Major vessel injury, 49
Malignant strictures, 54
Marginal artery of Drummond, 132
Margins, 198
Master class or dedicated fellowship courses, 10
Mechanical bowel preparation (MBP), 30, 36, 44
  with IV antibiotics, 36

Mechanical bowel preparation and preoperative oral antibiotic preparation (MBP/OAP), 35
Medial and lateral mobilization, 148
Medial to lateral dissection, 94–95
Mesenteric defect, 136–137
Mesenteric meandering artery, *see* Arc of Riolan
Mesocolic dissection, 141
Mesorectum, 15
Midclavicular line (MCL), 197
Middle colic artery (MCA), 14
Minilaparotomy; *see also* Laparoscopic sigmoid colectomy
  issues with, 186
  or convenient incision, 185
  for specimen extraction, 101
Minimal access surgery (MAS), 8
Minimally invasive surgery (MIS), 81, 196, 206
Minimally invasive techniques, 85
Minor bleeding, 52–53
Monopolar energy, 22
Monopolar hook or spatula, 21
MR defecography, 78
Mucocutaneous separation, 31
Mucosectomy, 106, 206
Multidisciplinary team tumor board (MDT), 214

N

Nasogastric tubes, avoidance of, 40
National Comprehensive Cancer Network (NCCN), 214
National Institue for Health and Care Excellence (NICE), 36
National Training Programme (NTP), 10
Natural orifice specimen extraction (NOSE), 185–186
  patient factors, 186–187
  potential factors, 187
  selection factors for, 186–187
Natural orifice transluminal endoscopic surgery (NOTES), 4, 6, 120
Natural orifice transumbilical surgery (NOTUS), 236
Near-infrared fluorescence (NIF), 121
Near infrared fluorescence imaging (NIR fluorescence imaging), 54
Necrotic appendicular base, 66
Neoadjuvant chemoradiation, 24
  selection of patients for, 166
Nerves, 198
Neurovascular bundles of Walsh (NVB), 219
Nonsteroidal anti-inflammatory drugs (NSAIDs), 40, 53

O

Obesity, 27–28
Obstructed bowel, 27
Obstructed defecation syndrome (ODS), 76, 78
Obstructed left sided colon cancers, 161
Obstructed tumors, 172
  clinical presentation, 172
  key steps for safe surgery, 176
  management, 172–173
  postoperative care and follow-up, 176–177
  treatment, 173–175
One-port umbilical surgery (OPUS), 236
One-stage IPAA, 105
Onlay mesh repair, 112
Operating room (OR), 8
Operative proctoscopes, 205–206

Optics, 206
Oral antibiotic prophylaxis, 36
Ostomy, 85
Oxford rectal prolapse grading system
    (ORPG), 76

P

Pain control, 46
Palanivelu, C., 3
Palliative resection, 176
Pancaking, 32
Pancreatic and gastric injury, 49
Pararectus, 111
Parastomal hernia (PH), 32, 109
    classifications, 110
    diagnosis, 110
    history of laparoscopy in stomal surgery,
        109–110
    incidence, 109
    indications and contraindications for
        surgery, 110
    intraperitoneal mesh repair, 112–113
    laparoscopic *vs.* open repair, 113
    onlay mesh repair, 112
    prevention of, 111
    prevention of parastomal hernia, 111
    recurrence, 113
    recurrent PH repair, 113
    risk factors, 110
    robotic PH repair, 113
    surgery for, 110–111
    techniques of repair, 112
Parenteral nutrition (TPN), 46
Partial rectal wall excision, 206
Pathologic complete response (pCR), 119
Patient-controlled analgesia (PCA), 46
Patient selection, 27–28
Pelvic dissection, 143, 148
Pelvic floor reconstruction after ELAPE, 156
Pelvic organ prolapse (POP), 77
Pelvic physiology studies, 78
Pericolonic vessels, 96
Perineal closure in ELAPE, 156
Peristomal skin excoriations and infections, 32
Peritoneal cavity, exploration of, 147
Peritoneal drains, 40
Peritoneal entry, 208
Phosphate enemas, 36
Physiological and Operative Severity Score for
        the Enumeration of Mortality and
        Morbidity (POSSUM), 44
Pneumoperitoneum, 134
    re-creation of, 102
Portal vein embolization (PVE), 182
Portal vein ligation (PVL), 182
Port placement philosophy, 92–93
Portsmouth-POSSUM (P-POSSUM), 44
Positive end-expiratory pressure (PEEP), 39
Positron emission tomography (PET), 179
Posterior colpotomy, *see* Vaginotomy
Posterior mobilization, 148
Posterior pelvic dissection, 142–143
Posterior relationships of colon, 16
Postoperative care, 151
Pouch anal anastomosis, 102–103
Pouch dysplasia/cancer, 105
Pouch failure, 104
Pouchitis, 103–104
Preceptorship, 10
Preoperative counselling and training, 38
Preoperative oral antibiotics, 30

Presacral bleeding, 50
Proctectomy, 162–163
Proctocolectomy, 163
Proctorship, 10
Prolapse, 31
ProMIS simulator, 9
Prone jackknife position (PJK position), 156
Prophylactic mesh, 111
Proximal diversion, 24
Pubococcygeus line on rest
        (PC line on rest), 78
Puborectalis contraction (PPC), 78
Pudendal nerve terminal motor latency testing
        (PNTML testing), 78

Q

Quality of life (QOL), 35
    issues, 158

R

Radiofrequency ablation, 182
Radiological imaging, 166
Rectal cancer, 119–120
    indications for extended lymphadenectomy
        in, 120
    technical evolution of rectal cancer
        surgery, 4
Rectal drains to preventing stoma, 31
Rectal malignancy, efficacy of minimal
        invasive surgery for, 119–120
Rectal mobilization, 97–99
Rectal prolapse, 4, 75
    types, 76
Rectal transection, 149
Recto-vaginal fistula, 209
Rectosigmoid cancer
    patient position and draping with
        placement of equipment and
        team, 140
    performing procedure, 140–144
    port placement and laparoscopic
        instrumentation, 140
    preoperative patient preparation, 139
Rectosigmoid colon, mobilization of lateral
        attachments of, 148
Rectourethral muscle (RUM), 219
Rectum
    embryological development, 12–13
    fascias of, 14–15
    lymphatic drainage, 14
    vascular anatomy, 13–14
Recurrence
    classification, 175–176
    risk factors for, 174–175
Recurrence, 113
Recurrent PH repair, 113
Recurrent tumors, 172
    clinical presentation, 172
    key steps for safe surgery, 176
    management, 172–173
    postoperative care and follow-up, 176–177
Renal and metabolic effect, 45
Rendez-vous, 217
Resection options, 206
Resection templates for left colon cancer,
        133–134
Respiratory system, effect on, 45
Restorative proctocolectomy (RPC), 90, 160;
        see also Total proctocolectomy
        (TPC); Minilaparotomy

Restorative proctocolectomy and ileal pouch
        anal anastomosis (RPC-IPAA),
        90, 162
    advantages, 92
    contraindications for, 91–92
    controversies, 105–106
    disadvantages, 92
    functional results, 105
    goals of surgery, 90–91
    indications for, 91
    operative principles of laparoscopic
        assisted RPC-IPAA, 92
    operative steps, 92–103
    postoperative care and usual recovery, 103
    postoperative complications, 103–105
    preoperative preparation, 92
    selection of patients, 91
    surgical options, 91
Retraction/flush stoma, 31
Retrograde appendectomy, 66
Right colic artery (RCA), 14
Right colon mobilization, 100–101
Right hemicolectomy, 123, 191–192
    indications, 123
    operative steps, 124–126
    operative technique, 123–124
    positioning and port placement, 123–124
    postoperative care, 126
    preoperative work up, 123
    SILS, 126
Risk evaluation, 38
Robot-assisted LR, *see* Da Vinci surgical
        system
Robot-assisted right hemicolectomy (RAC), 192
Robotic colectomy in era of complete
        mesocolic excision, 194–195
Robotic colonic cancer surgery, 190
    equipment, 190–191
    general principles, 191
    left and sigmoid colectomy, 192–194
    right hemicolectomy, 191–192
    robotic colectomy in era of complete
        mesocolic excision, 194–195
    transverse colectomy, 194
Robotic PH repair, 113
Robotic rectal cancer surgery, 158, 196
    advantages of robot-assisted TME for
        rectal cancer, 199
    cost, 199
    oncological outcomes, 199
    position, port placement, and
        instrumentation, 197
    preoperative preparation and precautions,
        196–197
    robotics in rectal cancer, 198–199
    steps of surgery, 197–198
Robotic rectopexy, 82
Robotic right hemicolectomy (RRH), 192
Robotic SILS, 237
Robotic surgery, 4
Robotic ventral mesh rectopexy (RVMR), 82
Rod lens system, 3

S

S-pouch, 106
Sacrectomy, 157
Sandwich repair, 112
Scottish Intercollegiate Guidelines Network
        (SIGN), 36
Severe active inflammatory bowel disease,
        27–28

Sexual dysfunction, 51–52, 105
Sigmoid colostomy, 86–87
Sigmoido/colonoscopy, 77
Sigmoid stoma reversal, 87
Single-access laparoscopic surgery (SALS), 236
Single-docking technique, 194
Single-incision laparoscopic anterior
  resection, 238
Single-incision laparoscopic appendectomy
  (SILA), 237
Single-incision laparoscopic colectomy
  (SILC), 237
Single-incision laparoscopic colorectal surgery
  ports and equipment, 236–237
  robotic SILS, 237
Single-incision laparoscopic left
  hemicolectomy, 237–238
Single-incision laparoscopic right
  hemicolectomy, 237
Single-incision laparoscopic total colectomy, 238
Single-incision robotic colectomy (SIRC), 194
Single-port access surgery (SPA surgery), 236
Single incision laparoscopic surgery (SILS), 4,
  6, 126
  appendicectomy, 66–67
  stoma, 88
Single laparoscopic incision transabdominal
  surgery (SLIT surgery), 236
Site selection, criteria for, 185
Small bowel and duodenal injury, 49
Small bowel obstruction (SBO), 50
Société Française de Chirurgie Digestive
  (SFCD), 36
Society of American Gastrointestinal and
  Endoscopic Surgeons (SAGES), 10, 36
Solid foods and milk, 38–39
Solitary rectal ulcer (SRUS), 76
Specimen removal, 149
Sphincter preservation, 155
Splenic flexure, 132–133, 148
  medial to lateral mobilization of, 148
  mobilization, 95–97, 135–136
Splenic injury, 49
Stapled vs. hand sewn pouch, 106
Staplers, 22, 65–66
Stenosis, 31
Stoma, 29
  anastomotic leak, 30
  care, 31–32
  closure and complications, 32
  complications, 31–32
  indications for temporary stoma, 30
  marking, counseling, and consenting, 29
  preoperative oral antibiotics and
    mechanical bowel preparation, 30
  role of rectal drains to preventing stoma, 31
Stoma care ostomy research (SCOR), 31
Stomal surgery, history of laparoscopy in,
  109–110
Stricture, 104
Strictures, 54
Subclinical leak, 53
Subtotal colectomy, 160
'Sugarbaker' technique, 112
Superior mesenteric artery (SMA), 12, 131

Superior mesenteric vein (SMV), 14
Surgical site infections (SSIs), 8, 35, 49–50, 186
Synchronous colon cancer, 160
Synchronous liver metastases, timing of
  resection for, 180
Systemic vascular resistance (SVR), 45

T

T4 tumor and pelvic exenteration for locally
  advanced tumors, 165
  clinical presentation, 165–166
  colonoscopy, 166
  in female patients, 169
  key differences in operative steps, 167–168
  key operative steps in routine laparoscopic
    colorectal surgery, 166–167
  laparoscopy and surgical technique, 166
  in male patients, 168
  preoperative evaluation, 166
  radiological imaging, 166
  selection of patients for neoadjuvant
    chemoradiation, 166
  special situations, 169
  specimen retrieval and formation of ileal
    conduit and stapler anvil head
    insertion, 168–169
Terminal ileum, 59–60
Three-stage IPAA, 105
Total abdominal colectomy with end
  ileostomy, 162
Total abdominal colectomy with ileorectal
  anastomosis (TAC-IRA), 162
Total colectomy (TC), 91, 160
Total laparoscopic colo rectal surgery
  (TLCR), 185
Total mesorectal excision (TME), 4, 14, 17, 51,
  119–120, 146, 166, 196, 211
Total proctocolectomy (TPC), 91, 160
  with end ileostomy, 162
Total proctocolectomy and ileal pouch anal
  anastomosis (TPC-IPAA), 4–5; see
  also Restorative proctocolectomy
  and ileal pouch anal anastomosis
  (RPC-IPAA)
Training
  of laparoscopic colorectal surgeon, 10–11
  in laparoscopic colorectal surgery, 18
  in specialized colorectal unit, 9
Transabdominal, 186
Transanal APR (taAPR), 216
Transanal dissection, 215–217
Transanal endoscopic microsurgery (TEM/
  TEMS), 4, 120, 204
Transanal minimally invasive surgery
  (TAMIS), 120, 204
  adaptable laparoscopic instruments, 206
  articulated stabilizing arm, 205–206
  complications, 208–209
  contraindications, 205
  indications, 204
  procedure, 206–208
  reach, 204
  resection options, 206
  risks, 204–205

Transanal TME (taTME), 4, 85, 211
  abdominal dissection, 215
  anastomosis, 217
  complications, 217–221
  history and results, 211–213
  operative approach, 214
  positioning, 214–215
  preoperative assessment, 214
  preoperative evaluation, 213–214
  Rendez-vous, 217
  transanal dissection, 215–217
Transanal transabdominal resections (TATA
  resections), 85
Transanal ultrasonography, 78
Transrectus, 111
Transvaginal/transanal specimen removal, 24
Transverse colectomy, 194
Transverse colon
  medial to lateral mobilization of, 148
  mobilization, 148
Transverse colon cancer
  anatomy, 128
  evidence of laparoscopic resection, 128
  preoperation preparation, 128–129
Transverse colostomy, 87
Transverses abdomonis release (TAR), 113
Transversus abdominis plane (TAP), 46, 217
Trephine, size of, 111
Two-stage IPAA, 105

U

Udwadia, T. E., 3
Ulcerative colitis (UC), 5, 90, 162
Ultrasonic energy, 22
Ultrasonography, 63
Ultrasound (US), 179
Unresectable liver metastasis, management
  of, 182
Upper gastrointestinal surgeries (UGI
  surgeries), 17–18
Ureteral injury, 50
Urethral injury, 51, 218–219
Urinary
  complications, 209
  dysfunction, 51
Urorectal septum, 12

V

Vaginotomy, 186
Vascular anatomy
  of colon and rectum, 13–14
  of left colon, 131–132
Vascularity, 198
Venous drainage, 14
Venous thromboembolism (VTE), 214
Ventral mesh rectopexy (VR), 75–76
Vertebral discitis, 81
Vessel sealing devices, 22
Virtual reality simulators, 9

W

Wound disruptions, 50

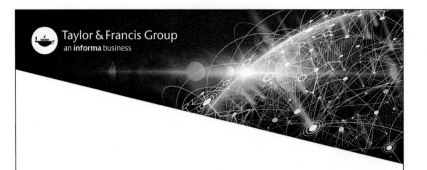